VISUAL CORTEX – CURRENT STATUS AND PERSPECTIVES

Edited by **Stéphane Molotchnikoff**
and **Jean Rouat**

Visual Cortex – Current Status and Perspectives
http://dx.doi.org/10.5772/3018
Edited by Stéphane Molotchnikoff and Jean Rouat

Contributors

José L. Bueno-López, Juan C. Chara, Juan L. Mendizabal-Zubiaga, Concepción Reblet, Alyssa A. Brewer, Brian Barton, Carole Peyrin, Benoit Musel, Athena Buckthought, Janine D. Mendola, Craig Aaen-Stockdale, Benjamin Thompson, Brendan D. Cameron, Gordon Binsted, Jackson E.T. Smith, Nicolas Y. Masse, Chang'an A. Zhan, Erik P. Cook, Claudio Castellanos Sánchez, Manuel Hernández Hernández, Pedro Luis Sánchez Orellana, Zhiyong Yang, Vincent de Ladurantaye, Jean Rouat, Jacques Vanden-Abeele, Ai-Ling Lin, Jia-Hong Gao, Peter T. Fox, Enrike G. Argandoña, Harkaitz Bengoetxea, Naiara Ortuzar, Susana Bulnes, Irantzu Rico-Barrio, José Vicente Lafuente, José Fernando Maya-Vetencourt, Matteo Caleo, Alessandro Sale, Nicoletta Berardi, Lamberto Maffei, Lyes Bachatene, Vishal Bharmauria, Stéphane Molotchnikoff, Shigeru Tanaka, I. Gerrikagoitia, B. Rienda, L. Martínez-Millán, Marina Arall, August Romeo, Hans Supèr

Published by InTech

Janeza Trdine 9, 51000 Rijeka, Croatia

Publishing Process Manager Sandra Bakic
Technical Editor InTech Prepress, Novi Sad
Cover InTech Design team

Additional hard copies can be obtained from orders@intechopen.com

Visual Cortex – Current Status and Perspectives,
Edited by Stéphane Molotchnikoff and Jean Rouat
p. cm.
ISBN 978-953-51-0760-6

For EU product safety concerns:
IN TECH d.o.o., Prolaz Marije Krucifikse Kozulić 3, 51000 Rijeka, Croatia,
info@intechopen.com or visit our website at intechopen.com.

Meet the editors

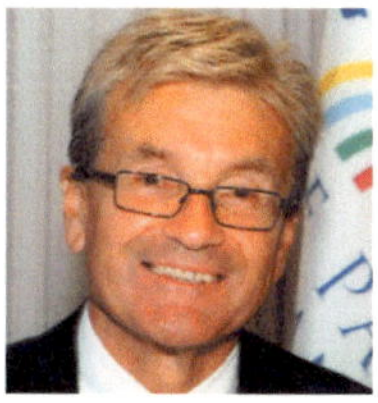

Prof. Dr. Stéphane Molotchnikoff following graduation from State University of New York (Buffalo), he joined the faculty as professor of physiology at the Département de Sciences Biologiques de l'Université de Montréal. Currently, he is also adjunct professor at the Engineering School of University of Sherbrooke. For the past several decades Professor Molotchnikoff taught courses in physiology from comparative physiology to neurosciences. Professor Molotchnikoff maintains an active laboratory and graduate research team that focuses on studying the mechanisms of the brain's visual system and more generally investigating the processes related to sensory functions in various vertebrate species. Presently two main themes are explored: adaptation-induced plasticity, and the modifications of connectomes induced by changes in the properties of visual targets. He was awarded the Purkyně medal from Charles University (Prague) and Chevalier de l'Ordre de la Francophonie et du Dialogue des Cultures de l'Assembléė Parlementaire de la Francophonie. His research has been continuously funded by Canadian research agencies.

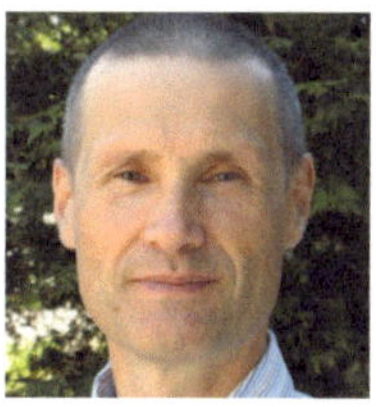

Prof. Jean Rouat holds a master degree in Physics from Université de Bretagne, France (1981), an E. & E. master degree in speech coding and speech recognition from Université de Sherbrooke (1984) and an E. & E. Ph.D. in cognitive and statistical speech recognition jointly with Université de Sherbrooke and McGill University (1988). His post-doc has been with the Medical Research Council, Applied Psychological Unit, Cambridge, UK and the Institute of Physiology, Lausanne, Switzerland. He is currently with Université de Sherbrooke where he founded the Computational Neuroscience and Intelligent Signal Processing Research group. He is also adjunct professor in the biological sciences department from Université de Montréal. His laboratory interests are in neurocomputational signal processing. He is an active member of scientific associations (Acoustical Society of America, Int. Speech Communication, IEEE, Int. Neural Networks Society, Association for Research in Otolaryngology, Society for Neuroscience and several others). He is a senior member of the IEEE and participates in many scientific committees.

Contents

Preface

The neurosciences have experienced tremendous and wonderful progress in many areas, and the spectrum encompassing the neurosciences is expansive. Suffice it to mention a few classical fields: electrophysiology, genetics, physics, computer sciences, and more recently, social and marketing neurosciences. Of course, this large growth resulted in the production of many books. Perhaps the visual system and the visual cortex were in the vanguard because most animals do not produce their own light and offer thus the invaluable advantage of allowing investigators to conduct experiments in full control of the stimulus. In addition, the fascinating evolution of scientific techniques, the immense productivity of recent research, and the ensuing literature make it virtually impossible to publish in a single volume all worthwhile work accomplished throughout the scientific world. The days when a single individual, as Diderot, could undertake the production of an encyclopedia are gone forever. Indeed most approaches to studying the nervous system are valid and neuroscientists produce an almost astronomical number of interesting data accompanied by extremely worthy hypotheses which in turn generate new ventures in search of brain functions.

Yet, it is fully justified to make an encore and to publish a book dedicated to visual cortex and beyond. Many reasons validate a book assembling chapters written by active researchers. Each has the opportunity to bind together data and explore original ideas whose fate will not fall into the hands of uncompromising reviewers of traditional journals. This book focuses on the cerebral cortex with a large emphasis on vision. Yet it offers the reader diverse approaches employed to investigate the brain, for instance, computer simulation, cellular responses, or rivalry between various targets and goal directed actions.

This volume thus covers a large spectrum of research even though it is impossible to include all topics in the extremely diverse field of neurosciences.

For a long time, university students have been taught that after the critical period following birth the brain remains relatively unchanged except for a gradual neuronal loss accompanying aging. As recent research demonstrates this latter view was a false perception of brain organization because indeed the adult brain is incredibly plastic. Thus it should not come as a surprise that this book contains several chapters dealing with adult brain modifications. Furthermore, thanks to recent advances in histological techniques, cellular membranes of neurons exhibit an extraordinary complexity, even though they constitute the structural unit membrane of the neuron. Bueno-Lopez and Chara et al. review subtypes of cerebral cortical principal cells and provide a detailed description of cellular partitions such as axon initial segments. Brewer and Barton expand our current understanding of the visual field map in human visual cortex organization and reciprocal connections as they relate to specific functions. Yet mapping comes with intrinsic problems, e.g., the coupling or uncoupling between neurovasculature and neurometabolic requirements. Ling and Gao et al., describe this challenge, adding an interesting historical note.

Plasticity in the adult brain constitutes the key theme of the majority of chapters since this particular field has seen remarkable development at all functional levels. Maya-Ventencourt and Caleo compellingly discuss processes of sensory deprivation in the visual system at intracellular signal transduction pathways which regulate changes of chromatin structure and gene expression patterns supporting these plastic phenomena. For many years plasticity was studied by deprivation, that is, eliminating or limiting visual inputs. Fortunately, recent experiments reversed this approach by introducing a novel experimental design that enriches the visual environment or by imposing particular stimuli. Sale and Berardi et al.'s chapter aims to review recent studies, mostly focusing on the effects of enriching the visual environment in promoting visual system development and in reopening neural plasticity windows in the adult brain. Special emphasis is given to excitation / inhibition balance, and to promoting functional recovery from pathological states of severe brain disability. Along this line Bachatene and Bharmauria et al., compellingly describe the change of functional connections between involved neurons following adaptation-induced plasticity. After forcefully adapting the same neurons to a desired stimulus feature, and using the cross correlogram approach, functional connections were established before and after adaptation between the same neurons recorded simultaneously in the primary visual cortex. The data show the network between them changed, reflecting on the ability of visual cortex for plastic modifications of its relationships between neurons following adaptation. Using brain optical imaging Tanaka is of the same opinion that the short-term single-orientation exposure can dramatically alter preferred orientations until postnatal 6 weeks, which is against the current consensus and reveals further complexity in orientation plasticity in cases where animals are exposed to a single orientation for a long time. Gerrikagoitial and Rienda et al. stress convincingly the importance of inhibitory factors regulating connections and sprouting capacity within the cortico-collicular network during plasticity processes.

Yet vision as it is processed in visual cortex is not by all means an end in itself as it initiates image perception that steers our behaviour. This book offers several chapters dealing with the topic.

Contextual influences should not be underestimated when investigating neuronal responses to visual stimuli. Arall and Romeo et al. describe findings showing that evoked responses in the primary visual cortex are modulated by surrounding stimuli. The role of extra-classical receptive field is highlighted in the figure-ground organization of an image. Peyrin and Musel aim to clarify the different attributes of the occipital cortex during scene perception. This suggests that the occipital cortex might serve as an"active blackboard"integrating the rapid analysis of low spatial frequency (LSF) carried out by higher order cortical areas and sent back via feedback connections to occipital areas to influence the subsequent analysis of high spatial frequencies (HSF) features. Concomitantly, the right occipital cortex is predominantly involved in the categorization LSF processing, while the left occipital cortex is chiefly involved in the categorization of HSF scenes. Buckthought and Mendola explain the methodological issues involved in perception investigations, showing that perceptual processing modalities can be conceptualized as a series of visual perceptual processing stages in occipital areas, as well as higher-level cognitive functions in parietal and frontal areas, involving stimulus selection, decision making, motor planning, memory, attention and conscious awareness. Stockdale and Thompson review comprehensively key aspects of visual motion perception with a particular emphasis on the cortical areas thought to be involved and the ability of the visual cortex to bind multiple features together into a coherent, stable visual percept. In addition, the effects of lesions and abnormal development affecting the cortical areas responsible for motion perception are described. Cameron and Binsted examine the relationship between vision and action, and survey evidence that regions of posterior parietal cortex are designed for directly transforming vision into action; interestingly, studies from patients and non-patients suggest that action processing can access visual information that perception does not. Smith and Masse et al. pose a challenging question: how does visual perception arise from the activity of neurons in visual cortex? The authors introduce the important concept of'behavioral sensitivity'neurons to answer this question that requires an understanding of how a visual cortical neuron's activity becomes correlated with the visually guided behavior of a subject.

The book ends with topics that are likely to blossom in the near future, i.e., modeling the complexity of brain functions. Castellanos-Sanchez and Hernandez et al. introduce the reader to bio-inspired models. Yang considers the brain as a statistical machine. The argument rests on the proposition that the statistics of the natural visual environment must be incorporated into the visual circuitry by successful behavior in the world over evolutionary and developmental time. Indeed, there is an almost infinite number of ways to model any given system, and this is particularly true if we are interested in something as complex as the human brain, including the visual cortex. By contrast Ladurantaye and Rouat et al. attempt in depth to regroup the different types of models into meaningful categories, to give the reader a fair overview of what is possible to achieve in terms of modeling biological vision. Each section of the chapter focuses on one of those categories and includes different implementation methods (i.e., specific models).

In closing it is our agreeable duty to express our gratitude to many anonymous reviewers who diligently revised the chapters. Finally, Mrs. Bakic is unreservedly thanked for her help during the tedious editing processes.

Prof. Dr. Stephane Molotchnikoff
Department of Biological Sciences, Faculty of Arts and Sciences, University of Montreal,
Canada

Prof. Jean Rouat
Department of Electrical and Computer Engineering, Faculty of Engineering,
University of Sherbrooke,
Canada

Projections, Partaken Circuits and Axon Initial Segments of Cortical Principal Neurons

José L. Bueno-López, Juan C. Chara,
Juan L. Mendizabal-Zubiaga and Concepción Reblet

Additional information is available at the end of the chapter

http://dx.doi.org/10.5772/50191

1. Introduction

The axon initial segment (AIS) is the portion of the neuron immediately distal to the axon hillock. The AIS has a specialized membrane that works for a manifold function. The first portion of the AIS membrane possess a collection of ion channels that allows for the modulation of the membrane potential of the parent cell whilst blocking the back propagation of the axon potential. The last portion of the AIS membrane possesses in addition voltage-dependent ion channels that are responsible for the ultimate display of the cell, that is, the generation of the axon potential. Much has been investigated recently on the ion channels that are embedded in the AIS membrane of nerve cells. Yet basic parameters such as the length and diameter of the AIS and, of no lesser importance, the number and distribution of boutons synapsing the AIS membrane remains largely unknown for distinct subpopulations of principal cells of cerebral cortex. Principal cells are heterogeneous in many anatomical, molecular and functional aspects but, in agreement with their distinctive possession of combinations of these aspects, they can be classified in different subpopulations. Taking as core features for this grouping the cell laminar address and the pattern of axon projection, this paper reviews subtypes of cerebral cortical principal cells and their AIS features. In doing so, this paper also presents an account of our past and present research on the AIS of principal cells in visual and other areas of cerebral cortex. Yet, aiming to furnish a background to the function of the AIS of cerebral cortical principal cells, we shall begin by reviewing the cellular types and circuits in cortex, and the axon projections arising from the cortex.

2. Cerebral cortical neurons

Spiny neurons are of an excitatory nature and most have extrinsic axons, that is, axons that project outside the cortical area where their somata lie. These cells employ glutamate or predominantly aspartate as a neurotransmitter (for percentages of aspartergic and glutamatergic cells out of projection cell subpopulations to several telencephalic and extratelencephalic targets, see [1]). By contrast, aspiny neurons are inhibitory, and most of their axons are intrinsic, i.e. they use gamma-amino-butyric acid (GABA) as a neurotransmitter and their axons remain within the cortical area in which the parent cell soma lies. They are usually named interneurons.

2.1. Interneurons

Interneurons are present in all cortical areas and layers and represent approximately 10%–20% of cortical neurons in rats [2] or 15%-30% of the total population in other species [3]. Interestingly, while in the occipital, parietal and frontal cortex of the rat the same proportion of GABAergic neurons among all neurons was found (15%, in [2]), the numerical density of all neurons in the frontal cortex (34,000 per cubic millimetre) was significantly lower than those in the occipital and parietal regions (52,000 per cubic millimetre and 48,000 per cubic millimetre, respectively) [2]. The fixed proportion of interneurons, irrespective of the number of neurons, is in keeping with the idea of the uniformity of cortical circuits. However, this does not exclude the possibility that the proportion of the different types of interneurons might vary in each cortical area, resulting in regional specialization of inhibitory circuits.

Interneurons show great morphological, biochemical and physiological diversity. However, interneurons with the same morphology may have different biochemical characteristics and connectivity [3]. Taken into account this consideration certain interneurons can be recognized by their unique morphological characteristics or they can be more generally divided in subgroups on the bases of their pattern of axonal arborization, synaptic connections (both with pyramidal cells or between themselves) and physiological and biochemical characteristics. One most accepted classification of interneurons is based on the domain of pyramidal neurons their axons target combined with the immunoreactivity for different calcium binding proteins and neuropeptides [4,5].

2.1.1. Axosomatic targeting interneurons

The axosomatic targeting interneurons are chandelier cells and basket cells. Chandelier cells target on the AIS of principal cells and basket cells target the somata and proximal portions of dendrites of principal cells. Both interneurons are likely to exhibit a greater impact on the direct output of postsynaptic neurons. An important number of them are fast-spiking interneurons, most of which being immunoreactive for the calcium binding protein parvalbumin. In turn, most parvalbumin-immunoreactive cells are fast spiking large basket cells and chandelier cells. Parvalbumin-immunoreactive cells in rodents account for 40%–50% of GABAergic neurons [6]. A much higher percentage (74%) was found in macaque visual cortex [7].

Chandelier cells. These cells are the only interneuron that shows clearly recognizable terminal axonal specializations, which form short vertical rows of terminal buttons, resembling candlesticks. These cells only synapse with the AIS of principal cells [8-10]. For this reason they were named axo-axonic cells. Chandelier cells have been found not only in the neocortex, but also in several areas of the mesocortex, paleocortex and archicortex, which include the piriform cortex, entorhinal cortex, subiculum, hippocampus, fascia dentata, cingulate cortex, claustrum and amygdala [5,11]. Chandelier cells are present in all cortical layers (except layer 1), most abundantly in layer 2/3 [5,12.13]. A single chandelier cell can innervate between 250 (in neocortex) and 1,200 (in hippocampus) principal cells, indicating the potential to synchronize many principal cells [5,14]. Thus, chandelier cells appear ideally suited to shut off entire groups of pyramidal cells, making them the ultimate cortical switches. Each chandelier-terminal innervates single AIS. Moreover, each AIS may be innervated by one or a few chandelier terminals (five or less), which may originate from the same or different chandelier cells (for a review, see [14]). Chandelier cells are parvalbumin-reactive and fast-spiking cells.

Basket cells. Basket cells are most difficult to classify for their somatodendritic variety and sizes. The term 'basket' comes from the basket-like appearance of their axonal terminals around pyramidal cell somata that results from convergent innervation by many basket cells. About 50% of all inhibitory interneurons are basket cells [12]. Basket cells target the somata (15%-30% of their synapses are on somata) and proximal dendrites of principal cells; yet basket cells also target somata and dendrites of interneurons, particularly other basket cells [5,15,16]. There are *small basket cells* with a dense local axonal arborization that targets more dendrites than somata of principal cells; these small basket cells predominate in infragranular layers. *Large basket cells* are the typical basket cells. They have an extensive horizontal axonal branching with few vertical types of collateral. They are therefore the primary source of lateral inhibition across the cortical columns. Large basket cell predominate in layer 2/3. There are intermediate sizes of basket cells too. Basket cells can be parvalbumin-immunoreactive and fast spiking cells [6,16,17]. Other subgroup of basket cells are regular spiking; large- and medium-size basket cells are cholecystokinin immunoreactive neurons; small basket cells are immunoreactive for other calcium binding protein, or the vasointestinal neuropeptide; all this depends on the species studied [6,12,17].

2.1.2. Dendritic targeting interneurons

The dendritic targeting interneurons are more suited to modify and gate incoming excitatory inputs. The dendritic targeting interneurons are the bipolar cells, Martinotti cells, neurogliaform cells and double-bouquet cells. The latter cells target dendrites and spines.

Double bouquet cells. The axon of a double bouquet cell forms a tight fascicular axonal cylinder that can extends across all layers, innervating distal dendrites and spines. The highly varicose collaterals that form these columnar bundles are unusually thicker than the axonal main stem. While the morphology and distribution of double bouquet cells are similar in the human and macaque neocortex, these cells are modified or less numerous in the neocortex of other species (e.g. the cat), and may even be absent (e.g. the mouse and rat). Thus, differences in the morphology, number and distribution of double bouquet cells may represent fundamental differences in cortical micro organization between primates and other species [3]. Double bouquet cells usually are calbindin-immunoreactive. Together with being calbindin-immunoreactive, they can be also calretinin-immunoreactive. Other double bouquet cells are vasointestinal-peptide-immunoreactive and still others, cholecystokinin-immunoreactive [3,5,12].

Martinotti cells have a prominent axonal projection to layer 1. They have many fine unmyelinated ascending axon collaterals, which fan out as they ascend, bearing 'en passant' boutons in intermediate layers; some of these collaterals reach and branch as well in layer 1. Many other interneurons have ascending axon collaterals, but the prominent axonal arbour in layer 1 distinguishes Martinotti cells. Martinotti cells lie in particular in the deep cortical layers but also in layer 3 [18]. The majority of Martinotti cells are somatostatin-immunoreactive.

Bipolar cells. These are small cells with spindle or ovoid somata and narrow bipolar (most often) or bitufted dendrites that extend vertically. These cells can be found in all layers but predominate in layer 2/3 and layer 6. Bipolar neurons can be excitatory by releasing only vasointestinal-peptide, or inhibitory by releasing mainly GABA (though inhibitory bipolar cells also express vasointestinal-peptide). Bipolar cells commonly express calretinin too. Their axon forms a narrow band that crosses all layers leaving a little proportion of terminals, mainly on the basal dendrites of principal cells [12].

Neurogliaform cells. These are small-sized 'button-type' cells with many fine, radiating dendrites that are short and aspiny, finely beaded and rarely branched. They form a highly symmetrical and spherical dendritic field. The axon can arise from any part of the soma or from the base of a dendrite, and shortly after its origin, it breaks up into a dense, intertwined arborization of ultra-thin axons with as many as ten orders of branching. Fine boutons are distributed on the axonal collaterals to form GABA synapses onto the dendrites of target cells. The molecular characteristics of neurogliaform cells are still not well understood [3,12].

2.2. Spiny neurons

In turn, the spiny group of cortical cell consists of several subgroups. Pyramidal neurons with upright somatodendritic orientation are by far the largest subgroup within the group of spiny cells. Upright pyramidal neurons are projecting cells of all cortical layers other than layer 1. Upright pyramidal neurons can be further subdivided (see below). In addition to upright pyramidal neurons, in layers 5-6 there is another collection of projection cells, of spiny nature too, the polymorphic-cell subgroup [19-23]. The spiny stellate neurons of layer 4 are an exception to the spiny-cell/extrinsic-projection correlation, because they are implicated in the canonical thalamo-cortical reciprocal circuit. They are directly innervated by thalamic axons and almost exclusively establish synaptic contact with the neighbouring layer 3. In this study we consider as a cerebral cortical principal cell any spiny neuron that extends an axon branch outside the cortical area where its soma is located.

2.2.1. Principal cells of intratelencephalic projection (inclusive of the type I cell, of striatal projection)

Principal neurons have been sub classified by the laminar position of the cell body, somatodendritic morphology, electrophysiology and axonal target [24]. For a review, see [25].

Concerning the axonal target, there are associative neurons of intracortical projection in the same hemisphere and commissural neurons that project to homotopic and heterotopic sites of the opposite hemisphere by way of the corpus callosum and anterior commissure. Principal cells of intratelencephalic projection encompass also those that can extend their axon to the striatum, claustrum, amygdala and other sites that are not out of the telencephalon.

Associative and commissural neurons exist in all layers but with differences concerning projection and species. A limited number of associative and commissural axons arise from spiny stellate cells of layer 4 and low layer 3 [26]. Most associative and commissural axons emerge from pyramidal cells sited in layers 2/3 and 5-6, and also from spiny inverted pyramidal cells and other polymorphic cells of layers 5-6 [23,27,28]. The axons of all these cells extend forward to innervate the layer 4 of cortical areas of higher-order hierarchy [23,27-30]. This is the so-called associative forward projection [31]. In turn, the associative backward projection arise from cells sited in layers 2/3 and 5-6 of higher-order areas to innervate layers 1 and, to a lesser extent, 3, 5 and 6 of areas of lesser-order hierarchy [23,27,32]. This layer-segregation of forward and backward projections indicates that they target very different neuronal elements in recipient regions [18].

Spiny inverted pyramidal cells are morphologically and numerically conspicuous among the cells of layers 5-6 furnishing the associative backward projection in rabbits and cats; these cells also originate an important proportion of commissural, cortico-claustral and cortico-striatal projections; they neglegeably project to extratelencephalic centres such as the geniculate nuclei, colliculi and pons [23,27,33]. See Table 1 for a summary and [28] for a review; see also Section 4 in this Chapter for more data on AIS of these cells.

Commissural axons result from a broad and anatomically diverse population of principal cells that are located primarily in layers 2/3, 5 and 6 of restricted areas; there are interspecies differences in the laminar address of commissural neurons; in ferrets, rabbits and rats the commissural neurons predominate in infragranular layers [23,26,27,34,35]. Commissural cells can be further defined based on patterns of collateral projections to the ipsi- and contralateral striata and cortices, as well as by the expression of combinations of molecular markers [36].

Despite having common morphologies and similar laminar distributions, the commissural and associative neurons have been reported to differ from each other in the rat, cat, and monkey neocortex; there, at least in adult animals, they constitute two separate populations of neurons that rarely have dual projections [26,34]. The expression of the orphan nuclear receptor Nurr1 is associated to layer 6 neurons projecting to the ipsilateral cortex, but not to those cells projecting to contralateral cortical regions [37]. Recent studies in mice motor cortex show that 4% of the commissural cells of layer 2/3 and 34% of layer 5 extends dichotomous axons to ipsilateral prefrontal cortex and contralateral motor cortex [38]. Also, in the rat sensory-motor cortex, there are bifurcated projections to associative and contralateral areas from cells of layers 5-6 [39].

Moreover, certain principal cells of layer 5 of rodents project to the striatum in addition to the ipsilateral and contralateral cortex [40-44]. Cells sited in layer 5 can also project to the ipsi- and contralateral claustra in rodents and rabbits [23,33,43]. These cortico-claustral cells may branch to the ipsilateral and contralateral cortical areas and striata, in addition to the claustra, but not to the thalamus [43]. By describing genes that identify molecularly distinct subpopulations of commissural neurons, a recent work has cast more light on the heterogeneity of these cells [45].

Projection type	Visual cortex	Auditory cortex	Retrosplenial cortex
Cortico-cortical intrahemispheric projection, total	25%	—	Not studied
Cortico-cortical intrahemispheric backward projection to primary cortex from columns across cortical layers of secondary cortex	26%	Not studied	Not studied
Cortico-cortical intrahemispheric backward projection to primary cortex from a horizontal, extended cell band along the layer 5/6 border of secondary and primary cortex*	82%	Not studied	Not studied
Cortico-cortical intrahemispheric forward projection to secondary cortex from columns across cortical layers of primary cortex	7.5%	42 %	Not studied
Cortico-cortical intrahemispheric lateral projection from columns across cortical layers of associative cortex	31%	30%	Not studied
Cortico-claustral projection from primary cortex	83%	Not studied	Not studied
Cortico-claustral projection from secondary cortex	23%	24%	Not studied
Cortico-claustral projection	—	—	10%
Cortico-striatal projection	< 20%	< 20%	Not studied
Cortico-thalamic projection to lateral and medial geniculate nuclei	Null	Null	Not studied
Cortico-collicular projection	Null	Null	Not studied
Cortico-pontine projection	< 1%	Not studied	Not studied

Table 1. Percentages of spiny inverted cells of layers 5-6 out of the total number of principal cells of layer 5-6 of identified projection in cerebral cortex of rabbits [23,27,33] (The commissural projection is not included in this Table, but see [23,27].) All but one* of these percentages were estimated taking into account all infragranular neurons within clear-cut columns of retrograde labelling that extended along the radial dimension of the cortex. (*) Spiny inverted neurons make up the majority of cells within a horizontal band of cells located at the border between layers 5 and 6 of primary and secondary visual cortex of projection to the ipsilateral primary visual cortex. This band of retrogradely labelled cells extends for millimetres in the secondary visual cortex from the sites of injection of retrograde tracer in the primary visual cortex. This band is particularly cell-populated in brains after multiple injections of tracer; with single injections, labelled cells lie scattered for millimetres in the border between layer 5 and layer 6 [27,28]. These findings have shown that there is a highly convergent yet diffuse projection from the layer 5/6-border principal cells of secondary visual cortex to discrete points of the primary visual cortex. Spiny inverted neurons are the principal source of this type of projection. This widespread projection is distinct from the backward cortico-cortical projection from secondary to primary visual cortex that originates in discrete columnar patches of cells.

All of these neurons of layer 2/3 and 5 that extend axons to telencephalic centres may be grouped in the type I principal cells upon the condition that they have branches to the striatum [44]. It should be noted, nevertheless, that this name (type I) had been chosen for the neurons of projection to extratelencephalic (or sub-cerebral centres) [1,46], which introduces confusion in the terminology.

2.2.2. *Principal cells of extratelencephalic projection*

The principal cells of extratelencephalic projection typically lie in layers 5-6. They include the projection cells to the thalamus and multiple sites in the brain stem and the spinal cord.

2.2.2.1. *Principal cells of extratelencephalic projection sited in layer 5 (type II multiple target principal cells and cortico-thalamic cells)*

Cortico-striatal axons of layer 5 cells can be collaterals not only of the type I [44] projection but also of the type II, extratelencephalic projection to regions such as the spinal cord, brain stem nuclei, pontine nuclei, colliculi, substantia nigra, zona incerta and subthalamic nucleus [20,40-44,47]. The latter projection arises from type II cells that in their origin may belong to the same kind of principal neuron with extensive sub-cortical projections that during development looses particularly some of them depending on the cortical area in which the parent soma lies, as it is the instance for the visual cortex [1]. As well, the type II projection leaves driver collaterals to the core cells of *higher-order nuclei* of the thalamus, which are parvalbumin-positive cells and in turn project to the cortical layer 4 [41,44,48]. Such a branching pattern has been demonstrated for the axonal pathways of visual, somatosensory, pre-limbic and motor cortex of rats, cats and monkeys [41,42,47-51]. The presynaptic boutons of the axon of type II cells of layer 5 are usually of a big size, typically bigger than those leaved by axons of type I intratelencephalic cells [44,51].

Although principal cells share numerous common features within layer 5, they are heterogeneous in their somatodendritic morphology [1,25,52]. Type II cells of layer 5 have a thick apical dendrite extending into cortical layer 1 with a prominent terminal tuft; these cells produce distinctive initial bursts of tonic firing in response to current injection [46,53-55]. Depending on the cell-body position in layer 5, type I cells are characterized by having an apical dendrite that can tuft in cortical layer 1 or ascend to this layer without tufting; type I cells tend to fire phasically [44,46,54-57]. In addition, cells of layer 5b of short apical dendrite may project to the thalamus and superior colliculus but not to the striatum [18].

Thus, at least three subtypes of principal cells of layer 5 can be tentatively classified in agreement to their projection: the type I cell of intratelencephalic projection; the type II cell of sub-cerebral projection with collaterals to the striatum and thalamus; finally, the cortico-thalamic cell of layer 5b, which can project to the superior colliculus but not to the striatum.

2.2.2.2. *Principal cells of extratelencephalic projection sited in layer 6*

It is well known that some cells of cortical layer 6 innervate the thalamus leaving collaterals to cortical layer 4. This cortico-thalamic projection is originated in pyramidal cells but not in spiny inverted or other polymorphic cells of layer 6 (Table 1) [23,28]. This projection is specific of the cortico-thalamo-cortical loop [5,51,58]. Remarkably, the cortico-thalamic projection of layer 6 cells can innervate both types of thalamic relay neurons, i.e. the first-order (core, parvalbumin-positive) and the higher-order (matrix, calbindin-positive) cells. Both types of relay neurons not only lie in *first-order relay nuclei* but also *higher-order or associative nuclei*—the relative number of first-order relay cells being predominant in first-order relay nuclei and vice-versa. Regardless their thalamic address, the first-order relay cells are driven by ascending axons to the thalamus and successively innervate the spiny stellate cells and small pyramidal cells of layers 4 and 3b of precise sites of corresponding cortical areas. The higher-order relay cells widely innervate principal cells of layers 1, 2 and 3a of several cortical areas [48,51]. The first-order relay neurons are driver cells to their innervated cortical cells whereas higher-order relay neurons would be modulator cells to their innervated cortical cells. In turn, cells of layer 6a of cortico-thalamic projection are modulatory cells to the core cells of *first-* and *higher order nuclei* of the thalamus whilst leaving collaterals to the thalamic reticular nucleus and cortical layer 4 cells. (It should be remembered here that the type II cells of layer 5 are driving cells to the core cells of the *higher-order nuclei* of the thalamus and do not leave collaterals to the thalamic reticular nucleus.) Layer 6b cells of cortico-thalamic projection innervate the core and matrix cells of *first-* and *higher order nuclei* of the thalamus and leave collaterals to cortical layer 5 and 6 layer. By this way, cortical output will influence the synchronous ascending first-order and high order thalamo-cortical pathways. In Ray W. Guillery's words, this is *"how anatomical pathways link perception and action"* [59]. At least in the visual primary area, the cortico-thalamic cells of layer 6a dominate numerically over cortico-thalamic cells of layer 6b. Cortico-thalamic cells of layer 6 have been estimated to be between 30%-50% of all cells of layer 6 neurons (see [60] for review).

3. Cortical intrinsic circuits

Principal cells. A solitary action potential in a single principal cell of layer 2/3 can trigger polysynaptic chains of activity, detected as excitatory postsynaptic potentials and inhibitory postsynaptic potentials in recorded neurons [61]. This reveals an extremely efficacious means of activity propagation in the cortical network. In human brain slices, a relatively high proportion of basket (20%) and chandelier (33%) neurons could be driven to threshold by a single principal cell spike, in stark contrast to an estimated 1% likelihood of finding polysynaptic events in rats [61,62]. The fact is that the intralaminar circuit of layer 2/3 is highly recurrent and dominates its own cells. Principal cells of layer 2/3 extend collaterals for several millimetres to form patchy connections in the layer in cats and monkeys [63,64]. On the contrary, the intralaminar circuit of layer 5 depends little of the input from its own layer [58]. Intralaminar circuits exist basically on all species studied. However, the weight of the layer 2/3 circuit could be lower in rodents and rabbits because they do not have a patchy pattern connection in layer 2/3 but in layer 5b-6a [27,65].

Only the type I of principal cells occurs in layer 2/3. These cells extend their axon to the cortex, striatum, claustrum and other telencephalic centres. The probability of reciprocal connections between projection subtypes of all of these intratelencephalic cells is similar [57]. In layer 5 there are several types of projection cells. Synapses occur reciprocally between cells of similar type, e.g., intratelencephalic with intratelencephalic cells, type II cells with type II cells, etc. There are connections between type I and type II cells of layer 5 too, but they are hierarchical, that is, projections from type I cells to type II cells are more probable than projections in opposite way [44,54-56]. Principal cells of layer 6 of intratelencephalic projection have a higher probability of extending reciprocal connections between one another than with other type of projection cells. Next, these cortico-cortical cells have a higher probability of extending collaterals to cortico-thalamic cells than vice-versa [60]. Cells of layer 6 receive collaterals from cells of any other layer except layers 2 and 4 and extend collaterals to cells of layers 5-6. The exception being the layer 6a cell of cortico-thalamic projection to the core cells of thalamic nuclei that also extend collaterals to the thalamic reticular nucleus. This cell originates cortico-cortical collaterals only to cortical layer 4 cells [60].

Considering all cortical layers, the weight of the local intrinsic circuit in cat and monkey neocortex is estimated to be 80%-85% of excitatory inputs on principal neurons [58,66] whereas the weight of short- and long-range cortico-cortical circuits are 15% and 3%; on the same cells, the weight of the cortico-thalamic and intriguing cortico-claustral circuits is 1.3% and 3% respectively [66]. Finally, although cells of layer 2/3 probably connect more with cells of the same layer, some cells of layer 2/3 send collaterals to both, type I and type II cells of layers 5 and 6.

Principal cells are approximately 80% of the total of cortical neurons; interneurons make up the remaining ≈20%. Over 71% of the synapses in the cortex are derived from principal cells. However, this number does not truly reflect the relative balance between excitation and inhibition in cortex. When the larger efficacy of inhibitory synapses is taken into account, the dominance of the principal cells is reduced to 24%. Thus, the spiny cells provide the basic framework of long-distance excitation in both the vertical and lateral dimensions of the cortex, which is moulded by local inhibitory neurons [67].

Interneurons. Cortical interneurons innervate mainly principal cells, but they also innervate interneurons [16]. Interneurons form distinct intralaminar and interlaminar networks [16,53]. The probability of reciprocal synaptic connections between principal cells and interneurons varies with the type of interneuron. The intralaminar reciprocal connections between fast-spiking interneurons (chandelier cells and basket parvalbumin-positive cells) and principal cells are significantly higher than the probability of reciprocal connections between non fast-spiking interneurons and principal cells [53]. On the contrary, the interlaminar reciprocal connection between principal cells and interneurons is more frequent with non fast-spiking interneurons [53].

Another distinctive feature of the network of interneurons is its coupling through gap junctions. Electrical coupling of neocortical interneurons is firmly established by anatomical studies and electrophysiological experiments since [68]. The coupling is generally between interneurons of the same type [69]. Chandelier cells are electrically coupled too, as disclosed recently [62]. However, neurogliaform cells are electrically coupled to other neurogliaform cells but also to basket cells, regular-spiking interneurons and chandelier cells, among others interneurons. Thus, the neurogliaform cell links networks of particular classes of interneurons, each network being in turn electrotonically coupled itself [70].

Fast-spiking interneurons target the somatic and perisomatic domains of the principal cell; thus, these interneurons strongly regulate the output of the principal cell [4,18]. Reciprocal connections between pyramidal cells and fast-spiking interneurons act as a recurrent feedback inhibition that can regulate the timings of pyramidal cell firing [5]. In turn, spike timings of fast-spiking interneurons are correlated with the local field potential in the network of principal neurons during gamma oscillations that depend on the electrical and chemical coupling between fast-spiking, parvalbumin-positive interneurons [17,71]. Parvalbumin-positive basket cells fire counter-phase with principal cells and in the same phase but slightly delayed to chandelier cells [17,72].

4. The axon initial segment

Electrically, the AIS bridges dendritic and axonal compartments, converting graded dendritic inputs into all-or-none action potentials. Molecularly, the AIS maintain neuronal polarity preserving the molecular distribution between the axonal and somatodendritic domains [73]. Recent studies have revealed an ever-expanding complexity in the molecular components and in the types and distribution of ion channels embedded in the AIS. This complexity underlies what is now being recognized as a highly dynamic structure [73]. AIS structure and composition vary considerably across, and even within, neuronal classes [74,75], seemingly tuned to the computational demands of the cell. A recent activity of the cell can affect AIS ion channel kinetics and availability, thus altering action potential waveform, timing, and probability. Over long timescales, even the location and size of the AIS can change to compensate for alterations in neuronal activity.

4.1. Ion channels, anchoring proteins and cytoskeletal components of the axon initial segment

Ion channels. Although multiple neuronal sites can support action potential generation, the high density of Na^+ channels inherent to the AIS makes it the lowest threshold site for it. Immunostaining, imaging of spike-dependent Na^+ flux and electrophysiological studies suggest a similar density of Na^+ channels throughout the AIS [73,76]. However, a recent study revealed that Na^+ channels at the distal AIS and the adjacent axon have a much lower half-activation voltage (up to 14 mV) than those at the proximal AIS and the soma [77]. Accordingly, the use of newly developed voltage imaging techniques combined with careful analysis of the site of initiation and propagation of the action potentials, show that they preferentially initiate at the distal end of the AIS [77-79]. Consistent with these electrophysiological data, immunostaining results revealed a segregation of two Na^+ channel subtypes at the AIS: high-threshold $Na_v1.2$ channels and low-threshold $Na_v1.6$ channels, targeted preferentially to the proximal and the distal AIS, respectively [77]. Immunostaining intensity of $Na_v1.6$ peaked at the distal end of the AIS, corresponding well to the action potential initiation zone (see [73] for review). Voltage-threshold for action potential initiation seems to be largely determined by the density of $Na_v1.6$, whereas $Na_v1.2$ channels in the proximal AIS support action potential back-propagation into the somato-dendritic compartment. Indeed, axonal action propagation fails to back propagate when the somatic membrane potential is hyperpolarized [77]. Spike-evoked Ca^{2+} influx in the AIS of different neurons in the SNC has been revealed by fluorescence imaging techniques [73]. These cells fire spike bursts typified by the recruitment of sub threshold Ca^{2+} influx through low voltage-activated Ca^{2+} channels, which include T- and R-type isoforms [80]. Traditionally, burst evoked Ca^{2+} influx was thought to be restricted to the dendrites. Indeed, these same low voltage-activated channels mediate Ca^{2+} influx in the AIS. Since low voltage-activated channels activate at hyperpolarized potentials, they contribute to sub threshold depolarization of the AIS. Thus, their activity can determine when and if a given stimulus evokes an action potential. Ca^{2+} influx through cartwheel cell T-type channels of the AIS, is down regulated by a type 3 dopamine receptor (D3R)-dependent pathway [81]. This neuromodulatory pathway is remarkably specific for just AIS T-type channels; neither dendritic T-type channels nor AIS Na^+ or K^+ channels were affected by D3R signalling [73]. $Serotonin_{1A}$ receptor mediates neuronal hyperpolarization by activating potassium channels in the AIS. In human and monkey neocortex the $serotonin_{1A}$ receptor have been reported to be highly concentrated in the membrane of the AIS of principal neurons [82,83].

Associated anchoring proteins and cytoskeletal components. The structure of the AIS of multipolar neurons possesses a dense layer of finely granular material undercoating the plasma membrane, scattered clusters of ribosomes and fascicles of microtubules. The fascicles of microtubules occur only in the axon hillock and initial segment. An undercoating of the plasma membrane of the axon occurs in the node of Ranvier [84-86]. Interestingly, the plasma membrane of AIS and nodes is surrounded by a large extracellular space containing dense material; this similarity between nodes and AIS is coincident with the presence of voltage gated channels and specialization of the cytoskeleton present therein [73,76]. In addition, the dense material undercoating the plasma membrane of the AIS is separated 15-25 microns from the internal surface of the AIS membrane [84]. The neuronal cytoskeleton, consisting of interacting spectrins and actins, forms the neuronal structural scaffold and is a spatial delimiter for neuronal membrane proteins; the membrane undercoating is a specialized cytoskeletal element, found only in the AIS. The ßIV isoform of spectrin (an actin-binding protein) and ankyrin G (a spectrin-binding protein) mutually confine each other to the AIS [14,76]. Ankyrin G provides a specific anchor for many AIS-specific proteins, including the Na^+ and K^+ channel subunits KCNQ2 and 3. PSD-93, other scaffold protein, binds to the K_v1 channels found at the AIS. In addition K_v1 channels are associated to the adhesion molecule Casppr2 in the layer 2/3 of the human cerebral cortex [76]. Silencing of PSD-93 expression in cultured hippocampal neurons blocks the recruitment of K_v1 channels to the AIS but not Na^+ channels [87]. The AIS is also enriched in the cell adhesion molecules Nr-CAM and Neurofascin-186, and the cytoskeletal linker ßIV spectrin [76]. Recruitment of these proteins to the AIS also depends on ankyrin G [73,88]. Together, these results point to ankyrin G as the master regulator of AIS assembly. Silencing of AIS proteins in mature neurons in culture reveals that as for development, ankyrin G is required to maintain ion channels at the AIS [89]. Intriguingly, these and other experiments also showed that ankyrin G functions not only to cluster and maintain ion channels, but also to maintain neuronal polarity [89].

4.2. Length of the axon initial segment

AIS-length of cortical principal cells ranges between 17-40 microns as counted from the axon hillock [76,84,86]. This AIS length approximately coincides with the electrophysiological zone of initiation of the action potential, estimated to be ≈35-50 microns from the soma [78,79,90,91]. Interneurons have a shorter AIS than principal cells [15]. Granule cells of the fascia dentata give rise to the smallest unmyelinated fibres of the CNS. In these cells the action potentials are initiated at the distal axon but at ≈5-15 microns from soma with Na^+ channel density specialized for robust action potential initiation and propagation with minimal current flow [91,92]. The length of the AIS of granule cells of the hippocampus resembled that of the large basket cells of the neocortex, which on average are 6 microns length although the axons of large basket cells are myelinated [15]. Hippocampal granule cells may be an exception because they are not connected between themselves as it occurs in all cortical neurons [5]. It would be of interest to explore if differences in the length of AIS are functionally relevant. In the AIS of hippocampal granule cells the $Na_v1.6$ channel is the predominant alfa-subunit whilst the $Na_v1.2$ cannot be detected [92]; this suggests that $Na_v1.6$ channels are enough to generate the axon potential, and therefore that the mechanisms governing this generation are different in the thin non-myelinated axon of the granule cell than in other myelinated or unmyelinated neurons having also a short AIS length.

5. Study with electron microscopy of the axon initial segment of the inverted variety of cerebral cortical principal cell (of intratelencephalic projections)

Our studies following the use of retrograde tracers in cerebral cortex of rats, rabbits and cats showed that spiny inverted neurons of layers 5 and 6 originate intra-telencephalic projections [23,27,28,33]. Spiny inverted neurons are odd because of having not only circumscribed projections and an inverse somatodendritic orientation but also for the sites from which their axon arises. As seen with Golgi-method impregnation, retrograde tracers and intracellular filling (for a review, see [28]), these cell sites may be (1) the basal surface of the soma, or even the basal dendrite portion next to the soma, (2) the (lateral) surface of the soma and (3) the apical dendrite, sometimes from a sector more remote from the soma than the emergence site of the first dendrite branching [23]. Of the 127 Golgi-impregnated spiny inverted neurons in the occipital and temporal cortices of rabbits which we examined, 29% of the axons arises from (1), 9.5% from (2) and 61.5% from (3) [23]. This distribution is similar to that in rat visual and sensory-motor cortices [28]: of 28 Golgi-impregnated spiny inverted neurons, 32% of the axons emerges from (1), 21.5% from (2) and 46.5% from (3). Hence, the probability of axon emergence from the apical dendrite is higher both in rabbits and rats. There, inputs on the apical dendrite and its branches can be more operational for the generation of cell outputs, as they do not pass the somatic robust inhibitory barrier; in turn, the back-propagation of a generated axon potential can more effectively result in changes of the membrane potential of the apical dendrite and its branches. Thus, two physically segregated input integrations may simultaneously operate in the cells in which the axon arises from the apical dendrite: one at the immediate apical-tree membrane domain, the other at the somatic and remaining dendritic membrane domain. In the cat visual cortex, the orientation of apical dendrites of a spiny inverted neuron depends on the position of the parent cell within the gyri [28]. Accordingly, the incidence of truly reversed spiny inverted neurons decreased from the top of the gyri to the bottom of the sulci, while that of almost horizontally orientated pyramidal neurons increased. Most axons were found to arise from the apical dendrite or from one of its first branches in cat spiny inverted neurons too.

We reconstructed by means of electron-microscopy serial photography the AIS of eleven spiny inverted neurons of unknown projection (though they probably were cortico-cortical. cortico-claustral, or cortico-striatal, see Table 1). The length of the AIS of these neurons ranged between 32.0 and 101.2 microns, and its thickness varied between 0.58 and 1.04 microns. The range of the AIS length described by others shows some variability, indicating that cells of different subtypes of projection neurons, or cells within the subtypes themselves, may have different AIS length; e.g. the commissural and cortico-thalamic cells show more variability in the length of the AIS than the cortico-cortical associative ones [86]. Importantly, the number of synaptic boutons received by the AIS of spiny inverted neurons was found to be 24.4 on the average, but the range was also wide (11-37 boutons). Analysis of the spiny inverted neurons as classified in terms of the emergence site of the axon revealed that AIS which proceed from the apical dendrite were the shortest, thinnest and less innervated, whereas AIS arising from the somatic flank were the longest, widest and most innervated. Thus, AIS originated on apical dendrites averaged a length of 38.8 microns (range 37.1—45.4 microns), a diameter of 6.0 microns (range 0.58–0.62 microns) and a number of 15 apposed boutons (range 11—18 boutons). AIS of lateral somatic emergence averaged a length of 95.5 microns (range 93.2–97.8), a diameter of 1.04 microns (range 1.04—1.04) and 34 boutons (range 31—37). In turn, six AISs of somatic basal emergence averaged 60.9 microns in length, 0.83 microns in diameter and 26 boutons (ranges being 32.0–101.2 microns, 0.71–0.96 microns and 21—29 boutons, respectively) [28]. These features of the AIS may support an output generation that is peculiar to subclasses of spiny inverted neurons. Work is currently in progress in our laboratory to refine to which extent differences in the number of synapses received by the AIS are related to the type of axon projection of spiny inverted cells.

6. Study with electron microscopy of the axon initial segment of the upright variety of cerebral cortical principal cell with experimentally identified backward ipsilateral and commissural projections in visual cortex

We present in the following a preliminary report on AIS of twelve pyramidal neurons of cortico-cortical projection to primary visual cortex; these cells, amid other projection cells, were recently studied in our laboratory [93]. All these twelve cells had a typical upright somatodendritic orientation; they sited in the lateral partition of secondary visual cortex of rats (Figure 1). The axons of six of these neurons projected to the ipsilateral primary visual cortex that bears the cortical representation of the vertical central meridian of binocular visual field. The axons of the remaining six neurons projected to the same region of primary visual cortex but contralaterally through the callosum. In each of these two groups, three neurons lay in layer 3 and the remaining three in layer 5. Thus, the neurons reported here were distributed in four subgroups in agreement with their layer address and cortico-cortical projection.

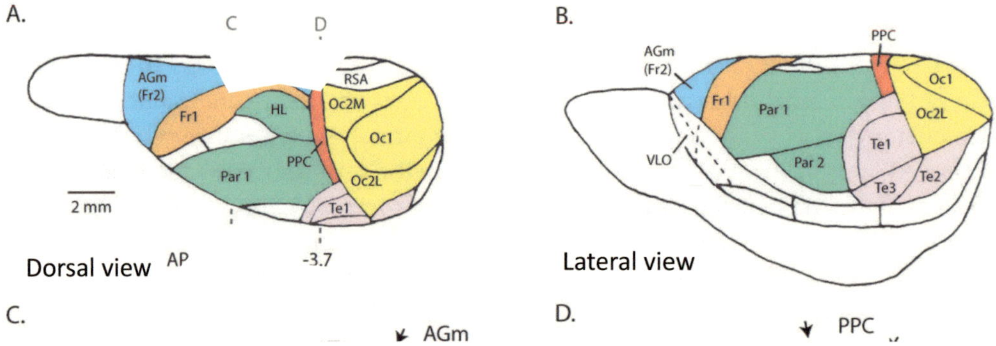

Figure 1. Schematic drawings of the dorsal view (A) and lateral view (B) of the left hemisphere of rat cerebral cortex. Oc1 corresponds with the primary visual area; Oc2M and Oc2L do so with the medial and lateral parts of the secondary visual area, respectively. The border between Oc1 and Oc2L is the cortical representation of the vertical central meridian of binocular visual field. Biotinylated dextran-amide (BDA) microinjections were placed in the Oc1 side of this border. Cells labelled with BDA by retrograde axon transport were taken from the ipsilateral Oc2L and homotopic contralateral border between Oc1 and Oc2L.

6.1. Material and methods

To study all these twelve neurons we combined axon track-tracing methods and serial electron microscopy. We injected biotinylated dextran-amide (BDA) in primary visual cortex, in order to identify projection pyramidal neurons under light microscopy (Figures 1, 2); then, we performed serial ultrathin-cutting and -photography to study anatomical parameters of labelled AISs under electron microscopy (Figures 3-5). Studied AIS parameters were length, thickness, and number of apposed synaptic boutons and distribution of these boutons along the AIS membrane. Student's t tests (p-value ≤ 0.05) and linear regressions statistics were used to compare measured AIS parameters (simple linear regression and non-parametric multiple tests; p-value ≤ 0.05).

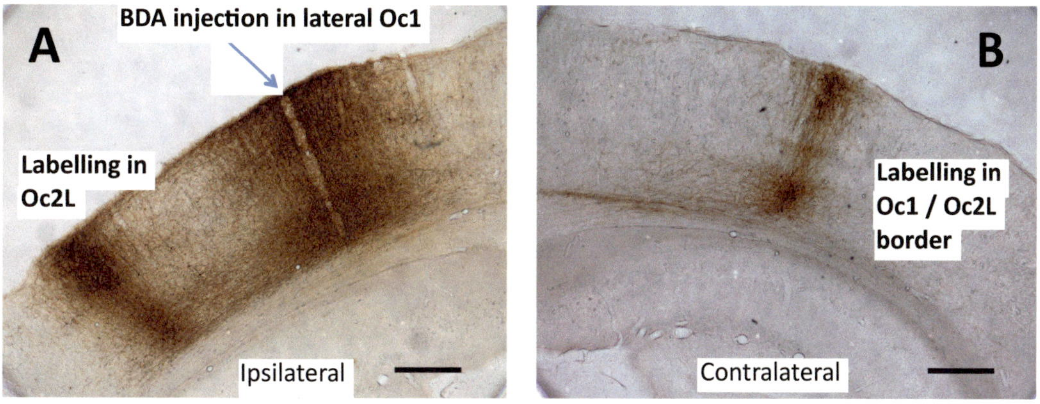

Figure 2. Microphotographs of paired coronal sections of left (A) and right (B) hemispheres of rat visual cerebral cortex. See columns of labelling in ipsilateral Oc2L (lateral partition of secondary visual area) and contralateral border between Oc2L and Oc1 after a biotinylated dextran-amide (BDA) microinjection (blue arrow) in Oc1 (primary visual area). Projection cells were selected for the present study among BDA-labelled cells of these or similar columns following comparable injections of BDA in other rats. Scale bars, 500 microns.

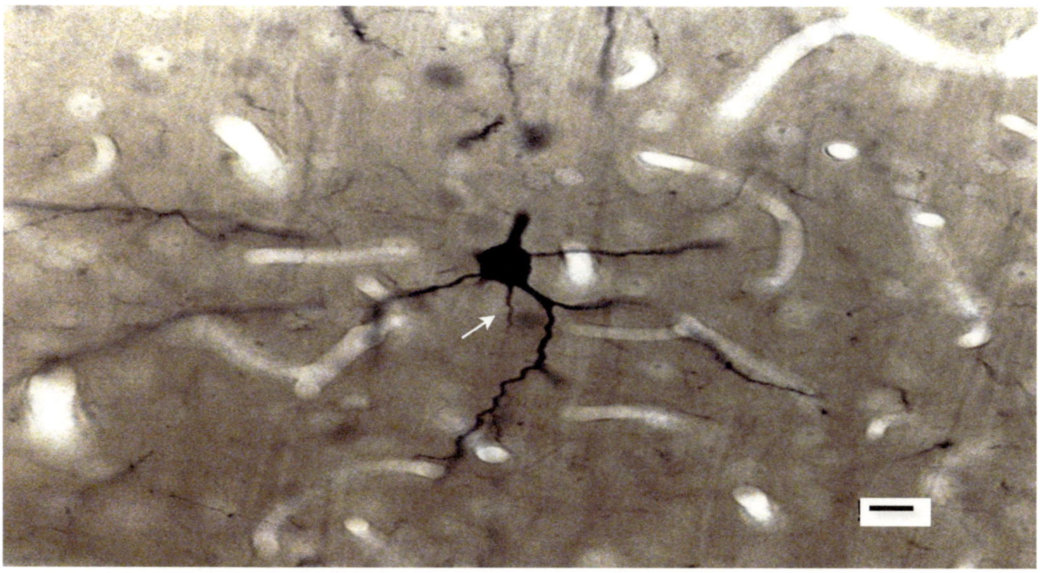

Figure 3. Microphotograph of a cell sited in layer 3 of Oc2L (lateral partition of secondary visual area); the cell was labelled after a biotinylated dextran-amide injection to ipsilateral Oc1 (primary visual area) in the cerebral cortex of a rat. The cell was flat embedded and the resultant slice was glued on top of a resin capsule. The axon initial segment (arrow) underwent serial ultrathin cutting and then it was examined under electronic microscopy. Scale bar, 15 microns.

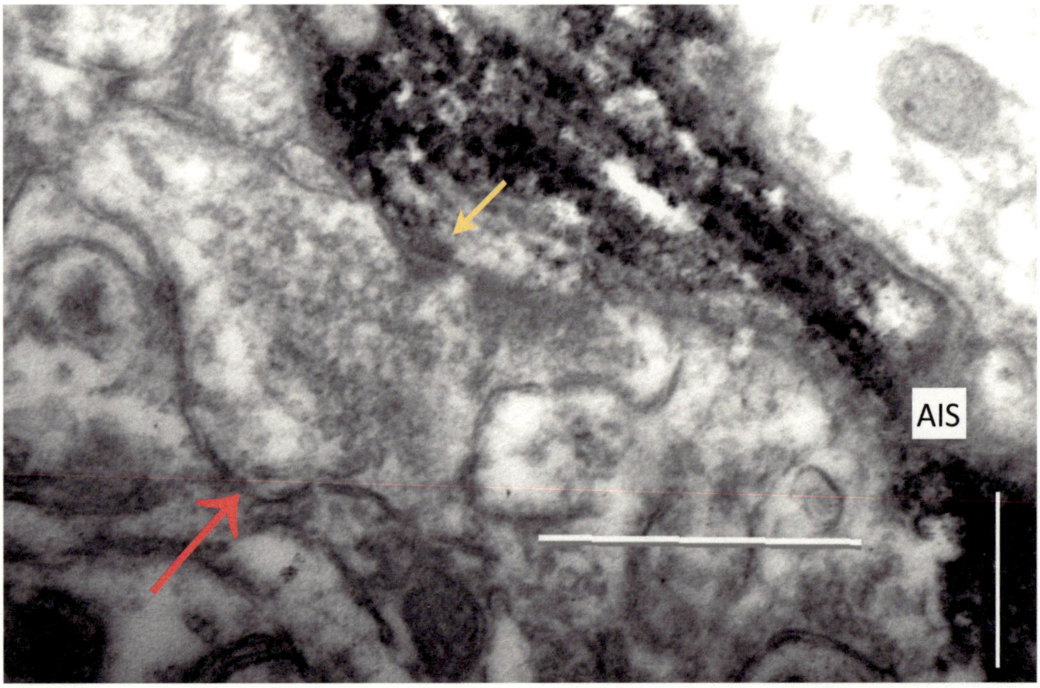

Figure 4. Electron-microscopy photograph of an axonal bouton (between red and yellow arrows) synapsing on the axon initial segment (AIS) of the cell shown in Figure 3. Most other boutons synapsing on this and other AIS contained flat vesicles. AIS was occupied by biotinylated dextran-amide, which gave it its black, grainy aspect. Notwithstanding this filling, see the pre- and postsynaptic densities, which are pointed at by the yellow arrowhead. Scale bar, 0.5 micron.

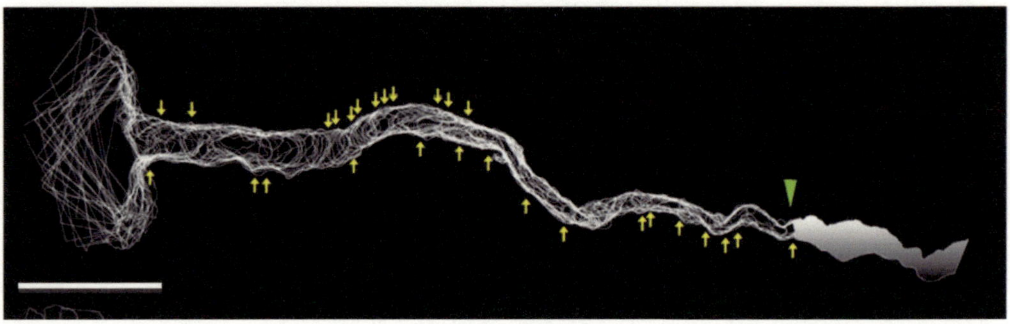

Figure 5. Electron-microscopy serial reconstruction of the axon initial segment (AIS) of the cell shown in Figures 3-4. The cell sited in layer 3 and furnished the associative backward projection to most-lateral (next to the border with lateral secondary cortex) primary visual cortex. The AIS was 22.27-micron-long, averaged a diameter of 0.93 microns and received 28 synaptic boutons (yellow arrows). Note the uneven distribution of these boutons along AIS: boutons were more abundant in the central tier and then in the distal one. Not all studied neurons in [93] and reported here had this bouton distribution along their AIS. The green arrowhead points to the site at which the myelin sheet begun. Scale bar, 5 microns.

6.2. Results

As a group, upright principal cells furnishing the associative backward projection from ipsilateral lateral secondary visual area to most-lateral primary visual area in the rat cerebral cortex had, on the average, shorter and thicker an AIS than similar cells of projection to the same area but through the callosum; these differences were however non-significant (Box 1). Importantly, AIS of cells of the associative backward projection averaged more synaptic boutons than AIS of cells of projection through the callosum; thus, the synaptic-bouton density per AIS length-unit was higher for AIS of cells of the associative backward projection; these differences were significant (Box 1).

Results also showed that the neurons sited in layer 3 had, on the average, shorter and thinner an AIS than the neurons sited in layer 5, these differences being non-significant except for the AIS-length comparison. Importantly, the AIS of layer 3 cells averaged more synaptic inputs than that of layer 5 cells; thus, the bouton density per AIS length-unit was higher for layer 3 cells. These differences were significant (Box 1).

AVERAGED VALUES OF PYRAMIDAL-NEURON AIS AND THEIR COMPARISON AS GROUPED BY AXON PROJECTION

Projection	Neurons	AIS Lenght (μm) ± Standard Deviation	AIS Ø (μm) ± Standard Deviation	Number of Boutons ± Standard Deviation	Syn. Bouton Density per AIS Lenght (μm)
Ipsilateral	6	**26.73 ± 5.08**	**0.98 ± 0.10**	**26 ± 5.25**	**1.02 ± 0.33**
Contralateral	6	**28.38 ± 4.41**	**0.96 ± 0.15**	**18 ± 3.10**	**0.66 ± 0.20**

AS GROUPED BY SOMA LOCATION

Location	Neurons	AIS Lenght (μm) ± Standard Deviation	AIS Ø (μm) ± Standard Deviation	Number of Boutons ± Standard Deviation	Syn. Bouton Density per AIS Lenght (μm)
Layer 3	6	**24.50 ± 4.01**	**0.92 ± 0.13**	**25.50 ± 5.75**	**1.06 ± 0.28**
Layer 5	6	**30.61 ± 2.91**	**1.02 ± 0.12**	**18.50 ± 3.62**	**0.62 ± 0.17**

Differences between values in gray boxes were statiscally significant (Student's t-test, $p < 0.05$)

Box 1. Averaged values of AIS parameters and their comparison as grouped by projection and layer address.

In human cortex, the length of AIS of layer 3 neurons ranges between 11-47 microns, as calculated by immunocytochemistry to ßIV spectrin, GAT-1 and Na^+ channels [76]. However the length of the AIS is not correlated with the size of the perykarion [84,86, but see 94]. By means of regression tests we compared (a) the lengths versus the diameters, and (b) the lengths versus the numbers of received synaptic boutons for the twelve separate AIS presented here. The first comparison revealed a linear and significant relation (p-value = 0.009), by which the AIS diameter variation explained the 52% the AIS length variation. The second comparison, i.e. the lengths versus the numbers of received synaptic boutons, revealed an inverse, non-significant relation (p-value = 0.136). With a non-parametric multiple regression test we compared for the twelve AIS, as taken separately, the numbers of received synaptic boutons versus the layer addresses of the parent cell somata and the projection of the on-going axons. Direct and highly significant correlations emerged from these comparisons (p-values being 9.3×10^{-5} and 0.00025, respectively). Thus, AIS with a high number of apposed synaptic boutons has up to 90% of probabilities of being part of a cell sited in layer 3, on the one hand, or projecting backwards to the primary visual cortex, on the other hand.

Though the number of measured cells in the present study is admittedly low, we believe it is satisfactory for an electron microscopy study. The numbers of synaptic boutons on AIS of upright principal cells of cortico-cortical projection reported here are in general agreement with others of different cortical areas and mammals, if differences between animals, area addresses and axon projections have to be taken into account. Major discrepancies are with cat visual cortex [85] and monkey sensory-motor cortex [95] (Table 2). It has to be said however that the number of boutons revealed for the cat visual cortex in [85] exceeds by a large amount the number of boutons found for the cat visual cortex in [96] and in [86]—though in [86] the layer address of the cells must be considered too. More quantitative studies on AIS innervation of subtypes of principal cells of identified axon projection in different animals and cerebral cortical areas are clearly needed.

Reference	**Animal**	**Type of cortex**	**Layer — projection**	**Cells**	**Boutons**
[96]	Cat	Visual	2/3 —unknown	18	24 (average)
[85]	Cat	Visual	2/3 — unknown	3	42-44
[86]	Cat	Area 17	2/3 — *a	18	16-28*a
[95]	Monkey	Sensory-motor	2/3 — callosal (2 cells) and unknown	8	2-52
[93]	Rat	Visual	2/3 — *b	6	19-34*b
[95]	Monkey	Sensory-motor	5 — unknown	8	2-26
[28]	Rat	Visual	5/6 — +	11	11-37+
[93]	Rat	Visual, secondary & primary	5/6 — *c	6	15-23*c
[97]	Rabbit	Visual	5 — **	1	10**
[86]	Cat	Visual	5 — ***	10	1-5***

Table 2. Comparison between numbers of synaptic boutons apposed to the AIS membrane as found in [93] and other studies. Note that the boutons seen on AIS of axons projecting to the thalamus and the colliculi are far fewer than those seen on AIS of axons projecting to intratelencephalic projections. Differences concerning types of projection: (*) cortico-cortical. (a) Contralateral projection from primary visual area to secondary visual area, 16-23 boutons; ipsilateral projection from primary visual area to secondary visual area, 22-28 boutons. (b) Contralateral projection from primary visual area to the border between primary visual area and lateral secondary visual area, 19-22 boutons; ipsilateral projection from lateral secondary visual area to the border between primary visual area and lateral secondary visual area, 28-34 boutons. (c) Contralateral projection from primary visual area to the border between primary visual area and lateral secondary visual area, 15-16 boutons; ipsilateral projection from lateral secondary visual area to the border between primary visual area and lateral secondary visual area, 20-23 boutons. ** Cortico-collicular projection. *** Cortico-thalamic projection. Difference concerning anatomical subtypes of principal cells: + Spiny inverted neuron AIS.

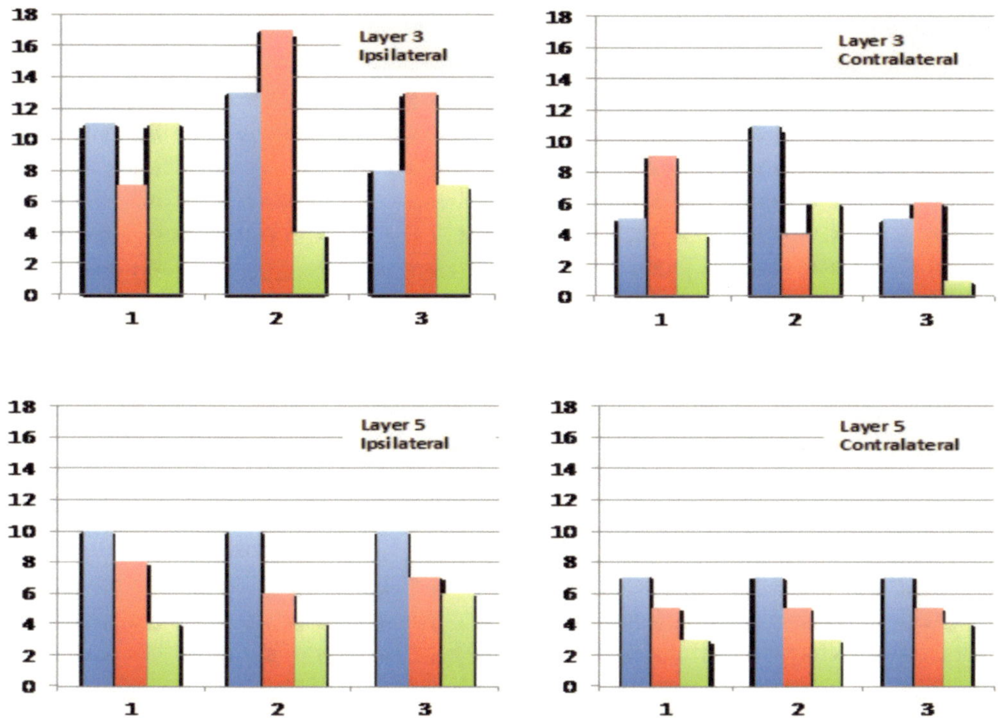

Figure 6. Distribution of synaptic boutons along each of twelve AIS of the present study [93]. Cells sited either in layer 3 or layer 5 and furnished either the associative backward (ipsilateral) projection or the callosal (contralateral) projection, both to primary visual cortex (3 neurons per layer and projection). Each AIS was divided into three segments of equal length (blue bars, closest tiers to the cell somata; green bars, closest tiers to the axon). X-axes show the bouton distribution for each AIS. Y-axes show the number of boutons counted per tier per AIS. Notice that, whilst all six AIS of layer 5 cells had a comparable decreasing pattern, AIS of layer 3 cells had uneven distributions even among cells of the same axon projection.

In order to know on the distribution of synaptic boutons along AIS, we divided each of the twelve AIS reported here in three equal longitudinal tiers and then we assigned boutons to tiers. As averaged for layer addresses and axon projection cell-subgroups, the distribution was decreasing towards the axon but for the subgroup of layer 3 cells of associative backward (ipsilateral) projection; there, the intermediate tier had more boutons (not shown). Most importantly, we compared one another the AIS of the twelve neurons (Figure 6). Then different patterns emerged not only for cells sited in layer 3 of ipsilateral projection but also for cells sited in layer 3 of commissural projection. Still, each cell sited in layer 5 had the decreasing pattern, notwithstanding if the cell was of ipsilateral or contralateral projection. Cells of layer 3 had uneven distributions, which can be tentatively grouped in two presumptive patterns: a 'reel' one, with more boutons apposed to the proximal and distal tiers of the AIS, and a 'barrel' type, with less boutons on the intermediate tier (Figure 6).

The variety in the distribution observed for the principal cells of layer 3 suggests either the presence in this cell group of examples of minor cell subpopulations occurring within those studied in [93], or activity-dependent AIS plasticity, or both. Ion channels composition at the AIS can vary considerably across different neuronal types [74] and diversity in the AIS length and position in the axon may also underlie interneuron variation in firing properties. For example, classes of retinal ganglion cells with different visual properties have initial segments that differ in length, and in their position within the axon [98]. In the avian magnocellularis and laminaris nuclei, which are respectively the second- and third-order nuclei in the auditory pathway [99], the length and the location of the AIS vary with the tuning frequency of neurons [100]. Activity-dependent AIS plasticity has been observed in cultured hippocampal neurons. Increasing chronically neuronal activity over 48 hours resulted in a significant shift in AIS position with the entire structure (ankyrin G, ßIV spectrin, and Na^+ channels) moving distally away from the soma [75]. Importantly, hippocampal AIS relocation is a bidirectional phenomenon because the AIS can shift proximally after neurons are returned to baseline activity conditions. In this way, on-going neuronal activity can fine-tune AIS position. Moreover, a lack of auditory input causes a change in AIS length of neurons of chick auditory nucleus magnocellularis [101]. All these studies showed that the AIS plasticity is coupled with changes in neuronal excitability. The distinct length of the AIS of hippocampal pyramidal neurons (≈30 microns) and the neurons of the nucleus magnocellularis (≈10 microns) has been suggested to be the cause of these different plastic changes in the AIS. Indeed, cell type-based variability in AIS plasticity is seen within hippocampal cultures, where GAD 65-expressing interneurons display little or no shift in AIS location upon high potassium stimulation [75]. Dopaminergic neurons in dissociated cultures of rat olfactory bulb show inverse AIS plasticity: their initial segments move proximally after 48 hours depolarization.

Although these plastic changes have not been shown for neocortical neurons to the best of our knowledge, nor is clear to which extent are associated with shifts on the distribution of presynaptic boutons apposed to the membrane of the AIS, it will be fascinating in the future to see how different types of neuron of diverse brain regions use different forms of AIS plasticity in response to perturbations in their electrical activity. Nonetheless, it follows from our study that at least for associative and commissural projections to primary visual cortex in the rat, the innervation of AIS of principal cells of typical somatodendritic orientation is steadier in layer 5 than in layer 3.

7. Conclusion

By presenting data on parameters such as the length and diameter of the AIS and, of no lesser importance, the number and distribution of presynaptic boutons apposed to the AIS membrane, this study advances the knowledge on the control of membrane potential and initiation of axon potential of visual cortex neurons, and particularly of the principal cells with cortico-cortical axon projection from layers 3 and 5 to primary visual area. It unveils that the bouton density on the AIS of principal cells would correlate significantly with the layer address and axon projection of the parent neuron rather than with the length and thickness of AIS proper. The present study additionally shows that there was a repeated decrease in the number of synaptic boutons apposed along the AIS of neurons of layer 5 but not of layer 3. It might be that neurons of layer 3 can be subdivided in subgroups within the groups of cortico-cortical ipsilateral or contralateral projection we have considered in the study. These subgroups might possess undisclosed structural and functional cell features associated to permanent or transitory synaptic-bouton distributions along the AIS.

Author details

José L. Bueno-López*, Juan C. Chara, Juan L. Mendizabal-Zubiaga and Concepción Reblet
Department of Neurosciences, School of Medicine and Dentistry,
The University of the Basque Country (UPV/EHU), Campus of Leioa (Bizkaia), Spain

Acknowledgement

This work was funded by grants GIU07/14 and UFI11/41 of UPV/EHU.

J.L.B.-L. and C.R. wish to lovingly dedicate this work to Laína H.B, Julia B.R. and Juan H.S. for leaving their mark on us ("*Todo pasa y todo queda, / pero lo nuestro es pasar, / pasar haciendo caminos, / caminos sobre el mar // ... // Caminante, son tus huellas / el camino y nada más; / caminante, no hay camino, / se hace camino al andar. // Al andar se hace camino / y al volver la vista atrás / se ve la senda que nunca / se ha de volver a pisar. // Caminante no hay camino / sino estelas en la mar...* ", Antonio Machado, Proverbios y Cantares, 1909).

8. References

[1] Molnár Z, Cheung, AFP. Classification of subpopulations of layer V pyramidal projection neurons. Neuroscience Research 2006; 55(2) 105–115, doi:10.1016/j.neures.2006.02.008

[2] Beaulieu C. Numerical data on neocortical neurons in adult rat, with special reference to the GABA population. Brain Research 1993; 609(1-2) 284–292, doi:10.1016/0006-8993(93)90884-P

[3] DeFelipe J, Alonso-Nanclares L, Arellano JI. Microstructure of the neocortex: comparative aspects. Journal of Neurocytology 2002; 31(3-5) 299-316, doi:10.1023/A:1024130211265

[4] DeFelipe J. Cortical interneurons: from Cajal to 2001. Progress in Brain Research 2002; 136(Chapter7) 215–238, doi:10.1016/S0079-6123(02)36019-9

[5] Somogyi P, Tamás G, Luján R, Buhl EH. Salient features of synaptic organisation in the cerebral cortex. Brain Research Reviews 1998; 26(2-3)113–35, doi:10.1016/S0165-0173(97)00061-1

[6] Burkhalter A. Many specialists for suppressing cortical excitation. Frontiers in Neuroscience 2008; 2(2) 155-167, doi:10.3389/neuro.01.026.2008

[7] DeFelipe J, González-Albo MC, Del Río MR, Elston GN. Distribution and patterns of connectivity of interneurons containing calbindin, calretinin and parvalbumin in visual

* Corresponding Author

areas of the occipital and temporal lobes of the macaque monkey. Journal of Comparative Neurology 1999; 412(3) 515–526, doi:10.1002/(SICI)1096-9861(19990927)412:3<515::AID-CNE10>3.0.CO;2-1

[8] Szentágothai J, Arbib MA. Conceptual models of neural organization. Neurosciences Research Program Bulletin 1974; 12(3) 306–510.

[9] Jones EG. Varieties and distribution of non-pyramidal cells in the somatic sensory cortex of the squirrel monkey. Journal of Comparative Neurology 1975; 160(2) 205–267, doi:10.1002/cne.901600204

[10] Somogyi P. A specific 'axo-axonal' interneuron in the visual cortex of the rat. Brain Research 1977; 136(-) 345–50.

[11] Inda MC, DeFelipe J, Muñoz A. Morphology and distribution of chandelier cell axon terminals in the mouse cerebral cortex and claustroamygdaloid complex. Cerebral Cortex 2009; 19(1) 41-54, doi:10.1093/cercor/bhn057

[12] Markram H, Toledo-Rodríguez M, Wang Y, Gupta A, Silberberg G, Wu C. Interneurons of the neocortical inhibitory system. Nature Reviews Neuroscience 2004; 5(-) 793–807, doi:10.1038/nrn1519

[13] Inda MC, DeFelipe J, Munoz A. The distribution of chandelier cell axon terminals that express the GABA plasma membrane transporter GAT-1 in the human neocortex. Cerebral Cortex 2007; 17(9) 2060-2071, doi:10.1093/cercor/bhl114

[14] Howard A, Tamás G, Soltesz I. Lighting the chandelier: new vistas for axo-axonic cells. Trends in Neurosciences 2005; 28(5) 310–316, doi:10.1016/j.tins.2005.04.004

[15] DeFelipe J, Hendry SHC, Jones EG. A correlative electron microscopic study of basket cells and large gabaergic neurons in the monkey sensory-motor cortex. Neuroscience 1986; 17(4) 991-1009, doi:10.1016/0306-4522(86)90075-8

[16] Kisvárday ZF, Beaulieu C, Eysel UT. Network of gabaergic large basket cells in cat visual cortex (area 18): implication for lateral disinhibition. Journal of Comparative Neurology 1993; 327(3) 398–415, doi:10.1002/cne.903270307

[17] Freund T. Interneuron diversity series: rhythm and mood in perisomatic inhibition. Trends in Neurosciences 2003; 26(9) 489-495, doi:10.1016/S0166-2236(03)00227-3

[18] Thomson AM, Bannister AP. Interlaminar connections in the neocortex. Cerebral Cortex 2003; 13(1) 5–14, doi:10.1093/cercor/13.1.5

[19] Ramón y Cajal S (1891) On the Structure of the Cerebral Cortex of Certain Mammals. (La Cellule 7: 125–176). In: DeFelipe J, Jones EG (trans. and eds.) Cajal on the Cerebral Cortex: An Annotated Translation on the Complete Writings (History of Neuroscience; Nº 1). New York: Oxford University Press; 1988, p23–54.

[20] Ramón y Cajal, S. (1911). Histologie du Systéme Nerveux de l'Homme et des Vertebrés. Paris: Maloine (Madrid: C.S.I.C. Facsimile Edition 1972). Chapters 24–35.

[21] Van der Loos H. The 'improperly' oriented pyramidal cell in the cerebral cortex and its possible bearing on problems of neuronal growth and cell orientation. Bulletin Johns Hopkins Hospital 1965; 117(-) 228–250.

[22] DeFelipe J, Jones EG. The Functional Histology of the Cerebral Cortex and the Continuing Relevance of Cajal's Observations. In: DeFelipe J, Jones EG (trans. and eds.)

Cajal on the Cerebral Cortex: An Annotated Translation on the Complete Writings (History of Neuroscience; Nº 1). New York: Oxford University Press; 1988, p557–621.
[23] Bueno-López JL, Reblet C, López-Medina A, Gómez-Urquijo S, Grandes P, Gondra J, Hennequet L. Targets and laminar distribution of projection neurons with inverted morphology in rabbit cortex. European Journal of Neuroscience 1991; 3(5) 415–430, doi:10.1111/j.1460-9568.1991.tb00829.x
[24] Larkman A, Mason A. Correlations between morphology and electrophysiology of pyramidal neurons in slices of rat visual cortex. I. Establishment of cell classes. Journal of Neuroscience 1990; 10(5) 1407–1414.
[25] DeFelipe J, Fariñas I. The pyramidal neuron of the cerebral cortex: morphological and chemical characteristics of the synaptic inputs. Progress in Neurobiology 1992; 39(6) 563–607.
[26] Innocenti GM. (1986). General Organization of Callosal Connections in the Cerebral Cortex. In: Jones EG, Peters A (eds) Cerebral cortex (vol. 5) Sensory-motor areas and aspects of cortical connectivity. Plenum Press, New York; 1986, p291–353.
[27] Reblet C, López-Medina A, Gómez-Urquijo SM, Bueno-López JL. Widespread horizontal connections arising from layer 5/6 border inverted cells in rabbit visual cortex. European Journal of Neuroscience 1992; 4(3) 221–234, doi:10.1111/j.1460-9568.1992.tb00870.x
[28] Mendizabal-Zubiaga JL, Reblet C, Bueno-López JL. The underside of the cerebral cortex: layer V/VI spiny inverted neurons. Journal of Anatomy 2007; 211(2) 223–236, doi:10.1111/j.1469-7580.2007.00779.x
[29] Casanovas-Aguilar C, Christensen MK, Reblet C, Martínez-García F, Pérez-Clausell J, Bueno-López JL. Callosal neurons give rise to zinc-rich boutons in the rat visual cortex. NeuroReport 1995; 6(3) 497-500.
[30] Casanovas-Aguilar C, Reblet C, Pérez-Clausell J, Bueno-López JL. Zinc-Rich afferents to the rat neocortex: projections to the visual cortex traced with intracerebral selenite injections. Journal of Chemical Neuroanatomy 1998; 72(2) 97–109, doi:10.1016/S0891-0618(98)00035-0
[31] Felleman DJ, Van Essen DC. Distributed hierarchical processing in the primate cerebral cortex. Cerebral Cortex 1991; 1(1) 1-47, doi:10.1093/cercor/1.1.1
[32] Coogan TA, Burkhalter A. Hierarchical organization of areas in rat visual cortex. Journal of Neuroscience 1993; 13(9) 3749-3772.
[33] Gutiérrez-Ibarluzea I, Acera-Osa A, Mendizabal-Zubiaga JL, Arana-Arri A, Bueno-López JL, Reblet C. Morphology and laminar distribution of cortico-claustral neurons in different areas of the rabbit cerebral cortex. European Journal of Anatomy 1999; 3(2) 101-109.
[34] Olavarría J, Van Sluyters RC. Organization and postnatal development of callosal connections in the visual cortex of the rat. Journal of Comparative Neurology 1985; 239(1) 1–26, doi:10.1002/cne.902390102
[35] Innocenti M, Manger PR, Masiello I, Colin I, Tettoni L. Architecture and callosal connections of visual areas 17, 18, 19 and 21 in the ferret (Mustela putorius). Cerebral Cortex 2002; 12(4) 411-422, doi:10.1093/cercor/12.4.411

[36] Molyneaux BJ, Arlotta P, Fame RM, MacDonald JL, MacQuarrie KL, Macklis JD. Novel subtype-specific genes identify distinct subpopulations of callosal projection neurons. Journal of Neuroscience 2009; 29(39) 12343–12354, doi:10.1523/ JNEUROSCI.6108-08.2009

[37] Arimatsu Y, Ishida M, Kaneko T, Ichinose S, Omori A. Organization and Development of Corticocortical Associative neurons expressing the orphan nuclear receptor Nurr1. Journal of Comparative Neurology 2003; 466(2) 180–196, doi:10.1002/cne.10875

[38] Mitchel BD, Macklis JD. Large-scale maintenance of dual projections by callosal and frontal cortical projection neurons in adult mice. Journal of Comparative Neurology 2005; 482(1) 17-32, doi:10.1002/cne.20428

[39] Veinante P, Deschênes M. Single-cell study of motor cortex projections to the barrel field in rats. Journal of Comparative Neurology 2003; 464(1) 98 –103, doi:10.1002/cne.10769

[40] Wilson CJ. Morphology and synaptic connections of crossed corticostriatal neurons in the rat. Journal of Comparative Neurology 1987; 263(4) 567-580, doi:10.1002/cne.902630408

[41] Levesque M, Charara A, Gagnon S, Parent A, Deschênes M. Corticostriatal projections from layer V cells in rat are collaterals of long range corticofugal axons. Brain Research 1996; 709(2) 311–315, doi:10.1016/0006-8993(95)01333-4

[42] Levesque M, Gagnon S, Parent A, Deschênes M. Axonal arborizations of corticostriatal and corticothalamic fibers arising from the second somatosensory area in the rat. Cerebral Cortex 1996; 6(6) 759–770, doi:10.1093/cercor/6.6.759

[43] Levesque M, Parent A. Axonal arborization of corticostriatal and corticothalamic fibers arising from prelimbic cortex in the rat. Cerebral Cortex 1998; 8(7) 602–613, doi:10.1093/cercor/8.7.602

[44] Reiner A, Hart NM, Lei W, Deng Y. Corticostriatal projection neurons—dichotomous types and dichotomous functions. Frontiers in Neuroanatomy 2010. 4(Article142) 1-15, doi:10.3389/fnana.2010.00142

[45] Shoemaker LD, Arlotta P. Untangling the Cortex: Advances in Understanding Specification and Differentiation of Corticospinal Motor Neurons. BioEssays 2010; 32(3) 197–206. Available online 27 January 2010; http://dx.doi.org/10.1002/bies.200900114

[46] Kasper EM, Larkman AU, Lübke J, Blakemore C. Pyramidal neurons in layer 5 of the rat visual cortex. III. Differential maturation of axon targeting, dendritic morphology and electrophysiological properties. Journal of Comparative Neurology 1994; 339(4) 495–518, doi:10.1002/cne.903390404

[47] Kita T, Kita H. The subthalamic nucleus is one of multiple innervation sites for long-range corticofugal axons: a single-axon tracing study in the rat. Journal of Neuroscience 2012; 32(17) 5990-5999, doi:10.1523/jneurosci.5717-11.2012

[48] Jones E.G. The thalamic matrix and thalamocortical synchrony. Trends in Neurosciences 2001; 24(10), 595-601, doi:10.1016/S0166-2236(00)01922-6

[49] Rockland KS. Convergence and branching patterns of round, type II corticopulvinar axons. Journal of Comparative Neurology 1998; 390(4) 515-536, doi:10.1002/(SICI)1096-9861(19980126)390:4<515::AID-CNE5>3.0.CO;2-3

[50] Veinante P, Lavallé P, Deschênes M. Corticothalamic projections from layer V of the vibrissal barrel cortex in the rat. Journal of Comparative Neurology 2000; 424(2) 197-204, doi:0.1002/1096-9861(20000821)424:2<197::AID-CNE1>3.0.CO;2-6
[51] Guillery RW, Sherman SM. Thalamic relay functions and their role in corticocortical communication: generalizations from the visual system. Neuron 2002; 33(2) 163-175, doi:10.1016/S0896-6273(01)00582-7
[52] Hallman LE, Schofield BR, Lin CS. Dendritic morphology and axon collaterals of corticotectal, cortico-pontine, and callosal neurons in layer V of the primary visual cortex of the hooded rat. Journal of Comparative Neurology 1990; 272(1) 149–160, doi:10.1002/cne.902720111
[53] Otsuka T, Kawaguchi Y. Cortical inhibitory cell types differentially form intralaminar and interlaminar subnetworks with excitatory neurons. Journal of Neuroscience 2009; 29(34) 10533-10540, doi:10.1523/jneurosci.2219-09.2009
[54] Brown SP, Hestrin S. Intracortical circuits of pyramidal neurons reflect their long-range axonal targets. Nature 2009; 457(-) 1133–1136, doi:10.1038/nature07658
[55] Kiritani T, Wickersham IR, Seung HS, Shepherd GMG. Hierarchical connectivity and connection-specific dynamics in the corticospinal-corticostriatal microcircuit in mouse motor cortex. Journal of Neuroscience 2012; 32(14) 4992-5001, doi:10.1523/jneurosci.4759-11.2012
[56] Morishima M, Morita K, Kubota Y, Kawaguchi Y. Highly differentiated projection-specific cortical subnetworks. Journal of Neuroscience 2011; 31(28) 10380-10391, doi:10.1523/jneurosci.0772-11.2011
[57] Otsuka T, Kawaguchi Y. Cell diversity and connection specifity between callosal projection neurons in the frontal cortex. Journal of Neuroscience 2011; 31(10) 3862-3870, doi:10.1523/jneurosci.5795-10.2011
[58] Binzegger T, Douglas RJ, Martin KAC. A quantitative map of the circuit of cat primary visual cortex. Journal of Neuroscience 2004; 24(39) 8441– 8453, doi:10.1523/jneurosci.1400-04.2004
[59] Guillery RW. Anatomical pathways that link perception and action. In: Progress in Brain Research. Elsevier BV. 2005; 149(Chapter 17) 235-256, doi:10.1016/S0079-6123(05)49017-2
[60] Thomson A.M. Neocortical layer 6, a review. Frontiers in Neuroanatomy 2010; 4(13) 4-14, doi:10.3389/fnana.2010.00013
[61] Molnár G, Oláh S, Komlósi G, Füle M, Szabadics J, Varga C, Barzo P, Tamás, G. Complex events initiated by individual spikes in the human cerebral cortex. PLoS Biology September 2008; 6(9):e222, doi:10.1371/journal.pbio.0060222
[62] Woodruff A, Yuste R. State-dependent function of neocortical chandelier cells. Journal of Neuroscience 2011; 31(49), 17872-17886, doi:10.1523/jneurosci.3894-11.2011
[63] Gilbert CD, Wiesel TN. Columnar specificity of intrinsic horizontal and corticocortical connections in cat visual cortex. Journal of Neuroscience 1989; 9(7), 2432–2442.
[64] Kisvárday ZF, Eysel UT. Cellular organization of reciprocal patchy networks in layer III of cat visual cortex area 17. Neuroscience 1992; 46(2) 275–286, doi: 10.1016/0306-4522(92)90050-C

[65] Burkhalter A. Intrinsic connections of rat primary visual cortex: laminar organization of axonal projections. Journal of Comparative Neurology 1989; 279(2) 171-186, doi: 10.1002/cne.902790202

[66] Markov NT, Misery P, Falchier A, Lamy C, Vezoli J, Quilodran R, Gariel MA, Giroud P, Ercsey-Ravasz M, Pilaz LJ, Huissoud C, Barone P, Dehay C, Toroczkai Z, Van Essen DC, Kennedy H, Knoblauch K. Weight consistency specifies regularities of macaque cortical networks. Cerebral Cortex 2011; 21(6) 1254—1272, doi: 10.1093/cercor/bhq201

[67] Douglas RJ, Martin KAC. Recurrent neuronal circuits in the neocortex. Current Biology 2007; 17(13) R496-R500.

[68] Galarreta M, Hestrin S. A network of fast-spiking cells in the neocortex connected by electrical synapses. Nature 1999; 402(-), 72–75, doi:10.1038/47029

[69] Fukuda T, Kosaka T, Singer W, Galuske RAW. Gap junctions among dendrites of cortical GABAergic neurons establish a dense and widespread intercolumnar network. Journal of Neuroscience 2006; 26(13) 3434 –3443, doi: 10.1523/jneurosci.4076-05.2006

[70] Simon A, Oláh S, Molnár G, Szabadics J, Tamás G. Gap-junctional coupling between neurogliaform cells and various interneuron types in the neocortex. Journal of Neuroscience 2005; 25(27) 6278-6285, doi:10.1523/jneurosci.1431-05.2005

[71] Bartos M, Vida I, Jonas P. (2007). Synaptic mechanisms of synchronized gamma oscillations in inhibitory interneuron networks. Nature Reviews Neuroscience 2007; 8(-) 45-56, doi:10.1038/nrn2044

[72] Klausberger T, Magill PJ, Márton LF, Roberts JD, Cobden PM, Buzsáki G, Somogyi P. Brain-state- and cell-type-specific firing of hippocampal interneurons in vivo. Nature 2003; 421(6925) 844-848.

[73] Grubb MS, Shu Y, Kuba H, Rasband MN, Wimmer VC, Bender, KJ. Short- and long-term plasticity at the axon initial segment. Journal of Neuroscience 2011; 31(45), 16049-16055, doi:10.1523/jneurosci.4064-11.2011

[74] Lorincz A, Nusser Z. Cell-type-dependent molecular composition of the axon initial segment. Journal of Neuroscience 2008; 28(53) 14329-14340, doi: 10.1523/jneurosci.4833-08.2008

[75] Grubb MS, Burrone J. Activity-dependent relocation of the axon initial segment fine-tunes neuronal excitability. Nature 2010; 465(-) 1070-1076, doi:10.1038/nature09160

[76] Inda MC, DeFelipe J, Muñoz A. Voltage-gated ion channels in the axon initial segment of human cortical pyramidal cells and their relationship with chandelier cells. PNAS 2006; 103(8) 2920-2925, doi:10.1073/pneas.05111971.03

[77] Hu W, Tian C, Yang M, Hou H, Shu Y. Distinct contributions of $Na_v1.6$ and $Na_v1.2$ in action potential initiation and backpropagation. Nature Neuroscience 2009; 12(-) 996-1002, doi:10.1038/nn.2359

[78] Palmer LM, Stuart GJ. Site of action potential initiation in layer 5 pyramidal neurons. Journal of Neuroscience 2006; 26(6) 1854–1863, doi: 10.1523/jneurosci.4812-05.2006

[79] Shu Y, Duque A, Yu Y, Haider B, McCormick, D. Properties of action-potential initiation in neocortical pyramidal cells: evidence from whole cell axon recordings. Journal of Neurophysiology 2007; 97(1) 746-760, doi:10.1152/jn.00922.2006

[80] Perez-Reyes E. Molecular physiology of low-voltage-activated t-type calcium channels. Physiological Reviews 2003; 83(1) 117-161, doi:10.1152/physrev.00018.2002

[81] Bender KJ, Ford CP, Trussell LO. Dopaminergic modulation of axon initial segment calcium channels regulates action potential initiation. Neuron 2010; 68(3) 500 –511, 10.1016/j.neuron.2010.09.026

[82] DeFelipe J, Hendry SH, Hashikawa T, Jones EG. Synaptic relationships of serotonin-immunoreactive terminal baskets on GABA neurons in the cat auditory cortex. Cerebral Cortex 1991; 1(2) 117-133.

[83] Dianne A, Cruz MS, Stephen M, Eggan BS, Efrain C, Azmitia Ph.D, David A, Lewis MD. Serotonin$_{1A}$ receptors at the axon initial segment of prefrontal pyramidal neurons in schizophrenia. American Journal of Psychiatry 2004; 161(4) 739–742, doi: 10.1176/appi.ajp.161.4.739

[84] Peters A, Proskauer CC, Kaiserman-Abramof IR. The small pyramidal neuron of the rat cerebral cortex. The axon hillock and initial segment. Journal of Cell Biology 1968; 39(3) 604-619.

[85] Somogyi P, Freund TF, Cowey A. The axo-axonic interneuron in the cerebral cortex of the rat, cat and monkey. Neuroscience 1982; 7(11) 2577–607, doi:10.1016/0306-4522(82)90086-0

[86] Fariñas I, DeFelipe J. Patterns of synaptic input on corticocortical and corticothalamic cells in the cat visual cortex. II. The axon initial segment. Journal of Comparative Neurology 1991; 304(1) 70-77, doi: 10.1002/cne.903040106

[87] Ogawa Y, Horresh I, Trimmer JS, Bredt DS, Peles E, Rasband MN. Postsynaptic density-93 Clusters K_v1 channels at axon initial segments independently of Caspr2. Journal of Neuroscience 2008; 28(22) 5731–5739, doi: 10.1523/jneurosci.4431-07.2008

[88] Davis JQ, Bennet V. Ankyrin binding activity shared by the neurofascin/L1/NrCAM family of nervous system cell adhesion molecules. Journal of Biological Chemistry 1994; 269(44) 27163-27166.

[89] Hedstrom KL, Ogawa Y, Rasband MN. AnkiyrinG is required for maintenance of the axon initial segment and neuronal plasticity. Journal of Cell Biology 2008; 183(4) 635-640, doi:10.1083/jcb.200806112

[90] Meeks JP, Mennerick S. Action potential initiation and propagation in CA3 pyramidal axons. Journal of Neurophysiology 2007; 97(5) 3460-3472, doi:10. 1152/jn.01288. 2006

[91] Schmidt-Hieber C, Bischofberger J. Fast sodium channel gating supports localized and efficient axonal action potential initiation. Journal of Neuroscience 2010; 30(30) 10233-10242, doi:10.1523/jneurosci.6335-09.2010

[92] Krees GJ, Dowling MJ, Meeks JP, Mennerick S. High threshold, proximal initiation, and slow conduction velocity of action potentials in dentate granule neuron mossy fibers. Journal of Neurophysiology 2008; 100(1) 281–291, doi:10.1152/jn.90295.2008

[93] Chara JC. Estudio paramétrico ultrastructural del segmento inicial del axon de las neuronas piramidales supra e infragranulares con proyección axonal identificada en la corteza visual de la rata. Tesis doctoral. Universidad del País Vasco (UPV/EHU); 2010.

[94] Sloper JJ, Powell TPS. A study of the axon initial segment and proximal axon of neurons in the primate motor cortex y somatic sensory cortices. Philosophical Transactions of the Royal Society of London 1979. Series B, Biological Sciences 285(1006) 173-197.

[95] DeFelipe J, Hendry SCH, Jones EG, Schmechel D. Variability in the terminations of GABAergic chandelier cell axons on initial segments of pyramidal cell axons in the monkey sensory-motor cortex. Journal of Comparative Neurology 1985; 231(3) 364-384, 10.1002/cne.902310307

[96] Fairén A, Valverde F. A specialized type of neuron in the visual cortex of the cat: a Golgi and electron microscope study of chandelier cells. Journal of Comparative Neurology 1980; 194(4) 761-779, doi:10.1002/cne.901940405

[97] Matute C, Contamina P, Martinez-Millán L. The axon initial segment of corticocollicular neurons in the rabbit visual cortex: An electron-microscope study with HRP. Histology and Histopathology 1987; 2(-) 147-151.

[98] Fried SI, Lasker ACW, Desail NJ, Eddington DK, Rizzo 3rd JF. Axonal sodium-channel bands shape the response to electric stimulation in retinal ganglion cells. Journal of Neurophysiology 2009; 10(4) 1972-1987, doi:10.1152/jn.91081.2008

[99] Konishi M. Coding of auditory space. Annual Review Neuroscience 2003; 26(-) 31–55, doi: 10.1146/annurev.neuro.26.041002.131123

[100] Kuba H, Ishii TM, Ohmori H. Axonal site of spike initiation enhances auditory coincidence detection. Nature 2006; 444(-) 1069-1072, doi:10.1038/nature05347

[101] Kuba H, Oichi Y, Ohmori H. Presynaptic activity regulates Na^+ channel distribution at the axon initial segment. Nature 2010; 465(-) 1075-1078, doi:10.1038/nature09087

Chapter 2

Visual Field Map Organization in Human Visual Cortex

Alyssa A. Brewer and Brian Barton

Additional information is available at the end of the chapter

http://dx.doi.org/10.5772/51914

1. Introduction

The search for organizing principles of visual processing in cortex has proven long and fruitful, demonstrating specific types of organization arising on multiple scales (e.g., magno-cellular / parvo-cellular pathways [1] and ocular dominance columns [2]). One of the more important larger scale organizing principles of visual cortical organization is the visual field map (VFM): neurons whose visual receptive fields lie next to one another in visual space are located next to one another in cortex, forming one complete representation of contralateral visual space [3]. Each VFM subserves a specific computation or set of computations; locating these VFMs allows for the systematic exploration of these computations across visual cortex [4, 5]. It has been suggested that this retinotopic organization of VFMs allows for efficient connectivity between neurons that represent nearby locations in visual space, likely necessary for such processes as lateral inhibition and gain control [6-9]. This chapter will discuss the primary neuroimaging techniques used for measuring human VFMs, our current understanding of the organization of visuospatial representations across human visual cortex, the present state of our knowledge of white matter connectivity among these representations, and how these measurements inform us about the functional divisions of visual cortex in human.

2. Neuroimaging methods for measuring human visual field maps

VFMs are routinely measured in the *in vivo* human brain using functional magnetic resonance imaging (fMRI) (e.g., [10-15]). The fMRI paradigms for these measurements take advantage of knowledge gleaned from electrophysiological measurements of visual cortex in animal models about the structure and stimulus preferences of VFMs. In monkey, as in human, visual information travels from the retina through the lateral geniculate nucleus (LGN) of the thalamus to primary visual cortex (area V1) in the posterior occipital lobe [16].

Primate visual cortex has been parcellated into multiple visual areas defined by their unique cytoarchitectonic structures, connectivity, functional processing, and visual field topography [14, 17-20]. In the more anterior areas of the occipital lobe and in the parietal and temporal lobes, the definitions and functions of many of these areas are still being investigated. These areas were first demonstrated in monkey, and it has been possible to identify several homologous visual areas in human posterior occipital cortex (e.g., [12, 21]).

In human measurements, the most compelling evidence for visual areas is the VFMs, also commonly called retinotopic maps. In short, a VFM is a visual area with a complete representation of visual space, where neurons that represent adjacent locations on the retina (and visual space) are also adjacent in cortex [12]. Because many computations are required to create our visual experience, our brains have many specialized VFMs which perform one or more of those computations across the entire visual scene (e.g., motion perception happens throughout our visual field, not just in the upper left quadrant). By taking advantage of the knowledge of the retinotopic organization of visual input, multiple cortical VFMs can be measured using fMRI with respect to the two orthogonal dimensions needed to identify a unique location in visual space: eccentricity and polar angle. This chapter will review two of the most powerful fMRI techniques for very detailed measurements of VFM in individual subjects: travelling wave retinotopy (TWR) [10] and population receptive field (pRF) modeling [22].

2.1. The standard paradigm: Travelling wave retinotopy

TWR has been the gold standard for visual field mapping since its development in the mid 1990's (**Figure 1**) [10, 23-26]. This technique uses two types of periodic stimuli that move smoothly across a contiguous region of visual space to measure the orthogonal dimensions of polar angle and eccentricity. One stimulus is designed to elicit each voxel's preferred polar angle by presenting a high-contrast, flickering checkerboard stimulus shaped like a wedge that spans the fovea to periphery along a small range of specific polar angles (**Figure 2A**). The wedge stimulus rotates either clockwise or counterclockwise in discrete even steps around the central fixation point to sequentially activate distinct polar angle representations of visual space. The second stimulus is designed to elicit each fMRI voxel's preferred eccentricity by presenting a stimulus shaped like a ring, which expands or contracts in discrete even steps between the central fovea and the periphery (**Figure 2B**). The measurement of these *two, orthogonal* dimensions is vital for the correct definition of VFMs, as these two measurements allow for the unique mapping of the responses of the neurons within a single voxel in cortex to a unique location in visual space. If only a single dimension is measured, the cortical response can only be localized to a broad swath of visual space, which does not allow for accurate delineation of VFM boundaries, as discussed further below.

These traveling-wave stimuli are typically comprised of a set of high contrast checkerboard patterns that are designed to maximally stimulate primary visual cortex and generally elicit an fMRI signal modulation on the order of 1%–3% (**Figures 1-2**). This modulation is typically 15–20 standard deviations above the background noise. Stimuli comprised of other shapes (e.g., faces, objects) have also been used in studies interested in measuring the retinotopic organization of higher order visual cortex, but the high contrast checkerboard stimulus has proven to drive even these regions well in many studies[26, 27].

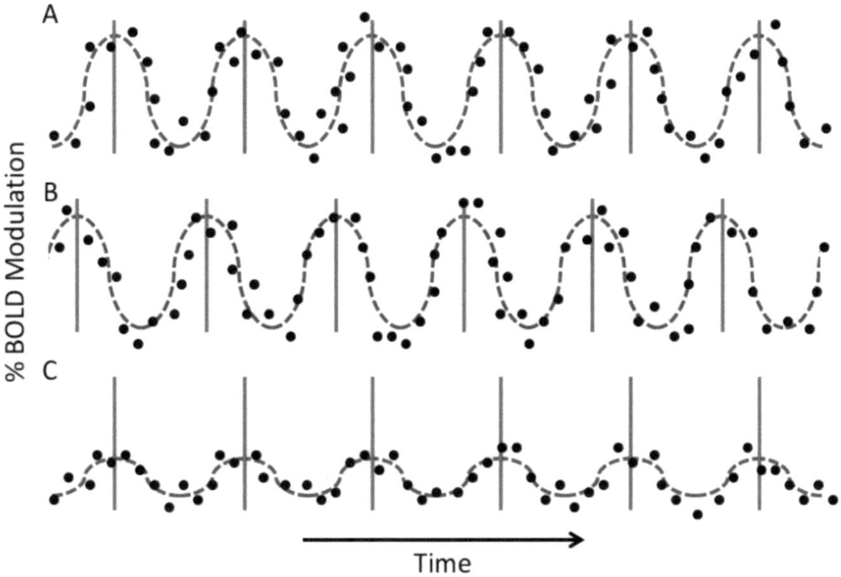

Figure 1. Visual Field Mapping Time Series Analysis. Each row represents the activity and analysis of a time series of a single 6-cycle scan of one type of experimental stimuli (expanding rings or rotating wedges) for a single voxel. Black dots indicate simulated raw data points of % blood oxygen level-dependent (BOLD) modulation. The red lines indicate the peak activations per cycle for an imaginary set of voxels, which are the measurements used by the traveling wave retinotopy (TWR) analysis. The blue dotted line represents a sinusoidal fit of the simulated data points, which are the measurements used by population receptive field (pRF) modeling. Rows (A) and (B) represent time series of voxels with identical %BOLD modulation, but different peak responses, which indicate different stimulus selectivity (different 'phases' of response). For example, (A) might represent a voxel with a preferred eccentricity tuning of 5° eccentric to fixation, whereas (B) might have a preferred tuning of only 2° eccentric to fixation. Rows (A) and (C) represent time series of voxels with identical peak responses, indicating identical stimulus selectivity. However, (C) has much lower %BOLD modulation than (A), which may be due to two primary factors: differences in local vasculature or broader receptive field tuning for (C) than (A).

In each scan, only one stimulus is presented, and all of visual space is cycled through several times with each stimulus (**Figure 1**). Typically, several scans are then averaged together for each stimulus type to increase the fMRI blood oxygen level-dependent (BOLD) signal to noise ratio. These stimuli create a travelling wave of cortical activity that travels from one end of the VFM to the other along iso-angle or iso–eccentricity lines, giving TWR its name. Thus the time, or phase, of the peak modulation varies smoothly across the cortical surface. This phase defines the most effective stimulus eccentricity (ring) and polar angle (wedge) to activate that region of cortex, giving TWR its description as 'phase-encoded retinotopy.' In

TWR data, the phase of the response is represented as a color-coded overlay on anatomical data (**Figure 2**). It is important to note that these types of TWR stimuli are not only excellent for measuring cortical VFMs, but that they only produce activity in regions that are retinotopically-organized.

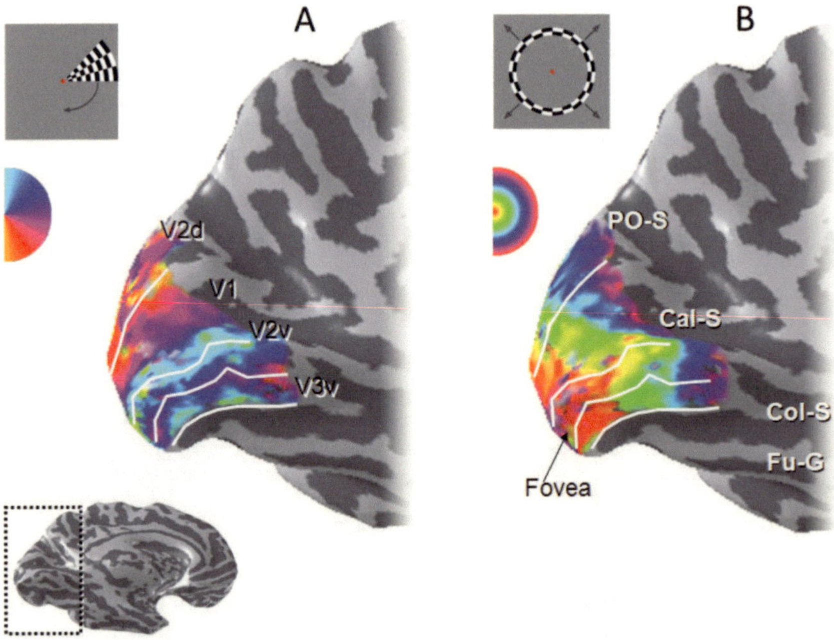

Figure 2. TWR Measurements. Traveling wave stimuli typically consist of a set of high contrast checkerboard patterns that move smoothly and periodically through a range of eccentricities (ring) or polar angles (wedge). The inflated cortical surface (inset) is labeled as follows: CC, corpus callosum; POS, parietal-occipital sulcus; CaS, calcarine sulcus. An expanded view of this surface near calcarine sulcus is overlaid with a color map showing the response phase at each location for polar angle (A) and eccentricity experiments (B) (see the colored legend insets). The stimuli covered the central 16° radius of visual space. The solid white lines indicate the boundaries of visual area V1 in the calcarine sulcus. For clarity, the colored visual responses are only overlaid on locations near the calcarine sulcus, and only voxels with a powerful response at a coherence ≥ 0.25 are colored.

The design of TWR presents all eccentricities or polar angles at a given frequency per scan (typically 6-8 cycles per scan), which allows the use of a Fourier analysis. TWR only considers activity that is at this signal frequency, excluding low-frequency physiological noise, among other things. The statistical threshold for cortical activity arising from the TWR stimulus is commonly determined by *coherence,* which is equal to the amplitude of the BOLD signal modulation at the frequency of stimulus presentation (e.g., 6 stimulus cycles per scan), divided by the square root of the power over all other frequencies except the first and second harmonic (e.g., 12 and 18 cycles per scan). These harmonic frequencies commonly can be considered signal in such analyses, but we often take a conservative approach and simply exclude their values from the calculation of coherence. Including these frequencies as noise would lead to an artificially high average for the noise frequencies in the Fourier analysis, incorrectly reducing overall coherence. For each stimulus condition (e.g., wedge or ring), each voxel is independently assigned a coherence value, thus measuring the strength of the response of that voxel to the stimulus. Only voxels with a coherence above a chosen threshold (typically 0.15 to 0.30 coherence) are further evaluated to determine the organization of cortical visuospatial representations into specific VFMs.

2.2. An innovative approach to measure the organization of human visual cortex: Population receptive field modeling

Once it became clear that there were limits to the ability of TWR to deal with VFMs with large RFs, researchers at Stanford University decided to improve VFM measurements by developing a new method that models the pRFs of each voxel within VFMs [22]. This model relies on the logic that, because VFMs are retinotopically organized, the population of RFs in each voxel of a VFM is expected to have similar preferred centers and sizes, allowing their combined pRF to be estimated as a single, two-dimensional Gaussian RF. Despite the fact that there is some variability in the neural RFs of each voxel in terms of their preferred centers and sizes, termed RF scatter, the pRF provides a good, if somewhat slightly larger, estimate of the individual neural RFs in the voxel. The advantages of the method are generally stated in comparison to TWR, as the field standard for measuring VFMs. The pRF method provides an accurate estimate of not only the preferred center for each voxel's pRF (as in TWR), but also its size (**Figures 3, 4**). In addition, the method does not require two distinct stimuli to measure orthogonal dimensions of visual space as in TWR, cutting down on the total number of scans necessary per subject.

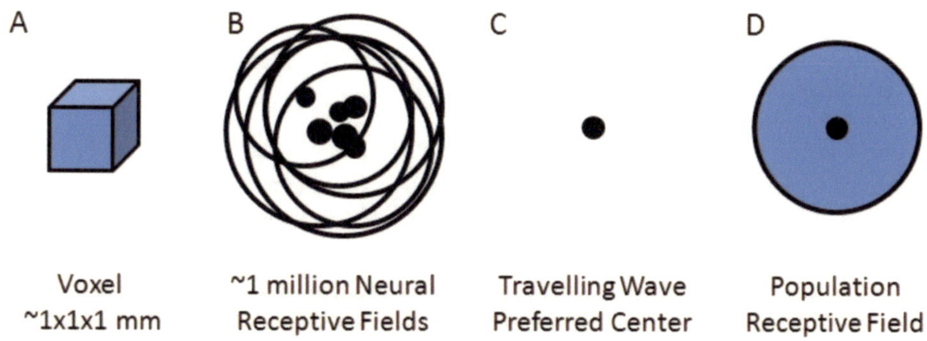

Figure 3. Measurements of an Individual Voxel. (A) A typical voxel recorded from a popular 3 Tesla MRI scanner is on the order of 1 mm^3, though often slightly larger (2-3 mm^3). (B) Within each typical voxel, there are on the order of ~1 million neurons, depending on the size of the voxel. For voxels in retinotopic visual cortex, the neurons each have similarly located spatial receptive fields (black outlines) with preferred centers (black dots). (C) Traveling wave retinotopy (TWR) takes advantage of the fact that nearby neurons in retinotopic cortex have similar preferred centers in order to estimate a population preferred center for the population of neurons in a given voxel. (D) Population receptive field (pRF) modeling takes advantage of the fact that nearby neurons in retinotopic cortex have similar receptive fields in order to estimate not only a preferred center, but also a pRF for the population of neurons in a given voxel.

To accomplish this, the pRF model first creates a very large database of possible pRF sizes and centers that cover the field of view of the stimulus (**Figure 4**). Then, the model convolves each of the pRF possibilities with a standard hemodynamic response function (HRF). Finally, the model uses a least-squares fitting method to iteratively test each of the pRF possibilities for each voxel independently against the actual data collected. Whichever pRF best fits the data is then assigned as the pRF for that voxel. Only voxels that contain activity above a chosen threshold of variance explained as determined by the model are included for further analysis.

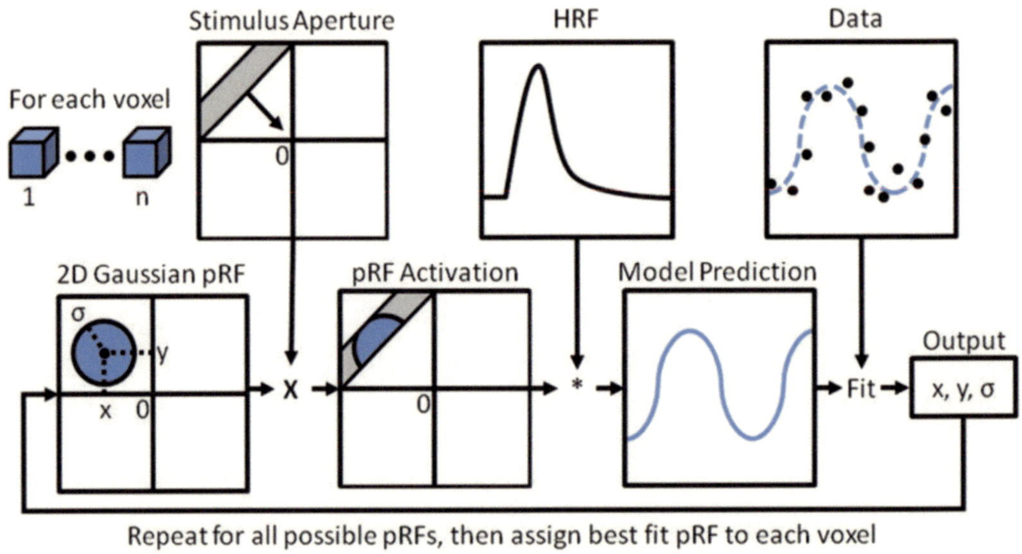

Figure 4. Population Receptive Field Modeling. The parameter estimation procedure for the population receptive field (pRF) model is shown as a flow chart. The example stimulus aperture is a moving bar stimulus. Adapted from Figure 2 in [22].

Although it is technically possible to use any stimulus that systematically traverses the entire field of view, typically the stimulus takes one of two forms. First is a slightly modified version of the TWR stimuli, in which neutral gray blank periods are inserted at an off-frequency from the stimulus frequency (i.e., 4 instead of 6-8 cycles/scan, so they are separable in the Fourier analysis). The second and increasingly common stimulus is a high-contrast flickering checkerboard bar stimulus that steps across the field of view in the 8 cardinal directions, again with several interspersed neutral gray blank periods. The neutral gray blank periods allow for an estimation of a voxel's response to any visual stimulus versus just the preferred visual stimulus, which is crucial for the accurate measurement of pRF sizes. In theory, one could also tile visual space using any stimulus of interest, if the aforementioned stimuli do not drive the area well. Since the checkerboard stimuli were designed to drive activity in early visual cortex, it is possible other stimuli containing more complex may perform better in higher-order VFMs.

The pRF method has the additional benefit of measuring other neuronal population properties, such as receptive field size and laterality. These pRF measurements can demonstrate differences in the internal receptive field structures between, for example, a hemifield map in primary visual cortex (V1) and a hemifield map in lateral cortex (e.g., LO-1; [28]). With the traveling wave method, both maps look very similar, as only the peak time series responses are measured. However, the underlying properties of the neuronal populations within these two maps are actually quite different, with finely tuned neurons in V1 and more broadly tuned neurons in lateral cortex. The models of the underlying neuronal properties from the pRF method can measure these receptive field differences, as well as the amount of input from ipsi- and contralateral visual fields (e.g., [29]). The human pRF size estimates for V1/V2/V3 reported by Dumoulin and Wandell [22] agree well with electrophysiological receptive field measurements at a range of eccentricities in corresponding locations within primate VFMs.

These pRF methods have successfully been used by a small group of labs to (1) investigate the normal organization of human visual cortex (e.g., [12, 29, 30]), (2) measure developmental plasticity in achiasmatic and sight recovery patients [31, 32], and (3) examine cortical reorganization in aged-related macular degeneration [33]. Because pRF Modeling has proven so successful, it is likely that it will eventually replace TWR as the standard method for measuring VFMs. Moreover, pRF modeling has an excellent future in the measurement of the details of pRFs, which is particularly important for the measurement of visual plasticity in humans. So far, the technique has primarily used a two-dimensional Gaussian profile for the pRF estimates, but researchers are working on the use of center-surround Gaussian pRFs, multiple location pRFs, and non-classical pRF shapes, which may allow for better pRF estimation as time continues. In the future, it is likely that pRF Modeling will be very successful when used in isolation, but also excellent to use in conjunction with other techniques.

2.3. Functional MRI data acquisition and analysis for individual subjects

The size of each VFM across the cortical surface varies significantly across individuals [22]. In fact, the size of primary visual cortex, V1, can vary by at least a factor of 3 in size, independent of overall brain size. This means that the locations of each specific VFM are necessarily shifted across individuals with respect to the underlying structural anatomy. This shift appears to be increasingly variable as measurements move anterior from primary visual cortex into regions of visual cortex that subserve higher-order computations (e.g., object recognition), the very regions that are also the most difficult to measure with TWR due to the larger RFs of the neurons here. Thus, averaging fMRI VFM data across subjects problematically blurs VFM data to a degree that should be unusable and may even obliterate VFM organization all together. Similarly, simply using coordinates from a standardized template (e.g., Talairach or MNI coordinates) to accurately estimate the location of any VFMs beyond area V1 in individual or group averaged data is not possible. The only accurate approach is to measure VFM in individual subjects. We will review here an example of one of several straightforward approaches for individual subject VFM data collection and analysis.

To optimize these VFM experiments, several types of fMRI scans are obtained for each subject. First, one acquires a high-resolution structural anatomy of the whole brain (e.g., 1 mm^3 resolution). Several types of pulse sequences are available, such as MPRAGE, a fast gradient echo T1- weighted inversion pulse sequence. The goal in this scan is to maximize the image contrast between white and gray cortical matter, important for the subsequent analysis. These anatomical data provide a basic coordinate frame for representing the fMRI data for each subject. Second, functional T2*-weighted BOLD contrast images are acquired for the VFM measurements. We commonly use a gradient echo pulse sequence with a SENSE factor of 1.5 that provides whole brain coverage with slices approximately parallel to the calcarine sulcus (home of V1) and a 1.8 x 1.8 x 3 mm slice resolution (no gap). Each functional scan typically lasts will approximately 3-4 minutes, and we acquire 4-8 scans per stimulus type (e.g., wedge, ring, bar) to average together. In addition, one lower resolution anatomical inplane image is acquired before each set of functional scans, with the same slice prescription as the functional scans but with a higher spatial resolution (e.g., 1 mm x 1 mm x 3 mm voxels). These T1-weighted slices are physically in register with the functional slices and can then be used to align the functional data with the high-resolution anatomy data [34].

For analysis of such functional imaging data for individual subjects, several neuroimaging software packages are available that can be used. We use a Matlab-based signal processing software package called *mrVista*, which was developed by the Wandell lab at Stanford University and is now widely used for such neuroimaging analysis [35, 36]; *mrVista* is open-source software and is publicly available online at http://white.stanford.edu/software/. With this software, the location of the cortical gray matter for each subject is identified ('segmented') in the high-resolution anatomical scan using the *mrVista* automated algorithm followed by hand-editing to minimize errors for individual subject analyses [36]. Gray matter is then grown from the segmented white matter to form a 3-4 mm layer covering the white matter surface. To improve sensitivity, only data from this identified gray matter are analyzed. The gray matter is then rendered in 3D close to the white matter boundary or unfolded into a continuous, flat sheet to allow visualization of functional activity within the sulci. During preprocessing of the functional data, linear trends are removed from the fMRI time series, but no spatial smoothing is applied to the data to better preserve the details of the VFM organization. Motion correction algorithms can then be applied between scans in each session as well as within individual scans (*mrVista* uses a mutual information motion correction algorithm [37]); however, motion correction algorithms may themselves create artifacts, so should not be routinely applied if not needed. If motion correction fails, then scans with motion artifact greater than one voxel can be discarded. After registration to the high-resolution anatomy, the functional activity can be visualized either in its original coordinate frame (inplanes), on the segmented gray matter in anatomical volume slices, or on inflated or flattened representations of the cortical surface to allow for optimal definition of VFM boundaries.

2.4. Defining visual field map boundaries

VFMs are defined by the following criteria: 1) both a polar angle and an eccentricity gradient must be present, 2) the polar angle and eccentricity gradients are orthogonal to one another, and 3) a VFM represents a complete contralateral hemifield of visual space (**Figure 5**; e.g., [5,

11]). The organization of retinotopic VFMs is typically determined by manually tracing the boundaries of quarter-field or hemifield representations (**Figure 2**). These boundaries are located at the position where the measurements of visual field angle reverse direction or, for regions on the end of visually responsive cortex, end at an angular meridian or at the periphery of a VFM [5, 11]. For boundaries in a reversal, the boundary is drawn to split the reversal evenly between the two maps, unless additional functional data (e.g., motion localizer) is present to suggest otherwise.

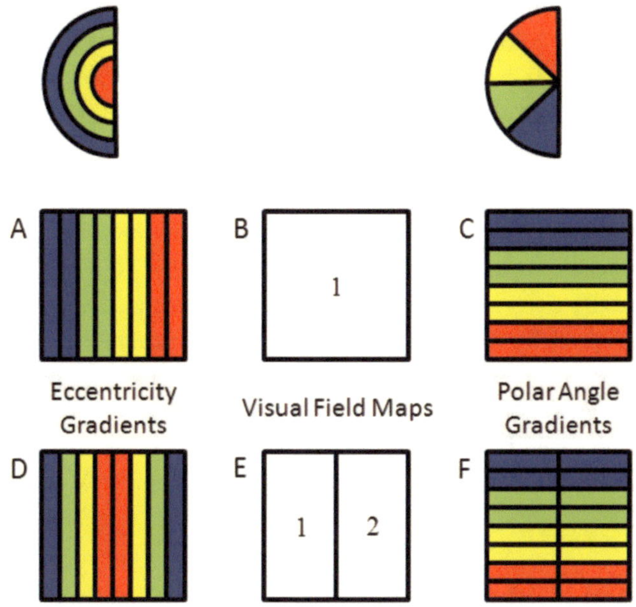

Figure 5. Orthogonal Dimensions of Visual Field Maps. Top Left: Eccentricity visual space legend. Each color represents an iso-eccentricity line in the left visual hemifield. Top Right: Polar angle visual space legend. Each color represents an iso-polar angle line in the left visual hemifield. (A) Eccentricity gradient for a visual field map (VFM). Note the gradient running from the center to more peripheral eccentricities runs from right to left. This gradient would be orthogonal to the polar angle gradient in (C), such that each iso-eccentricity line has a representation of the full range of polar angles. (B) A VFM. The combination of the orthogonal gradients in (A) and (C) form one complete representation of a hemifield of visual space. This forms one half of a complete VFM, the corresponding half being located in the opposite hemisphere of the brain. Because the hemifield represented is the left, this map would be located in the right hemisphere. The black outer border indicates that each of the two gradients is located in the same portion of cortex. (C) Polar angle gradient for a VFM. Note that the colors of the cartoon in (C) are inverted with respect to the polar angle visual space legend at top. The inverted cartoon is meant to more accurately represent the inverted representation of visual space in early visual cortex. For example, in primary visual cortex (V1), the lower quarterfield of visual space is represented on the dorsal (upper) surface of the occipital lobe, and vice versa. (D) Two adjacent eccentricity gradients running in opposite directions, with adjacent representations of the central visual hemifield. (E) When the gradients in (D) are combined with adjacent polar angle gradients such as that in (F), two complete representations of the hemifield of visual space are formed. (F) Two adjacent polar angle gradients running in the same direction, with each iso-polar angle line for each gradient lying adjacent to one another. Note that if one only measured polar angle information, one would not have the corresponding eccentricity information to know whether that portion of cortex truly contained one (as in (B)), two (as in (E)), or more complete representations of that hemifield of visual space.

In addition to expert manual definition of VFMs, one can also use an automated tool to help give an objective definition of the boundary reversals between VFMs. Only a few of these tools are currently available, however. One such algorithm identifies VFMs by minimizing the error between an expected visual map (atlas) and the observed data [38]. In this tool, the atlas is coarsely aligned with the data and then elastically deformed. The search algorithm minimizes the weighted sum of deviations between the predicted and measured maps and the force of the elastic deformation. This algorithm is applied to both angle and eccentricity maps simultaneously to obtain a fit between these retinotopic measurements and templates of the two expected VFMs. This automated approach thus give more objective determinations of the boundaries of hemifield and quarter field visual angle representations or of the periphery edge of eccentricity representations, which can then be used to define specific VMFs.

In cortical regions that have undetermined or ambiguous maps, this algorithm can be used to try a variety of possible templates of map organization (i.e., quarterfield map vs. hemifield map). Further, larger scale patterns of the organization of VFM across regions of cortex can be tested. By determining the error between the atlas template prediction and the actual angle and eccentricity measurements, the best fit template of VFM organization for a particular region can be estimated [11]. These atlas estimates can also be used to average map data across our subjects within a particular region of visual cortex [28]. The fitted atlas template additionally provides definitions of iso-angle and iso-eccentricity lines within each map, which can further be examined to compare patterns of VFM organization across the subject population [5, 11, 39].

3. Multiple visual field maps span human visual cortex

This section will review current human VFM organization and some of the controversies surrounding these measurements.

3.1. Visual field maps in medial occipital cortex

Three hemifield representations of visual space known as V1, V2, and V3 occupy the medial wall of occipital cortex in humans (**Figures 2, 5, 6**; for a review, see [12]). V1 is very reliably located in the calcarine sulcus, bounded on either side by the unique split-hemifield representations of V2 and V3 on the cuneus and lingual gyrus. V1 is known as "primary visual cortex," because it receives direct input from the retino-geniculate pathway and is the first place in the retino-geniculo-cortical pathway where information from the two eyes is combined. Not only that, but V1 is an important site of basic calculations of orientation, color, and motion. Each computation is performed across the entire visual field, yet V1 appears at the level of fMRI measurements to be a single, smooth representation of visual space. One can think of V1 as several VFMs laid on top of one another, each of which performs a single computation (one overlapping map each for color, orientation, and motion). To accomplish this organization, a very intricate mosaic of neurons subserving these computations allows for each computation to be performed over each portion of visual space. These mosaics, including ocular dominance columns, pinwheel orientation columns, and blobs/interblobs have been the subject of much study and argument (e.g., [2, 40, 41]). It remains to be seen how many maps throughout the visual hierarchy have similarly complex mosaics.

V1, V2, and V3 each contain a foveal representation positioned at the occipital pole, with progressively more peripheral representations extending into more anteromedial cortex, forming complete eccentricity gradients (**Figure 2**; e.g., [12, 13, 15, 23]). The region where the individual foveal representations meet at the occipital pole is commonly referred to the as the *foveal confluence* [42]. Despite the apparent merging of these foveal representations into one confluent fovea in fMRI measurements of eccentricity gradients, distinct boundaries between V1, V2, and V3 have been shown to be present even within this most central foveal representation [42, 43].

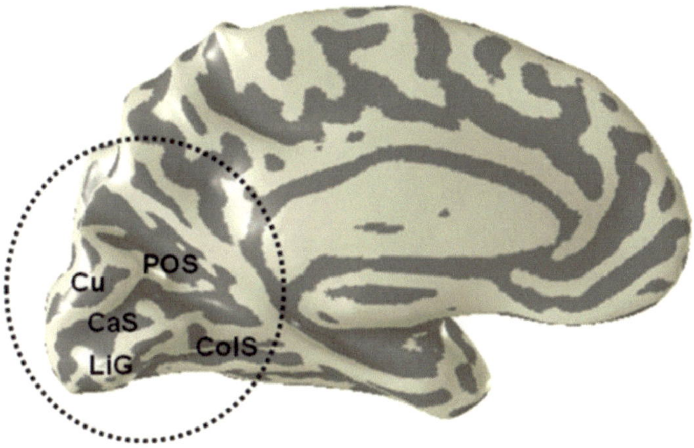

Figure 6. Medial Occipital Cortex. The anatomical region containing early visual areas V1, V2, and V3 is shown within the black dotted circle on an inflated rendering of the cortical surface of a single left hemisphere from one subject. Gray represents sulci, and white represents gyri. Cu, cuneus; CaS, calcarine sulcus; LiG, lingual gyrus; POS, parieto-occipital sulcus; ColS, collateral sulcus.

The boundaries between each map are delineated by reversals in polar angle gradients (**Figure 2, 5**; e.g., [12, 13, 15, 23]). V1 has a contiguous polar angle gradient. In contrast, V2 and V3 have split-hemifield representations (quarterfields), which are denoted by their locations dorsal or ventral to V1 (V2d, V2v, V3d, V3v). For each map, the lower visual quarterfield is represented on the dorsal surface, and the upper visual quarterfield is represented on the ventral surface. The quarterfields of V2 and V3 are connected at the fovea for each map, but are otherwise distinct. Although some details differ between the macaque and human V1, V2, and V3 maps (for example, the surface area of macaque V1 is roughly half that of human V1), they are arguably the most similar between the species in terms of structure and function [14, 17, 19, 20, 44, 45]. Beyond these three maps, even as early as hV4, the anatomical and topographical details of the maps diverge [11, 46]. As a practical matter, due to their relatively consistent anatomical locations and unique concentric organization, these three maps form the first landmarks identified in visual field mapping analyses [10, 13]. However, as noted above, these three maps can differ significantly in size across individuals. While V1 is always positioned along the calcarine sulcus in normal individuals, an increase in V1 size will necessarily shift the locations of V2 and V3 with respect to the specific underlying anatomy.

3.2. Visual field maps in ventral occipitotemporal cortex

Beyond V3v, the organization of VFMs in human cortex no longer follows that of macaque. This divergence should not be surprising given that the two species diverged from a common ancestor approximately 25 million years ago [47]. While the fourth visual area of

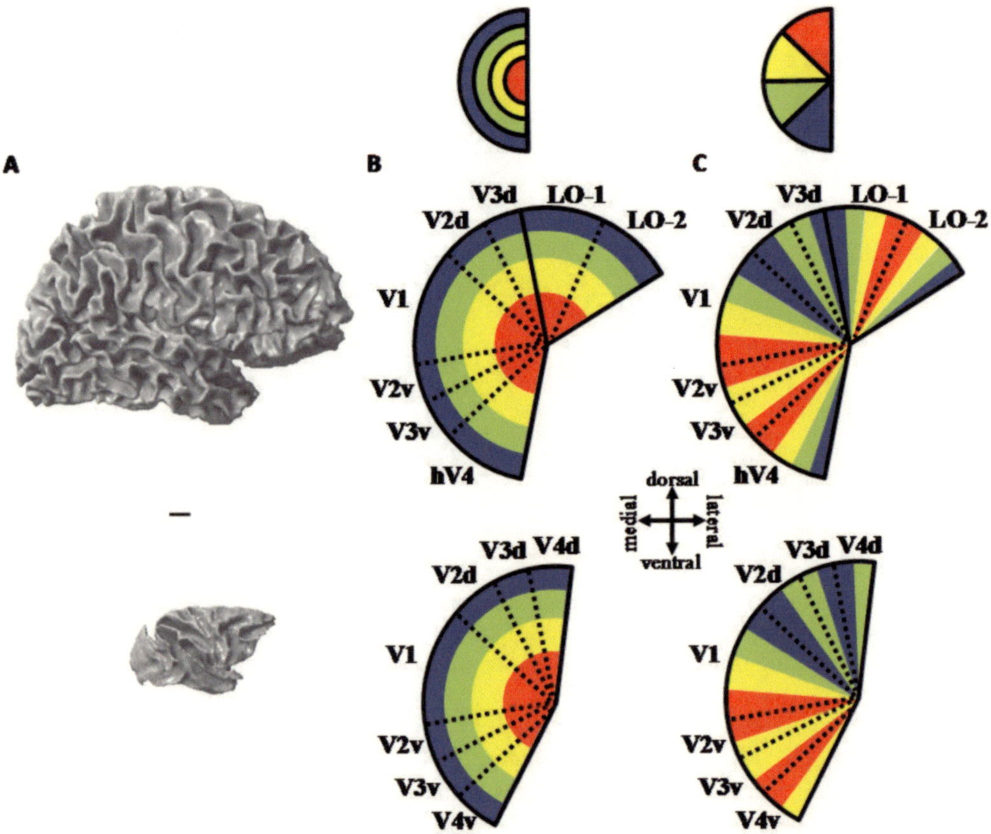

Figure 7. Comparison of Human and Macaque Monkey Occipital Cortex. (A) 3D renderings of human (top) and macaque monkey (bottom) cortex are shown for a single right hemisphere. Cortical sheet is rendered at the white-gray boundary to allow visualization into the sulci. Hemispheres are scaled to relatively match in size. Scale bar is 1 cm. (B) Cartoon representations of flattened sections of cortex are centered on the occipital pole and show eccentricity gradients of human (top) and macaque (bottom) for visual field maps (VFMs) in posterior occipital cortex. Black lines denote boundaries between VFMs. Each color represents the location in visual space that best drives this region of cortex (see color legend inset for left visual field eccentricity). (C) Cartoon representations now show polar angle gradients of human (top) and macaque (bottom) for VFMs in posterior occipital cortex. Each color represents the location in visual space that best drives this region of cortex (see color legend inset for left visual field polar angle). Arrows (center) depict the approximate anatomical orientation for the cartoon representations in (B) and (C).

macaque remains a split-hemifield adjacent to area V3, human V4 (designated hV4 because of the unclear homology to macaque V4) is positioned as a complete hemifield on the ventral occipital surface adjacent to V3v (**Figure 7**). Several additional VFMs containing representations of complete, contiguous hemifields lie anterior to hV4 roughly along the fusiform gyrus (**Figure 11**). These maps are named and numbered for their anatomical locations: VO-1 and VO-2, for ventral-occipital, and PHC-1 and PHC-2, for parahippocampal cortex (**Figure 8**).

The differences between human and macaque organization at the fourth visual area initially led to much controversy in the field regarding the organization of V4 in human, as some researchers sought a similar pattern of organization for the fourth visual area between human and macaque. To understand this controversy, it is important to review some of the history of measurements in this region.

One of the early lines of investigation into the ventral surface focused on measurements of both color and retinotopic organization. Zeki and colleagues measured responses to an isoluminant pattern modulated in chromatic contrast in two regions of ventral occipitotemporal cortex: V4 and V4 alpha [48, 49]. McKeefry and Zeki [50] then demonstrated that the posterior color-responsive region of V4 was at least coarsely retinotopically organized and represented the entire contralateral hemifield. However, they did not locate this map with respect to other neighboring VFMs.

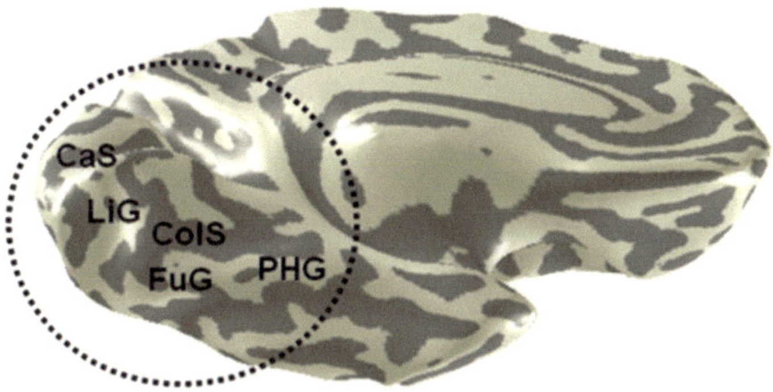

Figure 8. Ventral Occipitotemporal Cortex. The anatomical region containing ventral visual areas V2v, V3v, hV4, VO-1, VO-2, PHC-1, and PHC-2 is shown within the black dotted circle on an inflated rendering of the cortical surface of a single left hemisphere from one subject. CaS, calcarine sulcus; LiG, lingual gyrus; ColS, collateral sulcus; FuG, fusiform gyrus; PHG, parahippocampal gyrus. Other details as in **Figure 6**.

Hadjikhani et al. [51] also measured retinotopic and color organization along this region, describing two ventral retinotopic regions. The first was an upper quarterfield map, which they referred to as V4v. This putative V4v abutted the central visual field representation of V3v with an eccentricity map parallelingV1/V2/V3. Unlike the measurements of McKeefry and Zeki [50], they saw no adjacent lower quarterfield map that would form a complete contralateral hemifield. Instead, they described a hemifield map with an eccentricity representation that ran perpendicular to the putative V4v quarter field and called this VFM

V8. Using harmonic stimuli that alternated in luminance and chrominance, they also showed color responsivity within V8, although this stimulus type also would stimulate regions responsive to variations in luminance. Following the model of macaque cortex, Tootell and Hadjikhani [21] searched for a quarterfield map in dorsal occipital cortex to pair with their putative V4v. They failed to find the map and concluded that it did not exist. They did not resolve why an isolated quarterfield map would exist, a strange organization which would necessitate that whatever computation was subserved by putative V4v was only performed on one quarterfield of visual space.

With improvements in measurement techniques, we clarified the retinotopic organization of this ventral region [11, 46]. Our experiments defined three VFMs in ventral occipital cortex: hV4, VO-1, and VO-2, which we showed to be involved in the color and object processing pathways. HV4 is a hemifield map on the posterior fusiform gyrus that directly abuts the upper hemifield representation of V3v and shares a common eccentricity orientation with the confluent foveal representations of V1, V2, and V3 (**Figures 7, 8**). Anterior to the peripheral representation of hV4 is a distinct group of VFMs with a shared foveal representation separate from that of V1, V2, V3, and hV4. We have termed this organization of a discrete group of VFMs a *'clover leaf' cluster*, as described in more detail in **Section 4** below. This 'clover leaf' cluster contains at least two full hemifield representations of visual space: VO-1 and VO-2. The posterior portion of VO-1 is adjacent to the relatively peripheral visual field representation of hV4 and also abuts the peripheral V3v representation on the lingual gyrus. The posterior border of VO-1 represents the lower vertical meridian, and the anterior region represents the upper vertical meridian. This anterior upper vertical meridian reverses into the VO-2 hemifield map. The eccentricity gradient of VO-1 and VO-2 runs from the shared foveal representation on the fusiform gyrus anteromedially towards the more peripheral representation along the collateral sulcus and more anterior fusiform gyrus. Our recent measurements have suggested that additional maps (e.g., VO-3, VO-4) may be identified within this 'clover leaf' cluster in the future [52-54].

Our findings regarding hV4 and its neighbors have since been supported by measurements from several independent studies [28, 29, 39, 55-58]. Hansen et al. [57] initially continued the search for a hV4 organization more homologous to the split-hemifield of macaque V4 by proposing that a small section of dorsal lateral occipitotemporal cortex represented the inferior vertical meridian of hV4. This organization then left an hV4 division on the ventral surface that represented the full upper visual quarterfield adjacent to V3v plus some additional part of the visual field into the lower visual quarterfield. However, this organization conflicts with the now widely accepted dorsal occipitotemporal organization of LO-1 and LO-2 described below [28, 29, 39]. Further, additional measurements have now repeatedly confirmed 1) the full hemifield span of the ventral hV4 hemifield and 2) demonstrated that artifacts from a regional draining vein may in some subjects interfere with the accurate measurement of this section of hV4 [30].

Beyond hV4, VO-1, and VO-2, Arcaro et al. [55] defined two additional VFMs in this region that overlap with the parahippocampal place area, PHC-1 and PHC-2. Like the VFMs of the VO cluster, PHC-1 and PHC-2 also share a distinct foveal representation and appear in our data to be two VFMs within another distinct ventral 'clover leaf' cluster [52]. PHC-1 is located just anterior to VO-2, running from the fusiform gyrus into the parahippocampal gyrus (**Figure 8**). Both PHC-1 and PHC-2 represent a full contralateral hemifield of visual space, with the representation of the upper vertical meridian denoting the boundary between PHC-1 and PHC-2.

3.3. Visual field maps in lateral occipitotemporal cortex

In contrast to the posterior medial occipital VFMs, the lateral occipital cortex, with the object-responsive lateral occipital complex (LOC), has been much more difficult to measure in terms of retinotopic organization (**Figure 9**). This region was initially thought to be non-retinotopic or only to contain an 'eccentricity bias' (e.g., [21, 59, 60]). Recently, two VFMs, called LO-1 and LO-2 for 'lateral occipital', were described along the dorsal aspect of the LOC (**Figure 11**). LO-1 lies just anterior to V3d, reversing from the upper vertical meridian representation at the boundary into its representation of a full hemifield of visual space [28, 61]. LO-2 is located just inferior to LO-1, with the lower vertical meridian represented at the shared boundary of these two maps. The foveal representations of these two VFMs are located with the confluent foveal representations of V1, V2, V3, and hV4 on the occipital pole.

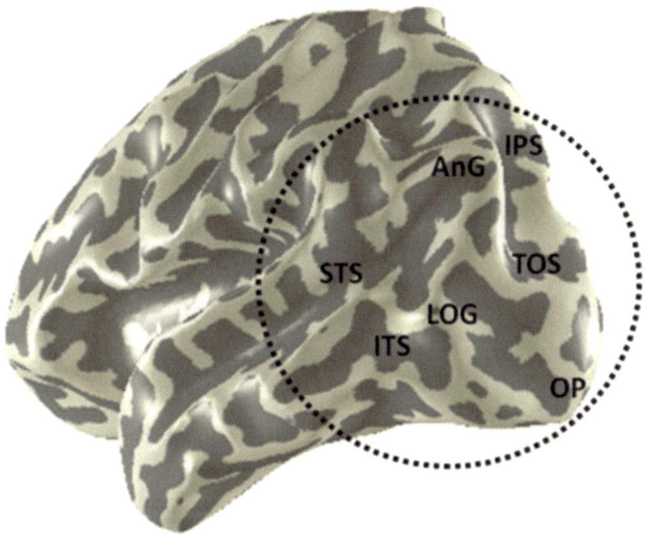

Figure 9. Lateral Occipitotemporal Cortex. The anatomical region containing lateral visual areas LO-1, LO-2, and the hMT+ cluster is shown within the black dotted circle on an inflated rendering of the cortical surface of a single left hemisphere from one subject. STS, superior temporal sulcus; ITS, inferior temporal sulcus; LOG, lateral occipital gyri; AnG, angular gyrus; IPS, intraparietal sulcus; TOS, transverse occipital sulcus; OP, occipital pole. Other details as in **Figure 6**.

In addition, regions just inferior to these maps have been shown to be responsive to lateralized visual stimuli, but have not yet been divided into specific VFMs [27, 62-64]. In macaque, there has been increasing electrophysiological evidence that neurons in homologous regions may maintain a high degree of retinotopic sensitivity [65]. It is important to note again that the presence of organized representations of visual space in this region can still allow for the stimulus size and position invariance frequently described across the object-responsive LOC. PRF sizes are expected to be large across this region, but may maintain just enough dispersion of pRF centers to allow for slightly different preferred tuning of responses to visual space. Thus, the responses to object stimuli from this cluster could remain both invariant to stimulus size and position over a wide field of view while retaining visuospatial information. With LO-1 and LO-2, the definition of additional VFMs spanning LOC would form the lateral half of an occipital pole 'clover leaf' cluster and would provide a concrete, visuospatial framework for reliably localizing specific computational regions within lateral object-responsive cortex [5, 12, 66, 67]. This inferior region of the LOC merges with the most lateral lower vertical meridian representation of hV4 [11] and is also subject to issues with the 'venous eclipse' fMRI artifact due to the presence of a draining vein here that has a somewhat variable position across subjects within this region [30]. This artifact has likely significantly contributed to the difficulties in measuring organized VFMs within this region.

Anterior to LOC, along the banks of the inferior temporal sulcus, lies the TO cluster, also known as hMT+ (**Figure 9**). Amano et al. [29] were able to provide the first clear measurements of VFMs in the human motion-selective MT complex (hMT+) using the pRF methods described above [68]. They named these two new hemifield VFMs TO-1 and TO-2, for temporal-occipital areas 1 and 2. These maps are positioned just anterior to the LO maps and share another distinct foveal representation. The representations of visual of space across these maps run anteriorly from the lower vertical meridian at the posterior border of TO-1, to the shared upper vertical meridian at the border of TO-1 and TO-2, to the lower vertical meridian at the anterior border. Following measurements by Huk et al. [68] that demonstrated retinotopic organization within the MT subdivision and differentiated human MT and human MST using dissociable motion stimuli, it is likely that TO-1 is the same as human MT, and TO-2 is the same as human MST.

Recently, Kolster et al. [39] verified that both TO-1 and TO-2 represent full, organized hemifields of visual space, but used a naming scheme homologous to macaque with MT and 'putative' MST (pMST). They also expanded the VFM measurements of this region, showing that the TO/hMT+ cluster contains four full hemifields of visual space. The two additional hemifields of visual space merge at the confluent fovea of TO-1 and TO-2 and are located just inferior to TO-1 and TO-2. They suggest that these VFMs correspond to macaque FST and V4t. Human 'putative' FST (pFST) is positioned anterior to human 'putative' V4t (pV4t), and the two VFMs meet an upper vertical meridian representation. Around this cluster, MT/V5 (TO-1) then shares a lower vertical meridian border with pV4t, and pMST (TO-2) shares a lower vertical meridian border with pFST. A similar clustered organization of these motion responsive VFMs in macaque has also recently been demonstrated by Kolster et al. [69]. We confirm these measurements with data showing the 'clover leaf' cluster organization for this group of VFMs in the human MT+ complex [5, 11, 12, 66, 67]. Because the homology to monkey has not yet been verified, we prefer the anatomy-based terminology TO-1, TO-2, TO-3, and TO-4 for these VFMs; these would correspond to Kolster et al.'s [39] MT, pMST, pFST, and pV4t, respectively.

Amano et al. [29] and Kolster et al. [39] disagreed, however, on the specific organization of the eccentricity gradients between the LO VFMs and the TO/hMT+ VFMs [29, 39]. Amano et al. [29] described LO-2 and TO-1 as positioned as a strip of VFMs on the lateral occipital surface, with hemifield representations sharing meridian boundaries from V3d, to LO-1, to LO-2, to TO-1, to TO-2. In this organization, LO-2 and TO-1 would share a boundary that represents the lower vertical meridian. TO-1 and TO-2 would still meet at a discrete foveal representation that runs only from the foveal representation to a more superior peripheral representation that merges only superiorly with that of LO-2. In contrast, Kolster et al. [39] describe the TO maps as a distinct cluster anterior to LOC and the LO maps, which do not share any meridian boundaries. With this cluster organization, it is the peripheral representation that is shared between the LO and TO maps. Our measurements confirm those of Kolster et al. [5, 11, 39, 66, 67]. The four TO maps form a complete 'clover leaf' cluster that merges with the eccentricity gradients of the LO VFMs at their peripheral eccentricity representations. This VFM definition can be seen in the data in Figure 1 of Amano et al. [29], but was differently interpreted prior to the measurements of the full TO 'clover leaf' cluster.

Finally, Kolster et al. [39] describe an additional putative new cluster of two VFMs inferior to the TO/hMT cluster they term putative human PIT (phPIT) based on possible homology to macaque PIT [39]. These are the first measurements of these VFMs in human and have not yet been verified by other labs. As techniques improve and we learn more about the effects of the venous eclipse artifact in this region [30], we expect that multiple VFMs will be measured by multiple labs in this and surrounding regions in future measurements [53, 66, 67].

3.4. Visual field maps in posterior parietal cortex

Beyond the medial part of the dorsal lower vertical meridian representation of human V3d, lies a series of hemifield VFMs running from the transverse occipital sulcus (TOS) up along the medial wall of the intraparietal sulcus (IPS) (**Figures 10, 11**; e.g., [12, 70]). The first maps bordering V3d are V3A and V3B [71-73]. These two maps share another discrete foveal representation within the TOS, forming a complete 'clover leaf' cluster [5]. V3A has some similarities to macaque V3A and is thought to play a role in motion processing; the computations subserved by V3B are not yet known [71, 72, 74, 75]. V3B was originally described Smith et al. [72] as at least a quarterfield of visual space next to V3A. This definition was expanded to cover a while hemifield of visual space by Press et al. [71], who noted that this region of V3A had a full hemifield polar angle gradient with an eccentricity gradient expanding concentrically from a central position within this hemifield. Such an organization necessitates that two representations of visual space are represented; thus, V3A and V3B were described in Press et al. [71]as a cluster of two VFMs sharing a distinct fovea. In comparing the initial V3B definitions from Smith et al. [72] and later definitions of LO-1 [27-29], which is just lateral and inferior to V3B, it is possible that the original V3B definitions were measuring a part of what was later called LO-1 and not the same hemifield that was described in Press et al. [71] as V3B. The field now generally considers V3A and V3B as the cluster of two VFMs in the TOS, and LO-1 and LO-2 as the dorsal aspect of the LO [12, 27-29].

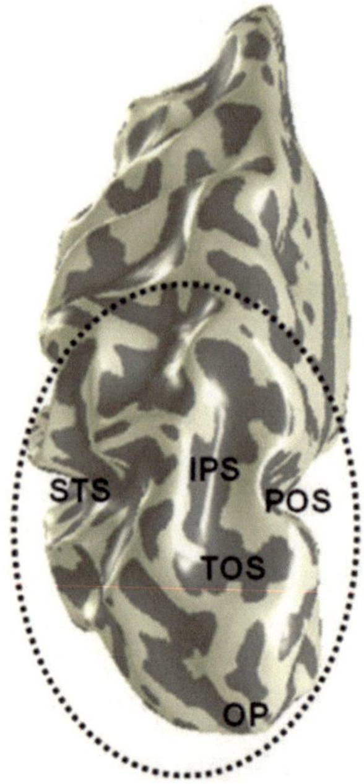

Figure 10. Posterior Parietal Cortex. The anatomical region containing dorsal posterior parietal cortex visual areas V3A, V3B, and the IPS maps is shown within the black dotted circle on an inflated rendering of the cortical surface of a single left hemisphere from one subject. STS, superior temporal sulcus; IPS, intraparietal sulcus; POS, parieto-occipital sulcus; TOS, transverse occipital sulcus; OP, occipital pole. Other details as in **Figure 6**.

Entering into the IPS, the next VFM anterior to the V3A/V3B cluster is IPS-0 (formerly called V7) [75, 76]. IPS-0 has a foveal representation distinct from the V3A/V3B cluster and represents a full hemifield of contralateral visual space, running from the lower vertical meridian representation at the posterior border to the upper vertical meridian representation anteriorly. Beyond IPS-0, a series of polar angle representations extends from IPS-0 along the medial wall of the IPS. All these polar angler representations have been primarily measured using attentionally demanding traveling wave stimuli, consistent with the description of this parietal region as having a role in spatial attention [74-79]. These representations have primarily been described as reversing smoothly through a strip of several hemifield representations from IPS-0 to IPS-5 [70, 76-78, 80-82].

It is important here to differentiate "polar angle representations" from complete "VFMs." For the initial part of the IPS, VFM IPS-0 (V7) has been relatively well characterized [76, 83]. However, VFMs IPS-1 through IPS-5 as well as human LIP (a possible homologous region to macaque LIP which has been suggested to align with IPS-1 or IPS-2) have been exclusively presented in the literature to date as only polar angle maps [70, 76-82, 84, 85], except for the one example we have found of an eccentricity representation in two hemispheres of one subject (see Figure 4 in [81]). Swisher et al. [81] note, for example, that "we reliably find a continuous gradient of eccentricity response phase along the V7(IPS-0)/ IPS-1 border," but that "the eccentricity representation in IPS-3/4 is less clear." Some of these studies have reported that eccentricity mapping was used in the VFM definitions, but failed to our knowledge, with the one exception, to show anything but the polar angle responses in the published data (main or supplemental).

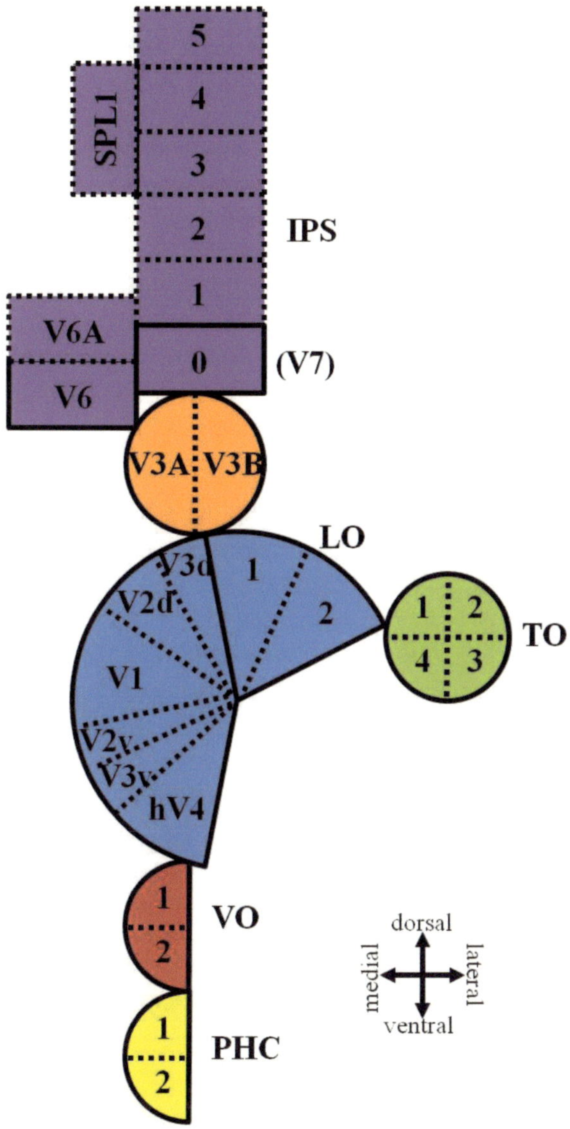

Figure 11. The Current State of Contiguous Visual Field Maps in Occipital, Parietal, and Temporal Lobes of Human Cortex. The figure depicts a cartoon overview of hemifield representations of visual field maps (VFMs) in a single right hemisphere if the cortical sheet of that hemisphere were removed from its usual position and laid flat. The center of the blue region is centered on the occipital pole, while the purple region is in parietal cortex, the red and yellow regions are on the ventral surface of the occipital and temporal lobes, and the green region is on the lateral surface of the temporal lobe. Each color except purple represents a likely or confirmed 'clover leaf' cluster of VFMs. Solid black lines indicate the borders between 'clover leaf' clusters and dotted lines indicate the borders between hemifield representations within clusters. In the purple region, the organization is much less clear, particularly for maps outlined in dotted rather than solid black lines (IPS-1, IPS-2, IPS-3, IPS-4, IPS-5, SPL1, and V6A). See main text for more details.

While polar angle representations (i.e., IPS-1/2/3/4/5) are excellent indicators that one or a number of VFMs may exist in a given location, they do not provide evidence of a unique, complete VFM. In the case of the IPS polar angle gradients, there could be any number of reversals of eccentricity representations along the polar iso-angle lines. Without obtaining clear, reliable orthogonal maps of both dimensions, it is impossible to know exactly how to divide up a region into multiple representations of visual space. We encountered such a division of what had appeared to be a single hemifield polar angle represenation into multiple VFMs given a central foveal representation previously in the segregation of human V3A into the 2-map cluster with V3B [71]. In those measurements, what had appeared to simply be a large single hemifield representation of V3A, we showed to actually be divided into two full hemifield maps of visual space along the centrally positioned foveal representation [5]. Current work is suggesting that the parietal cortex anterior to the V3A/V3B cluster may also in fact contain several additional 'clover leaf' clusters with VFMs that share several confluent, discrete foveae along the IPS [86, 87].

The medial wall of the parietal lobe has also been shown to contain at least three additional retinotopically organized regions. One VFM called V6 lies along the parieto-occipital sulcus just anterior to the peripheral representation of V3d [88, 89]. V6 represents the contralateral hemifield, with an inferior upper vertical meridian running superiorly to the lower vertical meridian representation and a distinct eccentricity gradient that extends far into the periphery. V6 has been shown to be involved in particular types of motion processing, such as pattern and self motion [89]. Adjacent to V6 is another VFM termed V6A [88-90]. Both areas are named to represent their expected homology to macaque. Human V6A has primarily been measured using visual stimuli that activate the far periphery and is likely involved in visuomotor integration [88, 89]. V6A contains at least a coarse representation of the contralateral hemifield and a very peripheral eccentricity gradient with expansion the representation of > 35° visual angle. The last retinotopic region so far measured here is named SPL1 (for superior parietal lobule 1) and is located just medial to the series of maps running along the IPS [70, 82, 85]. Although its position appears somewhat variable across subjects and publications with respect to the specific IPS maps it borders, it appears to be primarily located adjacent to IPS-2, IPS-3 and/or IPS-4. The polar angle gradient of SPL1 runs from its lower vertical meridian border along these IPS maps inferiorly to its upper vertical meridian border. To our knowledge, no eccentricity gradients for this region have yet been demonstrated in the literature. Like the other maps along the IPS, SPL1 may also play a role in spatial attention.

3.5. Visual field maps in frontal cortex

Several topographically organized representations of the contralateral hemifield have also been demonstrated in frontal cortex by a few studies using a variety of stimuli including TWR, visual spatial attention tasks, and memory-guided saccade tasks [70, 78, 79, 84, 85, 91]. These topographic representations of the polar angle of visual space arise in the frontal eye fields (FEF), the supplementary eye fields (SEF), dorsolateral prefrontal cortex (DLPFC), and precentral cortex (pre-CC), regions involved in complex visual processing of spatial attention and eye movement control (**Figure 12**). Like many of the measurements shown for the IPS region, these frontal regions also lack measurements of orthogonal eccentricity representations. It remains to be seen whether these attentional regions contain only very coarse eccentricity gradients that is difficult to measure or whether future measurements will unveil more detailed eccentricity gradients and possibly multiple VFMs within each topographic region.

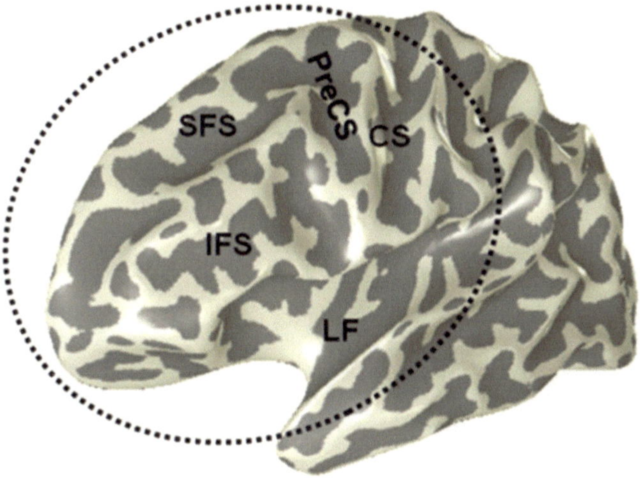

Figure 12. **Frontal Cortex.**SFS, superior frontal sulcus; IFS, inferior frontal sulcus; PreCS, precentral sulcus; CS, central sulcus; LF, lateral fissure. Other details as in **Figure 6**.

It is important to note that the stimulus paradigms used to define these regions do not differentiate between retina-centered (retinotopic) and head-, gaze-, body-, or world-centered (spatiotopic) topographic organization. While the VFMs in the occipital lobe have been shown to be retinotopically organized [92], there is more controversy regarding if and where the visual system transforms from retinotopic to spatiotopic organization. Spatiotopic representations have been suggested to be present in some visuo-motor pathways (for review, see [93]), but have also been shown to not be necessary for such transformations [94]. Similarly, the native coordinate system of spatial attention has been shown to be retinotopic [95, 96], suggesting that retina-centered visuospatial information is propagated throughout the visual system.

4. Organizational patterns of visual field maps across human cortex

As increasing numbers of VFMs have been defined in human visual cortex, one question that has arisen is whether there is an organizing principle for the distribution of these maps across visual cortex [5, 11, 58, 60, 69, 97, 98]. A basic approach that has worked for early visual cortex has been to define strings of VFMs along contiguous strips of occipital cortex, with adjacent portions of the maps representing similar portions of visual space, but performing different computations [3]. This configuration of maps again allows for more efficient connections between neurons in different maps, such that for a given portion of space, the length of the axons between neurons performing different sets of computations in the process of building the visual percept is minimized [6, 7, 99]. As additional VFMs have been defined in higher order visual cortex, more complex organizing principles for visual cortex have been proposed [5, 11, 58, 60, 69, 97, 98, 100, 101]. One such principle describes VFMs as organized into roughly circular clusters that we have termed 'clover leaf clusters' (**Figure 13**) [5, 11, 66, 67]. These clusters are hypothesized to each contain multiple VFMs which share similar processing properties across that cluster [5, 11, 69]. Several clusters have been partially described, and two have been repeatedly mapped in full: V3A/V3B and TO/hMT+ clusters [5, 11, 12, 29, 39].

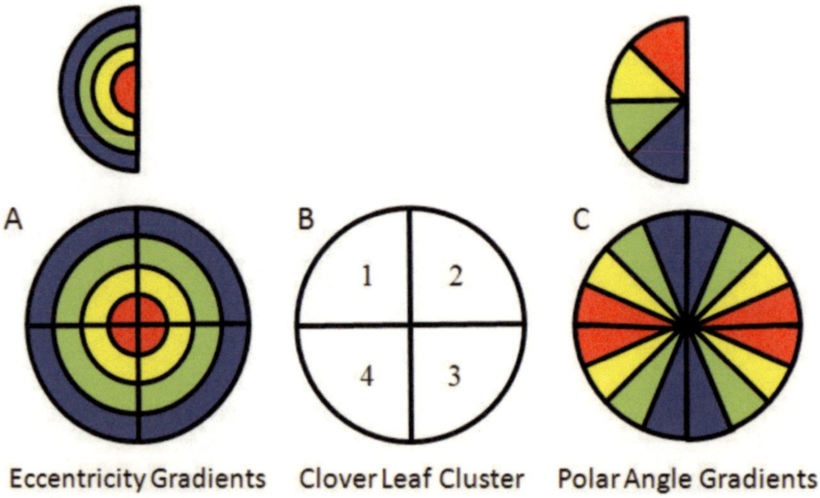

Figure 13. Orthogonal Dimensions of 'Clover Leaf' Clusters. Top Left: Eccentricity visual space legend. Each color represents an iso-eccentricity line in the left visual hemifield. Top Right: Polar angle visual space legend. Each color represents an iso-polar angle line in the left visual hemifield. (A) Eccentricity gradients of a typical 'clover leaf' cluster, containing 4 complete representations of the left visual hemifield. Each eccentricity gradient from the center to periphery of visual space runs physically from the center to the periphery of the cluster, such that iso-eccentricity lines form concentric circles about the center of the cluster. (B) A typical 'clover leaf' cluster with 4 complete representations of a hemifield of visual space. Note that, due to the radially orthogonal organization of 'clover leaf' clusters, each individual map must be shaped like a piece of pie. (C) Polar angle gradients of a typical 'clover leaf' cluster. Each iso-polar angle line runs from the center to periphery of the cluster like a 'spoke of the wheel' of the cluster, such that each polar angle gradient runs from one 'spoke of the wheel' of the cluster around to another 'spoke'. Note that, due to the fact that polar angle reversals (adjacent spokes with the same polar angle preference) denote the boundaries between hemifield representations within a 'clover leaf' cluster, there must always be an even number of hemifield representations in each 'clover leaf' cluster. To have an odd number would necessarily require a discrete jump in polar angle representation between hemifield representations, which has so far not been observed in human visual field mapping.

The VFMs within a 'clover leaf' clusters are organized such that the central fovea is represented in the center of the cluster, with more peripheral representations of space represented in more peripheral positions in the cluster in a smooth, orderly fashion. The representation of any given polar angle of space for any given VFM extends out from the center to the periphery of the cluster, effectively spanning the radius of the cluster like a spoke on a wheel. We refer to this type of organization – one dimension of space (polar angle) represented radially from center to periphery of a cluster and the other dimension (eccentricity) represented in concentric, circular bands from center to periphery – as being radially orthogonal. Furthermore, we expect that these clusters have consistent locations relative to one another, but that the maps within each cluster may be oriented somewhat differently. Finally, VFMs within each 'clover leaf' clusters are proposed to perform similar types of computations. This broad scale organizational pattern of VFM is currently under investigation by several groups [5, 7, 12, 39, 66, 67, 69], and we expect it to extend across human visual cortex.

5. Additional measurements to refine human visual field map definitions

5.1. White matter connectivity among human visual field maps

In order to fully investigate visuospatial processing in the human brain, it is important to measure not only patterns of functional VFM organization across cerebral cortex, but also the organization of the white matter tracts connecting these functional regions. Feedforward and feedback information from each VFM must be passed on to other maps up and down the hierarchy of visual processing [18]. The retinotopic human visual system processes portions of visual space in parallel, requiring connections for one type of processing in any particular location of the visual field to be passed to the same location of visual space in the next VFM for the next step in visual processing [102]. An elegant solution to this connectivity problem would be to maintain visuospatial organization in the white matter tracts between clusters. Such a solution allows for molecular cues to guide and maintain the relative structure of VFMs. Any other solution would necessarily require a breakdown of

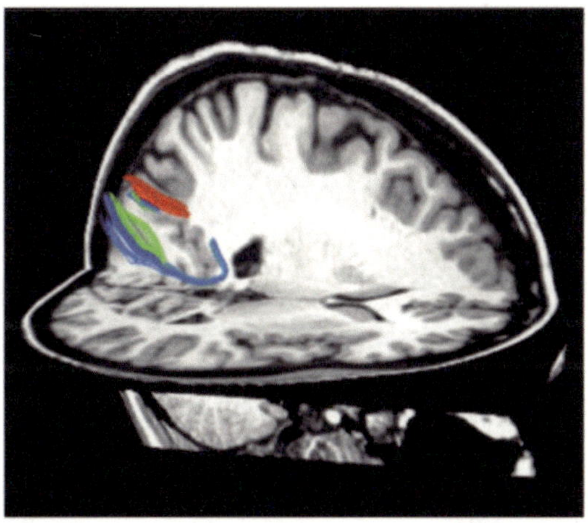

Figure 14. White matter connections in human visual cortex. (a) An example of separate sets of diffusion tensor imaging fibers estimated among maps in parietal cortex. Fibers originated from a 5 mm seed point located in the dorsal polar angle gradients IPS-1. Fibers colored red illustrate intra-hemispheric U-fibers connecting neighboring locations in left intraparietal sulcus (IPS). Blue and green fibers depict 2 subsets of a group of inter-hemispheric fiber tracks that connect to the contralateral IPS.

the organization inherent in connections coming out of a cluster into some other organization, and a rebuilding of the organization inherent in connections going into the next cluster, which is more costly, difficult, and complicated. The MR protocol of diffusion tensor imaging (DTI) is beginning to provide such measurements of connectivity among VFMs early in the visual processing hierarchy (**Figure 14**).

DTI is based upon a computer-assisted analysis of multiple diffusion-weighted images and uses a Gaussian model of diffusion, called an ellipsoid or 'tensor', to measure the mobility of water molecules within human tissue [103]. Traditional DTI measurements include fractional anisotropy (FA) and mean diffusivity (MD); custom software packages allow one to now also estimate the shapes, properties and destinations of white matter fiber tracts from DTI data (e.g., [104, 105]; http://white.stanford.edu/software/). The combination of DTI and fiber-tracking algorithms that combine tensors with similar principal diffusion directions can produce estimates of the major fiber bundles in the brain of individual subjects [106, 107]. FA, MD, and estimated fiber track locations and densities can be compared across individuals and between groups of subjects [108].

DTI has now successfully been used to measure the organization of the human optic tracts and optic radiations from the retina to the LGN to V1 [50, 109]. These measurements of the initial visual tracts match those measured by other methods [12, 110] and are now being used in studies examining how the optic radiations differ in specific patient populations (e.g., [32]). In cortex, DTI measurements have further demonstrated that the retinotopic organization of V1 is maintained in connections between homologous VFMs across hemispheres, with upper and lower visual field sections running together through the splenium of the corpus callosum [108, 111, 112]. These emerging measurements of white matter connectivity among VFMs will aid us both in refining our definitions of specific VFM boundaries throughout the visual processing hierarchy, especially in regions with more ambiguous VFM measurements, and in expanding our understanding of specific computational pathways.

5.2. Integration of visual field maps with other functional measurements in human visual cortex

The findings from combined structural and functional measurements have a profound impact on the study of vision in the brain. Any visual area that is organized retinotopically is subject to the constraints common to all VFMs in the human brain. Many areas of the brain have been considered "non-retinotopic" or containing only an "eccentricity bias," because laboratories using the field standard TWR were not able to demonstrate complete, precise retinotopic organization (e.g., [21, 97, 113]). Typically, this has been interpreted to mean that the early portion of the visual system is the only part that is retinotopic, and, at some point midway in the hierarchy, there must be a fundamental change in the way that the visual system is constructed. Not only is this a major theoretical claim, which would require a potentially complex transformation from a retinotopic framework to some other non-spatial organization, but it side-steps the basic fact that properties such as retinal-size-invariant object recognition can occur in VFMs without any cost. It is possible that the majority of higher order visual areas are retinotopic, maintaining retinotopically organized, dispersed receptive field centers despite increasingly large receptive field sizes. Why would we evolve an entirely different way to deal with one type of visual information when the simple solution of using large receptive fields and population codes within VFMs does not require a change in organization or connectivity? We contend that any failure to demonstrate retinotopic responses in a visually responsive area must be first carefully evaluated as a failure of the measurement methodology. This is a question whose answer is vital to understanding higher-order cognition, which need not abandon the visuospatial knowledge gained from low-level visual processing.

6. Conclusion

Our understanding the visuospatial organization of human visual cortex is crucial for our further exploration of the computations subserved by these visual pathways. Because every human brain shares common functional topography that is somewhat variably located anatomically, it is vital to correctly localize common functional areas in individual subjects in order to then study which specific computations are carried out by each area. The widespread technique of mapping anatomy to a common atlas not only destroys information about individual subjects, but also blurs data from adjacent areas within each subject, making it impossible to differentiate computations in adjacent areas.

This chapter has reviewed the primary measurement techniques for investigating the organization of human visual cortex as well as the present state of knowledge of the visuospatial representations across cortex. Until recently, the best technique for localizing visual field maps was TWR, which is excellent at identifying the centers of pRFs in fMRI voxels. Now, that technique has been surpassed by pRF modeling, which measures not only pRF centers, but the spread of each pRF. Both techniques have been used to successfully localize numerous visual field maps, most of which have been confirmed by numerous laboratories. However, it would be a mistake to assume that the current organizational model is entirely correct or complete. Some polar angle gradients still need to have eccentricity gradients measured in order to correctly determine the number of VFMs in parts of cortex such as posterior parietal cortex. Other maps simply need confirmation in the form of replication by independent laboratories. Perhaps most importantly, the current organizational model will need to be reconsidered in the face of evidence that VFMs are organized into 'clover leaf' clusters. These data will surely be updated as additional measurements both expand the known retinotopic representations in human visual cortex and clarify the current VFM definitions.

Author details

Alyssa A. Brewer and Brian Barton
Department of Cognitive Sciences, University of California, Irvine, USA

Acknowledgement

This work was supported by University of California, Irvine, startup funds to A.A.B.

7. References

[1] W. H. Merigan and J. H. Maunsell, "How parallel are the primate visual pathways?," *Annu Rev Neurosci,* vol. 16, pp. 369-402, 1993.

[2] D. L. Adams, L. C. Sincich, and J. C. Horton, "Complete pattern of ocular dominance columns in human primary visual cortex," *J Neurosci,* vol. 27, pp. 10391-403, Sep 26 2007.

[3] B. A. Wandell, S. O. Dumoulin, and A. A. Brewer, "Visual cortex in humans," in *Encyclopedia of Neuroscience.* vol. 10, L. R. Squire, Ed., ed Oxford: Academic Press, 2009, pp. 251-257.

[4] J. H. Kaas, "Topographic Maps are Fundamental to Sensory Processing," *Brain Research Bulletin,* vol. 44, pp. 107–112, 1997.

[5] B. A. Wandell, A. A. Brewer, and R. F. Dougherty, "Visual field map clusters in human cortex," *Philos Trans R Soc Lond B Biol Sci,* vol. 360, pp. 693-707, Apr 29 2005.

[6] G. Mitchison, "Neuronal branching patterns and the economy of cortical wiring," *Proc Biol Sci,* vol. 245, pp. 151-8, Aug 22 1991.

[7] D. B. Chklovskii and A. A. Koulakov, "Maps in the brain: what can we learn from them?," *Annu Rev Neurosci,* vol. 27, pp. 369-92, 2004.

[8] R. Shapley, M. Hawken, and D. Xing, "The dynamics of visual responses in the primary visual cortex," *Prog Brain Res,* vol. 165, pp. 21-32, 2007.

[9] F. Moradi and D. J. Heeger, "Inter-ocular contrast normalization in human visual cortex," *J Vis,* vol. 9, pp. 13 1-22, 2009.

[10] S. A. Engel, D. E. Rumelhart, B. A. Wandell, A. T. Lee, G. H. Glover, E. J. Chichilnisky, and M. N. Shadlen, "fMRI of human visual cortex," *Nature,* vol. 369, p. 525, Jun 16 1994.

[11] A. A. Brewer, J. Liu, A. R. Wade, and B. A. Wandell, "Visual field maps and stimulus selectivity in human ventral occipital cortex," *Nat Neurosci,* vol. 8, pp. 1102-9, Aug 2005.

[12] B. A. Wandell, S. O. Dumoulin, and A. A. Brewer, "Visual field maps in human cortex," *Neuron,* vol. 56, pp. 366-83, Oct 25 2007.

[13] M. I. Sereno, A. M. Dale, J. B. Reppas, K. K. Kwong, J. W. Belliveau, T. J. Brady, B. R. Rosen, and R. B. Tootell, "Borders of multiple visual areas in humans revealed by functional magnetic resonance imaging," *Science,* vol. 268, pp. 889-93., 1995.

[14] D. C. Van Essen, J. W. Lewis, H. A. Drury, N. Hadjikhani, R. B. Tootell, M. Bakircioglu, and M. I. Miller, "Mapping visual cortex in monkeys and humans using surface-based atlases," *Vision Res,* vol. 41, pp. 1359-78, 2001.

[15] E. A. DeYoe, G. J. Carman, P. Bandettini, S. Glickman, J. Wieser, R. Cox, D. Miller, and J. Neitz, "Mapping striate and extrastriate visual areas in human cerebral cortex," *Proc Natl Acad Sci U S A,* vol. 93, pp. 2382-6, Mar 19 1996.

[16] D. C. Van Essen, "Behind the optic nerve: an inside view of the primate visual system," *Trans Am Ophthalmol Soc,* vol. 93, pp. 123-33, 1995.

[17] D. C. Van Essen, W. T. Newsome, and J. H. Maunsell, "The visual field representation in striate cortex of the macaque monkey: asymmetries, anisotropies, and individual variability," *Vision Res*, vol. 24, pp. 429-48, 1984.

[18] D. J. Felleman and D. C. V. Essen, "Distributed hierarchical processing in the primate cerebral cortex," *Cerebral Cortex*, vol. 1, pp. 1-47, 1991.

[19] D. C. Van Essen, *Organization of visual areas in macaque and human cerebral cortex*. Boston: Bradford, 2003.

[20] D. C. Van Essen, D. J. Felleman, E. A. DeYoe, J. Olavarria, and J. Knierim, "Modular and hierarchical organization of extrastriate visual cortex in the macaque monkey," *Cold Spring Harb Symp Quant Biol*, vol. 55, pp. 679-96, 1990.

[21] R. B. Tootell and N. Hadjikhani, "Where is 'dorsal V4' in human visual cortex? Retinotopic, topographic and functional evidence," *Cereb Cortex*, vol. 11, pp. 298-311, Apr 2001.

[22] S. O. Dumoulin and B. A. Wandell, "Population receptive field estimates in human visual cortex," *Neuroimage*, vol. 39, pp. 647-60, Jan 15 2008.

[23] S. A. Engel, G. H. Glover, and B. A. Wandell, "Retinotopic organization in human visual cortex and the spatial precision of functional MRI," *Cereb Cortex*, vol. 7, pp. 181-92, Mar 1997.

[24] E. A. DeYoe, G. J. Carman, P. Bandettini, S. Glickman, J. Wieser, R. Cox, D. Miller, and J. Neitz, "Mapping striate and extrastriate visual areas in human cerebral cortex," *Proc. Natl. Acad. Sci. (USA)*, vol. 93, pp. 2382-2386, 1996.

[25] M. I. Sereno, C. T. McDonald, and J. M. Allman, "Analysis of retinotopic maps in extrastriate cortex," *Cerebral Cortex*, vol. 6, pp. 601-620, 1994.

[26] B. A. Wandell and J. Winawer, "Imaging retinotopic maps in the human brain," *Vision Res*, vol. 51, pp. 718-37, Apr 13 2011.

[27] R. Sayres and K. Grill-Spector, "Relating retinotopic and object-selective responses in human lateral occipital cortex," *J Neurophysiol*, vol. 100, pp. 249-67, Jul 2008.

[28] J. Larsson and D. J. Heeger, "Two retinotopic visual areas in human lateral occipital cortex," *J Neurosci*, vol. 26, pp. 13128-42, Dec 20 2006.

[29] K. Amano, B. A. Wandell, and S. O. Dumoulin, "Visual field maps, population receptive field sizes, and visual field coverage in the human MT+ complex," *J Neurophysiol*, vol. 102, pp. 2704-18, Nov 2009.

[30] J. Winawer, H. Horiguchi, R. A. Sayres, K. Amano, and B. A. Wandell, "Mapping hV4 and ventral occipital cortex: the venous eclipse," *J Vis*, vol. 10, p. 1, 2010.

[31] S. Prakash, S. O. Dumoulin, N. Fischbein, B. A. Wandell, and Y. J. Liao, "Congenital achiasma and see-saw nystagmus in VACTERL syndrome," *J Neuroophthalmol*, vol. 30, pp. 45-8, Mar 2010.

[32] N. Levin, S. O. Dumoulin, J. Winawer, R. F. Dougherty, and B. A. Wandell, "Cortical maps and white matter tracts following long period of visual deprivation and retinal image restoration," *Neuron*, vol. 65, pp. 21-31, Jan 14 2010.

[33] H. A. Baseler, A. Gouws, K. V. Haak, C. Racey, M. D. Crossland, A. Tufail, G. S. Rubin, F. W. Cornelissen, and A. B. Morland, "Large-scale remapping of visual cortex is absent

in adult humans with macular degeneration," *Nat Neurosci,* vol. 14, pp. 649-55, May 2011.

[34] F. Maes, A. Collignon, D. Vandermeulen, G. Marchal, and P. Suetens, "Multimodality image registration by maximization of mutual information," *IEEE Trans Med Imaging,* vol. 16, pp. 187-98, Apr 1997.

[35] B. A. Wandell, S. Chial, and B. T. Backus, "Visualization and measurement of the cortical surface," *J Cogn Neurosci,* vol. 12, pp. 739-52, Sep 2000.

[36] P. C. Teo, G. Sapiro, and B. A. Wandell, "Creating connected representations of cortical gray matter for functional MRI visualization," *IEEE Trans Med Imaging,* vol. 16, pp. 852-63, Dec 1997.

[37] O. Nestares and D. J. Heeger, "Robust multiresolution alignment of MRI brain volumes," *Magn Reson Med,* vol. 43, pp. 705-15, May 2000.

[38] R. F. Dougherty, V. M. Koch, A. A. Brewer, B. Fischer, J. Modersitzki, and B. A. Wandell, "Visual field representations and locations of visual areas V1/2/3 in human visual cortex," *J Vis,* vol. 3, pp. 586-98, 2003.

[39] H. Kolster, R. Peeters, and G. A. Orban, "The retinotopic organization of the human middle temporal area MT/V5 and its cortical neighbors," *J Neurosci,* vol. 30, pp. 9801-20, Jul 21 2010.

[40] E. Bartfeld and A. Grinvald, "Relationships between orientation-preference pinwheels, cytochrome oxidase blobs, and ocular-dominance columns in primate striate cortex," *Proc Natl Acad Sci U S A,* vol. 89, pp. 11905-9, Dec 15 1992.

[41] M. S. Livingstone and D. H. Hubel, "Anatomy and physiology of a color system in the primate visual cortex," *J Neurosci,* vol. 4, pp. 309-56, Jan 1984.

[42] M. M. Schira, C. W. Tyler, M. Breakspear, and B. Spehar, "The foveal confluence in human visual cortex," *J Neurosci,* vol. 29, pp. 9050-8, Jul 15 2009.

[43] M. M. Schira, C. W. Tyler, B. Spehar, and M. Breakspear, "Modeling magnification and anisotropy in the primate foveal confluence," *PLoS Comput Biol,* vol. 6, p. e1000651, Jan 2010.

[44] M. G. Rosa, "Visuotopic organisation of primate extrastriate cortex.," in *Cerebral Cortex.* vol. 12, K. J. Rockland KS, Peters A, Ed., ed New York: Plenum Press, 1997, pp. 127–203.

[45] M. G. Rosa and R. Tweedale, "Brain maps, great and small: lessons from comparative studies of primate visual cortical organization," *Philos Trans R Soc Lond B Biol Sci,* vol. 360, pp. 665-91, Apr 29 2005.

[46] A. R. Wade, A. A. Brewer, J. W. Rieger, and B. A. Wandell, "Functional measurements of human ventral occipital cortex: retinotopy and colour," *Philos Trans R Soc Lond B Biol Sci,* vol. 357, pp. 963-73, Aug 29 2002.

[47] S. B. Hedges and S. Kumar, "Genomic clocks and evolutionary timescales," *Trends in Genetics,* vol. 19, pp. 200-206, 2003.

[48] C. J. Lueck, S. Zeki, K. J. Friston, M.-P. Deiber, P. Cope, V. J. Cunningham, A. A. Lammertsma, C. Kennard, and R. S. J. Frackowiak, "The color center in the cerebral cortex of man," *Nature,* vol. 340, pp. 386-389, 1989.

[49] S. Zeki, J. D. G. Watson, C. J. Lueck, K. J. Friston, C. Kennard, and R. S. J. Frackowiak, "A direct demonstration of functional specialization in human visual cortex.," *J. Neuroscience,* vol. 11, pp. 641-649, 1991.

[50] D. J. McKeefry and S. Zeki, "The position and topography of the human colour centre as revealed by functional magnetic resonance imaging," *Brain,* vol. 120, pp. 2229-42, 1997.

[51] N. Hadjikhani, A. K. Liu, A. M. Dale, P. Cavanagh, and R. B. Tootell, "Retinotopy and color sensitivity in human visual cortical area V8," *Nat Neurosci,* vol. 1, pp. 235-41, Jul 1998.

[52] S. A. Drew, D. E. Asher, B. Barton, and A. A. Brewer, "Pinwheel cartography: New visual field map cluster in the human posterior parahippocampal complex," presented at the Society for Neuroscience, San Diego, CA, 2010.

[53] D. E. Asher and A. A. Brewer, "Hemispheric differences of color responses in human ventral visual cortex," *Vision Sciences Society. Journal of Vision,* vol. 9, pp. 776-776, 2009.

[54] D. E. Asher, S. A. Drew, B. Barton, and A. A. Brewer, "Pinwheel cartography: Novel visual field map cluster within human ventro-lateral occipital cortex. ," presented at the Society for Neuroscience, San Diego, CA, 2010.

[55] M. J. Arcaro, S. A. McMains, B. D. Singer, and S. Kastner, "Retinotopic organization of human ventral visual cortex," *J Neurosci,* vol. 29, pp. 10638-52, Aug 26 2009.

[56] S. Kastner, P. De Weerd, M. A. Pinsk, M. I. Elizondo, R. Desimone, and L. G. Ungerleider, "Modulation of sensory suppression: implications for receptive field sizes in the human visual cortex," *J Neurophysiol,* vol. 86, pp. 1398-411, Sep 2001.

[57] K. A. Hansen, K. N. Kay, and J. L. Gallant, "Topographic organization in and near human visual area V4," *J Neurosci,* vol. 27, pp. 11896-911, Oct 31 2007.

[58] C. W. Tyler and A. R. Wade, "Extended concepts of occipital retinotopy," *Current Medical Imaging Review,* vol. 1, p. 3190329, 2005.

[59] U. Hasson, T. Hendler, D. Ben Bashat, and R. Malach, "Vase or face? A neural correlate of shape-selective grouping processes in the human brain," *J Cogn Neurosci,* vol. 13, pp. 744-53, Aug 15 2001.

[60] R. Malach, I. Levy, and U. Hasson, "The topography of high-order human object areas," *Trends Cogn Sci,* vol. 6, pp. 176-184, Apr 1 2002.

[61] J. Larsson, M. S. Landy, and D. J. Heeger, "Orientation-selective adaptation to first- and second-order patterns in human visual cortex," *J Neurophysiol,* vol. 95, pp. 862-81, Feb 2006.

[62] A. McKyton and E. Zohary, "Beyond retinotopic mapping: the spatial representation of objects in the human lateral occipital complex," *Cereb Cortex,* vol. 17, pp. 1164-72, May 2007.

[63] C. C. Hemond, N. G. Kanwisher, and H. P. Op de Beeck, "A preference for contralateral stimuli in human object- and face-selective cortex," *PLoS One,* vol. 2, p. e574, 2007.

[64] M. Niemeier, H. C. Goltz, A. Kuchinad, D. B. Tweed, and T. Vilis, "A contralateral preference in the lateral occipital area: sensory and attentional mechanisms," *Cereb Cortex,* vol. 15, pp. 325-31, Mar 2005.

[65] J. J. DiCarlo and J. H. Maunsell, "Anterior inferotemporal neurons of monkeys engaged in object recognition can be highly sensitive to object retinal position," *J Neurophysiol,* vol. 89, pp. 3264-78, Jun 2003.

[66] A. A. Brewer and B. Barton, "'Clover Leaf' Cartography: Connectivity Among Visual Field Map Clusters," presented at the Society for Neuroscience, Washington, D.C., 2011.

[67] B. Barton and A. A. Brewer, "Pinwheel cartography: A fundamental organizing principle of the human visual system," presented at the Society for Neuroscience, San Deigo, CA, 2010.

[68] A. C. Huk, R. F. Dougherty, and D. J. Heeger, "Retinotopy and functional subdivision of human areas MT and MST," *J Neurosci,* vol. 22, pp. 7195-205, Aug 15 2002.

[69] H. Kolster, J. B. Mandeville, J. T. Arsenault, L. B. Ekstrom, L. L. Wald, and W. Vanduffel, "Visual field map clusters in macaque extrastriate visual cortex," *J Neurosci,* vol. 29, pp. 7031-9, May 27 2009.

[70] M. A. Silver and S. Kastner, "Topographic maps in human frontal and parietal cortex," *Trends Cogn Sci,* vol. 13, pp. 488-95, Nov 2009.

[71] W. A. Press, A. A. Brewer, R. F. Dougherty, A. R. Wade, and B. A. Wandell, "Visual areas and spatial summation in human visual cortex," *Vision Res,* vol. 41, pp. 1321-32, 2001.

[72] A. T. Smith, M. W. Greenlee, K. D. Singh, F. M. Kraemer, and J. Hennig, "The processing of first- and second-order motion in human visual cortex assessed by functional magnetic resonance imaging (fMRI)," *J Neurosci,* vol. 18, pp. 3816-30, 1998.

[73] A. T. Smith, K. D. Singh, A. L. Williams, and M. W. Greenlee, "Estimating Receptive Field Size from fMRI Data in Human Striate and Extrastriate Visual Cortex," *Cereb Cortex,* vol. 11, pp. 1182-1190., 2001.

[74] R. B. Tootell, N. Hadjikhani, E. K. Hall, S. Marrett, W. Vanduffel, J. T. Vaughan, and A. M. Dale, "The retinotopy of visual spatial attention," *Neuron,* vol. 21, pp. 1409-22, Dec 1998.

[75] R. B. Tootell, J. D. Mendola, N. K. Hadjikhani, P. J. Ledden, A. K. Liu, J. B. Reppas, M. I. Sereno, and A. M. Dale, "Functional analysis of V3A and related areas in human visual cortex," *J Neurosci,* vol. 17, pp. 7060-78, Sep 15 1997.

[76] M. A. Silver, D. Ress, and D. J. Heeger, "Topographic maps of visual spatial attention in human parietal cortex," *J Neurophysiol,* vol. 94, pp. 1358-71, Aug 2005.

[77] M. I. Sereno, S. Pitzalis, and A. Martinez, "Mapping of contralateral space in retinotopic coordinates by a parietal cortical area in humans," *Science,* vol. 294, pp. 1350-4, Nov 9 2001.

[78] S. Kastner, K. DeSimone, C. S. Konen, S. M. Szczepanski, K. S. Weiner, and K. A. Schneider, "Topographic maps in human frontal cortex revealed in memory-guided saccade and spatial working-memory tasks," *J Neurophysiol,* vol. 97, pp. 3494-507, May 2007.

[79] A. P. Saygin and M. I. Sereno, "Retinotopy and attention in human occipital, temporal, parietal, and frontal cortex," *Cereb Cortex,* vol. 18, pp. 2158-68, Sep 2008.

[80] D. Schluppeck, P. Glimcher, and D. J. Heeger, "Topographic organization for delayed saccades in human posterior parietal cortex," *J Neurophysiol,* vol. 94, pp. 1372-84, Aug 2005.
[81] J. D. Swisher, M. A. Halko, L. B. Merabet, S. A. McMains, and D. C. Somers, "Visual topography of human intraparietal sulcus," *J Neurosci,* vol. 27, pp. 5326-37, May 16 2007.
[82] C. S. Konen and S. Kastner, "Representation of eye movements and stimulus motion in topographically organized areas of human posterior parietal cortex," *J Neurosci,* vol. 28, pp. 8361-75, Aug 13 2008.
[83] T. Z. Lauritzen, M. D'Esposito, D. J. Heeger, and M. A. Silver, "Top-down flow of visual spatial attention signals from parietal to occipital cortex," *J Vis,* vol. 9, pp. 18 1-14, 2009.
[84] D. J. Hagler, Jr. and M. I. Sereno, "Spatial maps in frontal and prefrontal cortex," *Neuroimage,* vol. 29, pp. 567-77, Jan 15 2006.
[85] S. M. Szczepanski, C. S. Konen, and S. Kastner, "Mechanisms of spatial attention control in frontal and parietal cortex," *J Neurosci,* vol. 30, pp. 148-60, Jan 6 2010.
[86] A. A. Brewer and B. Barton, "Pinwheel cartography: Visual field map clusters in posterior parietal cortex that subserve visual attention and working memory," presented at the Society for Neuroscience, San Diego, CA, 2010.
[87] H. Kolster, R. Peeters, and G. A. Orban, "Ten retinotopically organized areas in human parietal cortex," presented at the Society for Neuroscience, Washington, D.C., 2011.
[88] S. Pitzalis, C. Galletti, R. S. Huang, F. Patria, G. Committeri, G. Galati, P. Fattori, and M. I. Sereno, "Wide-field retinotopy defines human cortical visual area v6," *J Neurosci,* vol. 26, pp. 7962-73, Jul 26 2006.
[89] S. Pitzalis, M. I. Sereno, G. Committeri, P. Fattori, G. Galati, F. Patria, and C. Galletti, "Human v6: the medial motion area," *Cereb Cortex,* vol. 20, pp. 411-24, Feb 2010.
[90] P. Dechent and J. Frahm, "Characterization of the human visual V6 complex by functional magnetic resonance imaging," *Eur J Neurosci,* vol. 17, pp. 2201-11, May 2003.
[91] D. J. Hagler, Jr., L. Riecke, and M. I. Sereno, "Parietal and superior frontal visuospatial maps activated by pointing and saccades," *Neuroimage,* vol. 35, pp. 1562-77, May 1 2007.
[92] J. L. Gardner, E. P. Merriam, J. A. Movshon, and D. J. Heeger, "Maps of visual space in human occipital cortex are retinotopic, not spatiotopic," *J Neurosci,* vol. 28, pp. 3988-99, Apr 9 2008.
[93] D. C. Burr and M. C. Morrone, "Spatiotopic coding and remapping in humans," *Philos Trans R Soc Lond B Biol Sci,* vol. 366, pp. 504-15, Feb 27 2011.
[94] A. P. Batista, C. A. Buneo, L. H. Snyder, and R. A. Andersen, "Reach plans in eye-centered coordinates," *Science,* vol. 285, pp. 257-60, Jul 9 1999.
[95] J. D. Golomb, M. M. Chun, and J. A. Mazer, "The native coordinate system of spatial attention is retinotopic," *J Neurosci,* vol. 28, pp. 10654-62, Oct 15 2008.
[96] J. D. Golomb, A. C. Marino, M. M. Chun, and J. A. Mazer, "Attention doesn't slide: spatiotopic updating after eye movements instantiates a new, discrete attentional locus," *Atten Percept Psychophys,* vol. 73, pp. 7-14, Jan 2011.
[97] U. Hasson, I. Levy, M. Behrmann, T. Hendler, and R. Malach, "Eccentricity bias as an organizing principle for human high-order object areas," *Neuron,* vol. 34, pp. 479-90, Apr 25 2002.

[98] H. P. Op de Beeck, J. Haushofer, and N. G. Kanwisher, "Interpreting fMRI data: maps, modules and dimensions," *Nat Rev Neurosci,* vol. 9, pp. 123-35, Feb 2008.

[99] A. A. Koulakov and D. B. Chklovskii, "Orientation preference patterns in mammalian visual cortex: a wire length minimization approach," *Neuron,* vol. 29, pp. 519-27, Feb 2001.

[100] J. Kaas, "Theories of visual cortex organisation in primates," in *Cerebral Cortex, vol 12. Extrastriate cortex in primates*. vol. 12, K. J. Rockland KS, Peters A, Ed., ed New York: Plenum Press, 1997, pp. 91–125.

[101] K. Grill-Spector and R. Malach, "The human visual cortex," *Annu Rev Neurosci,* vol. 27, pp. 649-77, 2004.

[102] D. C. Van Essen, W. T. Newsome, and J. L. Bixby, "The pattern of interhemispheric connections and its relationship to extrastriate visual areas in the macaque monkey," *J Neurosci,* vol. 2, pp. 265-83, 1982.

[103] P. J. Basser and C. Pierpaoli, "Microstructural and physiological features of tissues elucidated by quantitative-diffusion-tensor MRI," *J Magn Reson B,* vol. 111, pp. 209-19, Jun 1996.

[104] A. Sherbondy, D. Akers, R. Mackenzie, R. Dougherty, and B. Wandell, "Exploring connectivity of the brain's white matter with dynamic queries," *IEEE Trans Vis Comput Graph,* vol. 11, pp. 419-30, Jul-Aug 2005.

[105] A. J. Sherbondy, R. F. Dougherty, M. Ben-Shachar, S. Napel, and B. A. Wandell, "ConTrack: finding the most likely pathways between brain regions using diffusion tractography," *J Vis,* vol. 8, pp. 15 1-16, 2008.

[106] T. E. Conturo, N. F. Lori, T. S. Cull, E. Akbudak, A. Z. Snyder, J. S. Shimony, R. C. McKinstry, H. Burton, and M. E. Raichle, "Tracking neuronal fiber pathways in the living human brain," *Proc Natl Acad Sci U S A,* vol. 96, pp. 10422-7, Aug 31 1999.

[107] P. J. Basser, S. Pajevic, C. Pierpaoli, J. Duda, and A. Aldroubi, "In vivo fiber tractography using DT-MRI data," *Magn Reson Med,* vol. 44, pp. 625-32, Oct 2000.

[108] R. F. Dougherty, M. Ben-Shachar, R. Bammer, A. A. Brewer, and B. A. Wandell, "Functional organization of human occipital-callosal fiber tracts," *Proc Natl Acad Sci U S A,* vol. 102, pp. 7350-5, May 17 2005.

[109] A. J. Sherbondy, R. F. Dougherty, S. Napel, and B. A. Wandell, "Identifying the human optic radiation using diffusion imaging and fiber tractography," *J Vis,* vol. 8, pp. 12 1-11, 2008.

[110] E. A. DeYoe and D. C. Van Essen, "Concurrent processing streams in monkey visual cortex," *Trends Neurosci,* vol. 11, pp. 219-26, May 1988.

[111] K. S. Rockland and D. N. Pandya, "Topography of occipital lobe commissural connections in the rhesus monkey," *Brain Res,* vol. 365, pp. 174-8, Feb 12 1986.

[112] M. Saenz and I. Fine, "Topographic organization of V1 projections through the corpus callosum in humans," *Neuroimage,* vol. 52, pp. 1224-9, Oct 1 2010.

[113] E. Halgren, A. M. Dale, M. I. Sereno, R. B. Tootell, K. Marinkovic, and B. R. Rosen, "Location of human face-selective cortex with respect to retinotopic areas," *Hum Brain Mapp,* vol. 7, pp. 29-37, 1999.

Chapter 3

On the Specific Role of the Occipital Cortex in Scene Perception

Carole Peyrin and Benoit Musel

Additional information is available at the end of the chapter

http://dx.doi.org/10.5772/48438

1. Introduction

In recent years there has been mounting scientific excitement about the perception of scenes containing more realistic and complex stimuli than simple objects or drawings. Visual recognition of scenes is a fast, automatic and reliable process. Experimental studies have shown that complex natural scenes can be categorized in a very short time (under 150 ms [1]), suggesting a simple and efficient coding process. Many studies have attested to the importance of the Fourier components of images in scene categorization. In terms of signal representation, an image can be expressed in the Fourier domain as amplitude and phase spectra [2-5]. The amplitude spectrum highlights the dominant spatial scales (spatial frequencies) and the dominant orientations of the image, while the phase spectrum describes the relationship between spatial frequencies. It is now well established that the primary visual cortex is mainly dominated by complex cells which respond preferentially to orientations and spatial frequencies [6-8]. Simulation and psychophysical experiments have shown that information from low/medium frequencies of the amplitude spectrum is sufficient to enable scene categorization [9, 10]. These data support current influential models of scene perception [11-14].

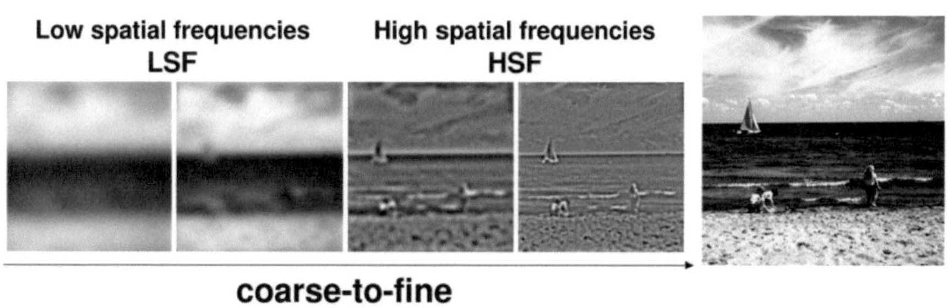

Figure 1. Coarse-to-fine sequence of spatial frequency processing (from low-to-high spatial frequencies) during scene perception

On the basis of convergent data from the functional neuroanatomy of magnocellular and parvocellular visual pathways [15], neurophysiological recordings in primates [12], and psychophysical results in humans [3, 4], these models have speculated that spatial frequency content may impose a specific temporal hierarchy on the processing of visual inputs. According to these models, visual analysis starts with the parallel extraction of different elementary attributes at different spatial frequencies, in a predominantly coarse-to-fine (low-to-high spatial frequencies) sequence which favours low spatial frequencies (LSF) in the initial stages of visual processing and high spatial frequencies (HSF) in the later stages (Figure 1). The LSF in a scene, conveyed by fast magnocellular visual channels, might therefore activate visual pathways and subsequently reach high-order areas in the dorsal stream (parietal and frontal) more rapidly than HSF, allowing an initial perceptual parsing of visual inputs prior to their complete propagation along the ventral stream (inferotemporal cortex) which ultimately mediates object recognition. This initial low-pass visual analysis might serve to refine the subsequent processing of HSF, which are conveyed more slowly by parvocellular visual channels to the ventral stream.

The majority of current visual models are, therefore, based on the neurophysiological properties of spatial frequency processing. However exactly how spatial frequencies are processed within the occipital cortex remains unclear. Initially, on the basis of neurophysiological recordings in nonhuman primates, Bullier [12] proposed that rapid LSF analysis, which takes place predominantly in the dorsal visual stream, might be "retro-injected" through feedback signals into low-level areas (e.g., primary visual cortex, V1), where it would influence subsequent HSF analysis and guide further processing through the ventral visual stream. The occipital cortex might therefore serve as an "active blackboard" integrating computations carried out by higher order cortical areas. Secondly, the issues of cerebral asymmetries and/or retinotopic organization of spatial frequency processing within the occipital cortex are still being debated in the literature. Many studies reveal retinotopic organization of spatial frequency processing in the occipital cortex [16-18]. HSF sinusoidal grating processing, for example, activates the foveal representation in all retinotopic areas (such as V1) of the occipital cortex, and LSF sinusoidal grating processing activates more peripheral representations in the same cortical areas. Despite studies showing retinotopic mapping of spatial frequency processing in the occipital cortex, many experimental arguments assume a certain hemispheric specialization of spatial frequency processing in the occipital cortex. The right occipital cortex appears to be preferentially specialized for LSF information processing, while the left occipital cortex seems to be preferentially specialized for HSF information processing [19-21]. It is, therefore, essential to determine whether hemispheric specialization and retinotopic processing can co-occur in the occipital cortex. While addressing this issue, the present chapter also aims to clarify the different attributes of the occipital cortex during scene recognition.

2. Coarse-to-fine analysis in visual perception

Results from various neurophysiological, computational, and behavioral studies all indicate that the totality of visual information is not immediately conveyed, but that information analysis follows a predominantly coarse-to-fine processing sequence (LSF are extracted first, followed by HSF). The first experimental evidence in support of this type of coarse-to-fine processing sequence in human vision comes from psychophysical studies using hierarchical stimuli (global forms composed of several local elements [22, 23]). Usually, these forms represent a large global letter form made up of small local letters. The subject's task is to identify a target letter either at global level, at local level, or at both levels. Using this paradigm, two main findings have emerged. Firstly, global form identification is faster than local form identification. This phenomenon is known as the global precedence effect. Secondly, while inconsistent global information slows down local information identification, the identification of local information has no effect on global identification. This asymmetrical effect is known as the global interference effect. However, these effects decrease or even vanish when the hierarchical forms are high-pass filtered (i.e. LSF are cut off). They are also affected by a subject's adaptation to a given frequency band (low vs. high), suggesting that LSF carry global information, whereas HSF carry local information [24-26]. Based on the assumption that global information is preferentially conveyed by LSF, and that local information is conveyed by HSF, the global-to-local processing sequence has been interpreted as reflecting a fundamental principle of the coarse-to-fine processing sequence.

Additional evidence of a coarse-to-fine processing sequence was provided by psychophysical studies using more ecological stimuli, such as natural scenes and faces [14, 27-30]. Schyns and Oliva [14], for example, used hybrid stimuli consisting of two superimposed images of natural scenes, taken from different semantic categories and containing different spatial frequencies (e.g., a highway scene in LSF superimposed on a city scene in HSF). The perception of these hybrid scenes was dominated by LSF information when presentation time was very brief (30 ms). However when presentation time was longer (150 ms), perception was dominated by HSF information, suggesting precedence of LSF over HSF in the visual processing time-course. Furthermore, when two successive hybrids displayed a coarse-to-fine sequence for a given scene (e.g., the highway scene in LSF in the first hybrid and then in HSF in the second hybrid) and a fine-to-coarse sequence simultaneously for another scene (e.g., the city scene in HSF in the first hybrid and then in LSF in the second hybrid), scene perception was more frequently based on a coarse-to-fine rather than a fine-to-coarse sequence.

Quite exactly how and where in the brain LSF and HSF information is differentially analyzed and eventually merged during visual processing remains an unresolved question. Traditional models have generally assumed that different visual cues are combined at successive stages along the cortical hierarchy [31, 32], and suggest that LSF and HSF might converge only in higher-level visual areas in the inferior temporal cortex (such as the fusiform or parahippocampal cortex [33, 34]). However, drawing on evidence from neurophysiological recordings in nonhuman primates [35], Bullier [12] proposed that rapid LSF analysis, predominantly carried out in the dorsal visual stream, might be "retro-injected" through feedback signals into low-level areas (e.g., primary visual cortex) where it would influence subsequent HSF analysis, and guide further processing through the ventral visual stream. The occipital cortex might therefore serve as an "active blackboard" integrating computations made by higher-order cortical areas. However, to date, the neural architecture and temporal dynamics of such top–down mechanisms have never been systematically investigated via direct testing of the preferential coarse-to-fine processing sequence during visual scene perception in humans.

3. Neural basis of the retro-injection mechanism during scene perception

In order to test the coarse-to-fine processing sequence and to identify its neural substrates in the human brain, we presented in rapid succession sequences of two spatial frequency-filtered scenes, with either an LSF image followed by an HSF image (coarse-to-fine sequence), or an HSF image followed by an LSF image (fine-to-coarse sequence) during fMRI and ERP recordings on the same participants [36]. Each scene in a sequence belonged to one of three categories (city, beach, or indoor). Half of the sequences displayed two scenes from the same category, and the other half displayed two scenes from different categories. Participants had to judge whether the two successive scenes belonged to the same category. This study also addressed the crucial issue of delayed "retro-injection" and spatial frequency integration in the occipital cortex.

Examination by fMRI showed selective increases in coarse-to-fine sequences (relative to fine-to-coarse sequences) in early-stage occipital areas, as well as in frontal and temporo-parietal areas. ERP topography and source analyses highlighted a similar network of cortical areas, but were in addition able to determine the time-course of activation in these regions, involving either LSF or HSF images in the different sequences. Higher-order areas in frontal and temporo-parietal regions responded more to LSF stimuli when these were presented first, whereas the occipital visual cortex responded more to HSF presented after LSF. More specifically, our results demonstrate that LSF in scenes (conveyed by fast magnocellular channels) can rapidly activate high-order areas, providing spatial (via the frontal eye fields) and semantic information (via the left prefrontal cortex and temporal areas), as well as attentional signals (via the temporo-parietal junction), all of which may promote the ongoing perceptual organization and categorization of visual input. This first coarse analysis may possibly be refined by further processing in the visual cortices of HSF in scenes (conveyed more slowly by the parvocellular channels). In order for this to occur, feedback from the first low-pass computations carried out in frontal and temporo-parietal areas might be "retro-injected" into lower level areas, such as the occipital cortex, at the level of the primary visual cortex, with a view to guiding the high-pass analysis and selecting the relevant finer details necessary for the recognition and categorization of scenes. These results provide critical support for recent models of vision, and for the retro-injection mechanism proposed by Bullier [12]. They also highlight the necessity for further investigation of the neural mechanisms of spatial frequency processing in the occipital cortex.

The majority of visual models assume, therefore, a predominantly coarse-to-fine sequence of spatial frequency processing in the whole brain, based on the functional properties of the visual cortex. However, many studies have highlighted the fact that in humans, the left and right hemispheres do not deal with all aspects of visual information processing with equal ability. The two hemispheres might in fact make complementary contributions to the processing of LSF and HSF.

4. Hemispheric specialization of spatial frequency processing during scene perception

Many experimental arguments assume that spatial frequency processing is shared between the two hemispheres, with right hemispheric predominance for LSF processing and left hemispheric predominance for HSF processing. This hemispheric specialization has been observed either through behavioral studies on healthy subjects [21, 37-48] and neurological patients [49-51], or through functional neuroimaging studies [19, 20, 52-65]. However, the hemispheric asymmetries in question were largely inferred from studies assessing hemispheric specialization in global and local processing.

4.1. Behavioral arguments

Using hierarchical visual stimuli consisting of a global form made up of several local elements [22, 23] displayed either in the left or right visual field, Sergent [46] demonstrated that global forms were identified more quickly when they were presented in the left visual hemifield, projecting directly to the right hemisphere, while recognition of local forms was faster when they were presented in the right visual hemifield, projecting directly to the left hemisphere [52] (see also [38]). These results suggest right hemispheric dominance for the recognition of global forms, and left hemispheric dominance for the recognition of local forms. Since global processing can be considered to be mediated by low-pass spatial analysis, and local processing by high-pass spatial analysis [24-26], the hemispheric specialization patterns observed in global and local processing have been interpreted as reflecting the hemispheric specialization of LSF and HSF, respectively [46].

Unfortunately, the relationship between local and global information and spatial frequencies in hierarchical forms is far from univocal [66]. Global information could, for example, be conveyed not only by LSF but also by HSF. The hypothesis of hemispheric asymmetry in spatial frequency processing was subsequently directly tested by making explicit changes in the spatial frequency spectrum of stimuli, using sinusoidal gratings as stimuli [40-42], or more complex visual stimuli such as images of natural scenes [21, 43, 44]. It should be noted that hierarchical forms do not allow this type of manipulation, because low-pass filtering cancels out the local form, thus rendering execution of the task impossible. In a series of behavioral studies conducted by our team [21, 43, 44], we evaluated hemispheric asymmetry in healthy subjects using natural scenes, while manipulating the spatial frequency components of the scenes, which were presented in divided visual fields. In the princeps study [43], participants were asked to recognize either an LSF or an HSF filtered target scene (a city or a highway), displayed in either the left or the right visual field. Results showed that LSF filtered scenes were recognized more quickly when they were presented in the left visual hemifield, projecting directly to the right hemisphere, while recognition of the HSF filtered scenes was faster when these were presented in the right visual hemifield, projecting directly to the left hemisphere. This study clearly demonstrated right hemispheric superiority for LSF and left hemispheric superiority for HSF processing, and therefore supports Sergent's assumption [46] that visual tasks which require the processing of LSF information (such as global letter identification in hierarchical forms) would result in a left visual field/right hemisphere advantage, whereas tasks requiring the processing of HSF information (such as local letter identification in hierarchical forms) would result in right visual field/left hemisphere superiority.

Following this, we examined whether the temporal characteristics of spatial frequency analysis (i.e. the temporal precedence of LSF over HSF as postulated by the coarse-to-fine processing sequence) might interfere with hemispheric specialization. We did this by manipulating the exposure duration of filtered natural scene images (30 vs. 150 ms [44]). Results showed the classical hemispheric specialization pattern for brief exposure duration (the right hemisphere was predominantly involved in LSF scene processing and the left in HSF scene processing), and a tendency towards right hemisphere advantage, irrespective of the spatial frequency content for longer exposure durations. These results suggest that the hemispheric specialization pattern for visual information processing ought to be considered as a dynamic system, within which the superiority of one hemisphere over the other could change according to the level of temporal constraints. The higher the temporal constraints of the task, the more the hemispheres become specialized in spatial frequency processing. In a subsequent study [21], we provided evidence for hemispheric specialization in spatial frequency processing in men, but not in women. These results are consistent with studies showing that the functional cerebral organization of women is less lateralized than that of men [67, 68].

4.2. Neural correlates of hemispheric specialization

Neuropsychological and neuroimaging studies conducted on hierarchical visual stimuli have reported conflicting results on which cortical structures present hemispheric specialization. Robertson and collaborators [51] showed, for example, that unilateral damage of the temporo–parietal junction could impair patients' performance in the hierarchical form paradigm. Patients with a lesion in the left superior temporal gyrus thus exhibited a slowing down in local form identification, whereas the performance of patients with a lesion situated in the right temporo–parietal region was impaired during global form identification. These data suggest that two independent perceptual sub-systems may be involved; the right temporo–parietal junction which emphasizes global information, and the left temporo–parietal junction which emphasizes local information. However, using positron emission tomography, Fink and collaborators [53-55] reported cerebral asymmetries in the occipital cortex. The right lingual gyrus was more highly activated during the processing of global as opposed to local forms, while the left inferior occipital gyrus was more highly activated during the processing of local rather than global forms. Using electroencephalographic recordings, Heinze and collaborators [57, 60] failed to demonstrate cerebral asymmetries in first-stage visual areas. Instead, their results, based on event-related potentials (ERPs), showed long latency asymmetries (260-360 latency range) for global versus local processing, suggesting that hemispheric specialization was present only in the higher levels of visual analysis.

Furthermore, some functional imaging data have revealed an attentional cortical mechanism which exerts control over the perceptual processes involved in global and local processing [50, 51, 53-55, 63-65]. This mechanism operates on the attentional selection of information presented either at global level, at local level, or at both levels depending on task constraints. This mechanism is located in the temporo-partial junction. Using Using ERPs, Yamaguchi and collaborators [65] investigated the neural substrates of attentional allocation to global and local components of a hierarchical form. For this purpose ERPs were recorded while participants shifted their attention to the global or local level of a hierarchical form. Shift direction was controlled by a preceding cue stimulus. Hemispheric asymmetries arose not only during the task in which global–local processing was actually being performed, but also in the time interval during which attention was directed towards global or local levels by the cues. Therefore, in addition to hemispheric asymmetry during "bottom-up" processing, this study demonstrated the existence of neural substrates for a top-down mechanism of hemispheric asymmetry in global and local selection. ERPs to the cue showed greater amplitude in the right hemisphere during attentional allocation at global level, and greater amplitude in the left hemisphere during attentional allocation at local level. The neural activity in question was located in the right temporo-parietal junction for the global shift, and in the left temporo-parietal junction for the local shift. These electrophysiological results provided an asymmetrical neural basis for the "top-down" allocation of attention to global and local features, and revealed the contribution of the temporal-parietal cortex to this attentional mechanism.

On the whole, the imaging studies mentioned previously have provided conflicting results on hemispheric specialization using hierarchical stimuli. By directly manipulating the spatial frequency content of stimuli, subsequent studies revealed hemispheric specialization in certain occipito-temporal areas [19, 20]. In one fMRI study [20], we investigated the neural correlates and the hemispheric specialization of spatial frequency processing during the perception of scene stimuli which allowed an explicit change in the spatial frequency spectrum. For this purpose, we used a categorization task of small LSF and HSF scene images (at a visual angle of 4°).

By comparing LSF to HSF scene categorization (Figure 2a), we observed significant activation in the right anterior temporal cortex and the right parahippocampal gyrus. As these regions are known to be involved in scene processing, these results suggest that scene recognition is based mainly on LSF extraction and analysis, following a coarse-to-fine processing sequence. Significant activation was also obtained in the right inferior parietal lobule, and this probably reflects attentional modulation during spatial frequency selection. Compared to HSF scene recognition, LSF scene recognition also activated the bilateral posterior part of the superior temporal cortex. This result contradicts neuropsychological studies [49-51], which have shown specialization of the right superior temporal cortex in the perceptual processing of global (LSF) information, and specialization of the left superior temporal cortex in the perceptual processing of local (HSF) information. Finally, comparisons between HSF and LSF scene categorization failed to show any significant activation, suggesting a bias towards the processing of LSF information.

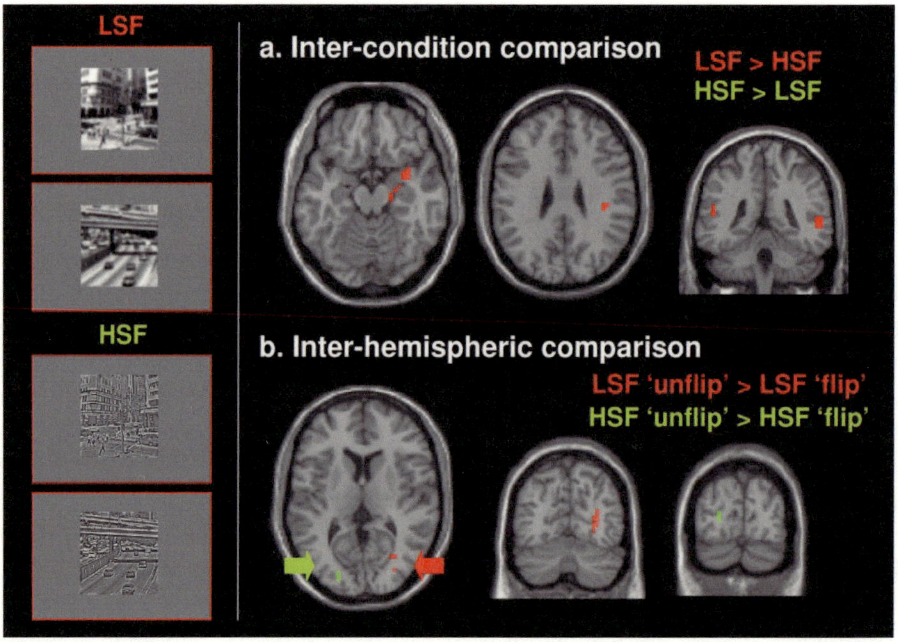

Figure 2. Hemispheric specialization of spatial frequency processing during scene perception

Based on behavioural experiments in which direct comparisons were made between the performances of the two visual fields [21, 40-44, 46], we suggested that any assessment of visual cerebral asymmetries must make direct comparisons between activation in the two hemispheres. In order to do so, we created a new method of fMRI data analysis. The method of direct inter-hemispheric comparison examines contrasts between "unflipped" and "left–right flipped" functional images from the same experimental condition (Figure 3), in order to compare activity in one hemisphere with activity in homologous regions of the other hemisphere [19, 20, 69, 70]. Using this method, we demonstrated higher levels of activation in the right middle occipital gyrus than in the left during the recognition of LSF scenes, and higher levels of activation in the left middle occipital gyrus than in the right during the recognition of HSF scenes (Figure 2b).

This result provides supplementary evidence for hemispheric specialization in the early stages of visual analysis when spatial frequencies are being processed. Another important point was that when analysing the fMRI data using a more traditional approach which contrasts spatial frequencies to one another, we observed stronger cerebral activation for LSF than for HSF scenes, while the reverse contrast did not reveal any significant activation. Results therefore differ according to the method of data analysis applied. A direct inter-hemispheric method of comparison seems more appropriate for the assessment of cerebral asymmetries, since it allows the cancelling out of any main effect deriving from spatial frequency bias (i.e. stronger global cerebral activation for LSF than for HSF scenes).

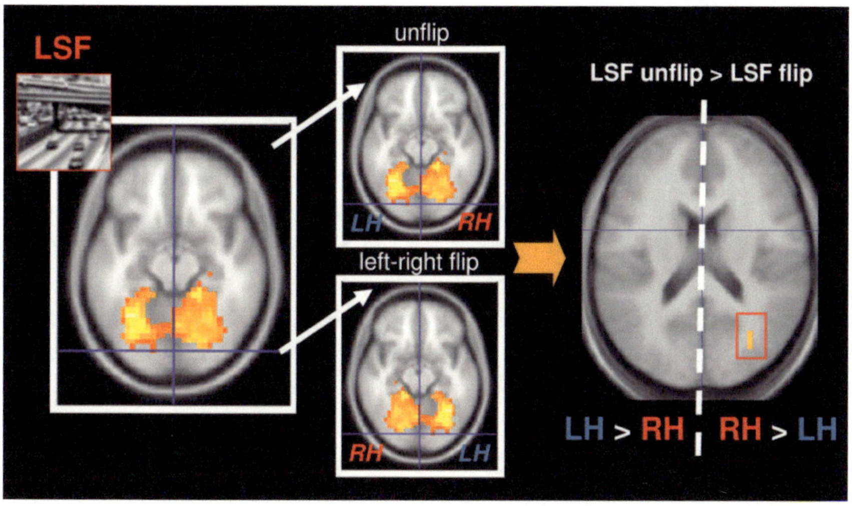

Figure 3. The method of direct inter-hemispheric comparison. In this method, two sets of functional volumes, obtained from functional scans, are compared at both individual and group level. One set is represented by functional volumes in accordance with neurological convention (the left hemisphere - LH appears on the left side of images) and the other set is represented by the same functional volumes this time in accordance with radiological convention (the right hemisphere – RH appears on the left side of images). Images from the second set were "flipped" by 180° in the midsagital plane, thus providing "mirror" images of the first set. Contrasts between "unflipped" and "left-right flipped" images were then calculated for each of the spatial frequency components of natural scenes. In order to assess hemispheric predominance during the perception of LSF scenes, for instance, the following contrast was calculated: LSF unflip > LSF flip. Regions which were statistically more highly activated in the left hemisphere than in the right hemisphere appear on the left side, and regions which were statistically more highly activated in the right hemisphere than in the left hemisphere appear on the right side.

Using a neuropsychological approach [21], we further investigated the role of the right occipital cortex in LSF processing in a female neurological patient with a focal lesion in this region following the embolization of an arterioveinous malformation. As a result, she suffered from a left homonymous hemianopia. The study was conducted 1 week before and 6 months after the surgical intervention. As expected, after the embolization, LSF scene recognition was more severely impaired than HSF scene recognition. These data support the hypothesis of a preferential specialization of the right occipital cortex for LSF information processing, and suggest more generally a hemispheric specialization in spatial frequency processing in females, although this is difficult to demonstrate behaviourally in healthy women.

4.3. Cerebral asymmetries during coarse-to-fine analysis of scenes

What is important here is that although LSF information may be perceptually available before HSF, this does not necessarily imply that it is always used first to support visual recognition in all tasks. Indeed, the global precedence effect can be turned into a local precedence effect by simple experimental manipulation (e.g., by changing the visual angle [22, 71] or the number of local elements [72]). In Schyns and Oliva's experiments [14], a substantial proportion (29%) of hybrid sequences were in fact categorized in accordance with a fine-to-coarse, rather than a coarse-to-fine sequence. Although the coarse-to-fine processing sequence appears to be the predominant way of operating, the processing sequence of spatial scale information has been found to be relatively flexible, and dependent on task demands [14, 29, 30]. A subsequent study by Schyns and Oliva [29] showed that the spatial scale preferentially processed in hybrid images can be constrained by a phase of prior sensitization which implicitly "primes" visual processing in favor of a particular scale (coarse or fine). After initial exposure to LSF information, the subsequent categorization of hybrid images was preferentially performed following LSF cues, whereas it was biased towards HSF information after priming by HSF. By using hybrid faces instead of scenes, Schyns and Oliva [30] showed that HSF information was preferentially used to determine whether a face was expressive or not, whereas LSF information was preferentially used to categorize emotion (e.g., happy, angry). The demands of a categorization task may, therefore, determine which range of spatial frequencies is extracted, and subsequently processed, from hybrid stimuli (even when using brief presentation times, such as 45 ms). In all, these studies suggest that all spatial frequencies were available at the beginning of categorization, and that both types of processing sequence may coexist in the visual system. The selection of spatial frequencies during the recognition of natural scenes may depend on dynamic interactions between the information requirements of a given recognition task and the perceptual information available. While a coarse-to-fine sequence of spatial frequency processing may preferentially arise for normal visual inputs containing both LSF and HSF information, our visual system should nonetheless be able to prioritize the processing of HSF in certain situations, such as when searching for a target known to be defined by specific local features rather than global visual properties (e.g., find something with a striped texture).

The cerebral occipital asymmetries observed in spatial frequency processing raise the fundamental question of the legitimacy of the coarse-to-fine sequence in the whole brain. It remains unclear whether coarse-to-fine analysis is used in both hemispheres and/or whether this sequence predominates in only one hemisphere. In an event-related fMRI experiment, we wondered whether hemispheric specialization of spatial frequency processing might underlie the flexibility of the temporal sequence used for spatial frequency analysis during scene perception [70]. In order to constrain spatial frequency processing according to different time-courses, we asked healthy participants to perform a matching task between two successive images of natural scenes (LSF or HSF), which were displayed either in a coarse-to-fine sequence (LSF scene presented first followed by HSF scene), or in a reverse fine-to-coarse sequence. Our direct inter-hemispheric comparison of the neural responses evoked by each spatial frequency sequence revealed greater activation in the right occipito-temporal cortex than in the left for the coarse-to-fine sequence, and greater activation in the left occipito-temporal cortex than in the right for the fine-to-coarse sequence. These fMRI results therefore indicate that the hemisphere functionally specialized in the processing of the visual sequence of different spatial frequency inputs is the same hemisphere that is specialized in the processing of the first spatial frequency-band appearing in this sequence (i.e. right hemispheric dominance for coarse-to-fine, but also for LSF information analysis when presented alone; and conversely, left hemispheric dominance for fine-to-coarse, but also for HSF information analysis alone). This pattern suggests that the hemisphere preferentially engaged during the sequential processing of different spatial frequencies might be determined by the initial spatial frequency-band appearing in this sequence, and that both a coarse-to-fine and fine-to-coarse analysis might take place independently in both hemispheres. Our findings indicate that the visual system might be equipped with two types of cortical apparatus which are able to support scene perception differentially and flexibly, according to task demands or input sequence. The apparatus in the right occipital cortex would give priority to LSF analysis and the one in the left occipital cortex would give priority to HSF analysis. However, although a considerable number of studies postulate hemispheric specialization of spatial frequency processing in the occipital cortex, others highlight retinotopic processing of spatial frequencies.

5. Retinotopic organization of spatial frequency processing during scene categorization

The distribution of retinal photoreceptors and retinal ganglion cells is nonhomogeneous throughout the visual system [73, 74]. The density of cones and midget ganglion cells, which are used to process HSF information, is greatest in the fovea, while the density of rods and parasol ganglion cells, which are used to process LSF information, increase with foveal eccentricity. Different imaging data obtained from patients with cerebral lesions [75, 76] and from healthy participants [77, 78] show that the human primary visual cortex is retinotopically organized. Representation of the visual field ranges from the posterior to the anterior visual cortex, and shifts from the centre to the periphery. Since the fovea is represented in the posterior areas of the visual cortex, it could well be that HSF information (conveyed by the parvocellular pathway to the visual cortex) is predominantly processed in these areas, which are devoted to foveal vision. Similarly, since the peripheral retina is represented in progressively more anterior areas of the visual cortex, LSF information (conveyed by the magnocellular pathway to the visual cortex) might well be predominantly processed in these areas, which are devoted to peripheral vision.

5.1. Spatial frequency tuning in retinotopic visual areas

A large number of neurophysiological studies performed on cats [79, 80], primates [6, 81-84] and humans [16-18] have mapped representations of the different spatial frequencies in retinotopic areas. Using retinotopic encoding with achromatic sinusoidal gratings, Sasaki and collaborators [17] have, in particular, shown that LSF are mapped in occipital areas in accordance with the cortical representation of the peripheral visual field, whereas HSF are mapped in accordance with the central visual field. Other studies have demonstrated that more complex cognitive functions, such as visual spatial attention, are also mapped consistently by cortical retinotopy [17, 85-89]. Using very large hierarchical visual stimuli in a block design fMRI study, Sasaki and collaborators [17] found evidence for retinotopic mapping of global and local attention in the occipital cortex. During "attend global" blocks, participants were required to deliberately focus their attention on the global form (at a visual angle of 29.4°) involving their peripheral vision, while during "attend local" blocks, they had to focus on local elements (at a visual angle of 2.4°), involving more foveal vision. FMRI data were analyzed using a traditional approach based on comparisons between local and global levels. Results showed that when attention was directed at local level (as opposed to global level), activation was consistent with the cortical representation of the fovea, which is also sensitive to HSF gratings. When attention was directed at global level (as opposed to local level), activation was consistent with the cortical representation of the periphery, which is also sensitive to LSF gratings.

The studies mentioned previously either postulate retinotopic processing of spatial frequencies [17], or demonstrate hemispheric specialization of spatial frequency processing in the occipital cortex [19, 20]. We conducted an fMRI study to reconcile the fact that spatial frequency processing could not only be retinotopically mapped, it could also be lateralized between both hemispheres.

5.2. How can retinotopy and cerebral asymmetries for spatial frequencies be reconciled?

The results obtained by Sasaki and collaborators [17] showed no hemispheric specialization for spatial frequency processing. However, the authors used a traditional method of data analysis, comparing global and local experimental conditions to one another, rather than the direct inter-hemispheric comparison method that we had used previously [20], and which had produced different results.

In a recent fMRI study, we used a categorization task (indoors vs. outdoors) of natural scenes filtered in LSF and HSF scenes, in order to evaluate, on the one hand the retinotopy, and on the other hand, functional lateralization in spatial frequency processing. With this aim in mind, we used larger scene images (at a visual angle of 24° x 18°) than in our previous studies (which used scenes with a visual angle of 4° x 4° [20, 21, 36, 43, 44, 70]), covering as broad a visual field as had Sasaki and collaborators [17]. We used a block-design fMRI paradigm, in which large LSF or HSF were displayed in separate experimental blocks. The retinotopy of spatial frequency processing was assessed using a traditional method of fMRI data analysis based on comparisons between LSF and HSF scene categorization. According to previous retinotopy studies, when processing spatial frequencies, the categorization of LSF scenes (compared to HSF) would recruit areas devoted to peripheral vision, whereas the categorization of HSF scenes (compared to LSF) would recruit areas devoted to foveal vision. Cerebral asymmetries were assessed using the inter-hemispheric comparison method. We expected a higher level of activation in right hemisphere than in the left during the processing of LSF, and more involvement of the left hemisphere during HSF processing.

Our results provided first of all evidence of retinotopic organization of spatial frequency processing in the human visual cortex. LSF (as opposed to HSF) scene categorization elicited medial occipital activation in the anterior half of the calcarine fissures in correspondence with the peripheral visual field, whereas HSF (as opposed to LSF) scene categorization elicited more lateral occipital activation in the posterior part of the occipital lobes in correspondence with the fovea, in accordance with retinotopic organization in visual areas (Figure 4a). By contrasting spatial frequency blocks to one another, we were, therefore, able to show that the processing of spatial frequencies is related to the organization of retinotopic eccentricity in the occipital cortex. In addition to the retinotopic activation obtained by contrasting spatial frequencies, cerebral asymmetries were also demonstrated. In order to identify cerebral asymmetries, we made direct comparisons between the two hemispheres by contrasting "unflipped" to "left-right flipped" functional images for each particular spatial frequency band (LSF and HSF). As expected from previous studies, and in accordance with our own previous results [20, 21], the inter-hemispheric method of comparison highlights occipital cortex predominance on the right (as opposed to on the left) for LSF scene categorization, and temporal cortex predominance on the left (as opposed to on the right) for HSF scene categorization (Figure 4b).

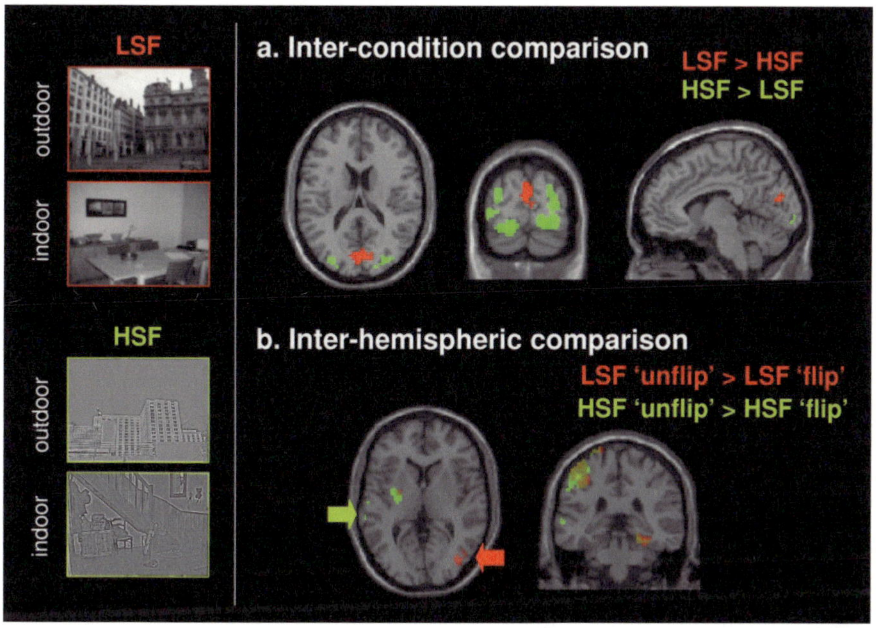

Figure 4. Retinotopic organization and hemispheric specialization of spatial frequency processing during scene perception

Using stimuli filtered in spatial frequencies covering a large part of the visual field, and depending on the method of data analysis used, we succeeded in showing that the processing of spatial frequencies is specifically organized in the visual areas of each hemisphere, as well as between the two hemispheres, according to functional lateralization. By using several different approaches on the same data, our results enabled us to reconcile for the first time retinotopic and lateralized processing of spatial frequencies in the human occipital-temporal cortex.

In addition to neuroimaging studies on healthy subjects, patients with retinal disorders constitute pathological models which enable the specific investigation of retinotopic mapping of spatial frequency processing in the occipital cortex through the relationship between the position of the lesion on the retina and the processing of spatial frequencies. We specifically explored the relationship between central retinal lesions in age-related macular degeneration (AMD) patients and the processing of spatial frequencies during scene categorization.

5.3. Scene perception and spatial frequency processing in age-related macular degeneration

AMD, characterized by a central vision loss caused by the destruction of macular photoreceptors [90], is the primary cause of vision loss in the elderly population [91-93]. Owing to the central position of the retinal lesion, and the neurophysiology of the parvocellular and magnocellular pathways, AMD patients would be expected to be deficient in the categorization of HSF scenes compared to age-matched healthy participants. Many studies have demonstrated impairment of low-level visual processes in AMD patients (e.g., contrast sensitivity in gratings [94-96]). However, research on the ability of AMD patients to process and recognize complex visual stimuli filtered in LSF and HSF is scarce. Recent studies have shown impairment of scene perception in AMD patients [97-99]. In face perception tasks, AMD patients were able to identify facial emotions when the decision was thought to be based on LSF processing [100]. Perception of details in facial emotions, conveyed by HSF, was impaired. However, in this study, the HSF processing deficit was inferred rather than clearly demonstrated, because the spatial frequency content of faces was not manipulated explicitly. In order to test this assumption, we recently conducted behavioural experiments [101], in which AMD patients and healthy age-matched participants performed categorization tasks of large scene images (indoors vs. outdoors) filtered in LSF and HSF. The results showed that AMD patients made more non-responses and had longer reaction times for the categorization of HSF than for that of LSF scenes, whereas healthy participants' performance was not differentially affected by the spatial frequency content of scenes.

Furthermore, retinal lesions caused by AMD induce a lack of stimulation in the part of the visual cortex which is devoted to the processing of the central visual field, suggesting a reorganization of the human cortex. If HSF processing activates the foveal representation in the occipital cortex, the specific impairment of HSF processing in AMD may result in atypical occipital activation. Using our categorization task of LSF and HSF scenes under fMRI, we recently investigated the functional cerebral reorganization of spatial frequency processing in an AMD patient. The patient showed a deficit in the processing of HSF, linked with hypoactivation in the occipital cortex, compared to age-matched healthy participants (Figure 5). However, LSF processing was relatively similar in the AMD patient and healthy participants, at both behavioural and neurobiological levels. The present findings point to a specific deficit in the processing of HSF information contained in photographs of natural scenes in AMD, linked with hypo-activation in the occipital cortex. LSF information processing was relatively well preserved. These results could also provide interesting perspectives for the diagnosis of AMD and monitoring of future treatments.

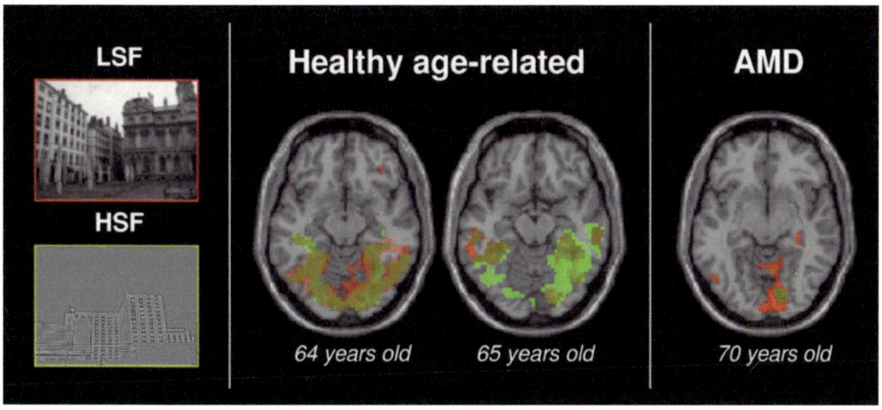

Figure 5. Hypoactivation in the occipital cortex during HSF scene perception in age-related macular degeneration (AMD)

6. Conclusion

Our findings demonstrate that LSF information may reach high-order areas rapidly to enable coarse initial parsing of the visual scene, which could then be retro-injected through feedback into the occipital cortex to guide a finer analysis based on HSF. Furthermore, spatial frequency processing may be retinotopically mapped and lateralized in the occipital cortex. Using stimuli filtered in spatial frequencies covering a large part of the visual field, and depending on the method of data analysis, we succeeded in showing that the processing of spatial frequencies is specifically organized in the visual areas of each hemisphere, as well as between the two hemispheres, according to functional lateralization. Critically, we provided evidence that a method of fMRI data analysis based on a direct inter-hemispheric comparison was more appropriate than the classical method of inter-condition comparison in the evaluation of hemispheric dominance. Using a method of inter-hemispheric comparison, we demonstrated greater activation in right occipital areas than in left during LSF scene perception, but greater activation in left than in right occipital areas during HSF scene perception, while the inter-condition comparison revealed retinotopic processing. HSF (compared to LSF) scenes activate the foveal representation in retinotopic areas of the occipital cortex, and LSF (compared to HSF) scenes activate more peripheral representations in the same cortical areas. Even if the hypothesis was not directly tested here, we suggest that retinotopic processing may result from bottom-up visual processes, while hemispheric specialization may be controlled by top-down attentional processes (in the temporo-parietal region). Finally, our findings indicate that in scene perception, the predominantly coarse-to-fine analysis seems to be preferentially performed in the right hemisphere, from the occipital to the inferior temporal cortex.

Our findings also demonstrate that pathology constitutes an interesting way of investigating cognitive models of spatial frequency processing, both at behavioural and cerebral levels. Future studies conducted in patients with visual field defects (following peripheral or cerebral damage) are needed to fully investigate spatial frequency processing in the occipital cortex. Behavioural studies in hemianopic patients following occipital lobe damage would specifically allow the investigation of hemispheric specialization in spatial frequency processing. Categorization of LSF scenes ought to be more impaired in patients with left hemianopic (right occipital lesion), while categorization of HSF scenes ought to be more impaired in patients with right hemianopic (left occipital lesion). In a complementary way, studies conducted on patients with contrasting retinal diseases (e.g., AMD patients characterized by a central vision loss, and retinitis pigmentosa characterized by a peripheral vision loss) would allow further investigation of the retinotopic processing of spatial frequencies. We would expect to observe a differential reorganization of the occipital cortex depending on the retinal lesion site which mirrors the dissociation of the visual disorder in question. According to the retinotopy of spatial frequency processing, if HSF processing activates the foveal representation in the occipital cortex, a specific impairment of HSF processing in AMD may result in atypical activation in occipital areas corresponding to the fovea (compared to age-matched healthy participants). Similarly, a specific impairment of LSF processing in patients with retinitis pigmentosa may result in atypical activation in occipital areas corresponding to the periphery.

On the whole, the results obtained suggest that the occipital cortex could be the point of convergence of both afferent connections from the thalamus, and feedback connections from high-order visual areas. Coarse visual information would be rapidly forwarded to high level visual areas, more specifically to the frontal and temporo-parietal areas, via the magnocellular visual pathways. This information would provide the spatial and semantic characteristics required for the identification of the visual scene. Feedback connections from frontal and temporo-parietal areas to occipital areas might then modulate the processing of fine information, slowly conveyed by the parvocellular pathway. In the occipital cortex, the hemisphere preferentially involved in visual processing may depend on the spatial frequency band required in the task. In coarse-to-fine sequence processing, the right occipital cortex would in that case be more involved than the left. Visual information would then be sent through the right ventral visual stream, from occipital to infero-temporal areas. In tasks requiring the use of fine details, visual information would be sent preferentially through the left ventral visual stream. A more advanced analysis of the scene would be performed at the very end of the ventral visual stream (e.g., in the parahippocampal place area [102]). In addition, spatial frequencies in scenes were also retinotopically mapped in the occipital cortex. However, additional studies on the time course of activation induced by spatial frequencies are necessary to specify whether retinotopic and lateralized representations emerge from ascendant or descendant processes.

Author details

Carole Peyrin and Benoit Musel
Laboratoire de Psychologie et NeuroCognition, France

Acknowledgement

This work was supported by a research grant from the Fyssen Foundation to Carole Peyrin, by a doctoral fellowship from the Région Rhone-Alpes to Benoit Musel and by the National Centre for Scientific Research in France. The authors extend warm thanks to the "Délégation à la Recherche Clinique et à l'Innovation" of the University Hospital of Grenoble for sponsoring their work. We thank Catherine Dal Molin for the English revision of the manuscript.

7. References

[1] Thorpe S, Fize D, Marlot C (1996) Speed of processing in the human visual system. Nature 381: 520-2.
[2] Field DJ (1987) Relations between the statistics of natural images and the response properties of cortical cells. J Opt Soc Am A 4: 2379-94.
[3] Ginsburg AP (1986) Spatial filtering and visual form perception. In: Boff K, Kauman L, Thomas J, editors. Hanbook of perception and human performance. NY: Wiley. pp. 1-41.
[4] Hughes HC, Nozawa G, Kitterle FL (1996) Global precedence, spatial frequency channels, and the statistic of the natural image. Journal of Cognitive Neuroscience 8: 197-230.
[5] Tolhurst DJ, Tadmor Y, Chao T (1992) Amplitude spectra of natural images. Ophthalmic Physiol Opt 12: 229-32.
[6] De Valois RL, Albrecht DG, Thorell LG.(1982) Spatial frequency selectivity of cells in macaque visual cortex. Vision Res 22: 545-59.
[7] De Valois RL, Yund EW, Hepler N (1982) The orientation and direction selectivity of cells in macaque visual cortex. Vision Res 22, 531-44.
[8] Poggio GF (1972) Spatial properties of neurons in striate cortex of unanesthetized macaque monkey. Invest Ophthalmol 11: 368-77.
[9] Guyader N, Chauvin A, Peyrin C, Herault J, Marendaz C (2004) Image phase or amplitude? Rapid scene categorization is an amplitude-based process. C R Biol 327: 313-8.
[10] Torralba A, Oliva A (2003) Statistics of natural image categories. Network 14: 391-412.
[11] Bar M (2003) A cortical mechanism for triggering top-down facilitation in visual object recognition. J Cogn Neurosci 15: 600-9.
[12] Bullier J (2001) Integrated model of visual processing. Brain Research Reviews 36: 96-107.
[13] Hegde J (2008) Time course of visual perception: coarse-to-fine processing and beyond. Prog Neurobiol 84: 405-39.
[14] Schyns PG, Oliva A (1994) From blobs to boundary edges: Evidence for time- and spatial-scale-dependant scene recognition. Psychol Sci 5: 195-200.

[15] Van Essen DC, DeYoe EA (1995) Concurrent processing in the primate visual cortex. In: Gazzaniga M, editor. The cognitive Neurosciences. Cambridge: Bradford Book. pp. 383-400

[16] Henriksson L, Raninen A, Nasanen R, Hyvarinen L, Vanni S (2007) Training-induced cortical representation of a hemianopic hemifield. J Neurol Neurosurg Psychiatry 78: 74-81.

[17] Sasaki Y, Hadjikhani N, Fischl B, Liu AK, Marret S, Dale AM, Tootell RBH (2001) Local and global attention are mapped retinotopically in human occipital cortex. Psychology 98: 2077-2082.

[18] Singh KD, Smith AT, Greenlee MW (2000) Spatiotemporal frequency and direction sensitivities of human visual areas measured using fMRI. Neuroimage 12: 550-64.

[19] Iidaka T, Yamashita K, Kashikura K, Yonekura Y (2004) Spatial frequency of visual image modulates neural responses in the temporo-occipital lobe. An investigation with event-related fMRI. Brain Res Cogn Brain Res 18: 196-204.

[20] Peyrin C, Baciu M, Segebarth C, Marendaz C (2004) Cerebral regions and hemispheric specialization for processing spatial frequencies during natural scene recognition. An event-related fMRI study. Neuroimage 23: 698-707.

[21] Peyrin C, Chokron S, Guyader N, Gout O, Moret J, Marendaz C (2006) Neural correlates of spatial frequency processing: A neuropsychological approach. Brain Res 1073-1074: 1-10.

[22] Kinchla RA, Wolfe JM (1979) The order of visual processing: "Top-down," "bottom-up", or "middle-out". Percept Psychophys 25: 225-31.

[23] Navon D (1977) Forest before trees: the precedence of global features in visual perception. Cognitive Psychology 9: 353-383.

[24] Badcock JC, Whitworth FA, Badcock DR, Lovegrove WJ (1990) Low frequency filtering and the processing of local-global stimuli. Perception 19:, 617-629.

[25] Lamb MR, Yund EW (1993) The role of spatial frequency in the processing of hierarchically organized stimuli. P Percept Psychophys 54: 773-84.

[26] Schulman G, Sulivan M, Gisch K, Sadoka W (1986) The role of spatial frequency channels in the perception of local and global structure. Perception 15: 259-273.

[27] Oliva A, Schyns PG (1997) Coarse blobs or fine edges? Evidence that information diagnosticity changes the perception of complex visual stimuli. Cognitive Psychology 34: 72-107.

[28] Parker DM, Lishman JR, Hughes J (1996) Role of coarse and fine spatial information in face and object processing. J Exp Psychol Hum Percept Perform 22: 1448-66.

[29] Schyns PG, Oliva A. (1997) Flexible, diagnosticity-driven, rather than fixed, perceptually determined scale selection in scene and face recognition. Perception 26: 1027-38.

[30] Schyns PG, Oliva A. (1999) Dr. Angry and Mr. Smile: when categorization flexibly modifies the perception of faces in rapid visual presentations. Cognition 69: 243-65.

[31] Biederman I (1995) Visual object recognition. In: Kosslyn SF, Osherson DN, editors. An invitation to cognitive science. Cambridge, MA: MIT Press. pp. 121–165.

[32] Riesenhuber M, Poggio T (1999) Hierarchical models of object recognition in cortex. Nat Neurosci 2: 1019-25.

[33] Bar M, Tootell RB, Schacter DL, Greve DN, Fischl B, Mendola JD, Rosen BR, Dale AM (2001) Cortical mechanisms specific to explicit visual object recognition. Neuron 29: 529-35.

[34] Rotshtein P, Vuilleumier P, Winston J, Driver J, Dolan R (2007) Distinct and convergent visual processing of high and low spatial frequency information in faces. Cereb Cortex 17: 2713-24.

[35] Hupe JM, James AC, Girard P, Lomber SG, Payne BR, Bullier J (2001) Feedback connections act on the early part of the responses in monkey visual cortex. J Neurophysiol 85: 134-45.

[36] Peyrin C, Michel CM, Schwartz S, Thut G, Seghier M, Landis T, Marendaz C, Vuilleumier P (2010) The neural substrates and timing of top-down processes during coarse-to-fine categorization of visual scenes: a combined fMRI and ERP study. J Cogn Neurosci 22: 2768-80.

[37] Chokron S, Bartolomeo P, Colliot P, Brickman AM, Tabert M, Wei T, Buchsbaum MS (2003) Selective attention, inhibition for repeated events and hemispheric specialization. Brain Cogn 53: 158-61.

[38] Chokron S, Brickman AM, Wei T, Buchsbaum MS (2000) Hemispheric asymmetry for selective attention. Brain Res Cogn Brain Res 9: 85-90.

[39] Hellige JB, Sergent J (1986) Role of task factors in visual field asymmetries. Brain Cogn 5: 200-22.

[40] Kitterle FL, Christman S, Hellige JB (1990) Hemispheric differences are found in the identification, but not the detection, of low versus high spatial frequencies. Percept Psychophys 48: 297-306.

[41] Kitterle FL, Hellige JB, Christman S (1992) Visual hemispheric asymmetries depend on which spatial frequencies are task relevant. Brain Cogn 20: 308-14.

[42] Kitterle FL, Selig LM (1991) Visual field effects in the discrimination of sine-wave gratings. Percept Psychophys 50: 15-8.

[43] Peyrin C, Chauvin A, Chokron S, Marendaz C (2003) Hemispheric specialization for spatial frequency processing in the analysis of natural scenes. Brain Cogn 53: 278-82.

[44] Peyrin C, Mermillod M, Chokron S, Marendaz C (2006) Effect of temporal constraints on hemispheric asymmetries during spatial frequency processing. Brain Cogn 62: 214-20.

[45] Sergent J (1982) Theoretical and methodological consequences of variations in exposure duration in visual laterality studies. Percept Psychophys 31: 451-61.

[46] Sergent J (1982b) The cerebral balance of power: confrontation or cooperation? J Exp Psychol Hum Percept Perfor 8: 253-72.

[47] Sergent J (1983) Role of the input in visual hemispheric asymmetries. Psychol Bull 93: 481-512.

[48] Sergent J, Hellige JB (1986) Role of input factors in visual-field asymmetries. Brain Cogn 5: 174-99.

[49] Lamb MR, Robertson LC, Knight RT (1990) Component mechanisms underlying the processing of hierarchically organized patterns: inferences from patients with unilateral cortical lesions. J Exp Psychol Learn Mem Cogn 16: 471-83.

[50] Robertson LC, Lamb MR (1991) Neuropsychological contributions to theories of part/whole organization. Cogn Psychol 23: 299-330.

[51] Robertson LC, Lamb MR, Knight RT (1988) Effects of lesions of temporal-parietal junction on perceptual and attentional processing in humans. J Neurosci 8: 3757-69.

[52] Buchsbaum MS, Buchsbaum BR, Chokron S, Tang C, Wei TC, Byne W (2006) Thalamocortical circuits: fMRI assessment of the pulvinar and medial dorsal nucleus in normal volunteers. Neurosci Lett 404: 282-7.

[53] Fink GR, Halligan PW, Marshall JC, Frith CD, Frackowiak RS, Dolan RJ (1996) Where in the brain does visual attention select the forest and the trees? Nature 382: 626-8.

[54] Fink GR, Halligan PW, Marshall JC, Frith CD, Frackowiak RS, Dolan RJ (1997) Neural mechanisms involved in the processing of global and local aspects of hierarchically organized visual stimuli. Brain 120: 1779-91.

[55] Fink R, Marshall JC, Halligan PW, Dolan RJ (2000) Neuronal activity in early visual areas during global and local processing: a comment on Heinze, Hinrichs, Scholz, Burchert Mangun. J Cogn Neurosci 12: 355-6.

[56] Han S, Weaver JA, Murray SO, Kang X, Yund EW, Woods DL (2002) Hemispheric asymmetry in global/local processing: Effects of stimulus position and spatial frequency. Neuroimage 17: 1290-1299.

[57] Heinze HJ, Hinrichs H, Scholz M, Burchert W, Mangun GR (1998) Neural mechanisms of global and local processing. A combined PET and ERP study. J Cogn Neurosci 10: 485-98.

[58] Kenemans JL, Baas JM, Mangun GR, Lijffijt M, Verbaten MN (2000) On the processing of spatial frequencies as revealed by evoked-potential source modeling. Clin Neurophysiol 111: 1113-23.

[59] Lux S, Marshall JC, Ritzl A, Weiss PH, Pietrzyk U, Shah NJ, Zilles K, Fink GR (2004) A functional magnetic resonance imaging study of local/global processing with stimulus presentation in the peripheral visual hemifields. Neuroscience 124: 113-20.

[60] Mangun GR, Heinze HJ, Scholz M, Hinrichs H (2000) Neural activity in early visual areas during global and local processing: a reply to Fink, Marshall, Halligan and Dolan. J Cogn Neuroscie 12: 357-359.

[61] Martinez A, DiRusso F, Anllo-Vento L, Sereno MI, Buxton RB, Hillyard SA (2001) Putting spatial attention on the map: timing and localization of stimulus selection processes in striate and extrastriate visual areas. Vision Res 41: 1437-57.

[62] Martinez A, Moses P, Frank L, Buxton R, Wong E, Stiles J (1997) Hemispheric asymmetries in global and local processing: evidence from fMRI. Neuroreport 8: 1685-9.

[63] Weissman DH, Woldorff MG (2005) Hemispheric asymmetries for different components of global/local attention occur in distinct temporo-parietal loci. Cereb Cortex 15: 870-6.

[64] Wilkinson DT, Halligan PW, Marshall JC, Buchel C, Dolan RJ (2001) Switching between the forest and the trees: brain systems involved in local/global changed-level judgments. Neuroimage 13: 56-67.

[65] Yamaguchi S, Yamagata S, Kobayashi S (2000) Cerebral asymmetry of the "top-down" allocation of attention to global and local features. J Neurosci 20: RC72.
[66] Palmer S (1993) Modern theories of gestalt perception. In: Humphreys GW, editor. Understanding Vision. Blackwell: Oxford. pp. 39-70.
[67] McGlone J, Kertesz A (1973) Sex differences in cerebral processing of visuospatial tasks. Cortex 9: 313-20.
[68] Voyer D (1996) On the magnitude of laterality effects and sex differences in functional lateralities. Laterality 1: 51-83.
[69] Cousin E, Peyrin C, Baciu M (2006) Hemispheric predominance assessment of phonology and semantics: a divided visual field experiment. Brain Cogn 61: 298-304.
[70] Peyrin C, Schwartz S, Seghier M, Michel C, Landis T, Vuilleumier P (2005) Hemispheric specialization of human inferior temporal cortex during coarse-to-fine and fine-to-coarse analysis of natural visual scenes. Neuroimage 28: 464-73.
[71] Lamb MR, Robertson LC (1990) The effect of visual angle on global and local reaction times depends on the set of visual angles presented. Percept Psychophys 47: 489-96.
[72] Martin M (1979) Hemispheric specialization for local and global processing. Neuropsychologia 17: 33-40.
[73] Curcio CA, Allen KA (1990) Topography of ganglion cells in human retina. J Comp Neurol 300: 5-25.
[74] Curcio CA, Sloan KR, Kalina RE, Hendrickson AE (1990) Human photoreceptor topography. J Comp Neurol 292: 497-523.
[75] Holmes G (1918) Disturbances of Vision by Cerebral Lesions. Br J Ophthalmol 2: 353-84.
[76] Horton JC, Hoyt WF (1991) The representation of the visual field in human striate cortex. A revision of the classic Holmes map. Arch Ophthalmol 109: 816-24.
[77] Engel SA, Glover GH, Wandell BA (1997) Retinotopic organization in human visual cortex and the spatial precision of functional MRI. Cereb Cortex 7: 181-92.
[78] Engel SA, Rumelhart DE, Wandell BA, Lee AT, Glover GH, Chichilnisky EJ, Shadlen MN (1994) fMRI of human visual cortex. Nature 369: 525.
[79] Everson RM, Prashanth AK, Gabbay M, Knight BW, Sirovich L, Kaplan E (1998) Representation of spatial frequency and orientation in the visual cortex. Proc Natl Acad Sci U S A 95: 8334-8.
[80] Issa NP, Trepel C, Stryker MP (2000) Spatial frequency maps in cat visual cortex. J Neurosci 20: 8504-14.
[81] Foster KH, Gaska JP, Nagler M, Pollen DA (1985) Spatial and temporal frequency selectivity of neurones in visual cortical areas V1 and V2 of the macaque monkey. J Physiol 365: 331-63.
[82] Gegenfurtner KR, Kiper DC, Levitt JB (1997) Functional properties of neurons in macaque area V3. J Neurophysiol 77: 1906-23.
[83] Tootell RB, Silverman MS, Hamilton SL, Switkes E, De Valois RL (1988) Functional anatomy of macaque striate cortex. V. Spatial frequency. J Neurosci 8: 1610-24.
[84] Xu X, Anderson TJ, Casagrande VA (2007) How do functional maps in primary visual cortex vary with eccentricity? J Comp Neurol 501: 741-55.

[85] Brefczynski JA, DeYoe EA (1999) A physiological correlate of the 'spotlight' of visual attention. Nat Neurosci 2: 370-4.
[86] Gandhi SP, Heeger DJ, Boynton GM (1999) Spatial attention affects brain activity in human primary visual cortex. Proc Natl Acad Sci U S A 96: 3314-9.
[87] Martinez A, Anllo-Vento L, Sereno MI, Frank LR, Buxton RB, Dubowi, DJ, Wong EC, Hinrichs H, Heinze HJ, Hillyard SA (1999) Involvement of striate and extrastriate visual cortical areas in spatial attention. Nat Neurosci 2: 364-9.
[88] Tootell RB, Hadjikhani N, Hall EK, Marrett S, Vanduffel W, Vaughan JT, Dale AM (1998) The retinotopy of visual spatial attention. Neuron 21: 1409-22.
[89] Watanabe T, Sasaki Y, Miyauchi S, Putz B, Fujimaki N, Nielsen M, Takino R, Miyakawa S (1998) Attention-regulated activity in human primary visual cortex. J Neurophysiol 79: 2218-21.
[90] Friedman DS, O'Colmain BJ, Munoz B, Tomany SC, McCarty C, de Jong PT, Nemesure B, Mitchell P, Kempen J (2004) Prevalence of age-related macular degeneration in the United States. Arch Ophthalmol 122: 564-72.
[91] Klein R, Peto T, Bird A, Vannewkirk MR (2004) The epidemiology of age-related macular degeneration. Am J Ophthalmol 137: 486-95.
[92] Vingerling JR, Dielemans I, Hofman A, Grobbee DE, Hijmering M, Kramer CF, de Jong PT (1995) The prevalence of age-related maculopathy in the Rotterdam Study. Ophthalmology 102: 205-10.
[93] Penfold PL, Madigan MC, Gillies MC, Provis JM (2001) Immunological and aetiological aspects of macular degeneration. Prog Retin Eye Res 20: 385-414.
[94] Faubert J, Overbury O (2000) Binocular vision in older people with adventitious visual impairment: sometimes one eye is better than two. J Am Geriatr Soc 48: 375-80.
[95] Kleiner RC, Enger C, Alexander MF, Fine SL (1988) Contrast sensitivity in age-related macular degeneration. Arch Ophthalmol 106: 55-7.
[96] Midena E, Degli Angeli C, Blarzino MC, Valenti M, Segato T (1997) Macular function impairment in eyes with early age-related macular degeneration. Invest Ophthalmol Vis Sci 38: 469-77.
[97] Boucart M, Despretz P, Hladiuk K, Desmettre T (2008) Does context or color improve object recognition in patients with low vision? Vis Neurosci 25: 685-91.
[98] Tran TH, Guyader N, Guerin A, Despretz P, Boucart M (2011) Figure ground discrimination in age-related macular degeneration. Invest Ophthalmol Vis Sci 52: 1655-60.
[99] Tran TH, Rambaud C, Despretz P, Boucart M (2011) Scene perception in age-related macular degeneration. Invest Ophthalmol Vis Sci 51: 6868-74.
[100] Boucart M, Dinon JF, Despretz P, Desmettre T, Hladiuk K, Oliva A (2008) Recognition of facial emotion in low vision: a flexible usage of facial features. Vis Neurosci 25: 603-9.
[101] Musel B, Hera R, Chokron S, Alleysson D, Chiquet C, Romanet JP, Guyader N, Peyrin C (2011) Residual abilities in age-related macular degeneration patients to process spatial frequencies during natural scenes categorization. Vis Neurosci 28: 529-541.
[102] Epstein RA, Kanwisher N (1998) A cortical representation of the local visual environment. Nature 392: 598-601.

Chapter 4

Neural Mechanisms for Binocular Depth, Rivalry and Multistability

Athena Buckthought and Janine D. Mendola

Additional information is available at the end of the chapter

http://dx.doi.org/10.5772/48446

1. Introduction

The purpose of this chapter is to present a review of recent functional neuroimaging (fMRI) studies of binocular vision, including binocular depth and rivalry, as well as a review of studies of perceptual multistability. As such, we will first emphasize the binocular aspects of binocular rivalry, while later emphasizing the rivalrous aspects. The interrelationship of binocular depth and rivalry, as well as multistability, will be described with reference to fMRI studies and single-unit recording studies in animals. These studies have provided provocative new evidence that the neural substrates for depth and rivalry, as well as other forms of multistability are remarkably similar. We will also describe our own research findings from two recent experiments, in which we performed (1) a direct comparison between binocular rivalry and depth, and (2) a direct comparison between binocular rivalry and monocular rivalry, a related form of bistability [1,2]. Our studies are unique in using both matched stimulation and comparable tasks, overcoming a limitation in the interpretation of many previous studies. As a result, these experiments are particularly relevant in delineating some of the global similarities and differences in the cortical networks activated in each of these different domains.

2. Binocular depth

Binocular depth perception arises as a consequence of the slightly displaced point of view of the two eyes. The horizontal displacement of image features in the two eyes (i.e. binocular disparities) makes it possible to reconstruct the depth relationships in the visual world. Binocular matching of local features in the retinal images may be used to obtain estimates of the absolute disparity (and distance) of objects or surfaces, as well as the relative disparity (or relative distances) between different objects. An example of an image with binocular depth is shown in Figure 1a. If the left and right images are cross-fused, the image appears to be tilted with the top coming forward. This occurs because the visual system interprets the greater shift in matched features at the top of the image as a displacement in front of the fixation plane. In general, crossed disparities, in which image features in the right image are shifted to the right, and image features in the left image are shifted to the left, are interpreted as in front of the fixation plane. Uncrossed disparities (with shifts in the opposite directions) are interpreted as behind the fixation plane. Absolute disparities are the total shift in front or behind the plane of fixation, while relative disparities can be computed as the difference in these absolute disparities for different objects. Thus the initial steps in recovering binocular depth relationships involve determining the horizontal shift in image features between the two eyes.

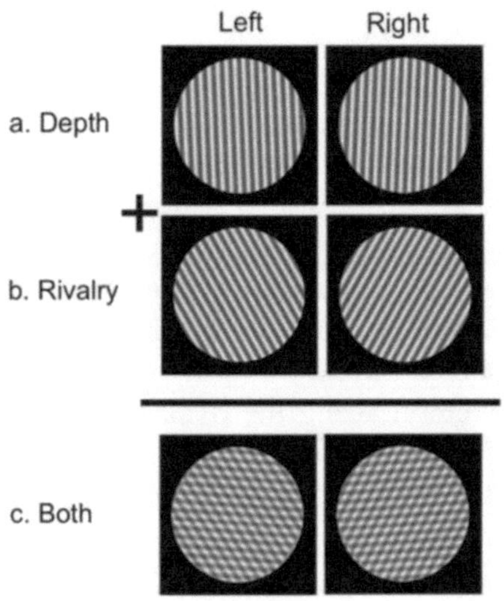

Figure 1. (a) Binocular depth and (b) rivalry. (c) Plaids in which both depth and rivalry are perceived.

The most prominent cortical areas which have been activated by binocular depth in previous studies have been superimposed on the right hemisphere of the human brain in Figure 2a. The brain areas highlighted in the Figure are occipital visual areas (V1, V2, V3, V4, V3A, V7 and lateral occipital cortex, LO), superior parietal cortex (SP), inferior parietal cortex/intraparietal sulcus (IP), temporoparietal junction (TPJ), ventral temporal cortex (VT), middle frontal gyrus (MF), inferior frontal gyrus (IF), premotor cortex (PM), supplementary motor area (SMA), frontal eye fields (FEF) and insula/frontal operculum (FO). The numeric labels refer to the number of fMRI studies which reported prominent activation at each cortical site (colour coded on a scale ranging from red to blue, from highest to lowest). Table 1 lists the studies which were used to compile these numbers. Note that if it was not absolutely clear that a particular area was reported, this is indicated with an asterisk in Table 1. It should be noted that some studies did not perform a whole brain analysis, or may not have had an interest in reporting activation in certain areas, so this may bias the numbers that appear in Figure 2 and Table 1. Some studies limited their analysis to occipital sites of activation only. Nevertheless, it is clear that the neural mechanisms for binocular

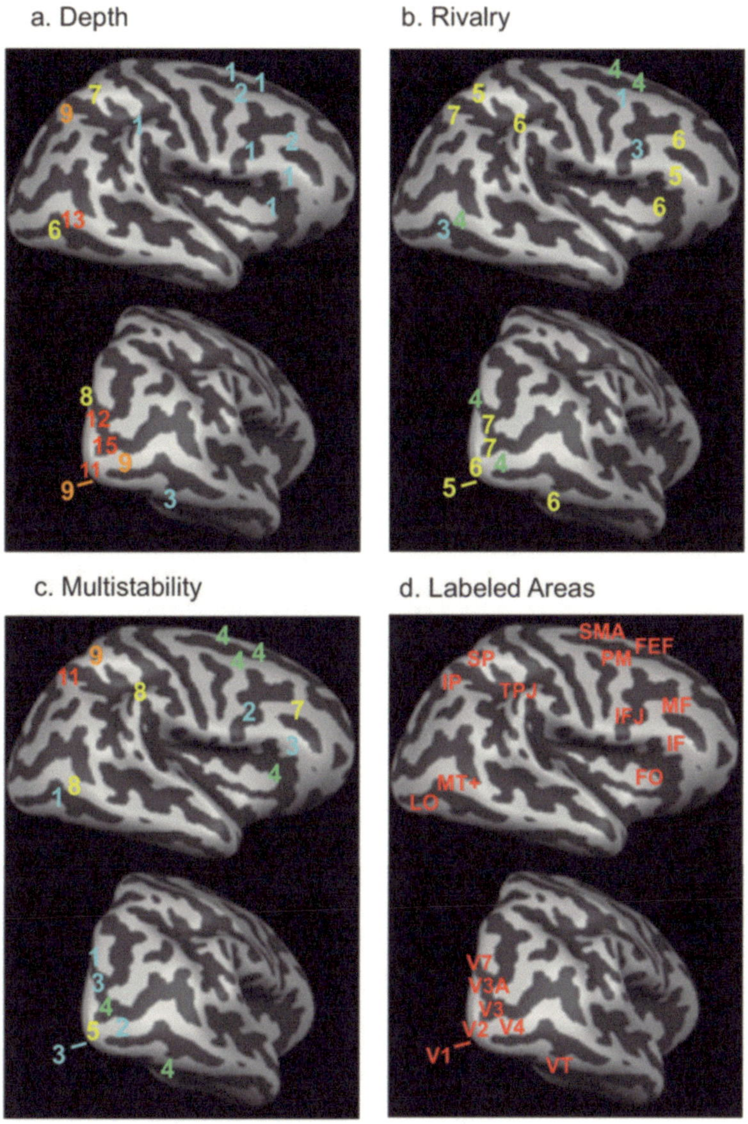

Figure 2. Brain areas highlighted in fMRI studies for (a) depth, (b) rivalry and (c) multistability.

depth perception involve a number of processing levels from early visual areas in the occipital lobe to higher-level occipito-parietal and frontal areas [3]. An early study of depth restricted the analysis to visual cortical areas, and found that disparity selectivity was present in areas V1, V2, V3, V3A and MT+ [4]. However, later studies which performed analysis over a larger number of visual areas found that the activation levels are highest in dorsal occipito-parietal areas, such as V3A, V7, V4d-topo and caudal intraparietal sulcus relative to others [3,5-8]. Moreover, considering all these studies together, the most consistent sites of activation for depth across many previous fMRI studies were V3A, V7, V4d-topo, or other lateral occipital areas, such as MT+, lateral occipital complex, and kinetic

	Depth	Rivalry	Multistability
Frontal eye fields	[2]	[1,19-21]	[1,19,29,30]
Anterior cingulate		[1,19,20]	[19,30-34]
Supplementary motor area	[2]	[1,2,20,22]	[1,33,35,36]
Primary motor cortex		[20,22]	[30,34]
Premotor cortex	[2,9]	[1]	[1,35-37]
Insula/frontal operculum	[2]	[1,2,19-22]	[1,19,30,36]
Ventrolateral prefrontal cortex	[2]	[1,2]	[1,30]
Inferior frontal gyrus	[2]	[2,19-22]	[1,19,33]
Inferior frontal junction	[2]	[1,2,19]	[1,19]
Middle frontal gyrus or Dorsolateral prefrontal cortex	[2,10]	[1,2,19-22]	[1,19,31,32,34-36]
Superior parietal lobe	[2,6-8,10-12]	[1,19-22]	[1,19,30,32,34-35,36*,37-38]
Inferior parietal lobe (intraparietal sulcus)	[2,3,5-11]	[1,2,5,19-21,23]	[1,19,29,30,32-35,36*,37-38]
Temporoparietal occipital junction	[2]	[1,2,19-22]	[19,29,30,32,33,35-37]
MT+	[2,4-15]	[1,2,19,21]	[19,30,32,33,35*, 36*, 37,38]
Lateral occipital complex	[5,6,8,9*,16,17]	[5,22,23]	[35*]
Ventral temporal cortex (fusiform)	[2,16,17]	[2,20-25]	[1,29,32,36*]
V7	[2,3,5-9,14]	[2,21*,22*,23]	[38]
Kinetic occipital area (KO)	[2,3,6,8,13,18]	[2]	[30]
V4	[2,3,5-7,13-15,18]	[2, 5,26,27]	[32,38]
V3A	[2-12,14]	[1,2,21*,22*,23,27, 28]	[1,32,38]
V3	[2-16]	[1,2,20,21,26-28]	[1,31,32,37]
V2	[2-7,10-12,14,15]	[1,2,21,26-28]	[1,31-33,37]
V1	[2-7,10,14,15]	[1,2,26-28]	[1,32,33]

Table 1. fMRI studies which highlighted particular brain areas for depth, rivalry and multistability.

occipital area [2,3,5,6,8,10,13], as well as intraparietal sulcus [2,3,6-12] and superior parietal lobe [2,6,7,8,10-12]. In addition, ventral temporal cortical areas, including the fusiform gyrus, have also been noted to be depth selective [2,16,17].

As reviewed in [3], single unit recording studies in the macaque monkey have also reported that a large percentage of neurons are sensitive to binocular disparity, disparity-defined 3D shape or 3-D surface orientation in many cortical areas (V1: 45%, V2: 65%, V3/V3A: 80%, VP:

52%, V4: 71%, MT: 95%, MST: 92%, caudal intraparietal sulcus: 78%, lateral intraparietal sulcus: 75%, TE: 78%, and frontal eye fields: 65%). Hence both fMRI and single unit recording studies indicate that binocular depth processing is not restricted to one cortical region but is processed in many areas, presumably subserving a wide range of different functions.

These studies indicate that a number of higher-level retinotopic visual areas are particularly prominent in depth processing, and yet the borders between these areas are sometimes difficult to distinguish across different studies. For example, V4d-topo has been defined as the human topographic homolog (topolog), an area situated (1) superior to V4v, (2) anterior to V3A, and (3) posterior to MT+, and should be distinguished from more ventral lateral occipital cortex [40]. V7 is an area adjacent and anterior to V3A that contains a hemifield map [40]. Hence V7 and V4d-topo both lie between V3A and area MT+, and the border between these areas is not always clear using conventional retinotopic mapping techniques, or retrospective review. Another region, referred to as the kinetic occipital area (KO), is particularly responsive to disparity edges, and appears to lie within V4d-topo [18]. Lateral occipital areas LO-1 and LO-2 also lie within KO [39].

2.1. Dorsal and ventral processing streams

The important depth processing areas can be subdivided into distinct dorsal and ventral processing streams, referred to as "what" and "where" pathways, related to the identification of objects, or actions relative to objects, respectively [7,10,14,23]. The dorsal stream is believed to project from the occipital visual areas to parietal areas, while the ventral stream projects from occipital to temporal areas [41]. More specifically, the ventral stream begins with V1, goes through visual area V2, then through visual area V4, and to the inferior/ventral temporal cortex, which includes lateral occipital cortex, fusiform gyrus and other ventral temporal areas, including the areas mentioned above for depth (Figure 2). The dorsal stream begins with V1, goes through area V2, then V3A, V6, V7 and MT+, and then to the posterior parietal cortex, including the parietal areas mentioned above (superior parietal lobe and intraparietal sulcus) for depth (Figure 2). The anatomical locations of some of these areas are also shown in Figure 3. The black contours superimposed on the top middle panel show locations for areas V1, V2, V3, V4d-topo, V3A, V7, lateral occipital cortex, and MT+ based upon retinotopic mapping and anatomical landmarks for one subject. (This Figure will also be discussed further below, in the discussion of rivalry and multistability).

The dissociation between dorsal and ventral areas has been most clearly delineated in single unit recording studies in the macaque [42]. In these studies, ventral areas have been found to have some of the properties necessary for object recognition, such as a detailed 3-D shape description of surface boundaries and surface content. In fact, specific responses are evoked only by binocular stimuli in which depth is perceived, but do not vary if depth is specified by different cues [42]. Conversely, dorsal areas (such as the intraparietal sulcus) have some of the properties necessary for making actions, such as selectivity for orientation in depth of surfaces and elongated objects. Moreover, their responses are invariant to changes in depth cues [42].

A dissociation between dorsal and ventral areas in human fMRI studies relates to greater selectivity for object recognition using shape defined by disparity in ventral areas [15,17,43-46]. One particular study took advantage of the fact that objects are more easily recognized if they lie in front of a background plane, than if they lie behind a plane [17]. The stimuli consisted of stereo-defined line drawings of objects that either protruded in front or behind a background plane. The activation in ventral and lateral occipital cortex, or lateral occipital complex (LOC), was greater for the objects which were located in front of the background plane, and the activity in these ventral stream areas was also strongly correlated with behavioral object recognition performance. Several other studies also found that activity in the lateral occipital complex could be related to the representation of shape from disparity by (1) making comparisons between object shapes with or without disparity [43], or (2) by comparisons between object shape conditions in which the 2-D monocular contour did not vary but the perceived 3-D shape differed [44]. The lateral occipital complex has also been found to be selective for convex and concave shapes defined by disparity, and is preferentially selective for convex shapes. This fits with behavioral measures since the visual system shows greater sensitivity for the perception of convex shapes [47]. A final study found that the lateral occipital complex combines disparity with perspective information to represent perceived three-dimensional shape [15].

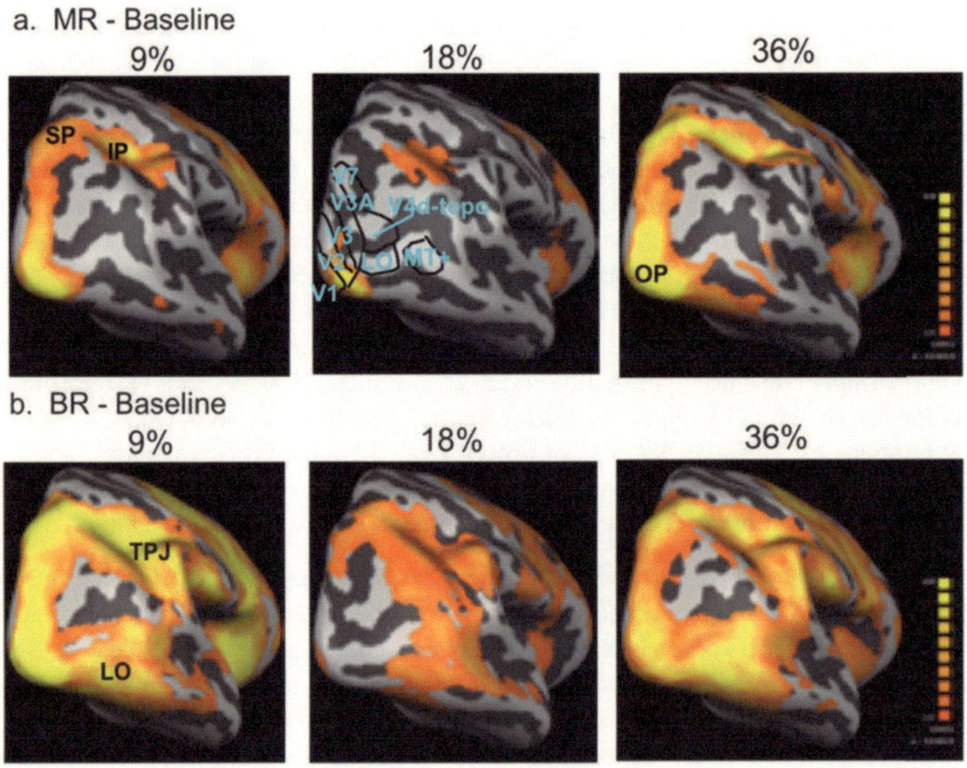

Figure 3. (a) Activation for monocular rivalry or (b) binocular rivalry above the blank baseline at three contrasts (9%, 18%, 36%).

Several other studies have found dissociations between the properties of dorsal and ventral areas with regards to the representation of disparity magnitude. One study found that when disparity was parametrically varied, the BOLD signal increased with disparity only in dorsal areas of the occipito-parietal cortex (i.e. V2, V3, V3A, as well as inferior and superior parietal lobe) [10]. Another study used a comparison of activation for correlated versus anticorrelated random dot stereograms (only the former case supports a depth percept) in order to assess depth selectivity across a number of areas [8]. Disparity selectivity was found in dorsal (visual and parietal) areas, including V3A, V7, MT+, intraparietal sulcus and superior parietal lobe, as well as ventral area LO (ventral lateral occipital cortex), but not in early (V1, V2) or intermediate ventral (V3v, V4) visual cortical areas. Furthermore, only dorsal areas were found to encode metric disparity (disparity magnitude), whereas ventral area LO appeared to represent depth position in a categorical manner (i.e., disparity sign). The findings suggest that activity in both dorsal and ventral visual streams reflects binocular depth perception but the neural computations may differ [8]. Consistent with these results, a third study measured the responses across a number of occipital and parietal areas to different magnitudes of binocular disparity [7]. Across all areas, there was an increase in BOLD signal with increasing disparity. However, the greatest modulation of response was found in dorsal visual and parietal areas, including V3A, MT+, V7, intraparietal sulcus and superior parietal lobe. These differences contrast with the response to the zero disparity plane stimulus, which is greatest in the early visual areas, smaller in the ventral and dorsal visual areas, and absent in parietal areas. These results illustrate that the dorsal stream can reliably represent and discriminate a large range of disparities [7]. Moreover, these findings indicate distinct computations performed in (possibly) different cortical areas, including fusional matching, metric depth, and categorical depth.

2.2. Posterior parietal cortex

The human parietal cortex is believed to extract three-dimensional shape representations that can support the ability to manipulate objects both physically and mentally (as reviewed in [6]). Lesions to the posterior parietal lobe can cause profound deficits in spatial awareness, including neglect of the contralateral half of visual space, inability to draw simple three-dimensional objects such as a cube, and inability to estimate distance and size [48]. The superior and inferior parietal areas of activation identified in human fMRI studies of binocular depth include several intraparietal sulcus (IPS) regions involved in 3D shape perception from disparity, dorsal IPS anterior (DIPSA) and dorsal IPS medial (DIPSM), ventral IPS (VIPS)/V7, and parieto-occipital POIPS [6,9,42]. These parietal regions extract 3D shape representations that can support motor functions, such as grasping hand movements or saccadic eye movements toward objects [42]. Regions DIPSM and DIPSA have been found to be sensitive to depth structure (i.e., spatial variations in depth along surfaces arising from disparity), but not position in depth, while a more posterior region, the ventral IPS (VIP) had a mixed sensitivity [6]. Regions DIPSM and DIPSA likely correspond to LIP and AIP in the monkey and process depth information necessary in order to make eye or hand movements, respectively [6,42]. These parietal areas (DIPSA and DIPSM) are also more strongly activated by curved surfaces than tilted surfaces. Hence these parietal areas (DIPSA, DIPSM and VIPS) show a full representation of a range of different 3D shapes from disparity, including frontoparallel, tilted and curved shapes [9]. Furthermore, these parietal areas appear to be involved in cue-invariant processing of 3D shape, including processing of monocular cues to depth (e.g., texture gradients, perspective, motion, shading) [6,42]. V7/VIPS is also an area sensitive to depth structure, depth position, as well as other cues which contribute to the representation of depth relationships, such as motion, 3D-structure from motion and 2D shape [6,9]. In previous fMRI studies, this area has also been described as showing activation strongly correlated with the magnitude of depth defined by disparity and was strongly correlated to the amount of depth perceived by subjects [9].

2.3. Questions for future study

The functional neuroimaging studies to date have broadly defined some of the functions of different areas in binocular vision, and delineated dorsal and ventral processing streams. There appears to be a progression in the dorsal pathway from more basic binocular processing in early visual areas, towards the metrical encoding of binocular depth in parietal areas, presumably to support eye or hand movements towards objects. Likewise, the ventral pathway appears to involve a progressive refinement towards depth encoding to support object recognition. However, in either case the processing stages are not understood. Important issues for future study will be to examine this in greater detail and draw stronger inferences in relating the functions of different areas. For example, a few studies have tried to compare the representation of relative and absolute disparity across a number of areas, with conflicting results, although there does appear to be a tendency for relative disparity to be encoded in ventral areas while both absolute and relative disparity are encoded in dorsal areas [3,10, 14]. The encoding of relative disparity is likely to be very important in object recognition, while both absolute and relative disparity may turn out to be important in perception for action. Future studies could explain more clearly how these different cues may be used in different contexts and with different tasks. Also, relatively few studies have examined the role of stereoscopic cues in complex object recognition. The absence of studies in this area may be related to the belief held by many investigators that binocular disparity is not critical in recognition of faces or other complex objects (for example, see [49,50]). However, ventral areas have selectivity to binocular disparity and hence it would be important to investigate further the role of these areas in binocular vision.

3. Binocular rivalry

If the images in the two eyes are not the same or similar, but rather incompatibly different, another distinctive perceptual state results. In binocular rivalry, incompatible images, such as left and right oblique oriented gratings, are presented to the two eyes. Observers typically perceive only one image at a time, and perception alternates between the left and right image every few seconds. An example of binocular rivalry is shown in Figure 1b. If the left and right images are cross-fused, alternations may be clearly perceived between the left oblique and right oblique oriented images. Because the retinal image stays constant, while the visual percept changes, this provides a popular method for studying conscious visual experience. Binocular rivalry has been modeled with interocular inhibition between monocular neurons representing the orthogonal left and right image components, as well as neuronal adaptation [51-54]. A monocular neuron may respond to a particular orientation (e.g. left oblique), and suppresses the response of neurons tuned to the opposite (i.e. right oblique) orientation. The neuron will continue to respond until adaptation or fatigue allows the other neurons to respond in turn to the opposite orientation. In the research lab, particularly robust binocular rivalry is created by presenting a number of different types of incompatible images to the two eyes, which may include simple gratings, contours or more complex images such as a face and house or other objects [51] (see also Figure 4(a-b) and 4(e-f)).

The interrelationship between binocular depth and rivalry has been a subject of longstanding debate and interest [51,55,56]. Generally, binocular rivalry ensues when the image features in the two eyes are too dissimilar to be reconciled, and depth cannot be recovered because the binocular disparities are too great. In our normal visual experience, there may be dissimilar features in the two eyes, but a strong sensation of binocular rivalry occurs only rarely. When unmatched rivalrous components are present in an image, this interferes with normal binocular depth perception [55]. Presumably this occurs because suppression from the unmatched components prevents binocular matching necessary for depth. Consistently, it has been proposed that binocular rivalry is the default outcome which arises when binocular fusion and depth fails [51,55]. However, recent studies have provided evidence that binocular rivalry and depth can be observed simultaneously over the same spatial location, which calls into question previous models and interpretations [2,57-58]. Moreover, there are a number of possible new interpretations which could reconcile these results. In particular, both binocular rivalry and depth involve mechanisms of binocular matching, to find correspondences between image features for depth or to detect larger, irreconcilable differences, in the case of binocular rivalry. The mechanisms for binocular rivalry may inhibit false matches at different orientations, effectively suppressing noise in neural responses and sharpening the tuning of orientational mechanisms, which can also be related to the phenomenon of dichoptic masking [59, 60]. Hence the strong inhibitory interactions which we are familiar with in the phenomenon of binocular rivalry may be fundamental in the resolution of ambiguity in binocular vision. Consequently, it has been found in fMRI studies that these processing mechanisms for depth and rivalry are closely related in many brain areas, and occur in parallel throughout the visual system [2, 3,5,20,61].

Models of binocular rivalry presume that binocular rivalry occurs as a consequence of interocular competition between monocular neurons, which would be expected to occur at early levels in the visual system [51-54]. This has been verified in a number of functional neuroimaging studies of binocular rivalry, which have reported eye-specific dominance and suppression in early visual areas in the occipital cortex (V1, V2, V3) [26,27,62], or the lateral geniculate nucleus (LGN) [63,64]. As expected from the theoretical models, a number of fMRI studies have also documented alternating response suppression, as well as neural

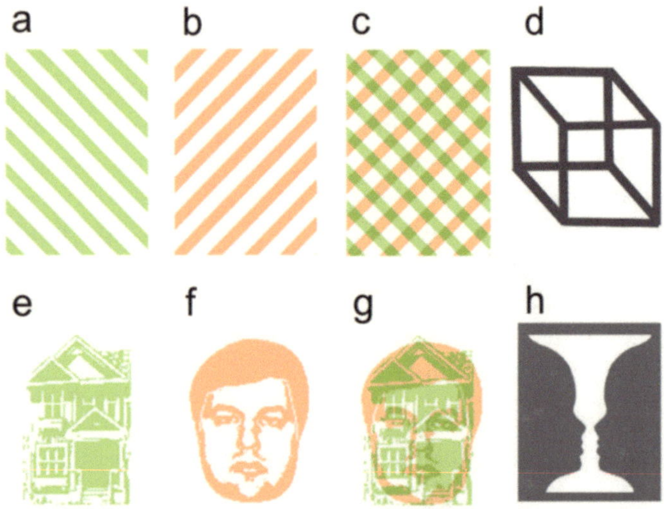

Figure 4. Examples of multistability. (a-b) Binocular rivalry (gratings), (c) monocular rivalry (gratings), (d) Necker cube, (e-f) binocular rivalry (face/house), and (g) monocular rivalry (face/house).

activation related to attentional monitoring and selection, at later stages in the visual pathway. A number of occipito-parietal areas (e.g. V3A, V7 and intraparietal sulcus) are again represented, as was the case for depth. The most important visual areas reported for rivalry include V1, V2, V3, V3A, V4d-topo, V7 [5], lateral occipital areas (MT+/lateral occipital complex) [1,2,5,19,21-23], and ventral temporal areas [2,20-25]. In addition to these visual cortical areas, a number of frontal and parietal sites of activation were reported, which have been associated with top-down control of attention, or stimulus-driven shifts of spatial attention [65-68]. These parietal areas include superior parietal lobe [1,19-22], intraparietal sulcus [1,2,5,19-21,23,61], and temporoparietal junction [1,2,19-22]. These frontal areas associated with attentional control or shifts of attention include middle frontal gyrus (or dorsolateral prefrontal cortex) [1,2,19-22], ventrolateral prefrontal cortex and inferior frontal gyrus [1,2,19-22], as well as insula/frontal operculum [1,2,19-22]. Additional areas were reported which could also be associated with attentional shifts or related to the preparation and execution of motor reports, such as supplementary motor area [1,2,20,22], frontal eye fields (FEF) and anterior cingulate [1,2,19-21]. The activation of some areas, such as FEF, could possibly be related to eye movements, but some studies used controls to verify that the activation is not related to eye movements, but more likely related to covert shifts of attention [20, 29].

Functional neuroimaging studies of early visual areas (V1, V2 or V3) have found that fMRI signal fluctuations during the perception of rivalry are generally lower than the signal fluctuations evoked by actual stimulus changes, in which the stimulus is physically replaced by the alternative [26-28]. However, much stronger correlations occur between subjective perception in binocular rivalry and activity in higher-level visual areas, such as functionally specialized extrastriate cortex [24]. For example, in binocular rivalry in which alternations are perceived between a face and house, signal fluctuations can be discerned in ventral temporal areas selective for faces and houses (i.e. fusiform face area and parahippocampal place area, respectively). The amplitudes of percept-related fMRI signal fluctuations during binocular rivalry in these visual areas are similar to those during actual stimulus alternations, suggesting that the conflict has been resolved at this stage, with no representation of the suppressed stimulus. Hence it appears that there is a progression from early visual areas towards higher-level areas in the magnitude of suppression, with the latter a closer match to the perceptual experience during binocular rivalry [53,69].

3.1. Functional interactions between cortical areas in rivalry

One fMRI study of binocular rivalry used analysis methods to detect whether temporal correlations were present in the activity in areas V2/V3 and other cortical areas during the perception of rivalry with no task [21]. Indeed, the results confirmed that many of the areas listed above for rivalry were related through a covariation of activity, indicating that these widespread, extrastriate ventral, superior and inferior parietal and prefrontal cortical areas comprise a network reflecting the changes in perception during rivalry. There was significant temporal modulation of activity in these areas that followed closely to the response patterns of human subjects indicating when perceptual alternations occurred. The results indicated that cooperative interactions between extrastriate visual and non-visual areas are important for conscious visual awareness, and that the prefrontal cortex may contribute to conscious vision. Another study of binocular rivalry inferred, using an event-related design, that activity in intraparietal sulcus preceded the onset of rivalrous alternations, providing evidence for a possible causal role for this area in initiating rivalry [61]. Intriguingly, the intraparietal sulcus was the only area identified in the event-related analysis in this study, and no frontal areas were implicated as playing a causal role in perceptual alternations.

3.2. Comparison of binocular depth and rivalry

The cortical areas activated by rivalry in previous fMRI studies are shown in Figure 2b and Table 1, for comparison with depth. Some of the differences between rivalry and depth can simply be accounted for by noting that there was a larger number of studies for depth than rivalry, particularly studies interested in reporting activation levels only in occipital areas. Nevertheless, the Figure makes it clear that parietal activation (i.e. intraparietal sulcus and superior parietal lobe) was prominently reported in both depth and rivalry studies. One exception to this is the temporoparietal junction, which was often reported as an activation site for rivalry but reported for depth only in one study, that actually employed a depth task [2]. This is consistent with our view that this area is usually active with stimulus-driven shifts of attention [65,67,70]. Overall, frontal activation was more prominent in rivalry than depth studies (such as dorsolateral and ventrolateral prefrontal cortex, middle frontal gyrus, inferior frontal gyrus, supplementary motor area, insula/frontal operculum), while occipital activation was relatively more prominent in depth studies (e.g. V3, V3A, V4d-topo, V7, lateral occipital complex and MT+). Some of these differences could be attributed to the more dynamic aspect of rivalry compared with depth, and the typical performance of a rivalry task, since these frontal and parietal areas have been associated with attention and working memory, as well as the performance of motor reports [65-68,70]. In particular, the anterior cingulate was reported for only rivalry but not depth.

If we step back and evaluate these patterns, then some caveats emerge. There appear to be some differences in the relative balance of frontal and occipital activation, comparing the results across depth and rivalry studies. However, it is challenging to compare the results across these studies because of substantial stimulus and task differences. Most studies of depth used (1) dynamic random dot stereograms (RDS) [4,8,10,11,13,14,17], (2) random dot dynamic checkerboards [3,10], (3) random dot sinusoidal corrugations at pedestal disparities [7], (4) random dot textured surfaces or shapes [9,16], (5) random line stimuli showing 3D depth structures [6], and (6) gratings or line drawings [17]. Rivalry studies have also used a variety of different stimuli, for example, (1) gratings [1,2,19,22,26-28], (2) faces/houses (1,24,26], (3) faces with differing emotional expressions [25], (4) tools, faces and textures [23], (5) slant rivalry [5,61], and (6) gratings/faces [20, 21]. The tasks used in depth and rivalry studies were also not comparable in terms of either the attentional demands or frequency of motor responses.

In order to address this issue, we performed a study designed explicitly to perform a direct whole-brain comparison of depth and rivalry with fMRI, with comparable stimulus patterns and tasks [2]. We used binocular plaid patterns in which depth is perceived from the near-vertical components and rivalry from the oblique components (Figure 1c). In Figure 1, the depth and rivalry components are added together to produce the plaids in which both depth and rivalry may be perceived. Subjects report that the percept of a rivalrous pattern is spatially superimposed on the tilted surface. The depth in the plaid stimulus changed every 3 s, between two possible percepts (top or bottom tilted forward). This was done in order to make a dynamic depth change that subjects could report, just as they reported dynamic changes in the rivalry task. For the depth task, subjects reported whether the top or bottom of the plaid stimulus pattern appeared to be tilted forward. The time interval of 3 s was chosen to match the mean time period between alternations for rivalry for the group of subjects. The depth change did not interfere with the rivalry percept, and subjects were able to perform a rivalry task with the identical plaid stimulus. This made it possible to compare conditions in which subjects perform either a depth or rivalry report task, while viewing identical plaid patterns, precisely matched for retinal stimulation. A comparison for the depth and rivalry task conditions would reveal the neural substrates for depth and/or rivalry.

3.3. Depth and rivalry task comparison

The most important comparison was that between the depth and rivalry task for identical plaid patterns. Our results showed that the whole brain network of activated cortical areas was remarkably similar for the rivalry task compared to the depth task when subjects viewed identical plaid patterns. These areas included the occipital, parietal, ventral temporal and frontal areas highlighted in Figure 2. Nevertheless, regions of superior and inferior parietal cortices (including temporoparietal junction and intraparietal sulcus) were activated more for the depth than the rivalry task, whereas a bias towards rivalry was seen in a lateral occipital region, calcarine, retrosplenial and ventral temporal areas. Thus, these results are important in showing that while parietal areas were clearly strongly activated by either depth or rivalry, consistent with previous studies (as discussed with reference to Figure 2 above), the activation levels were actually higher for depth when the two stimulus conditions had been equalized. This fits with an important role of these parietal areas in depth encoding in order to make hand or eye movements, which has been documented extensively (e.g. [6,9,42]). Conversely, lateral occipital area and ventral temporal areas were more specific for rivalry, consistent with a relatively greater number of studies which showed that these areas may be particularly relevant for the perception of rivalry [5,20-25].

Finally, in another manipulation, we included as a control, an orientation change task, which had similar stimulus features to the depth and rivalry tasks. In this case, the subject had to indicate with a key press which way the image was rotated. The orientation change condition required binocular fusion of matched features but evoked neither depth nor rivalry, serving to isolate those stages of binocular combination. This task was also matched to the depth and rivalry tasks in terms of the number of stimulus changes (which occurred every 3 s) and key presses. When the orientation change task was subtracted from either the depth or rivalry task, a lateral occipital area was highlighted, as well as V3A, V7, or ventral intraparietal sulcus (VIPS), and the kinetic occipital area (KO), including LO-1 and LO-2 [18]. This result indicated that these are areas active for either depth or rivalry, and may subserve a representation at the surface-level that would facilitate the grouping of features, and allow for more than one feature (i.e. depth or rivalry) to be coded at a spatial location [2].

3.4. Conclusions: Comparison of depth and rivalry

In conclusion, the combined results of fMRI and psychophysical studies indicate that depth and rivalry are processed in a similar network of cortical areas and are perceived simultaneously by coexisting in different spatial frequency or orientation channels (see [2,58] for further discussion of the latter point). An important aspect of the results reviewed was that the same frontal and parietal areas were prominently activated for both depth and rivalry. So by matching depth and rivalry for stimulus characteristics and task we found that globally similar sites would be activated, even though depth does not involve overt, endogeneous competition between alternate percepts. We confirmed that all of the prominent sites of activation for rivalry were also present for depth, including frontal (FEF, PM, SMA, MF, IF, IFJ, DLPF, VLPF, FO) and parietal areas (SP, IP and TPJ). These frontoparietal areas have traditionally been implicated in visual tasks requiring spatial shifts of attention and working memory [70]. Moreover, functional imaging experiments have shown that the superior parietal cortex is also engaged by successive shifts of spatial attention [71].

4. Multistability

Binocular rivalry is a specific example of a more general perceptual experience, multistability. Multistable images comprise important examples of conscious visual perceptual changes without any change in the stimulus being viewed. Multistability can be induced by using an ambiguous figure with more than one perceptual interpretation such as the Necker cube [72] or Rubin's vase/face [73] (Figure 4). For example, the image in Rubin's vase/face can be interpreted as either a vase or face, and formal observation shows that the perceptual organization changes between the face and vase over time. In a similar way, the Necker cube can be perceived with one face coming forward, or the other face forward and the percept fluctuates over time between these two possible organizations. As in the case of binocular rivalry, the retinal image stays constant, while the conscious percept changes. This lends itself to an investigation of visual conscious perception without a confounding stimulus change, as we have already seen for binocular rivalry. However, in comparison with binocular rivalry, observers do have somewhat greater voluntary control over their perception in these examples of multistability, and are better able to bias their interpretation towards one percept or the other [74]. Other examples of multistability include the rotating structure-from-motion sphere, which can be perceived to rotate in two different directions [36,38], and the apparent motion quartet, in which the perceived motion alternates between two different directions [19,33,75]. Another example of apparent motion is the spinning wheel, in which the perceived direction of rotation alternates between two directions [30]. Monocular (pattern) rivalry is yet another example of multistability in which a composite image is shown to both eyes, such as the sum of orthogonal gratings (Figure 4c) or a face/house composite (Figure 4g) [76]. These examples of monocular rivalry can be compared with examples of binocular rivalry in which either gratings or face/house pairs are shown to the left and right eyes (Figure 4a-b and e-f). Binocular rivalry can be perceived if (a-b) or (e-f) are cross-fused. Binocular rivalry can also be perceived for (c) and (g) if these are viewed using red-green stereoglasses. In monocular rivalry, the observer experiences perceptual alternations in which the two stimulus components (e.g. left and right oriented gratings) alternate in clarity or salience. The experience is similar to perceptual alternations in binocular rivalry, although the alternations are more difficult to perceive, because neither component is completely suppressed [69,77]. Thus in all these examples of multistability, the alternations between the different possible percepts are more subtle, compared with the near total suppression of one eye's image which occurs with binocular rivalry.

Recent functional neuroimaging studies of multistability have used a range of different image types, such as the (1) Necker cube [31,32,34,35,37], (2) Mach Pyramid, 3-D Triangle, Card, and Wave [31], (3) Rubins face/vase [29], (4) monocular rivalry with gratings [1], (5) rotating structure-from-motion sphere [36,38], and (6) apparent motion, which includes the spinning wheel [19,30], and (7) motion quartet [19,33]. There has been a remarkable congruence of findings across functional neuroimaging studies of multistability, despite the large variability in the images used to evoke changes in perceptual organization. For all image types, a distributed network of cortical areas is activated during the perception of multistability, which highlights occipito-parietal areas, as well as many interrelated areas of the occipital, parietal and frontal cortex, as was the case for depth and rivalry. The sites of activation which were most frequently reported included a number of frontal and parietal areas which have been associated with top-down control of attention, or stimulus-driven shifts of spatial attention, and working memory [65-68,70]. These parietal areas included superior parietal lobe [1,19,30,32,34-38], intraparietal sulcus [1,19,29,30,32-38] and temporoparietal junction [19,29,30,32,33,35-37]. The frontal sites of activation which also could be related to attention included dorsolateral prefrontal cortex or middle frontal gyrus [1,19,31,32,34-36], ventrolateral prefrontal cortex or inferior frontal gyrus [1,19,30,33]. Again, as was seen earlier for rivalry, a number of frontal areas were present which could be associated with attention or the preparation and execution of motor reports, such as frontal eye fields, anterior cingulate [1,19,29,30-34] and supplementary motor area [1,33,35,36]. These frontal and parietal areas were the most frequently reported sites of activation in these studies. However, several studies confirmed that activation also occurs in occipital areas, including ventral occipital (fusiform gyrus) [1,29,32,36], medial temporal areas (hMT+) [19,30,32,33,35-38] and areas V1, V2, V3, V3A or V4-d topo [1,5,31,32,37,38].

The overall global pattern of activation sites for depth, rivalry and multistability can be compared, in Figure 2 and Table 1. Parietal activation (i.e. superior parietal lobe and intraparietal sulcus) was prominently and equally reported in all three cases. However, an exception to this was the temporoparietal junction, which was reported for rivalry and multistability, but not for depth (with the exception of [2]), consistent for a role for this area in stimulus-driven shifts of attention [65,67,70]. Furthermore, there was overall more frontal activation (e.g. dorsolateral and ventrolateral prefrontal cortex, supplementary motor area, and insula/frontal operculum) for either rivalry or multistability, compared with depth. These frontal areas could be associated with top-down control of attention or stimulus-driven shifts of attention, as well as the planning and execution of motor responses. Conversely, there was greater emphasis on occipital areas (e.g. V7, V4d-topo, V3, V3A, lateral occipital complex, MT+), for depth compared with rivalry or multistability. In other words, the balance between frontal and occipital activation was in favour of frontal areas for multistability or in favour of occipital areas for depth, with rivalry falling in between. Again, part of these differences can be attributed to the fact that there were more depth studies that had an interest in reporting activation in occipital areas, but even taking this into consideration, the overall pattern shows that occipital activation was relatively more prominent in depth studies. In general, few previous depth studies performed a whole-brain analysis [2,3,5,7-12,16], and of these few, only three reported frontal activation [2,9,10]. It was not clear whether this was simply an absence of reporting, or due to the fact that there was no frontal activation because a task was not being performed in most of these studies. The areas reported in these few whole-brain studies were the usual set of prominent occipito-parietal areas we might expect, such as V2, V3, V3A, V4d-topo, V7, intraparietal sulcus and parietal lobe [2,3,5,7-12,16]. A useful area for future study would be more matched comparisons between depth and rivalry, in which dynamic changes in depth (and a task to report depth percepts) could be used to make a direct comparison to rivalry studies.

4.1. Comparison of monocular and binocular rivalry

As we have encountered before, there appears to be a global trend towards a slightly different distribution of frontal, parietal and occipital activation across binocular rivalry and other multistability studies. Yet, one of the difficulties in comparing results across rivalry and multistability studies is that the studies were not carried out with equivalent stimulus conditions, tasks or methodology, and functional imaging analyses. To address this, we carried out an fMRI study explicitly designed to perform a direct comparison between binocular rivalry and an example of multistability (monocular rivalry), using matched retinal stimulation and comparable tasks [2]. We used orthogonal gratings for binocular rivalry (left or right oblique grating in each eye) or monocular rivalry (sum of orthogonal gratings in each eye), as shown in Figure 4. Coloured stimuli were used in order to enhance the percept of monocular rivalry. As described earlier, the perceptual alternations in monocular rivalry are more subtle than those in binocular rivalry, reflecting less perceptual suppression [69,77].

A direct comparison of monocular and binocular rivalry using gratings is attractive as the same images with matched retinal stimulation can be used for both forms of bistability in order to isolate the effect of suppression, and to determine if they share common neural mechanisms. We anticipated that the effects of perceptual suppression would be evident in a lower BOLD signal for binocular compared with monocular rivalry in early visual areas, such as V1, V2 or V3. We also used so-called 'rivalry replay' conditions, in which the entire stimulus was physically changed between the two possible percepts, using the identical temporal sequences reported earlier during rivalry with button presses. This is intended to mimic rivalry in terms of stimulus changes and motor demands, and allows subtractions to be made between rivalry and replay in order to isolate the neural substrates which may be more directly related to the perception of rivalrous alternations.

Some results are shown in the form of brain activation maps, averaged across six subjects (Figure 3). The activation for monocular rivalry or binocular rivalry with grating stimuli above the baseline condition is shown at three contrasts (9%, 18%, 36%). A view from the back of the human brain is shown (right hemisphere only). The colour scale indicates statistically significant results ranging from t=2.35 to 8.00 (orange-yellow) (FDR, $p<0.05$). Compared to a blank screen, both binocular and monocular rivalry show a U-shaped function of activation as a function of stimulus contrast, i.e. higher activity for most areas at 9% and 36%. The sites of cortical activation for monocular rivalry included occipital pole (V1, V2, V3), ventral temporal cortex (including fusiform gyrus), superior parietal cortex, ventrolateral prefrontal cortex, dorsolateral prefrontal cortex, supplementary motor area, frontal eye fields, and insula/frontal operculum. Interestingly, the areas for binocular rivalry were more widespread, and also included lateral occipital regions, as well as inferior parietal cortex, including intraparietal sulcus and temporoparietal junction (TPJ). In particular, MT+, lateral occipital complex and V3A were more active for binocular than monocular rivalry for all contrasts. The comparison of binocular rivalry with the replay condition was particularly important in isolating the neural substrates for the perception of rivalry, and also highlighted these same regions of activation. The more widespread activation pattern for binocular than monocular rivalry may be consistent with the presence of neural competition at higher-level areas, as well as greater effects of attention. As anticipated, when binocular and monocular rivalry were directly compared, an interaction with stimulus contrast was found in early visual areas V1, V2, and V3. Binocular rivalry evoked greater activation than monocular rivalry for the low contrast images. However, at higher stimulus contrasts, where perceptual suppression was more complete, the response to binocular rivalry fell below that to monocular rivalry.

4.2. U-shaped function of activation

One of the important results of the study was that both binocular and monocular rivalry showed a U-shaped function of activation as a function of contrast. Current models and concepts regarding binocular rivalry can explain this pattern (e.g. [51-54,56,69]). Rivalry models include inhibitory neurons in addition to excitatory neurons to account for interocular inhibition and suppression. In addition, the contribution of inhibition and suppression would generally be expected to lower the BOLD signal. At high contrasts, we expect the activation to increase due to an increasing neuronal response gain, which also leads to faster alternation rates, explaining the increase from 18% to 36% contrast. The increase in activation at the lowest contrast can possibly be explained as reflecting disinhibition, assuming that the excitatory and inhibitory neurons have different thresholds. At low contrasts, inhibitory neurons would not be strongly activated, resulting in slower alternation rates. Thus the higher BOLD signal at 9% contrast might be due to a release from inhibition that accompanies slow alternation rates.

4.3. Role of parietal areas

An important result of the study was to show that in addition to the activation of visual areas presumed to be involved directly in competition between neural representations, there was also activity for either binocular or monocular rivalry in frontoparietal areas that are often implicated in attention, and previously identified for binocular rivalry [65-67,70]. The previous literature seems to indicate that the balance of frontal activation may have been slightly higher for multistability than rivalry (as shown in Figure 2). But in our study in which we matched binocular and monocular rivalry for stimulus features and used comparable tasks, the frontal and parietal activation was actually somewhat higher for binocular rivalry, and included temporoparietal junction (TPJ), which was not an area significantly activated for monocular rivalry. The TPJ is modulated by stimulus-driven attentional shifts to unexpected objects or events [65,67,70]. It is possible that the TPJ was less active for monocular rivalry since the perceptual changes did not signal a change in object identity, as in binocular rivalry. All the other forms of multistability studied in fMRI paradigms produced some TPJ activation, including ambiguous figures [29,32,35,37], apparent motion [19,30,33] or structure from motion [36]. Hence a change in object identity and stimulus-driven shifts to unexpected events may be very relevant to the perceptual experience of binocular rivalry and other forms of multistability.

4.4. Visuospatial attention in control of multistability

Two aspects of the deployment of attention in vision have been studied extensively using physiological methods: the effects of attention on modulating neural responses in early visual cortical areas, and the top-down control of attention from executive control regions of the brain [66,68]. The effect of visuospatial attention to a stimulus at a peripheral location (while maintaining central fixation) is to increase the cortical response associated with that stimulus in striate and extrastriate visual areas within the contralateral hemisphere compared to when that stimulus is not attended (e.g. [71]). This contralateral attention effect has been shown to operate on the precise retinotopic cortical representation of the attended stimulus. Visual attention can also operate by modulating the cortical responses to a given stimulus feature [71]. In contrast, the top-down control of spatial attention has been associated with activity in the dorsolateral prefrontal and posterior parietal cortex, including intraparietal sulcus and superior parietal lobe [68], and transient activity within these regions is thought to initiate a shift of attention between locations, features, or objects. Thus, the effect of attention is to modulate neural activity in visual areas, while the control of attention has been associated with transient activity in frontal and parietal cortex that occurs at the onset of attentional switches [65,70], in addition to sustained activity in these areas that maintains a given attentive state. Studies of the voluntary control of ambiguous figure reversals have also revealed transient frontoparietal activation, suggesting that there may be a common mechanism subserving the voluntary deployment of attention and voluntary control over perceptual bistability [32,34].

One pertinent study investigated whether the voluntary control of perceptual configuration in a multistable stimulus (Necker cube) is mediated by voluntary shifts of selective attention, using event-related functional imaging [32]. Two slightly different versions of the Necker cube display were used during attention and perception conditions. In the attention condition, participants were cued to shift attention between the squares in left and right hemifields. In the perception condition, corresponding corners of the squares were connected by horizontal lines producing a perceptually multistable Necker cube. Observers reported which of the two faces appeared forward in depth, and were provided with cues to induce voluntary perceptual reversals. Both the perception and attention conditions yielded increased activity in contralateral occipital visual areas (V1v, V2v, VP, V3, V3A, V4v, MT+, V1d, V2d). Furthermore, voluntary shifts of attention and voluntary shifts in perceptual configuration were associated with common activity in the posterior parietal cortex (superior parietal lobe and intraparietal sulcus), part of the frontoparietal attentional top-down control network [66]. These results support the hypothesis that voluntary shifts in perceptual bistability in the Necker cube are mediated by spatial attention [32].

4.5. Transitions between percepts in binocular rivalry or multistability

A recent study took a different approach in studying these issues, noting that a number of previous binocular rivalry studies have found a large network of frontal and parietal cortical areas (as in Figure 2) to be active around the time of perceptual transitions between interpretations [19]. As described earlier, some previous rivalry studies have used subtractions between rivalry and 'rivalry replay' conditions to isolate rivalry mechanisms, and these frontal and parietal activations were still present following these subtractions [2,20,22]. It is possible that this activation could be related to the difficulty in judging the transitions during real rivalry alternations. The investigators noted in particular that some transitions occur virtually instantaneously, with one percept abruptly suppressing the alternative percept, whereas other transitions comprise dynamic mixtures of both percepts for a period of time before one percept dominates completely. They studied the role of this frontoparietal activation, with specific interest in its relation to the temporal structure of transitions, which can be either instantaneous or prolonged by periods during which observers experience a mix of both perceptual interpretations. Using both bistable apparent motion and binocular rivalry, they found that transition-related frontoparietal activity is larger for transitions that last longer, suggesting that the frontoparietal activation remains throughout the duration of the transition. They also found that frontoparietal activity during binocular rivalry transitions exceeded activity during abrupt transitions simulated using rivalry replay, as was found previously in a number of studies [2,20,22]. However, they confirmed that this only occurs when perceptual transitions are replayed as instantaneous events. When replay depicts the transitions with the actual durations reported during rivalry, then transitions mimicked with replay and genuine rivalry produced equal activation levels in frontoparietal areas. The results are consistent with the view that at least a component of frontoparietal activation during bistable perception reflects a *response* to rivalrous (or replay) perceptual transitions rather than their *cause*. Hence the results shed light on the functional role of frontoparietal activity and the mechanisms underlying perceptual reorganizations during bistable perception. This activation could reflect the change in sensory experience and task demand that occurs during transitions, which fits well with the known role of these areas in attention and decision making [65-67,70,78,79].

5. Methodological issues in fMRI studies and role of frontal areas

Some of the differences in the results across depth, rivalry and multistability studies can be explained due to the use of differing methodology and functional imaging analysis methods. The majority of rivalry studies have used event-related designs which correlated activations in different brain areas to the start of each alternation [5,19,20,22,28,61], while a smaller number of rivalry studies used block designs in which stimulus blocks with rivalry were contrasted with blocks of rivalry replay [1,2,26]. One other rivalry study analyzed temporal correlations between cortical areas during passive viewing of rivalry [21]. In general, multistability studies have used methods which are quite similar to those used in rivalry studies. For example, a large number of multistability studies used event-related designs correlating brain activation to reversals [29,30,32,33,36], while others used block designs comparing multistability to baseline conditions [31,34,35,37], or multivariate pattern analysis to predict perceptual states [38].

In contrast to rivalry or multistability, the majority of depth studies have used block designs. In these studies, stimulus blocks showing images with depth were contrasted with blocks with no depth [2,3, 6,7,9-12,17], or correlated disparity versus anticorrelated disparity images [13]. Other depth studies used methods more similar to those used for binocular rivalry, such as multivoxel pattern analysis [8], event-related adaptation [15], event-related designs in which brain activation was correlated to changes in perceived depth [5,16], or adaptation in a block design to assess population responsiveness to different types of depth stimuli [14]. These differences in methodology also mean that subjects performed a task in rivalry or multistabiity studies using event-related designs [5,19,20,22,28-30,32,33,36], or block designs [1,2,26,31,34,35], but subjects did not perform tasks in depth studies [3,6,9-13,17], although there are a few exceptions to this generalization for depth [2,4,5,7,17]. Also, a few rivalry or multistability studies did not use a task [21,37,61], and some rivalry studies used fixation tasks unrelated to the perception of rivalry [23,28].

These differences in methodology are obviously related to current concepts of rivalry and multistability as essentially dynamic perceptual phenomena while depth is static, but it should also be acknowledged that these differences could systematically affect the outcome of these studies. In particular, the fact that subjects usually performed a task in rivalry or multistability studies but not depth studies could explain why frontoparietal activation was more likely to be reported for rivalry or multistability. However, this is not the whole story, as several studies have found that frontoparietal activation is present for passive viewing of rivalry (including areas SP, IP, PM, FEF, SMA, MF, IF and FO in Figure 2), even when there is no task [2,21]. However, we noted in our own study that although activation in these widespread areas was still present, the absolute levels were lower with no task [2]. One multistability study which used passive viewing found that the typical parietal activation was present (superior and inferior parietal areas including TPJ), as well as one frontal site of activation (i.e. premotor cortex), but no significant activation of any other frontal areas, notably there was no significant activation in middle or inferior frontal gyrus [37]. Hence, frontoparietal activation is still present when there is no task, but it is reduced.

Some other studies of multistability have used tasks involving spatial shifts of attention instead of the more typical motor responses. One particular study of multistability which used spatial shifts of attention between the two possible percepts but no motor reports found activation in parietal areas (SP, IP), and a smaller subset of frontal areas, including only SMA, PM, and MF [35]. As described above, a second study of multistability which used spatial shifts of attention between two possible percepts found voluntary shifts of attention associated with activation of essentially the same sets of areas (namely parietal areas, SP, IP) and a small subset of frontal areas, including SMA but no significant activation in MF, IF or prefrontal cortex [32]. Hence, the use of tasks involving spatial shifts of attention tends to restrict frontal activation, although the usual site of parietal activation (i.e. SP, IP) are still present.

The use of an event-related design also has an impact on results. Studies of multistability which used block designs reported overall less frontal activation, although parietal activation was consistently reported in these studies [31,34,35,37]. This could be because frontal area fluctuations only occur at the onset of alternations and sum to zero over the longer periods. Most binocular rivalry studies used event-related designs, so it is difficult to assess what effect this has on the results.

In comparing the results across the depth, rivalry and multistability studies, a few other trends are apparent. A number of occipital areas, notably V2, V3, V3A, V4d-topo, V7 and MT+, were more frequently reported in depth studies than either rivalry or multistabililty. These areas may not have been frequently reported in studies of multistability because the analysis methods (usually event-related designs) would not find large signal differences in low-level visual representations since the visual appearance of the stimulus barely changes during alternations. For example, multistability studies involving apparent motion usually did not report any activation in these visual areas (with the exception of MT+), likely because of the similarity in stimulus configuration between the two possible percepts [19,30,33]. Likewise, there may not have been large signal changes in these areas occurring at the onset of binocular rivalry alternations because the two alternative percepts would not selectively activate any of these areas. Some of the rivalry and multistability studies that did report activation in these areas had one stimulus aspect in common: there was a depth interpretation present in the stimulus alternatives (for example, rotating structure-from-motion sphere, or slant/perspective rivalry, [5,38]). In contrast, ventral temporal areas, including fusiform gyrus, were more likely to be active in studies which used faces as one of the two possible percepts, such as faces/grating stimuli [20,21,24,29]. Another stimulus difference which could explain trends is that a number of different examples of multistability which were used had a dynamic aspect (e.g. apparent motion), which was in addition to the multistable percept itself. In general, the frontal activation was greater and included a larger number of areas for the dynamic examples of multistability [19,30,33,36,37,38], compared with static examples [29,31,34,35].

6. Future research

A number of questions remain unanswered by the existing functional imaging studies on binocular depth, rivalry and multistability. Current models of binocular vision need to be revised in order to explain the interrelationship between depth and rivalry and explain why they are processed in parallel through a number of cortical areas [51-54,56]. It may be possible that the strong inhibitory interactions which we are familiar with in binocular rivalry may serve the purpose of resolving ambiguity in binocular vision. The mechanisms for binocular rivalry may be important in inhibiting false matches at different orientations, suppressing noise in neural responses and sharpening the tuning of orientational mechanisms [59,60]. A more general binocular vision model would incorporate these important inhibitory mechanisms, together with binocular matching which is necessary for depth perception. In addition, it is important to incorporate the finding that it is possible to perceive both depth and rivalry simultaneously at a single spatial location. There may be a representation at the surface-level that would facilitate the grouping of binocular depth and rivalry features, and allow for more than one feature to be coded at a spatial location [2].

A common set of frontoparietal cortical brain areas are activated during depth, rivalry or multistability, implying that there is an underlying cortical network with a complex interplay of neural processing between cortical brain areas, which is not yet understood. Such frontoparietal activations could reflect top-down processes that initiate a reorganization of activity in visual cortex during perceptual reversals. Alternatively, as a result of neural activity fluctuations in visual cortex, frontoparietal activations could merely reflect the feed-forward communication of salient neural events from visual cortex to higher-level areas. These two possibilities differ in the causal chain assumed to underlie changes in visual awareness, but it remains difficult to infer causality from correlative neurophysiological measures. Ideally, this would be addressed by probing the causal role of frontal and parietal areas using experimental lesion and microstimulation techniques. For example, a recent study which used transcranial magnetic stimulation (TMS) to create virtual lesions showed that particular frontal cortical areas (e.g. dorsolateral prefrontal cortex) were causally relevant for voluntary control over perceptual switches in a multistable structure-from-motion stimulus [80]. Other observations that activations in frontal and parietal areas precede activity associated with the sensory processing of perceptual switches also suggest that feedback signals from frontoparietal areas modulate visual processing [33,81].

However, other results reviewed earlier suggest that the ultimate resolution will be more nuanced and complicated than the dichotomy referred to above (e.g., [19,32,61]). One particularly appealing framework previously proposed suggests that the frontal and parietal areas form part of a sensorimotor continuum and are designed to periodically check or update the current perceptual organization in the visual system [82,83]. Hence this central control network would mediate between alternative perceptions for conscious awareness. This process may in fact occur all the time in natural vision, but would usually proceed unnoticed, resulting in a stable perception of the visual world. In any case, it will be important to carry out further studies in order to clarify the functional role of frontoparietal activity and determine the manner in which it relates to the mechanisms underlying perception in general, and reorganizations during bistable perception.

7. Conclusions

A review of recent functional neuroimaging studies indicates that binocular depth, rivalry and multistability are three perceptual processing domains which share neural substrates, including largely overlapping occipital, parietal and frontal cortical areas. All three of these perceptual processing modalities can be conceptualized as a series of visual perceptual processing stages in occipital areas, as well as higher-level cognitive functions in parietal and frontal areas, involving decision making, motor planning and execution, attention, awareness and memory. Current research will further study the manner in which these cortical areas interact, and the causal sequence of events which underlies each of these three perceptual processing modalities, recalling some of the most important themes of neuroscience in these overlapping and interrelated functions.

Author details

Athena Buckthought[*] and Janine D. Mendola
Department of Ophthalmology, McGill University, Montreal, Canada

Acknowledgement

This work was supported by NSERC and NIH R01 EY015219 grants, and a LOF grant from the Canadian Foundation for Innovation.

8. References

[1] Buckthought A, Jessula S, Mendola JD (2011) Bistable Percepts in the Brain: FMRI Contrasts Monocular Pattern Rivalry and Binocular Rivalry. PLoS One 6: e20367.
[2] Buckthought A, Mendola, JD (2011) A Matched Comparison of Binocular Rivalry and Depth Perception with FMRI. J Vis. 11: 1-15.
[3] Tsao DY, Vanduffel W, Sasaki Y, Fize D, Knutsen TA, Mandeville JB, Wald LL, Dale AM, Rosen BR, Van Essen DC, Livingstone MS, Orban GA, Tootell RBH (2003) Stereopsis Activates V3A and Caudal Intraparietal Areas in Macaques and Humans. Neuron 39: 555-568.
[4] Backus BT, Fleet DJ, Parker AJ, Heeger DJ (2001) Human Cortical Activity Correlates with Stereoscopic Depth Perception. J Neurophysiol. 86: 2054-2068.
[5] Brouwer GJ, van Ee R, Schwarzbach J (2005) Activation in Visual Cortex Correlates with the Awareness of Stereoscopic Depth. J Neurosci. 25: 10403-10413.
[6] Durand JB, Peeters R, Norman JF, Todd JT, Orban GA (2009) Parietal Regions Processing Visual 3D Shape Extracted from Disparity. Neuroimage 46: 1114-1126.
[7] Minini L, Parker AJ, Bridge H (2010) Neural Modulation by Binocular Disparity Greatest in Human Dorsal Visual Stream. J Neurophysiol. 104: 169-178.
[8] Preston TJ, Li S, Kourtzi Z, Welchman AE (2008) Multivoxel Pattern Selectivity for Perceptually Relevant Binocular Disparities in the Human Brain. J Neurosci. 28: 11315-11327.
[9] Georgieva S, Peeters R, Kolster H, Todd JT, Orban GA (2009) The Processing of Three-Dimensional Shape From Disparity in the Human Brain. J Neurosci. 29: 727-742.
[10] Rutschmann RM, Greenlee MW (2004) BOLD Response in Dorsal Areas Varies With Relative Disparity Level. Neuroreport 15: 615-619.
[11] Iwami T, Nishida Y, Hayashi O, Kimura M, Sakai M, Kani, K, Ito R, Shiino A, Suzuki M (2002) Common Neural Processing Regions for Dynamic and Static Stereopsis in Human Parieto-Occipital Cortices. Neurosci Lett. 327: 29-32.

[*] Corresponding Author

[12] Nishida Y, Hayashi O, Iwami T, Kimura M, Kani K, Ito R, Shiino A, Suzuki M (2001) Stereopsis-Processing Regions in the Human Parieto-Occipital Cortex. Neuroreport 12: 2259-2263.

[13] Bridge H, Parker AJ (2007) Topographical Representation of Binocular Depth in the Human Visual Cortex Using FMRI. J Vis. 7: 1-14.

[14] Neri P, Bridge H, Heeger DJ (2004) Stereoscopic Processing of Absolute and Relative Disparity in Human Visual Cortex. J Neurophysiol. 92: 1880-1891.

[15] Welchman AE, Deubelius A, Conrad V, Bulthoff HH, Kourtzi Z (2005) 3D Shape Perception From Combined Depth Cues in Human Visual Cortex. Nat Neurosci. 8: 820-827.

[16] Chandrasekaran C, Canon V, Dahmen JC, Kourtzi Z, Welchman AE (2007) Neural Correlates of Disparity-Defined Shape Discrimination in the Human Brain. J Neurophysiol. 97: 1553-1565.

[17] Gilaie-Dotan S, Ullman S, Kushnir T, Malach R (2002) Shape-Selective Stereo Processing in Human Object-Related Visual Areas. Hum Brain Mapp. 15: 67-79.

[18] Tyler CW, Likova LT, Kontsevich LL, Wade AR (2006) The Specificity of Cortical Region KO to Depth Structure. Neuroimage 30: 228-238.

[19] Knapen T, Brascamp J, Pearson J, van Ee R, Blake R (2011) The Role of Frontal and Parietal Brain Areas in Bistable Perception. J Neurosci. 31: 10293-10301.

[20] Lumer ED, Friston KJ, Rees G (1998). Neural Correlates of Perceptual Rivalry in the Human Brain. Science 280: 1930-1934.

[21] Lumer ED, Rees G (1999) Covariation of Activity in Visual and Prefrontal Cortex Associated with Subjective Visual Perception. Proc Natl Acad Sci U S A 96: 1669-1673.

[22] Wilcke JC, O'Shea RP, Watts R (2009) Frontoparietal Activity and Its Structural Connectivity in Binocular Rivalry. Brain Res. 1305: 96-107.

[23] Fang F, He S (2005) Cortical Responses to Invisible Objects in the Human Dorsal and Ventral Pathways. Nat Neurosci. 8: 1380-1385.

[24] Tong F, Nakayama K, Vaughan JT, Kanwisher N (1998) Binocular Rivalry and Visual Awareness in Human Extrastriate Cortex. Neuron 21: 753-759.

[25] Jiang Y, He S (2006) Cortical Responses to Invisible Faces: Dissociating Subsystems for Facial-Information Processing. Curr Biol. 16: 2023-2029.

[26] Lee S-H, Blake R (2002) V1 Activity is Reduced During Binocular Rivalry. J Vis. 2: 618–626.

[27] Polonsky A, Blake R, Braun J, Heeger DJ (2000) Neuronal Activity in Human Primary Visual Cortex Correlates with Perception During Binocular Rivalry. Nat Neurosci. 3: 1153-1159.

[28] Moradi F, Heeger DJ (2009) Inter-ocular Contrast Normalization in Human Visual Cortex. J Vis. 9: 1-22.

[29] Kleinschmidt A, Buchel C, Zeki S, Frackowiak RS (1998) Human Brain Activity During Spontaneously Reversing Perception of Ambiguous Figures. Proc Biol Sci. 265: 2427-2433.

[30] Sterzer P, Russ MO, Preibisch C, Kleinschmidt A (2002) Neural Correlates of Spontaneous Direction Reversals in Ambiguous Apparent Visual Motion. Neuroimage 15: 908-916.

[31] Raz A, Lamar M, Buhle JT, Kane MJ, Peterson BS (2007) Selective Biasing of a Specific Bistable-Figure Percept Involves FMRI Signal Changes in Frontostriatal Circuits: A Step Toward Unlocking the Neural Correlates of Top-Down Control and Self-Regulation. Am J Clin Hypn. 50: 137-156.

[32] Slotnick SD, Yantis S (2005) Common Neural Substrates for the Control and Effects of Visual Attention and Perceptual Bistability. Brain Res Cogn Brain Res. 24: 97-108.

[33] Sterzer P, Kleinschmidt A (2007) A Neural Basis for Inference in Perceptual Ambiguity. Proc Natl Acad Sci U S A 104: 323-328.

[34] Tracy JI, Flanders A, Madi S, Natale P, Goyal N, Laskas J, Delvecchio N, Pyrros A (2005) The Brain Topography Associated with Active Reversal and Suppression of an Ambiguous Figure. Eur J Cogn Psychol. 17: 267-288.

[35] Inui T, Tanaka S, Okada T, Nishizawa S, Katayama M, Konishi J (2000) Neural Substrates for Depth Perception of the Necker Cube; A Functional Magnetic Resonance Imaging Study in Human Subjects. Neurosci Lett. 282: 145–148.

[36] Raemaekers M, van der Schaaf ME, van Ee R, van Wezel RJA (2009) Widespread fMRI Activity Differences between Perceptual States in Visual Rivalry and Correlated with Differences in Observer Biases. Brain Res. 1252: 161-171.

[37] Schoth F, Waberski TD, Krings T, Gobbele R, Buchner H (2007) Cerebral Processing of Spontaneous Reversals of the Necker Cube. Neuroreport 18: 1335-1338.

[38] Brouwer GJ, van Ee R (2007) Visual Cortex Allows Prediction of Perceptual States During Ambiguous Structure-From-Motion. J Neurosci. 27: 1015-1023.

[39] Larsson J, Heeger DJ (2006) Two Retinotopic Visual Areas in Human Lateral Occipital Cortex. J Neurosci. 26: 13128-13142.

[40] Tootell RB, Hadjikhani NK, Vanduffel W, Liu AK, Mendola JD, Sereno MI, Dale AM (1998) Functional Analysis of Primary Visual Cortex (V1) in Humans. Proc Natl Acad Sci USA 95: 811– 817.

[41] Ungerleider LG, Mishkin M (1982) Two Cortical Visual Systems. In: Ingle DJ, Goodale MA, Mansfield RJW, editors. Analysis of Visual Behavior. Cambridge, Mass: MIT Press. pp. 549–86.

[42] Orban GA, Claeys K, Nelissen K, Smans R, Sunaert S, Todd JT, Wardak C, Durand JB, Vanduffel W (2006) Mapping the Parietal Cortex of Human and Non-Human Primates. Neuropsychologia 44: 2647-2667.

[43] Kourtzi Z, Bülthoff HH, Erb M, Grodd W (2002) Object-Selective Responses in the Human Motion area MT/MST. Nat Neurosci. 5:17–18.

[44] Kourtzi Z, Erb M, Grodd W, Bulthoff HH (2003) Representation of the Perceived 3-D Object Shape in the Human Lateral Occipital Complex. Cereb Cortex 13: 911-920.

[45] Mendola JD, Dale AM, Fischl B, Liu AK, Tootell RBH (1999) The Representation of Real and Illusory Contours in Human Cortical Visual Areas Revealed by FMRI. J Neurosci. 19: 8560–8572.

[46] Moore C, Engel SA (2001) Neural Response to Perception of Volume in the Lateral Occipital Complex. Neuron 29: 277–286.

[47] Haushofer J, Baker CI, Livingstone MS, Kanwisher N (2008) Privileged Coding of Convex Shapes in Human Object-Selective Cortex. J Neurophysiol. 100: 753-62.

[48] Thier P, Karnath HO (1997) Parietal Lobe Contributions to Orientation in 3D Space, Volume 25. Heidelberg: Springer-Verlag.

[49] Liu CH, Collin CA, Chaudhuri A (2000) Does Face Recognition Rely on Encoding of 3-D Surface? Examining the Role of Shape-From-Shading and Shape-From-Stereo. Perception 29: 729-743.

[50] Liu CH, Ward J (2006) The Use of 3D Information in Face Recognition. Vision Res. 46: 768-73.

[51] Blake R (1989) A Neural Theory of Binocular Rivalry. Psychol Rev. 96: 145-167.

[52] Dayan P (1998). A Hierarchical Model of Binocular Rivalry. Neural Comput. 10: 1119-1135.

[53] Freeman AW (2005) Multistage Model for Binocular Rivalry. J Neurophysiol. 94: 4412–4420.

[54] Wilson HR (2007) Minimal Physiological Conditions for Binocular Rivalry and Rivalry Memory. Vision Res. 47: 2741-2750.

[55] Blake R, Yang YD, Wilson HR (1991) On the Coexistence of Stereopsis and Binocular Rivalry. Vision Res. 31: 1191-1203.

[56] Hayashi R, Maeda T, Shimojo S, Tachi S (2004) An Integrative Model of Binocular Vision: a Stereo Model Utilizing Interocularly Unpaired Points Produces Both Depth and Binocular Rivalry. Vision Res. 44: 2367-2380.

[57] Andrews TJ, Holmes D (2011) Stereoscopic Depth Perception During Binocular Rivalry. Front Hum Neurosci. 5: 1-5.

[58] Buckthought A, Wilson HR (2007) Interaction Between Binocular Rivalry and Depth in Plaid Patterns. Vision Res. 47: 2543-2556.

[59] Macknik SL, Martinez-Conde S (2004) Dichoptic Visual Masking Reveals That Early Binocular Neurons Exhibit Weak Interocular Suppression: Implications for Binocular Vision and Visual Awareness. J Cogn Neurosci. 16: 1049-1059.

[60] van Boxtel JJ, van Ee R, Erkelens CJ (2007) Dichoptic Masking and Binocular Rivalry Share Common Perceptual Dynamics. J Vis. 7: 1-11.

[61] Brouwer GJ, Tong F, Hagoort P, van Ee R (2009) Perceptual Incongruence Influences Bistability and Cortical Activation. PLoS One 4: e5056.

[62] Tong F, Engel S (2001) Interocular Rivalry Revealed in the Human Cortical Blind-Spot Representation. Nature 411: 195–199.

[63] Haynes JD, Deichmann R, Rees G (2005) Eye-Specific Effects of Binocular Rivalry in the Human Lateral Geniculate Nucleus. Nature 438: 496-499.

[64] Wunderlich K, Schneider KA, Kastner S (2005) Neural Correlates of Binocular Rivalry in he Human Lateral Geniculate Nucleus. Nat Neurosci. 8: 1595-1602.
[65] Corbetta M, Kincade JM, Ollinger JM, McAvoy MP, Shulman GL (2000) Voluntary Orienting is Dissociated from Target Detection in Human Posterior Parietal Cortex. Nat Neurosci. 3: 292-297.
[66] Corbetta M, Shulman GL (2002) Control of Goal-Directed and Stimulus-Driven Attention in the Brain. Nat Rev Neurosci. 3:201-215.
[67] Kincade JM, Abrams RA, Astafiev SV, Shulman GL, Corbetta M (2005) An Event-Related Functional Magnetic Resonance Imaging Study of Voluntary and Stimulus-Driven Orienting of Attention. J Neurosci. 25: 4593-4604.
[68] Yantis S, Serences JT (2003) Cortical Mechanisms of Spaced-Based and Object-Based Attentional Control. Curr. Opin. Neurobiol. 13: 187– 193.
[69] Freeman AW, Nguyen VA, Alais D (2005) The Nature and Depth of Binocular Rivalry Suppression. In: Alais D, Blake R, editors. Binocular Rivalry. Cambridge, MA: MIT Press. pp. 47-62.
[70] Corbetta M, Patel G, Shulman GL (2008) The Reorienting System of the Human Brain: From Environment to Theory of Mind. Neuron 58: 306-324.
[71] Corbetta M, Miezin FM, Dobmeyer S, Shulman GL, Petersen SE (1990) Attentional Modulation of Neural Processing of Shape, Color, and Velocity in Humans. Science 248: 1556–1559.
[72] Necker LA (1832) Observations on Some Remarkable Phenomena Seen in Switzerland, and an Optical Phenomenon Which Occurs on Viewing of a Crystal or Geometrical Solid. Philosophical Magazine 1: 329-337.
[73] Rubin E (1921) Visuell Wahrgenommene Figuren. Kobenhaven: Glydenalske Boghandel.
[74] Meng M, Tong F (2004). Can Attention Selectively Bias Bistable Perception? Differences Between Binocular Rivalry and Ambiguous Figures. J Vis. 4: 539-551.
[75] Ramachandran VS, Anstis SM (1985) Perceptual Organization in Multistable Apparent Motion. Perception 144: 135-143.
[76] Breese BB (1899) On Inhibition. Psychological Monographs 3: 1-65.
[77] O'Shea RP, Parker A, La Rooy D, Alais D (2009) Monocular Rivalry Exhibits Three Hallmarks of Binocular Rivalry: Evidence for Common Processes. Vision Res. 49: 671-681.
[78] Cole MW, Schneider W (2007) The Cognitive Control Network: Integrated Cortical Regions with Dissociable Functions. Neuroimage 37: 343-360.
[79] Pastor MA, Day BL, Macaluso E, Friston KJ, Frackowiak RS (2004) The Functional Neuroanatomy of Temporal Discrimination. J Neurosci. 24: 2585-2591.
[80] de Graaf TA, de Jong MC, Goebel R, van Ee R, Sack AT (2011) On the Functional Relevance of Frontal Cortex for Passive and Voluntarily Controlled Bistable Vision. Cereb Cortex 21: 2322-2331.

[81] Britz J, Pitts MA, Michel CM (2011) Right Parietal Brain Activity Precedes Perceptual Alternation During Binocular Rivalry. Hum Brain Mapp. 32:1432-1442.

[82] Leopold DA, Logothetis NK (1999) Multistable Phenomena: Changing Views in Perception. Trends Cogn Sci. 3: 254-264.

[83] Mendola JD, Conner IP, Sharma S, Bahekar A, Lemieux S (2006) FMRI Measures of Perceptual Filling-In in the Human Visual Cortex. J Cogn Neurosci. 18: 363-75.

Chapter 5

Visual Motion: From Cortex to Percept

Craig Aaen-Stockdale and Benjamin Thompson

Additional information is available at the end of the chapter

http://dx.doi.org/10.5772/50402

1. Introduction

A brown bear pads across a snowfield. It is watched (hopefully from a safe distance) by an observer. As the bear tramps through the snow, a bear-shaped patch of darkness is projected onto the back of the observer's eye. The motion of this image across the observer's otherwise brightly illuminated retina causes a series of changes in the activity of densely packed photoreceptors that are sensitive to changes in light intensity. The observer's visual system can, as the bear progresses, perform the remarkable feat of computing its speed and direction of motion – and the speed and direction of each of the bear's constituent parts - from many million changes in neural firing rate. This ability has clear evolutionary advantages, and as such it has been widely selected for in the animal kingdom.

Less common is the ability to detect motion that is not based on changes in luminance. To return to our wintery example, the force and direction of the wind or the presence of a smaller animal burrowing under the snow can be determined by detecting changes in the pattern of random flicker caused as flakes of snow on the ground are disturbed. Here, the changes in luminance do not, in themselves, signal any consistent speed or direction of motion, but the movement can clearly be seen.

In this chapter, we review key aspects of visual motion perception with a particular emphasis on the cortical areas thought to be involved. We begin with the integration of motion signals across extended regions of the visual field. This is central to the ability of the visual cortex to bind multiple features together into a coherent, stable visual percept. We then move on to the question of plasticity within the early cortical areas responsible for motion perception and review the brain regions thought to be involved in the processing of complex motion information such the motion signals that flow over the retina as an observer moves around in their environment. In the final two sections of the chapter we consider the mechanisms involved in the perception of motion in the absence of useful luminance information and the consequences of lesions and abnormal development affecting the cortical areas responsible for motion perception.

2. Cortical processing of visual information

Visual processing has often been thought of as being subdivided into two parallel processing streams known as the parvocellular (also known as ventral) and magnocellular (also known as dorsal) pathways (Ungerleider & Mishkin, 1982; Goodale & Milner, 1992). This delineation begins at the level of retinal ganglion cells. Small (midget) and larger (parasol) ganglion cells project, respectively, to the distinct parvocellular ("P") and magnocellular ("M") layers of the lateral geniculate nucleus of the thalamus (LGN) (Derrington & Lennie, 1984; Merigan et al., 1991). In turn, these M and P LGN cells project to distinct sub-regions of layer 4c within the primary visual cortex (Hubel & Wiesel, 1972). According to the "dual pathway" model, the parvocellular pathway, primarily carrying high spatial frequency (fine detail) and colour information, then projects to ventral areas of the extrastriate cortex such as V4. Conversely, the magnocellular pathway, primarily carrying low spatial (coarse detail) and high temporal frequency information, innervates dorsal extrastriate regions such as the middle temporal visual area (MT) also known as V5 and the middle superior temporal visual area (MST). These projections are thought to produce cortical pathways specialized for form processing and spatial position/motion perception respectively (Ungerleider & Haxby, 1994). It is now clear that there is considerable crosstalk between these two pathways and that other connections exist between the retina and the brain that include the koniocellular layers of the LGN and other thalamic regions such as the superior colliculus and pulvinar (see de Haan & Cowey, 2011 for a recent review). However the concept of parallel processing has provided a useful framework for the investigation of motion perception and has inspired a large number of psychophysical studies in this area.

2.1. Local motion analysis – V1

The first port of call for the majority of visual information in the cortex is the primary visual cortex, or V1. It is also often referred to as the "striate cortex" due to its stratified appearance under the microscope. Thanks to the Nobel prize winning experiments by Hubel and Wiesel, we know that single striate cortex neurons in the cat (Hubel & Wiesel, 1959) and monkey (Hubel & Weisel, 1968) respond best to oriented lines and that some of these neurons are also selective for the direction in which a luminance-defined stimulus is moved across their receptive field. The neural architecture necessary to achieve luminance-based motion detection and discrimination is, therefore, already in place at the relatively low level of V1. Various computational theories have successfully modelled the detection of this type of luminance-based motion (Adelson & Bergen, 1985; van Santen & Sperling, 1985; Watson & Ahumada, 1985). The method common to all of these models is to combine the outputs of two neurons, one whose receptive field has an "odd" (sine phase) spatial profile and an "even" (cosine phase) temporal profile and another neuron whose receptive field has an even spatial profile and an odd temporal profile. By appropriately combining the outputs of non-directional V1 neurons whose spatial and temporal responses are 90° out-of-phase (often referred to as "quadrature pairs"), motion energy can be recovered (Adelson &

Bergen, 1985). Alternative models have been suggested based on inhibitory interactions between adjacent regions within the receptive field (Barlow & Levick, 1965), spatiotemporal differencing (Marr & Ullman, 1981) or spatiotemporal gradients (Johnston et al., 1992), but the motion energy model is currently the dominant model of V1 motion selectivity.

2.2. Global motion analysis – V3A and the middle temporal visual area (MT/V5)

The year 1985 was a seminal year for the study of visual motion (Burr & Thompson, 2011) seeing, as it did, publication of several influential models of local motion processing (Adelson & Bergen, 1985; van Santen & Sperling, 1985; Watson & Ahumada, 1985). Although it had taken a great leap forward, the race to understand the processing of visual motion was, however, far from over. It is one thing to understand how local motion selectivity arises in single neurons, but quite another to understand how these local motion signals are combined across space to give the perception of moving edges, surfaces and objects. The major hurdle (and it is a significant one) is that the output of individual local motion detectors, such as those present in V1 and those modelled in the literature mentioned above, is often *ambiguous.*

Since V1 neurons (or a hypothetical local motion detector) only "see" a small portion of the world, they do not respond maximally to a single stimulus form, but to a whole family of motions. This problem, referred to as the *aperture problem* is demonstrated in Figure 1.

By integrating the outputs of many motion detectors over larger and larger portions of the visual field, the visual system can disambiguate these signals and extract genuine motion from the inherently ambiguous local motion signals, a processing stage known as the extraction of *global motion.* Such a process is thought to occur in extrastriate cortical areas such as V3A and MT, both of which contain cells that respond to coherent global motion (Allman et al., 1985; Movshon et al., 1985; Newsome & Pare, 1988; Rodman & Albright, 1989; Salzman et al., 1992; Heeger et al., 1999; Braddick et al., 2001). Similar properties seem to be present in the human analogue of MT known as V5 or hMT+ (Beckers & Zeki, 1995; Tootell et al., 1995; Huk & Heeger, 2002; Cowey et al., 2006). For example, we have recently demonstrated (Figure 2) that inhibitory repetitive transcranial magnetic stimulation (rTMS) of human V5 can impair the combination of local motion signals into a global motion percept (Thompson et al., 2009). With such abundant evidence that this cortical region is crucial to the perception of global motion, a question still to be answered is what sort of combinatorial processes are actually occurring in V5?

Several models of local motion combination have been proposed. A widely cited early model is the *intersection-of-constraints* (Adelson & Movshon, 1982) in which local one-dimensional (1D) motions (see legend of Figure 1) are extracted from the two-dimensional (2D) visual stimulus, their respective constraint lines are computed and the motion of the pattern corresponds to the intersection of these constraint lines. The intersection-of-constraints is a geometrical solution to the aperture problem and therefore provides a useful point of comparison for psychophysical data and resulting models aiming to understand how global motion is computed within the brain. A number of psychophysical results have suggested that perception does not always follow the intersection of constraints rule (Ferrera & Wilson, 1990; Yo & Wilson, 1992) and, as such, alternative models have been developed. One key alternative is the *vector sum* model (Wilson et al., 1992; Wilson & Kim, 1994) in which global motion is computed as the sum of the local motion vectors.

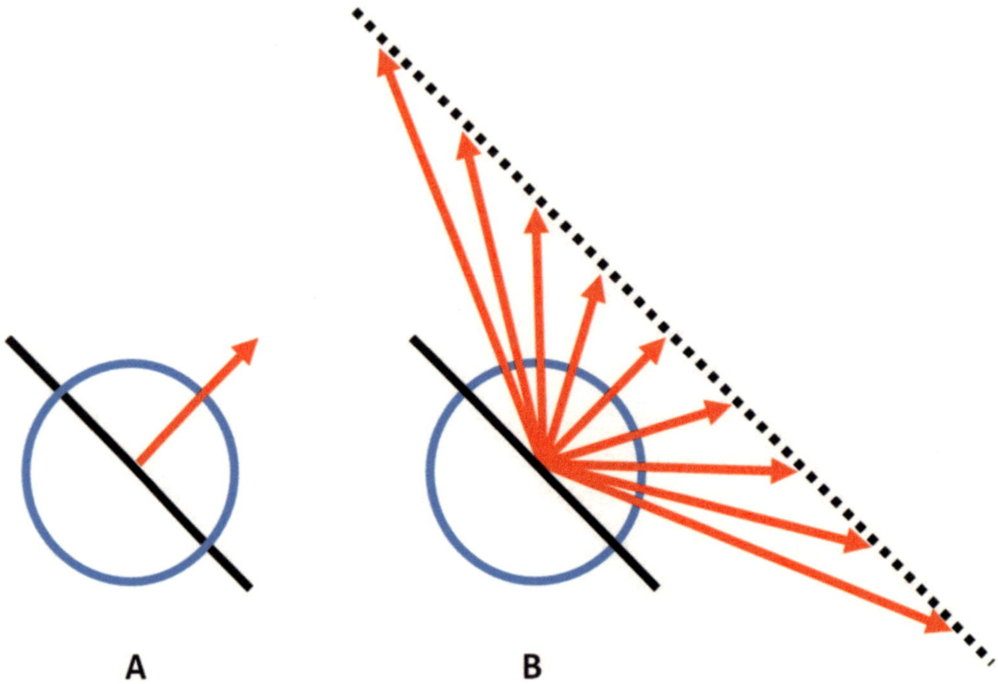

Figure 1. The aperture problem. A) An edge, represented by the black line, moves in a particular direction, at a particular speed, through the receptive field of a motion-sensitive neuron (blue circle). The direction in which the edge is moving is represented by the red arrow, and the speed at which it is moving is represented by the length of the arrow. Assume that the neuron is sensitive to stimuli of this particular orientation moving at this particular speed, and so fires. The aperture problem arises because exactly the same response can be achieved by moving another edge, oriented at the same angle, through the receptive field in a completely different direction, at a much faster speed. Since the edge is uniform and featureless, the neuron is unable to determine its direction and speed of motion. The *global motion* of the edge is therefore ambiguous. B) It turns out that exactly the same stimulus can be reproduced by a family of different combinations of speed and direction constrained by a *constraint line* (dashed line) perpendicular to the end point of the shortest (i.e. slowest) motion vector. As such, only motion perpendicular to a contour can be detected by a single detector. It is therefore referred to as *one-dimensional* motion.

Both of these models are, however, two-stage operations in which the 2D stimulus is decomposed into its local 1D motions and then reconstructed according to a mathematical rule. There are a number of psychophysical results that are not consistent with this decomposition-recombination approach. The ability to discriminate the direction of motion of a plaid appears to depend critically upon the speed of the 2D features or "blobs" in the

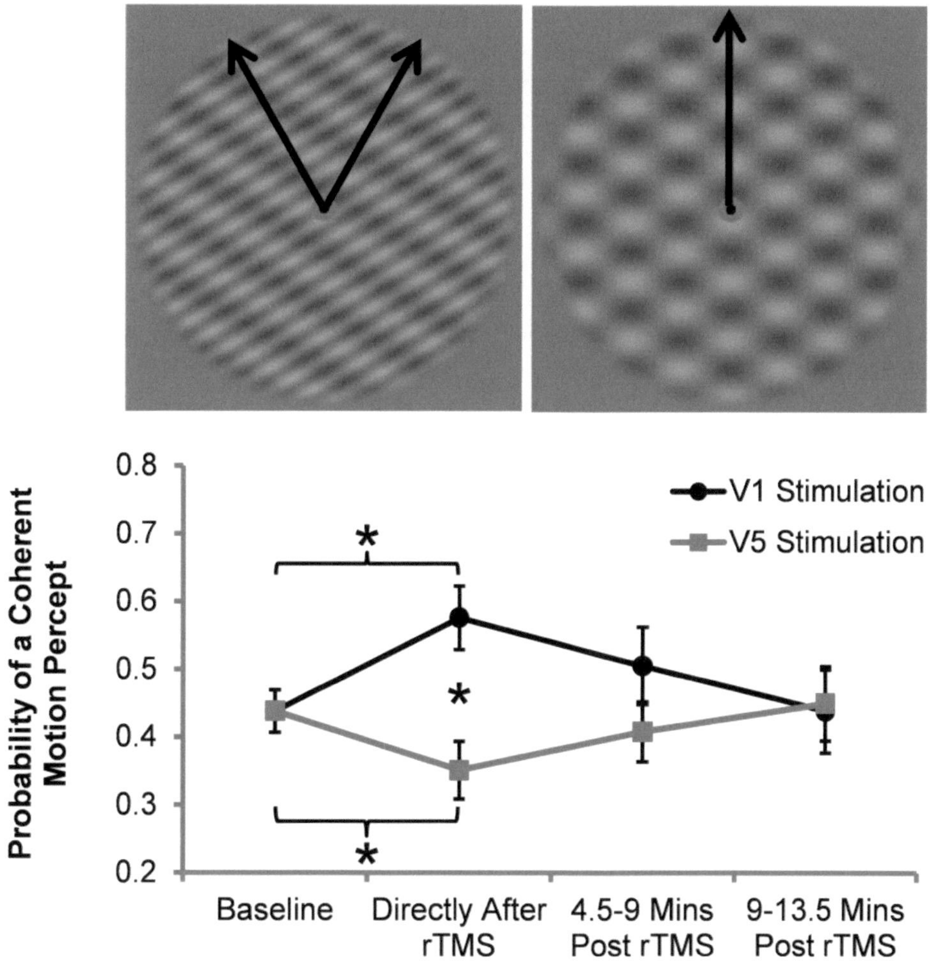

Figure 2. Evidence for the role of human V5 in the processing of global motion. The top panel depicts plaid stimuli that are constructed from two gratings moving in different directions within a circular aperture. If the spatial properties of the gratings are sufficiently dissimilar then the two gratings are seen to drift over one another in directions orthogonal to their orientation due to the aperture problem described above (top-left image). However, if the gratings are similar to one another they may be perceived as a coherent patterned surface moving globally in a different direction from either of the component gratings (top-right image). The lower panel shows average data from 11 participants who viewed ambiguous plaid patterns that could be perceived as either coherent or incoherent before and after inhibitory repetitive transcranial magnetic stimulation of either V1 or V5. The probability of perceiving the stimuli as moving coherently is shown for three different time points after stimulation. rTMS of V5 significantly reduced the probability that participants would perceive plaids as moving coherently directly after stimulation, suggesting that this area is centrally involved in global motion perception. Stimulation of V1 had the opposite effect. Data re-plotted from (Thompson et al., 2009).

stimulus, not the speed of its components (Derrington & Badcock, 1992; Wright & Gurney, 1992). In addition, the size and number of blobs within plaid stimuli influence the perceived motion direction and the direction of the associated motion after-effects (Alais et al., 1994;

Alais et al., 1996; Alais et al., 1997). Furthermore, physiological data show that motion-selective cells in V1, that have broad orientation-tuning, respond to the motion of 2D features in the stimulus (Tinsley et al., 2003) and presumably feed this information forward to MT/V5, where it is combined with 1D local motion signals to influence perception. The visual system has for some time been likened to a Fourier analyser, that breaks down the complicated visual stimulus into its simpler 1D components, then recombines it (Campbell & Robson, 1968). The work of Tinsley et al. and Alais and colleagues is by no means fatal to the two-stage conception of global motion analysis, but rather reminds us that the first-stage is not a straightforward global Fourier analysis. In addition, these data suggest that the visual system may shift between different strategies for combining local motion based on the task demands and available information (Nishida, 2011).

2.2.1. Spatial suppression

Centre-surround antagonism is a common feature of the visual system that begins at the level of the retina and assists segmentation of the visual image into objects and background. Briefly, stimulation in a neuron's central receptive field causes excitation, whilst stimulation in the receptive field surround results in inhibition. These two signals may cancel each other out if stimulation of the centre and surround is uniform. This results in neurons that are selective for discontinuities in the visual image. At the level of the cortex, excitatory and inhibitory regions are organised in such a way that neurons show selectivity for a variety of properties such as orientation, spatial frequency or motion within their receptive field centres. These are sometimes referred to as the "classical" receptive field. Many other cortical neurons also show a substantial inhibitory surround whose stimulus selectivity is antagonistic to the receptive field centre. It has been argued that this fundamental property of the visual system may give rise to some curious psychophysical correlates, including one well-known motion-based perceptual effect termed "spatial suppression."

As the retinal size of a stimulus increases, one would expect motion detection and discrimination to improve according to spatial summation of contrast resulting from the recruitment and integration of progressively larger numbers of motion sensors. Contrary to this idea, Tadin et al. (2003) noted that observers got *worse* at discriminating the direction of motion as the size of a high contrast stimulus was increased. Spatial summation occurred as expected only if the patch was low contrast, resulting in *better* performance as size increased. Tadin et al. proposed that their psychophysical results were a perceptual correlate of centre-surround antagonism in motion-selective neurons in cortical visual area V5, and have recently reported TMS findings to support this view (Tadin et al., 2011). The rationale is that large, high contrast stimuli activate *both* the excitatory centre and inhibitory surround of cells in V5, resulting in a less robust neural representation of motion. Further, this effect does not occur for low contrast stimuli, as the inhibitory surround requires high contrasts to become active.

It was subsequently reported that older observers (over 60 years of age) showed weaker spatial suppression, which paradoxically led to *better* performance than younger observers in the high contrast conditions (Betts et al., 2005). The authors proposed that this weaker spatial suppression in older observers is a perceptual correlate of age-related changes in GABA-mediated inhibitory processes in the brain (Leventhal et al., 2003). Similar claims regarding a weakening (or not) of centre-surround antagonism in cortical areas have since been made using the same psychophysical technique for observers with schizophrenia (Tadin et al., 2006), depression (Golomb et al., 2009) and migraine (Battista et al., 2010).

However, the proposed correlation of this psychophysical effect to centre-surround antagonism in cortical area V5, and the connection with age- or psychiatric-related changes in the GABA inhibitory system, has been criticised on the basis that the evidence to date is circumstantial (Aaen-Stockdale et al., 2009; Wallisch & Kumbhani, 2009).

Chen and colleagues propose that spatial suppression is indeed a consequence of centre-surround antagonism, but that this surround inhibition is not occurring in V5 (Chen, 2011). They argue that the simple gratings or 100% coherent dot stimuli used in previous studies of these effects would primarily activate earlier motion-sensitive areas such as V1, that also show centre-surround antagonism. Rather than use these types of stimuli, they instead used a variable-coherence random dot stimulus. This sort of stimulus requires the involvement of integration and segregation mechanisms found at higher levels of visual cortex, and would result in greater activation of V5. Using this global motion stimulus, Chen et al. tested a group of schizophrenic participants and found that, contrary to previous studies, the influence of the surround was *stronger* in schizophrenics (Chen et al., 2008) not *weaker*, suggesting that these patients have weaker inhibitory mechanisms in early visual cortex, not V5.

The data from migraineurs are also difficult to explain purely on the basis of centre surround interactions in V5. Migraineurs show stronger than normal spatial suppression, rather than the weaker suppression found in depressives and schizophrenics (Battista et al., 2010). This is unexpected considering that one of the dominant theories of migraine proposes that it results from cortical hyperexcitability caused by reduced cortical inhibition, a theory for which there is some physiological (Aurora et al., 2005; Chadaide et al., 2007; Brighina et al., 2009) and psychophysical (Palmer et al., 2000) support. The psychophysical results of Battista et al. using the spatial suppression paradigm (Tadin et al., 2003) would therefore seem to be at odds with the reduced inhibition model of migraine. This contradiction could be resolved if migraine resulted from primary neural hyperexcitability, but it is unclear whether this is the case (Aurora & Wilkinson, 2007; Coppola et al., 2007).

With regard to the weaker spatial suppression reported in older observers (Betts et al., 2005), subsequent studies have failed to replicate this effect (Karas & McKendrick, 2011) and other studies, again using stimuli designed to selectively target V5, have concluded that any motion deficits in older observers are primarily a result of contrast sensitivity loss (Allen et al., 2010). Intrigued by the counterintuitive idea that older observers were performing better than their younger counterparts, we carried out a series of experiments in which we reproduced a "suppressive" effect in younger observers very similar to that of Tadin et al., and we also showed that this effect was absent in older observers, akin to the study of Betts et al. (Aaen-Stockdale et al., 2009). However, we also obtained contrast thresholds for all observers at all stimulus sizes and calculated the suprathreshold contrast for each stimulus. In this analysis, we found that the "suppressive" effect (and its absence in older observers) was entirely predictable from the observer's contrast threshold. This explanation of psychophysical spatial suppression based on low-level visual mechanisms has however been disputed (Glasser & Tadin, 2010).

The prevailing interpretation of psychophysical spatial suppression rests upon the idea that surround-inhibition is weaker at low contrasts. However, induced motion, an illusion in which the motion of a central patch is biased by the motion of its surround – a phenomenon which is almost certainly mediated by centre-surround antagonism – is *stronger* at low contrasts rather than weaker (Hanada, 2010). On the balance of it, whether centre-surround antagonism in V5 is directly to blame for paradoxical psychophysical results or whether other factors are responsible or contribute to the effect remains unresolved.

2.2.2. Perceptual learning

A number of psychophysical studies have demonstrated that specific aspects of motion perception can improve with repeated exposure, a phenomena known as perceptual learning (Fine & Jacobs, 2002). For example, repeated practise of a task that involves discrimination of the motion direction of a field of moving dots, results in significant improvements in task performance (Ball & Sekuler, 1982; Ball & Sekuler, 1987). The fact that such improvements are often highly specific for particular aspects of the trained stimulus such as motion direction and location within the visual field led to the suggestion that learning, and the associated neural plasticity, takes place at a relatively early stage of visual motion processing such as MT. There is additional evidence supporting the idea that MT plays a causal role in perceptual learning of motion tasks. Lesions of MT in monkeys result in an inability to demonstrate perceptual learning for tasks involving the detection of a coherent motion within a random dot kinematogram (Rudolph & Pasternak, 1999). This particular stimulus consists of two populations of moving dots, one moving in a coherent (signal) direction and the other moving in random (noise) directions. The task is to identify the signal direction and task difficulty is manipulated by varying the signal to noise ratio within the stimulus (Newsome & Pare, 1988). In addition, it has been demonstrated psychophysically that perceptual learning of a challenging motion orientation discrimination task is impaired or absent when the ability of MT neurons to encode the motion signal is compromised (Lu et al., 2004). This was achieved by constraining the local motion of pairs of dots within the training stimulus to be equal and opposite. The theory was that this would activate suppressive motion opponent mechanisms within MT (Qian & Andersen, 1994), which would interfere with the global processing of the stimulus and disrupt perceptual learning. In support of this concept, it was subsequently found that while the motion opponent stimulus impaired learning, simply removing the motion opponency from the stimulus by altering the phase of local dot motions resulted in pronounced perceptual learning (Thompson & Liu, 2006). It has also been reported that patients who have hemianopia due to V1 lesions that do not extend to MT are able to learn a motion coherence task in their blind hemifield (Huxlin et al., 2009). This raises the intriguing possibility that V1 may not be necessary for perceptual learning of specific types of motion stimuli.

It would appear, therefore, that MT is centrally involved in perceptual learning of motion-based tasks. However, the available neurophysiological data, collected using random dot kinematogram stimuli, do not directly support the hypothesis that perceptual learning leads to long-term plastic changes within MT. For example, Zohary et al (1994), found that neurons within MT and MST narrowed their directional tuning and increased their firing rate as monkeys improved their performance on a motion coherence task *within* a single training session. However these changes did not persist *across* multiple training sessions. More recent neurophysiological work, also in monkeys, has implicated the lateral intraparietal area in perceptual learning of coherent motion perception (Law & Gold, 2008). This suggests that perceptual learning of specific types of motion stimuli may rely on changes in the way that the responses of cells within MT are 'read out' by higher level extrastriate areas. Whether this is the case for the human brain and for other types of motion tasks is yet to be established.

2.3. Complex motion analysis – the middle superior temporal area (MST) and V6

Still higher cortical areas respond to *complex motion* signals such as global expansion, contraction and rotation. These types of motion are particularly interesting, because they are generated by the interaction between an observer and the environment. For example, radial patterns of motion such as expansion and contraction occur on the retina when objects approach or recede from an observer, respectively. These patterns of motion could be caused by motion of the object, the head and body or both. Similarly, rotational patterns of motion can be caused either by tilting of the head or physical rotation of an object. In other words, neurons selective for these motion patterns could encode "optic flow" and allow us to navigate in the world (Gibson, 1950).

Physiological work has shown that the medial superior temporal area, MST (Saito et al., 1986; Tanaka et al., 1986; Tanaka et al., 1989; Tanaka & Saito, 1989; Duffy & Wurtz, 1991b; Duffy & Wurtz, 1991a; Britten & van Wezel, 1998) is selective for such translational, radial and rotational motion patterns over wide areas of the visual field. Neuroimaging has demonstrated the presence of a human homologue of MST in what has become known as the hMT+ complex or V5, which also includes area MT (Morrone et al., 2000; Dukelow et al., 2001; Huk et al., 2002). The extraction of patterns of complex motion such as radial and rotational motion, has been modelled from the combined outputs of MT neurons (Perrone, 1992; Grossberg et al., 1999). Recently, a second visual area responsive to wide-angle flow fields has been identified (Pitzalis et al., 2010) and is thought to be a homologue of macaque area V6 (Galletti et al., 1996). Although most work on optic flow has concentrated on area MST, neurons in this second region have many similar characteristics and the two areas are strongly connected. Pitzalis et al. propose that MST and V6 work in concert, the former analysing the motions of objects in the world and the latter extracting self-motion.

Whether MST neurons are responsive to only the cardinal motion directions (radial, rotational and translational) as suggested by some psychophysical work (Morrone et al., 1999; Burr et al., 2001), or whether other intermediate forms of motion such as spiral motion are encoded directly, is still a matter of some debate. In support of the direct detection of spiral motions, it has been suggested that summation of mechanisms tuned to purely cardinal motion directions is insufficient to explain the psychophysical data (Snowden & Milne, 1996; Meese & Harris, 2001; Meese & Anderson, 2002) and some physiological work seems to have identified neurons tuned to spiral motions (Graziano et al., 1994; Geesaman & Andersen, 1996). A particularly interesting study found that continuously-changing flow stimuli, obtained by morphing one flow field into the next, lead to a continuum of responses in MST (Paolini et al., 2000). This supports the "generalised spiral" model of MST, in which the tuning of MST neurons is a continuum from pure contraction, though clockwise-contraction, to clockwise-rotation, to clockwise-expansion, to pure expansion, and so on.

2.4. Biological motion perception – the superior temporal sulcus (STS)

Human observers are acutely sensitive to the complex pattern of motion trajectories generated by other people and animals known as biological motion (Johansson, 1973; Mather & West, 1993). Investigations of biological motion often use stimuli constructed from dots or "point lights" that represent the joints of an actor (Troje, 2002). When stationary, these displays appear as an elongated group of dots, however when set in motion, a vivid percept of a person moving is generated. Sufficient information can be extracted from dynamic point light stimuli to allow for identification of a wide range of complex attributes such as gender (Mather & Murdoch, 1994) and mood (Dittrich et al., 1996), and observers are sensitive to these stimuli in both the central and peripheral visual field (Thompson et al., 2007). Although point light stimuli contain both motion information and configural, form-based cues (the relative position of the points), motion cues do appear to be centrally involved in the processing of biological motion. For example, observers can still perform above chance on a walking direction discriminating task when the relative positions of each of the dots representing the joints of an actor are scrambled (Troje & Westhoff, 2006). Interestingly, simply inverting the dots representing the feet of walking humans or animals disrupts discrimination of walking direction suggesting that the characteristic local motion cues specific to biological motion, may be processed by dedicated "life detector" mechanisms (Troje & Westhoff, 2006).

Initial insights into the regions of the visual cortex involved in biological motion perception were provided by the neurophysiological investigations of Oram and Perrett (1994) in the monkey. Cells were found within the superior temporal polysensory area, a region anterior to MT and MST within the superior temporal sulcus, that were sensitive to biological motion stimuli. Subsequently, a large number of neuroimagaing studies have been conducted in humans with the aim of identifying the cortical areas involved in biological motion perception. It is now apparent that biological motion perception recruits a distributed neural circuit in humans which includes the posterior region of the superior temporal sulcus (Grossman et al., 2000; Grezes et al., 2001; Servos et al., 2002; Grossman et al., 2005; Pelphrey et al., 2005; Peelen et al., 2006) and may also involve "mirror neurons" in the ventral premotor cortex (Saygin et al., 2004) along with a range of additional visual areas including the posterior middle temporal gyrus and regions known as the extrastriate and fusiform body areas (Jastorff & Orban, 2009). A recent meta-analysis of neuroimaging data in humans has emphasised the importance of the pSTS in processing motion cues from biological motion stimuli and also identified a region within the hMT+ complex that may play a role in the perception of human body movement (Grosbras et al., 2012).

2.5. Structure-from-motion – the lateral occipital sulcus (LOS) and the intraparietal sulcus (IPS)

As well as being able to extract biologically relevant information from motion patterns, the visual system is also able to extract three-dimensional (3D) structure from moving two-dimensional stimuli, often referred to as the "kinetic depth effect" or "structure-from-motion" (SFM) (Wallach & O'Connell, 1953). Several models have been developed to explain how the visual system achieves this remarkable feat, some based on the tracking of local positional cues (Ullman, 1984; Grzywacz & Hildreth, 1987; Shariat & Price, 1990; Snowden et al., 1991) and others based on the use of local motion information (Clocksin, 1980; Longuet-Higgins & Prazdny, 1980; Koenderink & van Doorn, 1986; Husain et al., 1989; Hildreth et al., 1995). The weight of evidence currently seems to suggest that motion rather than positional information is crucial to extracting SFM (Andersen & Bradley, 1998; Farivar, 2009; Farivar et al., 2009).

SFM is usually investigated by using random dot stimuli in which the dots are randomly distributed across the image, but are projected onto an "invisible" object, which is then rotated with the direction and speed of the dots being dictated by their position on the object. Provided that the dot density is high enough, SFM can be perceived with very short, two-frame displays in which dots simply jump from one position to another (Lappin et al., 1980). SFM is not perceived if a very small number of dots are used. However, periodically re-positioning a similarly small number of dots across the stimulus, allows the surface of the object to be reconstructed via interpolation (Husain et al., 1989; Treue et al., 1995). Functional magnetic resonance imaging (fMRI) suggests that SFM is carried out in a network of cortical regions: V5, lateral occipital sulcus (LOS) and several sites along the intraparietal sulcus (IPS) (Orban et al., 1999; Peuskens et al., 2004).

3. Second-order motion

The preceding discussion has dealt mainly with the processing of luminance-based motion, often called *first-order* motion. However, at the input stage, motion can also be defined by characteristics other than luminance, such as flicker, texture and contrast. To return to our snowfield example, the force and direction of the wind or the presence of a small animal burrowing under the snow can be detected visually by detecting changes in the pattern of random flicker caused as flakes of snow on the ground are disturbed. Motion that is defined by modulation of a property other than luminance is referred to as *second-order* motion

(Cavanagh & Mather, 1989) and second-order motion is invisible to first-order, i.e. luminance-based, motion sensors (Chubb & Sperling, 1988).

3.1. Local second-order motion

Currently, it is a mystery how the visual system detects second-order motion, as the primary input to the visual system represents changes in retinal illumination. The visual system has a small compressive non-linearity, probably at the level of the photoreceptors (Scott-Samuel & Georgeson, 1999) that could transform second-order information into a weak luminance signal. This weak *internal* artefact could mean that second-order motion is actually detected by first-order mechanisms and could explain the (usually) weaker performance for purely second-order motion stimuli. However, the distortion product measured by Scott-Samuel & Georgeson is only detectable in high speed, high contrast modulation stimuli. Since second-order motion is still visible in slow moving, or low-modulation, stimuli, the early non-linearity is unlikely to be able to fully explain many of the experimental results. Figure 3 shows a schematic wiring diagram of the motion processing hierarchy and the dotted orange arrow shows the presence of these "pseudo-second-order" motion signals.

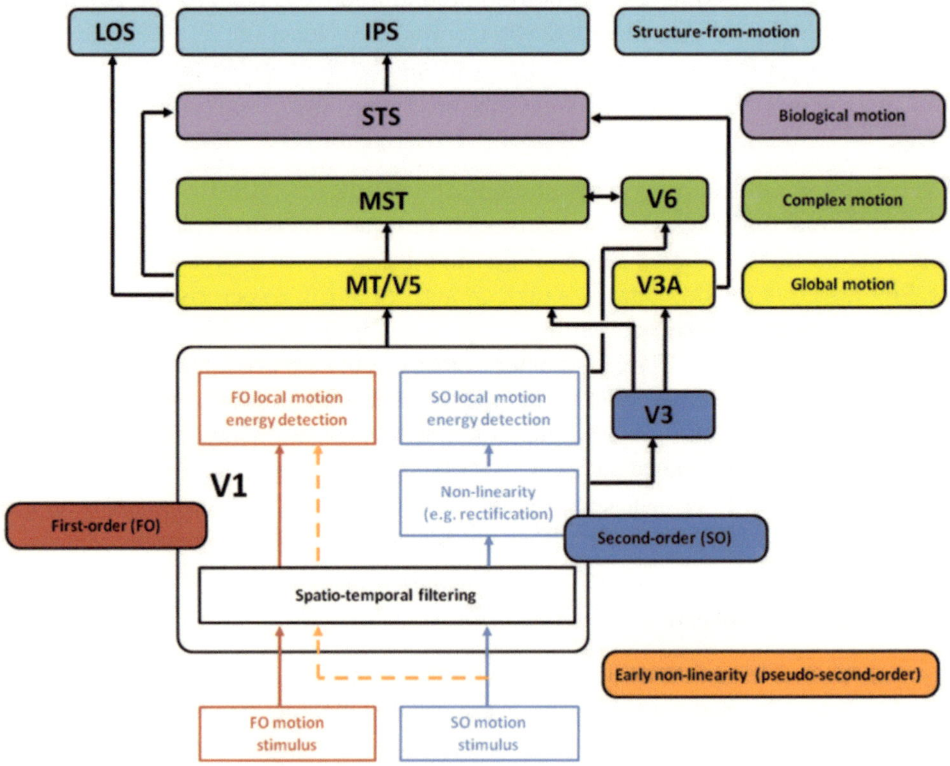

Figure 3. A schematic view of the orthodox model of motion processing in the cortex. FO = first order, SO = second order, MT = middle temporal visual area, MST middle superior temporal visual area, STS = superior temporal sulcus, IPS = intraparietal sulcus, LOS = lateral occipital sulcus. See text for further details.

If second-order motion was ultimately detected by first-order mechanisms, we might expect the two types of stimuli to interact. This does not seem to be the case for local motion. Temporally interleaving first- and second-order stimuli in alternate frames of a motion stimulus fails to generate the percept of smooth motion, suggesting that the two systems do not interact at this level (Ledgeway & Smith, 1994). Adaptation to one type of motion does not impair detection of the other type (Nishida et al., 1997), and the second-order system does not seem to be able to discriminate the direction of motion at detection threshold, unlike the first-order system (Smith & Ledgeway, 1997), which can discriminate motion direction as soon as motion is detected. It is therefore likely that first- and second-order motion are initially analysed in parallel by separate processing streams (shown in figure 3 in red and blue, respectively).

Several neuroimaging studies have investigated the possibility that some cortical areas may be selective for second order motion, as predicted by the dual-pathway hypothesis. To date, however, the results from these studies have been mixed. Second-order specific responses have been reported in areas such as V3 (Smith et al., 1998), but other studies have found either substantial overlap of first and second-order motion responses throughout the visual cortex (Dumoulin et al., 2003) or no anatomical segregation of areas responsive to first- and second-order motion (Nishida et al., 2003; Seiffert et al., 2003; Ashida et al., 2007). The idea of an anatomically distinct second-order pathway may be rescued if different neurons in the same anatomical area responded selectively to different types of motion, or if the same neurons responded to both first- and second-order motion, but had different spatial/temporal tuning for first-order motion than for second-order motion. This latter contention is supported by some neurophysiological investigations of MT in the primate (O'Keefe & Movshon, 1998) and areas 17 and 18 in the cat (Mareschal & Baker, 1998). However, the idea that different neuronal populations for first- and second-order motion exist, but share common anatomical locations has also found support in a human neuroimaging study using fMRI adaptation (Ashida et al., 2007). In this technique, repeated presentation of similar stimuli causes a reduction of the blood oxygen level–dependent (BOLD) response in cortical regions containing neurons that cannot differentiate between the stimuli, whereas little or no reduction occurs if the different stimuli activate distinct populations of neurons. Ashida et al. found direction-selective fMRI adaptation for stimuli of the same type, but no cross-adaptation between first- and second-order motion. These fMRI results provide persuasive evidence that neural populations differentially selective for first- and second-order motion co-exist in motion sensitive regions of the human brain such as V3a, MT and MST.

3.2. Higher level second-order motion

Assuming segregation of first- and second-order motion at early stages of visual motion processing, at what point in the visual motion hierarchy are the two types of motion combined? Models of the mammalian visual motion processing hierarchy (Wilson et al., 1992; Lu & Sperling, 1995; Lu & Sperling, 2001) usually integrate first- and second-order streams at, or before, the level of global motion analysis (see Figure 3) and insensitivity to such low-level stimulus characteristics, termed "cue-invariance", has been found in neurons at the level of MT (Albright, 1992; O'Keefe & Movshon, 1998) and MST (Geesaman & Andersen, 1996). The argument that extrastriate areas are cue-invariant has also been supported by a TMS study in humans (Cowey et al., 2006).

There is, however, plenty of counter-evidence to the presence of cue-invariance at MT and MST in the physiological literature (Olavarria et al., 1992; Churan & Ilg, 2001) and some human psychophysical studies have suggested that the two processing streams could remain segregated at even higher levels than MT. For example, Badcock and colleagues have shown that the addition of second-order noise dots to either a first-order global motion stimulus or complex motion stimulus does not impair detection and discrimination of the first-order signal (Edwards & Badcock, 1995; Badcock & Khuu, 2001; Cassanello et al., 2011). Several studies have suggested that the contribution of the second-order pathway to mechanisms responsible for extraction of structure-from-motion is weak or non-existent (Dosher et al., 1989; Mather, 1989; Landy et al., 1991; Hess & Ziegler, 2000), while research on whether second-order motion can support biological motion has produced differing results (Mather et al., 1992; Ahlstrom et al., 1997; Bellefeuille & Faubert, 1998).

Although these findings are certainly of interest, it seems counterintuitive that the visual system would maintain two separate pathways for the analysis of different types of high-level motion stimuli that differ only in terms of their local characteristics. Some recent studies by ourselves and our collaborators support the conventional concept of a functional integration of first- and second-order motion at higher levels of the motion hierarchy. Ledgeway, et al. (2002) and Aaen-Stockdale et al. (forthcoming) have argued that the relative visibility of the first- and second-order dots in the stimuli used by Badcock and colleagues may not have been equalised (Edwards & Badcock, 1995; Badcock & Khuu, 2001). Although the *static* first- and second-order dots were highly visible, their relative visibility to first- or second-order motion sensors (which have different spatio-temporal characteristics) (Derrington et al., 1993; Ledgeway & Hess, 2002) may not have been equal. Ledgeway, Hess & McGraw (2002) demonstrated that reducing the visibility of the luminance-modulated (first-order) dots resulted in interactions between first- and second-order dots in global motion stimuli consistent with a combination of the two motion cues within extrastriate visual areas. Aaen-Stockdale et al. (forthcoming) showed that these visibility-dependent interactions also occurred with complex (radial and rotational) motion stimuli and that weakening the first-order signal by increasing the size of dot displacements between frames resulted in similar interactions. This latter study also pitted opposing first- and second-order motion signals against each other to demonstrate that impairments of first-order motion discrimination caused by the inclusion of second-order dots within the stimulus was genuinely a result of a cue-invariant motion system attempting to integrate these separate signals, and not simply the result of increased noise. Subsequent work by us has used these same techniques to show that other types of higher-order motion perception are similarly cue-invariant. For example we (Aaen-Stockdale, et al., 2008) found that when relative stimulus visibility was varied, first- and second-order elements interacted to mask biological motion of the opposite class suggesting that biological motion perception is cue invariant. Similarly, it had been proposed that the contribution of the second-order pathway to structure-from-motion mechanisms was weak or non-existent (Dosher et al., 1989; Mather, 1989; Landy et al., 1991; Hess & Ziegler, 2000), but reducing the relative visibility of the first-order elements in structure-from-motion displays results in almost linear summation between first- and second-order mechanisms, suggesting that this modality may also be cue-invariant (Aaen-Stockdale et al., 2010). These findings have highlighted the importance of ensuring that local first-order and second-order motion signals are of equal strength when comparing the two systems.

4. Abnormalities of motion processing

4.1. Akinetopsia

The first widely accepted report of akinetopsia or "motion blindness" due to bilateral lesions affecting the hMT+ complex but sparing the primary visual cortex, was reported by Zihl and colleagues (Zihl et al., 1983; Zeki, 1991). This patient, LM, did not have a scotoma (region of blindness) as would be expected from damage to the primary visual cortex; however LM exhibited a severe and selective impairment of motion perception. Subsequent work with this patient indicated that LM could perceive motion direction and structure from motion under certain circumstances as long as the stimuli did not contain noise elements such as static or randomly moving dots. However, as soon as noise was introduced into the stimulus, task performance was dramatically reduced (Baker et al., 1991; Rizzo et al., 1995). This pattern of deficits is similar to that reported by Rudolph and Pasternak (Rudolph & Pasternak, 1999) who studied the effects of MT lesions in macaque monkeys. Immediately after the lesions the animals exhibited a pronounced and general impairment in motion perception. However, over time, performance on motion tasks that did not include noise elements recovered, whereas performance for tasks requiring signal/noise segregation, such as those involving RDKs, did not recover. As a whole, these data from both humans and primates suggest that MT and MST may have a particular specialization for the detection of motion in a noisy environment.

4.2. A motion deficit in amblyopia?

Deficits in motion perception have also been reported for patients with a developmental disorder of the visual cortex known as amblyopia (or "lazy eye"). Unilateral amblyopia occurs when the images seen by each eye are poorly correlated during early visual development due to a chronically blurred image in one eye (anisometropia), a turned eye (strabismus) or less commonly a congenital cataract (Holmes & Clarke, 2006). This can result in abnormal development of the visual cortex and a visual impairment in the affected eye that is not due to a problem with eye itself, but is the result of abnormal processing of inputs from the amblyopic eye within the visual cortex (Hubel & Wiesel, 1965; Barnes et al., 2001) and possibly the lateral geniculate nucleus (Hess et al., 2009; Li et al., 2011).

Although amblyopia is typically regarded as a disorder of spatial vision, a number of studies have identified deficits in motion perception that appear to be independent of impairments of form perception (see Thompson et al., 2011 for a recent overview). Many of the motion deficits that have been reported are consistent with abnormalities at the level of hMT+ complex. For example, patients with amblyopia exhibit elevated motion coherence thresholds when viewing random dot kinematograms, even when abnormal contrast sensitivity is taken into account (Simmers et al., 2003; Constantinescu et al., 2005; Simmers et al., 2006). These deficits are present across spatial scale (Aaen-Stockdale & Hess, 2008), include both first- and second-order motion stimuli (Aaen-Stockdale et al., 2007), may involve deficits in spatial summation (Thompson et al., 2011) and appear to be related to the segregation of signal from noise (Mansouri & Hess, 2006; Thompson et al., 2008b). In agreement with these psychophysical findings, it has recently been reported that cells within MT of monkeys made experimentally strabismic are less direction selective and less tolerant of noise (El-Shamayleh et al., 2011). It would appear, therefore, that motion sensitive areas such as MT are susceptible to abnormal sensory experience during development and that this can result in specific deficits in motion perception.

In this context we were surprised to find that patients with amblyopia did not show pronounced impairments in the perception of coherent plaid stimuli (Thompson et al., 2008a). As described above, plaid stimuli have been used extensively to investigate the integration of local motion signals within the visual cortex and cells have been found within MT that respond selectively to the integrated "pattern motion" direction of coherent plaids. We therefore expected to find reduced levels of coherent motion perception in patients with amblyopia as would be predicted by deficient processing within MT. In contrast to this we found that within the small region of the parameter space where amblyopes did exhibit differences from controls, these differences were characterised by an increased probability of coherent motion perception (Thompson et al., 2008a). Since a similar change in plaid perception can be induced in the normal visual system when inhibitory rTMS is delivered over V1 (Thompson et al., 2009) (figure 2), the differences between amblyopic observers and controls in plaid perception may be due to abnormal processing within V1 rather than MT.

This seemingly anomalous result has recently been further explored using fMRI (Thompson et al., 2012). Coherent and incoherent plaid stimuli that were perceived in exactly the same way by control observers and amblyopes, activated distinct networks of brain areas when the plaids were viewed by non-amblyopic eyes vs. amblyopic eyes. For controls and patients viewing through their non-amblyopic eye, the hMT+ complex was differentially activated by coherent and incoherent plaids consistent with previous fMRI studies (Castelo-Branco et al., 2002) and the idea that this area is centrally involved in motion integration. However this was not the case for amblyopic eye viewing for which there appeared to be a selective loss of response within hMT+ to incoherent plaid motion. In patients for whom the hMT+ complex could be subdivided into MT and MST, this loss was apparent in both areas. It would appear, therefore, that areas other than hMT+ were involved in the normal perception of plaid patterns for amblyopic eye viewing. The fMRI data provided preliminary evidence for a preserved response to incoherent motion within the pulvinar complex of the patients with amblyopia. This area has previously been shown to be involved in the processing of pattern motion (Merabet et al., 1998; Villeneuve et al., 2005) and has extensive reciprocal connections with extrastriate brain areas including MT (Casanova, 2004). These results in humans with amblyopia raise the intriguing possibility that alternate brain areas may play a role in motion perception if the function of hMT+ is sub-optimal or compromised. If this were to be the case, the current psychophysical data from patients with amblyopia and both humans and monkeys with MT lesions (described above) imply that this compensatory processing is highly sensitive to noise such as the random dots present in RDK stimuli.

5. Conclusion

The cortical mechanisms involved in the perception of visual motion represent one of the most widely studied and well-understood processes in neuroscience, however there are still many questions left to answer. Over the last few decades a picture has emerged of a motion processing system that is rigidly hierarchical, yet possesses considerable redundancy, and plasticity. In general terms, progressively higher-level areas of the brain integrate the outputs of areas below them in order to detect and discriminate increasingly complicated stimuli. However, with apologies to the Reverend William Paley, the visual brain is not an organ that has been designed, but one that has evolved over the millennia, and which demonstrates all the adaptations and redundancies that implies. A very much open question relates to the evolutionary origins of specialised forms of motion perception, such as second-order motion, structure-from-motion or biological motion; assuming that there actually are dedicated mechanisms for these type of motion, a question which is by no means settled.

Author details

Craig Aaen-Stockdale
Department of Optometry and Visual Science, Buskerud University College, Norway

Benjamin Thompson
Department of Optometry and Vision Science, University of Auckland, New Zealand

Acknowledgement

Craig Aaen-Stockdale is supported by an *Yggdrasil* international mobility grant from the Research Council of Norway (*Forskningsrådet*). Benjamin Thompson is supported by grants from the Health Research Council of New Zealand, the Marsden Fund, the University of Auckland and the Neurological Foundation of New Zealand.

6. References

Aaen-Stockdale, C. & Hess, R.F. (2008). The amblyopic deficit for global motion is spatial scale invariant. *Vision Res, 48* (19), 1965-1971.

Aaen-Stockdale, C., Ledgeway, T., & Hess, R.F. (2007). Second-order optic flow deficits in amblyopia. *Invest Ophthalmol Vis Sci, 48* (12), 5532-5538.

Aaen-Stockdale, C.R., Farivar, R., & Hess, R.F. (2010). Co-operative interactions between first- and second-order mechanisms in the processing of structure from motion *Journal of Vision, 10* (13), 6.

Aaen-Stockdale, C.R., Ledgeway, T., McGraw, P.V., & Hess, R.F. (forthcoming). Integration of first- and second-order motion at, above and beyond MT/V5. *Vision Research,*

Aaen-Stockdale, C.R., Thompson, B., Hess, R.F., & Troje, N.F. (2008). Biological motion perception is cue-invariant. *Journal of Vision, 8* (8), 6.

Aaen-Stockdale, C.R., Thompson, B., Huang, P.C., & Hess, R.F. (2009). Low-level mechanisms may contribute to paradoxical motion percepts. *Journal of Vision, 9* (5)

Adelson, E.H. & Bergen, J.R. (1985). Spatiotemporal energy models for the perception of motion. *J Opt Soc Am A, 2* (2), 284-299.

Adelson, E.H. & Movshon, J.A. (1982). Phenomenal coherence of moving visual patterns. *Nature, 300* (5892), 523-525.

Ahlstrom, V., Blake, R., & Ahlstrom, U. (1997). Perception of biological motion. *Perception, 26* (12), 1539-1548.

Alais, D., Burke, D., & Wenderoth, P. (1996). Further evidence for monocular determinants of perceived plaid direction. *Vision Res, 36* (9), 1247-1253.

Alais, D., Wenderoth, P., & Burke, D. (1994). The contribution of one-dimensional motion mechanisms to the perceived direction of drifting plaids and their after effects. *Vision Res, 34* (14), 1823-1834.

Alais, D., Wenderoth, P., & Burke, D. (1997). The size and number of plaid blobs mediate the misperception of type-ii plaid direction. *Vision Res, 37* (1), 143-150.

Albright, T.D. (1992). Form-cue invariant motion processing in primate visual cortex. *Science, 255* (5048), 1141-1143.

Allen, H.A., Hutchinson, C.V., Ledgeway, T., & Gayle, P. (2010). The role of contrast sensitivity in global motion processing deficits in the elderly. *J Vis, 10* (10), 15.

Allman, J., Miezin, F., & McGuinness, E. (1985). Direction- and velocity-specific responses from beyond the classical receptive field in the middle temporal visual area (MT). *Perception, 14* (2), 105-126.

Andersen, R.A. & Bradley, D.C. (1998). Perception of three-dimensional structure-from-motion. *Trends in Cognitive Sciences, 2* (6), 222-228.

Ashida, H., Lingnau, A., Wall, M.B., & Smith, A.T. (2007). fMRI adaptation reveals separate mechanisms for first-order and second-order motion. *J Neurophysiol, 97* (2), 1319-1325.

Aurora, S.K., Barrodale, P., Chronicle, E.P., & Mulleners, W.M. (2005). Cortical inhibition is reduced in chronic and episodic migraine and demonstrates a spectrum of illness. *Headache, 45* (5), 546-552.

Aurora, S.K. & Wilkinson, F. (2007). The brain is hyperexcitable in migraine. *Cephalalgia, 27* (12), 1442-1453.

Badcock, D.R. & Khuu, S.K. (2001). Independent first- and second-order motion energy analyses of optic flow. *Psychol Res, 65* (1), 50-56.

Baker, C.L., Jr., Hess, R.F., & Zihl, J. (1991). Residual motion perception in a "motion-blind" patient, assessed with limited-lifetime random dot stimuli. *J Neurosci, 11* (2), 454-461.

Ball, K. & Sekuler, R. (1982). A specific and enduring improvement in visual motion discrimination. *Science, 218* (4573), 697-698.

Ball, K. & Sekuler, R. (1987). Direction-specific improvement in motion discrimination. *Vision Res, 27* (6), 953-965.

Barlow, H.B. & Levick, W.R. (1965). The mechanism of directionally selective units in rabbit's retina. *J Physiol, 178* (3), 477-504.

Barnes, G.R., Hess, R.F., Dumoulin, S.O., Achtman, R.L., & Pike, G.B. (2001). The cortical deficit in humans with strabismic amblyopia. *J Physiol, 533* (Pt 1), 281-297.

Battista, J., Badcock, D.R., & McKendrick, A.M. (2010). Centre-surround visual motion processing in migraine. *Investigative Ophthalmology & Visual Science, 51* (11), 6070-6076.

Beckers, G. & Zeki, S. (1995). The consequences of inactivating areas V1 and V5 on visual motion perception. *Brain, 118 (Pt 1)*, 49-60.

Bellefeuille, A. & Faubert, J. (1998). Independence of contour and biological-motion cues for motion-defined animal shapes. *Perception, 27* (2), 225-235.

Betts, L.R., Taylor, C.P., Sekuler, A.B., & Bennett, P.J. (2005). Aging reduces center-surround antagonism in visual motion processing. *Neuron, 45* (3), 361-366.

Braddick, O.J., O'Brien, J.M., Wattam-Bell, J., Atkinson, J., Hartley, T., & Turner, R. (2001). Brain areas sensitive to coherent visual motion. *Perception, 30* (1), 61-72.

Brighina, F., Palermo, A., & Fierro, B. (2009). Cortical inhibition and habituation to evoked potentials: Relevance for pathophysiology of migraine. *J Headache Pain, 10* (2), 77-84.

Britten, K.H. & van Wezel, R.J. (1998). Electrical microstimulation of cortical area MST biases heading perception in monkeys. *Nat Neurosci, 1* (1), 59-63.

Burr, D.C., Badcock, D.R., & Ross, J. (2001). Cardinal axes for radial and circular motion, revealed by summation and by masking. *Vision Res, 41* (4), 473-481.

Burr, D.C. & Thompson, P. (2011). Motion psychophysics: 1985-2010. *Vision Res, 51* (13), 1431-1456.

Campbell, F.W. & Robson, J.G. (1968). Application of fourier analysis to the visibility of gratings. *J Physiol, 197* (3), 551-566.

Casanova, C. (2004). The visual functions of the pulvinar. In: L.M. Chalupa & J.S. Werner (Eds.), *The Visual Neurosciences* (pp. 592-608). Cambridge, USA: The MIT Press.

Cassanello, C.R., Edwards, M., Badcock, D.R., & Nishida, S. (2011). No interaction of first- and second-order signals in the extraction of global-motion and optic-flow. *Vision Res, 51* (3), 352-361.

Castelo-Branco, M., Formisano, E., Backes, W., Zanella, F., Neuenschwander, S., Singer, W., & Goebel, R. (2002). Activity patterns in human motion-sensitive areas depend on the interpretation of global motion. *Proc Natl Acad Sci U S A, 99* (21), 13914-13919.

Cavanagh, P. & Mather, G. (1989). Motion: The long and short of it. *Spat Vis, 4* (2-3), 103-129.

Chadaide, Z., Arlt, S., Antal, A., Nitsche, M.A., Lang, N., & Paulus, W. (2007). Transcranial direct current stimulation reveals inhibitory deficiency in migraine. *Cephalalgia, 27* (7), 833-839.

Chen, Y. (2011). Abnormal visual motion processing in schizophrenia: A review of research progress. *Schizophr Bull, 37* (4), 709-715.

Chen, Y., Norton, D., & Ongur, D. (2008). Altered center-surround motion inhibition in schizophrenia. *Biol Psychiatry, 64* (1), 74-77.

Chubb, C. & Sperling, G. (1988). Drift-balanced random stimuli: A general basis for studying non-fourier motion perception. *J Opt Soc Am A, 5* (11), 1986-2007.

Churan, J. & Ilg, U.J. (2001). Processing of second-order motion stimuli in primate middle temporal area and medial superior temporal area. *J Opt Soc Am A Opt Image Sci Vis, 18* (9), 2297-2306.

Clocksin, W.F. (1980). Perception of surface slant and edge labels from optical flow: A computational approach. *Perception, 9* (3), 253-269.

Constantinescu, T., Schmidt, L., Watson, R., & Hess, R.F. (2005). A residual deficit for global motion processing after acuity recovery in deprivation amblyopia. *Invest Ophthalmol Vis Sci, 46* (8), 3008-3012.

Coppola, G., Pierelli, F., & Schoenen, J. (2007). Is the cerebral cortex hyperexcitable or hyperresponsive in migraine? *Cephalalgia, 27* (12), 1427-1439.

Cowey, A., Campana, G., Walsh, V., & Vaina, L.M. (2006). The role of human extra-striate visual areas V5/MT and V2/V3 in the perception of the direction of global motion: A transcranial magnetic stimulation study. *Exp Brain Res, 171* (4), 558-562.

de Haan, E.H. & Cowey, A. (2011). On the usefulness of 'what' and 'where' pathways in vision. *Trends Cogn Sci, 15* (10), 460-466.

Derrington, A.M. & Badcock, D.R. (1992). Two-stage analysis of the motion of 2-dimensional patterns, what is the first stage? *Vision Res, 32* (4), 691-698.

Derrington, A.M., Badcock, D.R., & Henning, G.B. (1993). Discriminating the direction of second-order motion at short stimulus durations. *Vision Res, 33* (13), 1785-1794.

Derrington, A.M. & Lennie, P. (1984). Spatial and temporal contrast sensitivities of neurones in lateral geniculate nucleus of macaque. *J Physiol, 357*, 219-240.

Dittrich, W.H., Troscianko, T., Lea, S.E., & Morgan, D. (1996). Perception of emotion from dynamic point-light displays represented in dance. *Perception, 25* (6), 727-738.

Dosher, B.A., Landy, M.S., & Sperling, G. (1989). Kinetic depth effect and optic flow--I. 3D shape from fourier motion. *Vision Res, 29* (12), 1789-1813.

Duffy, C.J. & Wurtz, R.H. (1991a). Sensitivity of MST neurons to optic flow stimuli. I. A continuum of response selectivity to large-field stimuli. *J Neurophysiol, 65* (6), 1329-1345.

Duffy, C.J. & Wurtz, R.H. (1991b). Sensitivity of mst neurons to optic flow stimuli. II. Mechanisms of response selectivity revealed by small-field stimuli. *J Neurophysiol, 65* (6), 1346-1359.

Dukelow, S.P., DeSouza, J.F., Culham, J.C., van den Berg, A.V., Menon, R.S., & Vilis, T. (2001). Distinguishing subregions of the human MT+ complex using visual fields and pursuit eye movements. *J Neurophysiol, 86* (4), 1991-2000.

Dumoulin, S.O., Baker, C.L., Jr., Hess, R.F., & Evans, A.C. (2003). Cortical specialization for processing first- and second-order motion. *Cereb Cortex, 13* (12), 1375-1385.

Edwards, M. & Badcock, D.R. (1995). Global motion perception: No interaction between the first- and second-order motion pathways. *Vision Res, 35* (18), 2589-2602.

El-Shamayleh, Y., Kiorpes, L., Kohn, A., & Movshon, J.A. (2011). Visual motion processing by neurons in area MT of macaque monkeys with experimental amblyopia. *J Neurosci, 30* (36), 12198-12209.

Farivar, R. (2009). Dorsal-ventral integration in object recognition. *Brain Res Rev,*

Farivar, R., Blanke, O., & Chaudhuri, A. (2009). Dorsal-ventral integration in the recognition of motion-defined unfamiliar faces. *J Neurosci, 29* (16), 5336-5342.

Ferrera, V.P. & Wilson, H.R. (1990). Perceived direction of moving two-dimensional patterns. *Vision Res, 30* (2), 273-287.

Fine, I. & Jacobs, R.A. (2002). Comparing perceptual learning tasks: A review. *J Vis, 2* (2), 190-203.

Galletti, C., Fattori, P., Battaglini, P.P., Shipp, S., & Zeki, S. (1996). Functional demarcation of a border between areas V6 and V6a in the superior parietal gyrus of the macaque monkey. *Eur J Neurosci, 8* (1), 30-52.

Geesaman, B.J. & Andersen, R.A. (1996). The analysis of complex motion patterns by form/cue invariant MSTd neurons. *J Neurosci, 16* (15), 4716-4732.

Gibson, J.J. (1950). Perception of the visual world. Boston: Houghton Mifflin.

Glasser, D.M. & Tadin, D. (2010). Low-level mechanisms do not explain paradoxical motion percepts. *J Vis, 10* (4), 20 21-29.

Golomb, J.D., Beck, J.R., Ruf, B.M., Chen, J.I., Saricicek, A., Maloney, K.H., Hu, J., Chun, M.M., & Bhagwagar, Z. (2009). Enhanced visual motion processing in major depressive disorder. *Journal of Neuroscience, 29* (28), 9072-9077.

Goodale, M.A. & Milner, A.D. (1992). Separate visual pathways for perception and action. *Trends Neurosci, 15* (1), 20-25.

Graziano, M.S., Andersen, R.A., & Snowden, R.J. (1994). Tuning of MST neurons to spiral motions. *J Neurosci, 14* (1), 54-67.

Grezes, J., Fonlupt, P., Bertenthal, B., Delon-Martin, C., Segebarth, C., & Decety, J. (2001). Does perception of biological motion rely on specific brain regions? *Neuroimage, 13* (5), 775-785.

Grosbras, M.H., Beaton, S., & Eickhoff, S.B. (2012). Brain regions involved in human movement perception: A quantitative voxel-based meta-analysis. *Hum Brain Mapp, 33* (2), 431-454.

Grossberg, S., Mingolla, E., & Pack, C. (1999). A neural model of motion processing and visual navigation by cortical area MST. *Cereb Cortex, 9* (8), 878-895.

Grossman, E.D., Battelli, L., & Pascual-Leone, A. (2005). Repetitive TMS over posterior STS disrupts perception of biological motion. *Vision Res, 45* (22), 2847-2853.

Grossman, E.D., Donnelly, M., Price, R., Pickens, D., Morgan, V., Neighbor, G., & Blake, R. (2000). Brain areas involved in perception of biological motion. *J Cogn Neurosci, 12* (5), 711-720.

Grzywacz, N.M. & Hildreth, E.C. (1987). Incremental rigidity scheme for recovering structure from motion: Position-based versus velocity-based formulations. *J Opt Soc Am A, 4* (3), 503-518.

Hanada, M. (2010). Differential effect of luminance contrast reduction and noise on motion induction. *Perception, 39* (11), 1452-1465.

Heeger, D.J., Boynton, G.M., Demb, J.B., Seidemann, E., & Newsome, W.T. (1999). Motion opponency in visual cortex. *J Neurosci, 19* (16), 7162-7174.

Hess, R.F., Thompson, B., Gole, G., & Mullen, K.T. (2009). Deficient responses from the lateral geniculate nucleus in humans with amblyopia. *Eur J Neurosci, 29* (5), 1064-1070.

Hess, R.F. & Ziegler, L.R. (2000). What limits the contribution of second-order motion to the perception of surface shape? *Vision Res, 40* (16), 2125-2133.

Hildreth, E.C., Ando, H., Andersen, R.A., & Treue, S. (1995). Recovering three-dimensional structure from motion with surface reconstruction. *Vision Res, 35* (1), 117-137.

Holmes, J.M. & Clarke, M.P. (2006). Amblyopia. *Lancet, 367* (9519), 1343-1351.

Hubel, D.H. & Weisel, T.N. (1968). Receptive fields and functional architecture of monkey striate cortex. *J Physiol, 195* (1), 215-243.

Hubel, D.H. & Wiesel, T.N. (1959). Receptive fields of single neurones in the cat's striate cortex. *J Physiol, 148*, 574-591.

Hubel, D.H. & Wiesel, T.N. (1965). Binocular interaction in striate cortex of kittens reared with artificial squint. *Journal of Neurophysiology, 28* (6), 1041-&.

Hubel, D.H. & Wiesel, T.N. (1972). Laminar and columnar distribution of geniculo-cortical fibers in the macaque monkey. *J Comp Neurol, 146* (4), 421-450.

Huk, A.C., Dougherty, R.F., & Heeger, D.J. (2002). Retinotopy and functional subdivision of human areas MT and MST. *J Neurosci, 22* (16), 7195-7205.

Huk, A.C. & Heeger, D.J. (2002). Pattern-motion responses in human visual cortex. *Nat Neurosci, 5* (1), 72-75.

Husain, M., Treue, S., & Andersen, R.A. (1989). Surface interpolation in three-dimensional structure-from-motion perception. *Neural Computation, 1*, 324-333.

Huxlin, K.R., Martin, T., Kelly, K., Riley, M., Friedman, D.I., Burgin, W.S., & Hayhoe, M. (2009). Perceptual relearning of complex visual motion after V1 damage in humans. *J Neurosci, 29* (13), 3981-3991.

Jastorff, J. & Orban, G.A. (2009). Human functional magnetic resonance imaging reveals separation and integration of shape and motion cues in biological motion processing. *The Journal of Neuroscience, 29* (22), 7315-7329.

Johansson, G. (1973). Visual perception of biological motion and a model for its analysis. *Attention, Perception, & Psychophysics, 14* (2), 201-211.

Johnston, A., McOwan, P.W., & Buxton, H. (1992). A computational model of the analysis of some first-order and second-order motion patterns by simple and complex cells. *Proc R Soc Lond B Biol Sci, 250* (1329), 297-306.

Karas, R. & McKendrick, A.M. (2011). Age related changes to perceptual surround suppression of moving stimuli. *Seeing Perceiving,* EPub ahead of print.

Koenderink, J.J. & van Doorn, A.J. (1986). Depth and shape from differential perspective in the presence of bending deformations. *J Opt Soc Am A, 3* (2), 242-249.

Landy, M.S., Dosher, B.A., Sperling, G., & Perkins, M.E. (1991). The kinetic depth effect and optic flow--II. First- and second-order motion. *Vision Res, 31* (5), 859-876.

Lappin, J.S., Doner, J.F., & Kottas, B.L. (1980). Minimal conditions for the visual detection of structure and motion in three dimensions. *Science, 209* (4457), 717-719.

Law, C.T. & Gold, J.I. (2008). Neural correlates of perceptual learning in a sensory-motor, but not a sensory, cortical area. *Nat Neurosci, 11* (4), 505-513.

Ledgeway, T. & Hess, R.F. (2002). Failure of direction identification for briefly presented second-order motion stimuli: Evidence for weak direction selectivity of the mechanisms encoding motion. *Vision Res, 42* (14), 1739-1758.

Ledgeway, T., Hess, R.F., & McGraw, P.V. (2002). Masking effects between local first-order and second-order motions in the extraction of global-motion direction depend critically on stimulus visibility. *Perception, 31* (ECVP Abstract Supplement)

Ledgeway, T. & Smith, A.T. (1994). Evidence for separate motion-detecting mechanisms for first- and second-order motion in human vision. *Vision Res, 34* (20), 2727-2740.

Leventhal, A.G., Wang, Y., Pu, M., Zhou, Y., & Ma, Y. (2003). GABA and its agonists improved visual cortical function in senescent monkeys. *Science, 300* (5620), 812-815.

Li, X., Mullen, K.T., Thompson, B., & Hess, R.F. (2011). Effective connectivity anomalies in human amblyopia. *Neuroimage, 54* (1), 505-516.

Longuet-Higgins, H.C. & Prazdny, K. (1980). The interpretation of a moving retinal image. *Proc R Soc Lond B Biol Sci, 208* (1173), 385-397.

Lu, H., Qian, N., & Liu, Z. (2004). Learning motion discrimination with suppressed MT. *Vision Res, 44* (15), 1817-1825.

Lu, Z.L. & Sperling, G. (1995). The functional architecture of human visual motion perception. *Vision Res, 35* (19), 2697-2722.

Lu, Z.L. & Sperling, G. (2001). Three-systems theory of human visual motion perception: Review and update. *J Opt Soc Am A Opt Image Sci Vis, 18* (9), 2331-2370.

Mansouri, B. & Hess, R.F. (2006). The global processing deficit in amblyopia involves noise segregation. *Vision Res, 46* (24), 4104-4117.

Mareschal, I. & Baker, C.L., Jr. (1998). Temporal and spatial response to second-order stimuli in cat area 18. *J Neurophysiol, 80* (6), 2811-2823.

Marr, D. & Ullman, S. (1981). Directional selectivity and its use in early visual processing. *Proc R Soc Lond B Biol Sci, 211* (1183), 151-180.

Mather, G. (1989). Early motion process and the kinetic depth effect. *Quarterly Journal of Experimental Psychology, 41A* (1), 183-198.

Mather, G. & Murdoch, L. (1994). Gender discrimination in biological motion displays based on dynamic cues. *Proceedings of the Royal Society of London. Series B: Biological Sciences, 258* (1353), 273-279.

Mather, G., Radford, K., & West, S. (1992). Low-level visual processing of biological motion. *Proc Biol Sci, 249* (1325), 149-155.

Mather, G. & West, S. (1993). Recognition of animal locomotion from dynamic point-light displays. *Perception, 22* (7), 759-766.

Meese, T.S. & Anderson, S.J. (2002). Spiral mechanisms are required to account for summation of complex motion components. *Vision Res, 42* (9), 1073-1080.

Meese, T.S. & Harris, M.G. (2001). Independent detectors for expansion and rotation, and for orthogonal components of deformation. *Perception, 30* (10), 1189-1202.

Merabet, L., Desautels, A., Minville, K., & Casanova, C. (1998). Motion integration in a thalamic visual nucleus. *Nature, 396* (6708), 265-268.

Merigan, W.H., Katz, L.M., & Maunsell, J.H. (1991). The effects of parvocellular lateral geniculate lesions on the acuity and contrast sensitivity of macaque monkeys. *J Neurosci, 11* (4), 994-1001.

Morrone, M.C., Burr, D.C., Di Pietro, S., & Stefanelli, M.A. (1999). Cardinal directions for visual optic flow. *Curr Biol, 9* (14), 763-766.

Morrone, M.C., Tosetti, M., Montanaro, D., Fiorentini, A., Cioni, G., & Burr, D.C. (2000). A cortical area that responds specifically to optic flow, revealed by fMRI. *Nat Neurosci, 3* (12), 1322-1328.

Movshon, J.A., Adelson, E.H., Gizzi, M.S., & Newsome, W.T. (1985). The analysis of moving visual patterns. In: C. Chagass, R. Gattass, & C. Gross (Eds.), *Pattern Recognition Mechanisms* (pp. 117-151). Rome: Vatican Press.

Newsome, W.T. & Pare, E.B. (1988). A selective impairment of motion perception following lesions of the middle temporal visual area (MT). *J Neurosci, 8* (6), 2201-2211.

Nishida, S. (2011). Advancement of motion psychophysics: Review 2001-2010. *J Vis, 11* (5), 11.

Nishida, S., Ledgeway, T., & Edwards, M. (1997). Dual multiple-scale processing for motion in the human visual system. *Vision Res, 37* (19), 2685-2698.

Nishida, S., Sasaki, Y., Murakami, I., Watanabe, T., & Tootell, R.B. (2003). Neuroimaging of direction-selective mechanisms for second-order motion. *J Neurophysiol, 90* (5), 3242-3254.

O'Keefe, L.P. & Movshon, J.A. (1998). Processing of first- and second-order motion signals by neurons in area MT of the macaque monkey. *Vis Neurosci, 15* (2), 305-317.

Olavarria, J.F., DeYoe, E.A., Knierim, J.J., Fox, J.M., & van Essen, D.C. (1992). Neural responses to visual texture patterns in middle temporal area of the macaque monkey. *J Neurophysiol, 68* (1), 164-181.

Oram, M.W. & Perrett, D.I. (1994). Responses of anterior superior temporal polysensory (STPA) neurons to "biological motion" stimuli. *Journal of Cognitive Neuroscience, 6* (2), 99-116.

Orban, G.A., Sunaert, S., Todd, J.T., Van Hecke, P., & Marchal, G. (1999). Human cortical regions involved in extracting depth from motion. *Neuron, 24* (4), 929-940.

Palmer, J.E., Chronicle, E.P., Rolan, P., & Mulleners, W.M. (2000). Cortical hyperexcitability is cortical under-inhibition: Evidence from a novel functional test of migraine patients. *Cephalalgia, 20* (6), 525-532.

Paolini, M., Distler, C., Bremmer, F., Lappe, M., & Hoffmann, K.P. (2000). Responses to continuously changing optic flow in area MST. *J Neurophysiol, 84* (2), 730-743.

Peelen, M.V., Wiggett, A.J., & Downing, P.E. (2006). Patterns of fMRI activity dissociate overlapping functional brain areas that respond to biological motion. *Neuron, 49* (6), 815-822.

Pelphrey, K.A., Morris, J.P., Michelich, C.R., Allison, T., & McCarthy, G. (2005). Functional anatomy of biological motion perception in posterior temporal cortex: An fMRI study of eye, mouth and hand movements. *Cereb Cortex, 15* (12), 1866-1876.

Perrone, J.A. (1992). Model for the computation of self-motion in biological systems. *J Opt Soc Am A, 9* (2), 177-194.

Peuskens, H., Claeys, K.G., Todd, J.T., Norman, J.F., Van Hecke, P., & Orban, G.A. (2004). Attention to 3-d shape, 3-d motion, and texture in 3-d structure from motion displays. *J Cogn Neurosci, 16* (4), 665-682.

Pitzalis, S., Sereno, M.I., Committeri, G., Fattori, P., Galati, G., Patria, F., & Galletti, C. (2010). Human V6: The medial motion area. *Cereb Cortex, 20* (2), 411-424.

Qian, N. & Andersen, R.A. (1994). Transparent motion perception as detection of unbalanced motion signals. II. Physiology. *J Neurosci, 14* (12), 7367-7380.

Rizzo, M., Nawrot, M., & Zihl, J. (1995). Motion and shape perception in cerebral akinetopsia. *Brain, 118 (Pt 5)*, 1105-1127.

Rodman, H.R. & Albright, T.D. (1989). Single-unit analysis of pattern-motion selective properties in the middle temporal visual area (MT). *Exp Brain Res, 75* (1), 53-64.

Rudolph, K. & Pasternak, T. (1999). Transient and permanent deficits in motion perception after lesions of cortical areas MT and MST in the macaque monkey. *Cereb Cortex, 9* (1), 90-100.

Saito, H., Yukie, M., Tanaka, K., Hikosaka, K., Fukada, Y., & Iwai, E. (1986). Integration of direction signals of image motion in the superior temporal sulcus of the macaque monkey. *J Neurosci, 6* (1), 145-157.

Salzman, C.D., Murasugi, C.M., Britten, K.H., & Newsome, W.T. (1992). Microstimulation in visual area MT: Effects on direction discrimination performance. *J Neurosci, 12* (6), 2331-2355.

Saygin, A.P., Wilson, S.M., Hagler, D.J., Jr., Bates, E., & Sereno, M.I. (2004). Point-light biological motion perception activates human premotor cortex. *J Neurosci, 24* (27), 6181-6188.

Scott-Samuel, N.E. & Georgeson, M.A. (1999). Does early non-linearity account for second-order motion? *Vision Res, 39* (17), 2853-2865.

Seiffert, A.E., Somers, D.C., Dale, A.M., & Tootell, R.B. (2003). Functional MRI studies of human visual motion perception: Texture, luminance, attention and after-effects. *Cereb Cortex, 13* (4), 340-349.

Servos, P., Osu, R., Santi, A., & Kawato, M. (2002). The neural substrates of biological motion perception: An fMRI study. *Cereb Cortex, 12* (7), 772-782.

Shariat, H. & Price, K.E. (1990). Motion estimation with more than 2 frames. *IEEE Transactions on Pattern Analysis and Machine Intelligence, 12* (5), 417-434.

Simmers, A.J., Ledgeway, T., Hess, R.F., & McGraw, P.V. (2003). Deficits to global motion processing in human amblyopia. *Vision Res., 43*, 729-738.

Simmers, A.J., Ledgeway, T., Mansouri, B., Hutchinson, C.V., & Hess, R.F. (2006). The extent of the dorsal extra-striate deficit in amblyopia. *Vision Res, 46*, 2571-2580.

Smith, A.T., Greenlee, M.W., Singh, K.D., Kraemer, F.M., & Hennig, J. (1998). The processing of first- and second-order motion in human visual cortex assessed by functional magnetic resonance imaging (fMRI). *J Neurosci, 18* (10), 3816-3830.

Smith, A.T. & Ledgeway, T. (1997). Separate detection of moving luminance and contrast modulations: Fact or artifact? *Vision Res, 37* (1), 45-62.

Snowden, R.J. & Milne, A.B. (1996). The effects of adapting to complex motions: Position invariance and tuning to spiral motions. *Journal of Cognitive Neuroscience, 8*, 435-452.

Snowden, R.J., Treue, S., Erickson, R.G., & Andersen, R.A. (1991). The response of area MT and V1 neurons to transparent motion. *J Neurosci, 11* (9), 2768-2785.

Tadin, D., Kim, J., Doop, M.L., Gibson, C., Lappin, J.S., Blake, R., & Park, S. (2006). Weakened center-surround interactions in visual motion processing in schizophrenia. *J Neurosci, 26* (44), 11403-11412.

Tadin, D., Lappin, J.S., Gilroy, L.A., & Blake, R. (2003). Perceptual consequences of centre-surround antagonism in visual motion processing. *Nature, 424* (6946), 312-315.

Tadin, D., Silvanto, J., Pascual-Leone, A., & Battelli, L. (2011). Improved motion perception and impaired spatial suppression following disruption of cortical area MT/V5. *J Neurosci, 31* (4), 1279-1283.

Tanaka, K., Fukada, Y., & Saito, H.A. (1989). Underlying mechanisms of the response specificity of expansion/contraction and rotation cells in the dorsal part of the medial superior temporal area of the macaque monkey. *J Neurophysiol, 62* (3), 642-656.

Tanaka, K., Hikosaka, K., Saito, H., Yukie, M., Fukada, Y., & Iwai, E. (1986). Analysis of local and wide-field movements in the superior temporal visual areas of the macaque monkey. *J Neurosci, 6* (1), 134-144.

Tanaka, K. & Saito, H. (1989). Analysis of motion of the visual field by direction, expansion/contraction, and rotation cells clustered in the dorsal part of the medial superior temporal area of the macaque monkey. *J Neurophysiol, 62* (3), 626-641.

Thompson, B., Aaen-Stockdale, C., Koski, L., & Hess, R.F. (2009). A double dissociation between striate and extrastriate visual cortex for pattern motion perception revealed using rTMS. *Human Brain Mapping, 30* (10), 3115-3126.

Thompson, B., Aaen-Stockdale, C.R., Mansouri, B., & Hess, R.F. (2008a). Plaid perception is only subtly impaired in strabismic amblyopia. *Vision Res, 48* (11), 1307-1314.

Thompson, B., Hansen, B.C., Hess, R.F., & Troje, N.F. (2007). Peripheral vision: Good for biological motion, bad for signal noise segregation? *J Vis, 7* (10), 12 11-17.

Thompson, B. & Liu, Z. (2006). Learning motion discrimination with suppressed and un-suppressed MT. *Vision Res, 46* (13), 2110-2121.

Thompson, B., Richard, A., Churan, J., Hess, R.F., Aaen-Stockdale, C., & Pack, C.C. (2011). Impaired spatial and binocular summation for motion direction discrimination in strabismic amblyopia. *Vision Res, 51* (6), 577-584.

Thompson, B., Troje, N.F., Hansen, B.C., & Hess, R.F. (2008b). Amblyopic perception of biological motion. *J Vis, 8* (4), 22.21-2214.

Thompson, B., Villeneuve, M.Y., Casanova, C., & Hess, R.F. (2012). Abnormal cortical processing of pattern motion in amblyopia: Evidence from fMRI. *Neuroimage, 60* (2), 1307-1315.

Tinsley, C.J., Webb, B.S., Barraclough, N.E., Vincent, C.J., Parker, A., & Derrington, A.M. (2003). The nature of V1 neural responses to 2d moving patterns depends on receptive-field structure in the marmoset monkey. *J Neurophysiol, 90* (2), 930-937.

Tootell, R.B., Reppas, J.B., Kwong, K.K., Malach, R., Born, R.T., Brady, T.J., Rosen, B.R., & Belliveau, J.W. (1995). Functional analysis of human MT and related visual cortical areas using magnetic resonance imaging. *J Neurosci, 15* (4), 3215-3230.

Treue, S., Andersen, R.A., Ando, H., & Hildreth, E.C. (1995). Structure-from-motion: Perceptual evidence for surface interpolation. *Vision Res, 35* (1), 139-148.

Troje, N.F. (2002). Decomposing biological motion: A framework for analysis and synthesis of human gait patterns. *J Vis, 2* (5), 371-387.

Troje, N.F. & Westhoff, C. (2006). The inversion effect in biological motion perception: Evidence for a "Life detector"? *Curr Biol, 16* (8), 821-824.

Ullman, S. (1984). Maximizing rigidity: The incremental recovery of 3-d structure from rigid and nonrigid motion. *Perception, 13* (3), 255-274.

Ungerleider, L.G. & Haxby, J.V. (1994). 'What' and 'where' in the human brain. *Curr Opin Neurobiol, 4* (2), 157-165.

Ungerleider, L.G. & Mishkin, M. (1982). Two cortical visual systems. In: D.J. Ingle, M.A. Goodale, & R.J.W. Mansfield (Eds.), *Analysis of Visual Behavior* (pp. 549-586): MIT Press.

van Santen, J.P. & Sperling, G. (1985). Elaborated reichardt detectors. *J Opt Soc Am A, 2* (2), 300-321.

Villeneuve, M.Y., Kupers, R., Gjedde, A., Ptito, M., & Casanova, C. (2005). Pattern-motion selectivity in the human pulvinar. *Neuroimage, 28* (2), 474-480.

Wallach, H. & O'Connell, D.N. (1953). The kinetic depth effect. *J Exp Psychol, 45* (4), 205-217.

Wallisch, P. & Kumbhani, R.D. (2009). Can major depression improve the perception of visual motion? *Journal of Neuroscience, 29* (46), 14381-14382.

Watson, A.B. & Ahumada, A.J., Jr. (1985). Model of human visual-motion sensing. *J Opt Soc Am A, 2* (2), 322-341.

Wilson, H.R., Ferrera, V.P., & Yo, C. (1992). A psychophysically motivated model for two-dimensional motion perception. *Vis Neurosci, 9* (1), 79-97.

Wilson, H.R. & Kim, J. (1994). Perceived motion in the vector sum direction. *Vision Res, 34* (14), 1835-1842.

Wright, M.J. & Gurney, K.N. (1992). Lower threshold of motion for one and two dimensional patterns in central and peripheral vision. *Vision Res, 32* (1), 121-134.

Yo, C. & Wilson, H.R. (1992). Perceived direction of moving two-dimensional patterns depends on duration, contrast and eccentricity. *Vision Res, 32* (1), 135-147.

Zeki, S. (1991). Cerebral akinetopsia (visual motion blindness). A review. *Brain, 114 (Pt 2),* 811-824.

Zihl, J., von Cramon, D., & Mai, N. (1983). Selective disturbance of movement vision after bilateral brain damage. *Brain, 106 (Pt 2),* 313-340.

Zohary, E., Celebrini, S., Britten, K.H., & Newsome, W.T. (1994). Neuronal plasticity that underlies improvement in perceptual performance. *Science, 263* (5151), 1289-1292.

Chapter 6

Visual Processing in the Action-Oriented Brain

Brendan D. Cameron and Gordon Binsted

Additional information is available at the end of the chapter

http://dx.doi.org/10.5772/48461

1. Introduction

Visual processing does not occur in passive systems. We and our evolutionary ancestors are and were acting creatures, and our visual systems evolved to enable effective locomotion and action. Indeed, sensation of the external world is only evolutionarily meaningful to the extent that the sensing organism can respond to the input (accounting for the dearth of eyes in the plant kingdom), and if vision's purpose is action, our understanding of the visual brain is likely to be well served by studying vision in an action context. Even for our more sedentary activities, like reading, watching TV, or chatting with a friend, our eyes are in constant motion, actively gathering information. We are virtually incapable of passive vision. Our goals in this chapter are to highlight some of the ways in which seeing is coupled to action and to show that our understanding of visual processing can be enhanced by considering its relationship to action. To make our case, we will demonstrate that action has access to visual information that perception does not, and we will demonstrate that actions and action plans influence what we consciously perceive.

We will begin the chapter with an overview of cortical substrates for visuomotor processing and prevailing theories about the division of visual-processing labour in the cortex. We will then discuss findings from neuropsychological and behavioural studies and what they have taught us about the complex and sometimes counter-intuitive relationship between vision and action. Our approach might be considered ecological to the extent that it stresses vision's tight coupling with action processing. Indeed, our analysis focuses mainly on functions that are considered to be under the purview of the visuomotor 'dorsal stream' in the posterior parietal cortex and, as we discuss in the next section, this visual stream is thought to be involved in the direct transformation of vision into action. It has previously been suggested that the visual functions of the dorsal stream might be those for which an ecological approach to vision is appropriate, in contrast to the visual functions of the perceptual 'ventral stream,' for which a constructivist approach to vision may be more fitting [1]. We are sympathetic to this view and to the idea that a greater respect for vision's behavioural role will assist future vision science. And though we will not be endorsing Gibson's direct perception approach to vision [2] or declaring allegiance to a strictly ecological approach to vision, the spirit of our argument will echo J.J. Gibson's contention that vision relies on the moving, acting person in their environment.

2. Cortical substrates for visuomotor processing

In the human primary visual pathway, visual input from the retina proceeds, via the lateral geniculate nucleus, to primary visual cortex (V1), located in the occipital lobe. Visual information then proceeds to extrastriate visual areas in the occipital lobe, posterior parietal lobe, and temporal lobe. Our discussion will focus mainly on functional areas within the posterior parietal cortex (PPC), which are thought to be involved in the preparation and control of visually guided actions. Some of the areas of the PPC that will be particularly relevant to the discussion are the parietal-occipital junction (POJ), the superior parietal lobule (SPL), the intra-parietal sulcus (IPS), and the inferior parietal lobule (IPL). Studies in patient populations have shed light on the functions of these areas, and we address some of this work later in the section. First, however, we discuss three theories of cortical organization for visual processing that have significantly advanced our understanding of extrastriate processing: Mishkin, Ungerleider, and Macko's [3] two visual stream hypothesis, Goodale and Milner's [4,5] Perception-Action Model (PAM), and Glover's [6] Planning-Control Model (PCM). These theories all posit branching paths of visual output from V1, and their differences lie in the functions they assign to each visual processing stream. The PAM and the PCM are particularly relevant to our thesis, for they highlight regions of parietal cortex devoted to the translation of vision into action.

Mishkin, Ungerleider, and Macko [3] proposed that the primate visual system is divided into two cortical streams: a dorsal stream projecting from primary visual cortex to posterior parietal cortex (PPC) and a ventral stream projecting from primary visual cortex to inferior temporal cortex (IT). They suggested that the dorsal stream is responsible for processing visual information relating to object location ('where'), while the ventral stream is responsible for processing visual information relating to object identity ('what'). This functional division was supported by evidence from monkeys with lesioned PPC, who were impaired in their ability to select a target based on its relationship to a landmark object, and from monkeys with lesioned IT, who were impaired in their ability to select a target based on its shape and surface patterning.

Goodale and Milner [4,5] suggested an important modification to the two visual streams hypothesis. They argued that the functions of the two streams should be considered in terms of the purpose for which the visual information is being processed. According to the PAM the dorsal stream processes visual information for action ('how') and the ventral stream processes visual information for perception ('what' and 'perceptual where'). One of the key pieces of evidence for Milner and Goodale's model was the perceptual and motor performance of D.F., a patient with visual form agnosia. D.F.'s ability to identify objects and their shapes is dramatically impaired. However, her ability to reach to and grasp objects is largely preserved. For example, D.F. can accurately rotate a card to fit through a slot during a posting action, but will fail to perceptually report the orientation of the slot [7]. D.F. suffered damage to her lateral occipital cortex (LOC) [8] in the ventral stream but has a largely intact PPC, and Milner and Goodale [5] inferred that the PPC was responsible for her preserved visuomotor function. Milner and Goodale contrast D.F.'s preserved motor abilities and pattern of cortical damage with those of patients with optic ataxia (a condition we describe in more detail later), who experience impaired goal-directed action and tend to have lesions to areas within the PPC [5].

Additional support for the PAM was provided by studies in non-patient participants interacting with visual illusions, which were shown to fool perceptual reports but not goal-directed actions [e.g. 9,10]. For instance, when participants responded to the central circle in the Ebbinghaus illusion, a size-contrast illusion in which the central circle appears larger when surrounded by smaller circles, perceptual reports were more susceptible to the illusion than actions were [9]. These findings were consistent with the idea that the ventral stream considers relationships among objects, driving the size-contrast illusion effects, while the dorsal stream considers only the action-relevant parameters of the target object. However, conflicting findings across studies and issues relating to task differences among perceptual and reach tasks ultimately weakened – though may not have defeated – the case from the illusion literature, and we refer the reader elsewhere for an extensive discussion of the illusion controversy [11,12].

Milner and Goodale's [5] reformulation of the two visual streams hypothesis was possible thanks to a consideration of the relationship between action and vision. They shifted the focus from the *kinds* of visual information (spatial vs. identity) to the *behavioural role* of the visual information (acting vs. perceiving). Thus, Milner and Goodale's [5] model provides an example of how thinking about action advanced our understanding of vision.

Glover's [6] PCM, like the PAM, also emerged from a focus on the role of action in visual processing. Indeed, it shares much in common with the PAM; both models assign perceptual/cognitive and visuomotor processes to different cortical streams. Where the PCM differs from the PAM is in its proposal that different visual information is used for movement planning than for movement control and in its contention that distinct cortical areas serve as substrates for the two phases of action. To assist in clarifying the differences between the PCM and the PAM, we return, briefly, to the PAM and its view of movement preparation and control.

According to the PAM, the role of the ventral stream is to permit a high-level understanding of one's visual environment and the relationships among the objects within it. Information derived from ventral stream processing allows one to select, based on current goals, an object for action. Once this is done, control is passed to the dorsal stream, which carries out the specification of the movement parameters and monitors online performance. This action preparation and online control is, according to Milner and Goodale [5], carried out within the superior parietal lobe (SPL) and the intraparietal sulcus (IPS).

PCM's differences from the PAM are related primarily to what factors influence movement preparation and what cortical areas are responsible for different kinds of visuomotor processing. The PCM proposes a third stream, in the inferior parietal lobe (IPL), that is responsible for movement preparation. This stream, according to Glover [6], considers non-spatial target factors (e.g. object weight) and contextual elements (e.g. background motion), which inform -- and, in the case of visual illusions, fool -- the initial preparation of the movement. Whereas the PAM places both movement preparation and online control within the same 'how' stream in the SPL and IPS, Glover's PCM separates the initial phase of movement production (in the IPL) from real-time control (in the SPL), and argues that separate representations underlie each phase of the movement. One of the pieces of behavioural evidence for the PCM was a careful examination of the unfolding movement during actions towards visual illusions. Glover and Dixon [13] showed that the effect of an illusion on grip aperture was stronger at the start of the movement and diminished as the movement progressed, potentially indicating that movement planning and movement control were drawing upon different representations of the target and its environment.

Glover [6] is not alone in arguing for a third visual stream. Rizzolatti and Matelli [14] have argued for a division of labour within the dorsal stream: a dorsal-dorsal stream in the SPL that is responsible for online control and a ventral-dorsal stream in the IPL that is involved in both action and perception. Pisella et al. [15] have also argued for more than two visual streams. We will encounter some of the evidence for a divided dorsal stream in the section on optic ataxia.

2.1. Evidence from patient populations

We turn next to visual deficits in patients who have suffered damage to different areas of visual cortex. We have chosen to focus on three conditions: blindsight, because it provides a dramatic example of vision for action without conscious awareness; optic ataxia, because it involves damage to the PPC and is informative with regard to action processing in that region; and hemispatial neglect, because it provides an important contrast to optic ataxia and also provides insight into the role of attention in action.

2.2. Blindsight

The term 'blindsight' is typically used to describe the phenomenon in patients with lesioned V1 who report being unaware of objects in their blind visual field yet remain able to access some visual information about objects presented within it. For instance, patients can locate stimuli in their blind field for which they do not report any conscious awareness [16]. There has been considerable debate regarding the implications of blindsight for conscious visual processing and whether incomplete lesioning of V1 can explain performance in blindsight patients (see [17,18] for reviews). We will not outline the debate here; rather, we wish to highlight the important point that several of the behaviours observed in blindsight -- looking at a target [19], pointing to a target [16], or even reaching to post a letter through a slot [20] -- involve acting without consciously seeing. These behaviours provide examples of situations where action is able to access visual information that perception cannot. The phenomenon is analogous to the one described in the visual agnosia patient D.F., who can interact with objects of which she is perceptually unaware [5]. Indeed, Milner and Goodale [5] have previously drawn attention to the implications of blindsight for the PAM, and have suggested that projections from subcortical structures to areas in the PPC may permit the preserved action in blindsight. We refer the reader to that text for a more detailed discussion of the evidence.

A recent blindsight study by Whitwell et al. [21] does provide indirect support for Milner and Goodale's [5] PAM model. Whitwell et al. [21] examined real-time and delayed grasping performance in a blindsight patient (S.J.) when she reached to targets presented in her blind field. They found that S.J. scaled her grip aperture to target size when movements were initiated while the target was 'visible' (i.e., not occluded by the experimenter), but failed to scale her grip aperture when the target was occluded 2 seconds prior to the imperative stimulus. Furthermore, S.J. was incapable of perceptually reporting the size of the target presented in her blind field. These findings are consistent with Milner and Goodale's [5] suggestion that the dorsal stream has no memory and only processes currently available visual information; however, this inference does rely on the assumption that dorsal stream processing is preserved in S.J.

Independent of any dorsal/ventral considerations, blindsight studies show that goal-directed actions can uncover visual function that perceptual reports may not. Action's ability to tap into non-conscious vision has also been observed in non-patients: In a later section we describe a behavioural study [22] that reveals movement scaling to perceptually-inaccessible target size, an effect that mimics the non-conscious reach performance in blindsight. That study suggests that the putative dorsal-stream processing in blindsight patients naturally occurs in non-patient participants, whose visuomotor systems are able to see what perception cannot.

2.3. Optic ataxia

Optic ataxia is a motor disorder characterized by deficits in goal-directed reaching, and neuropsychological investigations of the brain lesions associated with optic ataxia have contributed considerably to our understanding of visuomotor processing. However, the nature of the disorder is complex, and some of its implications for our understanding of the visuomotor dorsal stream are not yet clear.

One of the main pieces of evidence presented by Milner and Goodale [5] for the PAM is the proposed double-dissociation between visual agnosia and optic ataxia. The preserved motor function and impaired object perception in D.F., who has lesioned ventral stream and intact PPC, contrasts with the impaired motor function and preserved object perception in patients with optic ataxia, who have intact ventral streams and lesioned PPC. Other researchers, however, have questioned the validity of this double-dissociation [15,6].

Part of the difficulty with interpreting performance in optic ataxia stems from the observation that motor performance to targets presented in central vision is often comparable to that of controls; major performance deficits appear only when targets are presented in the visual periphery [23]. In other words, when patients are able to fixate the target, they can accurately reach to it. However, there is evidence that subtle movement deficits can be detected when the target is in central vision. A study by Pisella et al. [24], for instance, showed that an optic ataxia patient, I.G., who has bilateral lesions to PPC was much slower and less fluid than controls in correcting her movements online when a target in central vision was displaced during a reach (though this effect, too, may be explained by the central/peripheral distinction, for the displacement moved the target away from fixation). Such findings have been taken to indicate that the dorsal stream may be more important for on-line movement control than it is for the initial parameterization of movements [25,6].

Milner and Goodale [26] have outlined some evidence that counters this view of an 'on-line only' dorsal stream, noting preparation deficits in optic ataxia as well as the preserved movement preparation, not just preserved on-line control, in the visual agnosia patient D.F. However, Milner and Goodale [26] do not directly address the central vs. peripheral vision discrepancy observed in optic ataxia [15,25] leaving the optic ataxia/visual agnosia double-dissociation question unresolved. At the very least, however, research on optic ataxia suggests that regions within the SPL are involved in transforming visual input to motor output. Whether the SPL's function is restricted to *on-line* visuomotor processing has yet to be determined.

More recently, Pisella et al. [27] have suggested that the evidence from optic ataxia indicates that one of the key functions of the dorsal stream is the spatial coding of targets in an eye-centered coordinate frame. Pisella et al. [27] assign this spatial coding function specifically to the parietal-occipital junction (POJ), a common lesion site in patients with optic ataxia. This account helps explain the peripheral target deficit observed in optic ataxia. Pisella et al. [27] further argue that dorsal stream function is important for both action *and* perception. This claim is supported by a recent study [28], which showed that optic ataxia patient I.G. was not only impaired in her on-line responses to a target displacement, but that she was also impaired in her perceptual report of the same target displacement.

Pisella et al. [27] also raise the important point that the dorsal stream probably has some role in perception for another reason: Areas within the dorsal stream are thought to be involved in attention orienting, which is fundamental to perceptual processing. Later in the chapter we address the important links between attention, perception, and action. In anticipation of that discussion, we provide first an overview of hemispatial neglect, a disorder of attention and spatial representation that, like optic ataxia, typically results from damage to regions within the parietal cortex.

2.4. Hemispatial neglect

Patients with hemispatial neglect suffer from a tendency to ignore half of their visual field, failing to acknowledge or interact with objects in the neglected field unless strongly encouraged to do so. Their performance deficits are generally considered distinct from those of optic ataxia patients, and the reaching deficits in optic ataxia are thought to be related to damage to the SPL or POJ, while the performance deficits in neglect are thought to be related to damage to the IPL [29].

Hemispatial neglect theoretically provides an interesting comparison to optic ataxia, for it should allow researchers to examine the relationship between attention and visuomotor control without the complicating visuomotor deficits present in optic ataxia. It also allows researchers to examine the impact, or lack thereof, of impaired visual awareness on motor function. However, one of the challenges researchers face when interpreting performance in neglect patients lies in ruling out the possibility that any visuomotor deficits observed in these patients arise from cortical damage that extends into visuomotor areas. For instance, Himmelbach and Karnath [30] have suggested that superior temporal cortex, rather than IPL, is directly responsible for the deficits of perceptual space representation found in neglect, and that the motor deficits found in some patients with neglect might stem from damage that extends to the IPL, a region they argue is involved in spatial coding for motor function, but which is not involved in the cognitive spatial coding that characterizes neglect. More recently, Himmelbach et al. [31] have argued that the neglect-specific effects of space representation are specifically linked to lesion sites at the superior temporal gyrus and temporo-parietal junction. They have also suggested that real-time motor control functions, such as those observed in optic ataxia, are supported by the POJ, an argument that aligns with Pisella et al.'s [27].

As mentioned earlier, the motor deficits of optic ataxia are particularly prominent when participants reach for targets presented in the visual periphery. This contrasts with the visuomotor performance of patients with neglect, who generally exhibit accurate motor performance to objects presented in their neglected field [31]. Although motor deficits have been observed in neglect patients, these tend to be relatively minor compared to the deficits of optic ataxia patients. One of the motor performance deficits that has been found in neglect patients is a delay in the initiation of reaching movements into their neglected visual field. Some studies also indicate minor impairments in online performance, whereas others show an absence of any deficits in online control (see [32] for a review). Himmelbach et al. [30,31] argue that when a proper control group is used (i.e., patients with parietal damage who do not exhibit neglect), hemispatial neglect is not associated with any impairments in movement control. However, a recent study by Rossit et al. [33] suggests that neglect patients may be slower to correct their movements online compared to both healthy controls and right hemisphere patients without neglect.

In the Rossit et al. [33] study, the authors applied a target jump design modeled after Pisella et al.'s [24] design, in which a participant is tasked with either going to a target when it is displaced at movement onset (location-go) or trying to stop their movement as soon as the target is displaced (location-stop). The location-stop condition allows the researcher to probe the automaticity of the online corrections; any deviations toward the target that occur in this condition can be attributed to automatic online control. In the location-go condition, neglect patients were slower than the control groups, by 80-100ms, to correct their movements online when the target jumped into their neglected field. Endpoint accuracy, however, was equivalent across the groups. In the location-stop condition, neglect patients exhibited an equivalent number of online corrections to the control groups. The neglect patients, in fact, had greater difficulty stopping their movements than the participants in the control groups. These results suggest that the 'automatic pilot' is intact in neglect patients. However, the results also suggest that visuomotor processing in the neglected field is slowed, perhaps as a result of impaired attention-for-action in that field.

Some authors have suggested that optic ataxia and hemispatial neglect represent a double dissociation (e.g. [31,32]). In support of this view, a recent case study showed that real-time grasping was preserved in a neglect patient's neglected field, whereas delayed grasping was dramatically impaired [34]. These outcomes are the inverse of those in optic ataxia patient I.G., who exhibits impaired real-time grasping but actually improves when asked to execute a delayed pantomime grasp [35].

The relative absence of major motor deficits in hemispatial neglect provides a further piece of evidence for action having access to visual information that perception does not. As noted at the outset of this section, patients with hemispatial neglect have a failure in the perceptual representation of part of their visual world. Their visuomotor system's preserved ability to reach to and grasp objects within this neglected field is suggestive of a perception/action dissociation, though it may not fall precisely along ventral/dorsal lines. A recent review by Harvey and Rossit [29] provides a comprehensive overview of visuomotor function in hemispatial neglect, and we direct the interested reader there for a fuller account of the syndrome's complexities and its implications for the functional organization of parietal and temporal cortex.

2.5. Section summary

We overviewed three theories of cortical organization for visual processing and discussed neuropsychological findings from blindsight, optic ataxia, and hemispatial neglect. The picture that emerges is one of a modularized PPC, with current evidence favouring the POJ and the SPL as key sites for real-time visuomotor computations. Critically, the visuomotor processing carried out by these areas appears to proceed automatically, without mediation by conscious visual processing. These sites are implicated in direct visual-to-motor transformations, and they are areas whose visual functions can only be probed by engaging participants in goal-directed movement tasks.

The visuomotor role of the IPL is somewhat less clear. It is a common lesion site in hemispatial neglect, which may implicate it in the orienting of attention. Glover [6] has argued that the IPL is important for movement planning, and neglect patients with damage to that area do tend to exhibit more motor deficits than neglect patients with undamaged IPL [30], which provides some support for Glover's assertion. At the same time, the breakdown in the cognitive spatial representation that is associated with damage to superior areas of the temporal cortex [31], a spatial deficit that does not appear to undermine action control, is consistent with Milner and Goodale's [5] argument for different spatial representations for perception and action.

The findings from patients with cortical lesions to visual areas support the idea that vision-for-action *can* proceed independently of vision-for-perception, though the possibility remains that the effects observed in patients do not represent the normal function of the preserved cortical areas. In the following section we examine converging evidence from non-patient participants for the idea that vision-for-action can access information that perception does not.

3. Action can proceed without perception: Evidence from cortically-intact participants

In this section we provide further evidence for action processing without visual awareness. We focus on studies in non-patients, which show that even when all areas of visual cortex are intact, visual information that drives action can elude conscious detection. This suggests that action's access to unperceived visual information is part of normal visual processing. We examine evidence from three different paradigms: backward masking, saccadic suppression of target displacement, and motor adaptation. In each case, motor responses to events are not only possible, but do not appear to suffer as a result of suppressed visual awareness.

3.1. Evidence from backward masking

One of the ways that non-conscious visual processing has been investigated is by masking a response-relevant stimulus and observing its impact on behaviour. When a stimulus is successfully masked, the participant does not report awareness of it. In metacontrast masking, for instance, the stimulus to be masked (the prime) is presented and then, shortly after, a larger stimulus (the mask) is presented around the prime. This sequence of stimuli can eliminate participants' awareness of the prime while influencing motor responses [36].

Taylor and McCloskey [37], for example, used metacontrast masking and showed that the reaction times for a motor task were influenced by the unseen prime. When a light was briefly flashed and then, 50ms later, 4 lights that closely surrounded the location of the first light were flashed, thereby producing a metacontrast mask, participants' reaction times were linked to the presentation of the initial stimulus, in spite of their having failed to consciously report its presence. Furthermore, Cressman et al. [38] have shown that movements that have already been initiated can be influenced by an unseen directional prime, such that participants adjust their movement online. In that study, a directional prime (left arrow, right arrow, or neutral stimulus) was presented at movement onset and then quickly masked with a larger arrow. Participants' movement endpoints were dictated by the mask, but the unseen directional primes triggered substantial trajectory deviations ahead of the explicit response to the mask.

These results suggest that the motor system can respond to visual information that is inaccessible to conscious awareness. However, this does not necessarily imply that the prime information is being processed by the dorsal stream. In fact, when the prime is a symbol that must be translated into a directional response (e.g. [36,38]), it is likely that ventral stream processing is involved. The perceptual representation of the shape may fail to reach awareness, but it is a representation that has the *potential* to be perceived, which, as Milner and Goodale [5] argue, should still be classified as ventrally-mediated.

However, when the masked stimulus is, itself, the target of the action, direct involvement of the dorsal stream is more likely. In a study by Binsted et al. [22], participants were tasked with making aiming movements directly to a masked target, the size of which was manipulated across trials. The study showed that movement times were scaled to the size of the target (shorter times for larger targets, longer ones for smaller targets), in accordance with Fitts' Law. Thus, even though participants did not consciously perceive any changes in the size of the target, their motor responses were appropriately tuned to it. This study showed that healthy participants could experience a blindsight-like ability to scale their visuomotor response to something they could not consciously see. Because the visual information that action is drawing upon in this instance is presumably the same information that it would be using in the absence of the mask, we can infer that visual processing for immediate action control is not normally mediated by conscious vision. Action may have access to sub-threshold conscious vision or it may draw upon different visual information altogether, as suggested by the PAM. Thus, either as a matter of *degree* of visual input to which they are sensitive or *kind* of visual input upon which they rely, vision-for-action and vision-for-perception clearly differ.

3.2. Evidence from reaches to saccadically-suppressed target displacements

We consider next a very robust dissociation between perception and control that occurs when people make simultaneous eye and hand movements. We will take up the perceptual effects of saccadic eye movements in more detail in a later section. For the current section, one need only know that when a target is displaced during a saccadic eye movement, the displacement is largely invisible. Surprisingly, people fail to notice a change in the target's location even when the displacement is as large as one third of the saccade magnitude [39].

Bridgeman et al. [40] showed that when participants pointed to a target that had been displaced during a saccade, they could accurately acquire it, even though they were unaware of the change in location. Goodale et al. [41] and Pelisson et al. [42] demonstrated that online responses of the motor system were also sensitive to saccadically-displaced targets. They showed that even when participants had initiated a reach towards a target's pre-saccadic location, the reach smoothly updated itself to acquire the displaced post-saccadic target location. This adjustment to the reach occurred in spite of participants having no vision of their hand and no awareness of the target displacement. This effect was also shown for targets that were displaced tangentially to the primary axis of the movement [43]. In sum, awareness of a target displacement is not needed for motor adjustments to the displacement.

3.3. Evidence from motor learning in response to unperceived visual changes

When people encounter an altered visual environment, they adapt their movements over the course of exposure to it, such that initially inaccurate movements gradually improve. For example, if one were to view the world through displacing prisms that shifted the visual world to the right, one's movements would initially err to the right of a reach target. Visual feedback would allow correction of this error over the course of multiple movements. Subsequent removal of the prisms would then produce motor errors in a leftward direction ('aftereffects') as a result of the newly acquired mapping between vision and motor output.

The interesting effect for the purposes of the current discussion is that people can acquire new visuomotor mappings without any awareness that their visual environment has changed. In fact, learning appears to be more robust if people do not know that the environment has been altered. Michel et al. [44], for instance, showed that gradually incrementing the amount of prism shift, such that participants were unaware of it, led to stronger aftereffects than the introduction of a large, consciously detectable prism shift.

People can also adapt to systematic, imperceptible changes in a target's location between the start and end of their movements. This adaptation can occur when the movement error is presented at the end of a reaching movement [45], but it can also occur when the target is displaced during the reaching movement, allowing for online corrections that eliminate any visual error at the end of the reach [46, cf. 47]. Furthermore, if participants are made aware of the target displacement, the amount of adaptation is considerably diminished [48].

The adaptation effect for reaching movements to displaced targets is similar to the adaptation that occurs for eye movements. Saccadic adaptation is a well-documented phenomenon in which the size of saccades gradually increases (or decreases) when people are repeatedly exposed to forward (or backward) displacements of the target [49]. This effect, like the one for reaching movements, is thought to draw upon the natural calibration of our movements that occurs throughout our everyday lives, a process that typically occurs without any awareness of the error in our movements.

3.4. Section summary

Conscious perception of changes in the visual environment is required for neither real-time control nor motor learning. In fact, motor learning may even be enhanced if one is unaware that a change has occurred. These findings do not necessarily imply that vision for perception and vision for action rely on separate cortical streams, but they do show that what action sees is not necessarily what perception sees. This is an important point, for it suggests that the principles governing vision for perception may differ from those governing vision for action. By measuring motor responses, not just perceptual reports, we can tap into a wealth of visual processing that we might otherwise miss.

4. Action influences visual attention and perception

So far, in discussing topics such as the PAM, blindsight, and masking studies in healthy participants, we have devoted much attention to the phenomenon of acting without consciously seeing. In this section we turn our attention to perception, and examine some of the ways that the intention to act changes what we see.

4.1. Saccades in action

Perhaps the most obvious example of the link between action and perception is eye movements. To pick up detailed information about the world around us, we constantly re-orient our gaze via movements of our eyes and head. Saccades, which are fast and largely ballistic, are the most common type of eye movement, and much of our internal representation of the visual world is constructed from the detailed snapshots they provide. While it is probably not surprising to many of us that saccades are constantly being used to shift our gaze and thus inform perception, saccades also influence perception in other more subtle ways.

One perceptually subtle (but experimentally dramatic) effect of saccades is their ability to mask large changes in the visual scene. As previously mentioned, saccade targets can be displaced by distances as large as a third of the saccade magnitude without the participant reporting any change [39]. Entire objects can be rotated or even deleted from a scene during a saccade, and participants will fail to notice the change [50]. In short, saccadic eye movements introduce periods of change blindness. This effect is thought to be partly due to our visual system's built-in assumption that the world is stable and that trans-saccadic changes in object locations are more likely to result from eye movement errors than they are to result from actual changes in the scene [51]. Ironically, then, the perceptual effect of saccadic suppression is a no-percept effect; suppression serves to keep the visual world stable and our conscious perception of it unperturbed. This demonstrates not only that oculomotor plans influence perception, but also that our action-driven visual system is carefully tuned to compensate for perturbations that are caused by internally generated movement.

4.2. Action goals dictate where our eyes go

When we reach to, pick up, and use objects to accomplish goals, our eyes precede our manual actions, orienting to the relevant parts of relevant objects. Land et al. [52] tracked people's eye movements as they carried out the actions of brewing a cup of tea in a kitchen, and the researchers observed that people's eye movements were tied to the behavioural goals; the eyes did not jump from one visually salient object to another but, rather, moved deliberately from one task-relevant object to the next. Detailed analysis of eye-hand coordination during object grasping and manipulation tells the same story: the eyes are drawn to contact points between the hand and the object and between the manipulated object and other objects [53,54].

Furthermore, the coupling between the eyes and the hand appears to be quite strong, and will resist conscious attempts to break it. For instance, when people are told to look and point to a target and then move their eyes to a new saccade target that appears while the hand is in flight, they fail to complete the saccade task. The eyes remain locked on the target of the reaching movement until the hand has landed [55]. Thus, the eyes strategically move to pick up relevant information for goal-directed action, and they are tightly bound to this task. The coupling between eye and hand is a perfect example of action's role in dictating where and when we acquire visual information from our environment.

As much as the eyes may want to lead the hand, it is possible to override the coupling by fixating the eyes in one location prior to initiating a reach to a peripheral target. The task requires some effort on the part of the performer, but it can be done (and is, in fact, well employed in laboratory settings when tight control over visual input is desired). You may have noticed, for instance, that you can reach for a cup of coffee while keeping your eyes on the book or screen before you, though at some cost to movement accuracy. As the next sections will show, however, even when the eyes remain locked in place during a manual task, visual attention does not; it is bound to action goals.

4.3. On the relationship between action and attention

Attention is vital to our experience of the visual world. Most of us have probably experienced the frustrating search through a crowded restaurant in which we only see our dinner companions after having already walked past them once or twice, or the search that happens at the open fridge door, where the item we want, and cannot find, has been in front of us all along. Controlled experiments have shown that people will reliably fail to see large objects that disappear and reappear in blinking scenes [56] or even fail to see a person in a gorilla suit walk through the middle of a scene [57]. Attention is the construct used to explain these effects. The idea is that there is far more information in the visual field than our brain can or wants to cope with at any one time. The brain, therefore, relies on attention to select a portion of visual information for analysis. And, as a result, if we do not attend to something, we are blind to it.

That attention is important for conscious perception is clear. When we consider, however, that the purpose of human information processing is not just perception but also action, it is also clear that attention systems should not be examined independently of action systems. One of the first to raise this point was Allport [58], who noted that the important constraint upon visual analysis of a scene may not be central processing limitations, but the need for action coherence. Allport's [58] argument was that motor systems need to be tied to one object at a time; if visual information about multiple objects is permitted access to these systems simultaneously, the action will fail. The hand, for example, cannot successfully grasp a cup if the information guiding the reach is also coming from the apple, the bottle, and pencil sitting next to the cup.

The importance of action to the allocation of attention has also been stressed by Rizzolatti et al. [59], who proposed a premotor theory of attention, in which eye-movement motor programs drive the spatial allocation of visual attention. Tipper et al. [60] have likewise emphasized the role of action in attention, proposing that attention operates within an action-centered representation of visual space. Schneider [61], meanwhile, has proposed the Visual Attention Model (VAM), a framework in which a central attention mechanism binds perceptual and action systems to the same object. Each of these perspectives on the relationship between attention and action will be examined next.

4.4. Premotor theory

The premotor theory of attention has probably been the most influential of the action-based theories of attention. As initially proposed [59], premotor theory attributed the control of attention to oculomotor programming; even when the eyes remained still while attention was shifted (covert orienting), the attention shift was purportedly due to the programming of an eye movement that was subsequently inhibited. Premotor theory was later modified to allow for goal-directed motor programming of any kind (e.g. reaching) to produce attention shifts [62], but the basic premise remained the same. The mechanism underlying this process was, according to Rizzolatti et al. [62], the activation of neurons in spatial pragmatic maps.

These pragmatic maps are proposed to reside in brain areas associated with action (e.g., parietal reach areas; parietal, frontal, or sub-cortical eye movement areas), and they code space only insofar as it is relevant to the action that they are involved in programming. Thus, according to premotor theory, there is no higher-level attention system. Rather, attention shifts simply result from the selective activation of pragmatic map neurons, and this activation only occurs when a movement is programmed to that region of space.

Some of the strongest support for premotor theory can be found in neurophysiological studies. Moore and Fallah [63], for instance, showed a causal link between activation of eye movement cortex and the allocation of attention. Moore and Fallah stimulated monkeys' frontal eye field (FEF), a cortical area involved in the control of voluntary eye movements. They began by stimulating a part of the FEF with enough current to trigger an eye movement. They then reduced the stimulation to a sub-threshold level (i.e., the stimulation was too low to trigger an eye movement). They found that this sub-threshold stimulation improved the monkey's ability to detect a change in the target stimulus when the stimulus fell within the region of the visual field corresponding to the destination of the eye movement that had previously been triggered by supra-threshold stimulation of the FEF. In a similar study investigating the attentional role of the superior colliculus (SC) (a subcortical area directly involved in the control of eye movements), Muller, Philiastides, and Newsome [64] found that sub-threshold stimulation of the SC also produced enhanced detection of the target stimulus. Both of these studies demonstrate covert orienting of attention resulting from activation of oculomotor areas of the brain, consistent with premotor theory.

4.5. Action-centered attention

An important step in understanding attention is determining the nature of the spatial representation upon which it operates. Premotor theory suggests that spatial pragmatic maps underlie the allocation of spatial attention (though it also states that attention emerges from these maps, rather than operating upon them). A related view, advanced by Tipper et al. [60], suggests that attention operates upon an action-centered representation. To get a better sense of what such a representation might be, we will first consider other kinds of spatial representation.

Tipper et al. [60] outline 4 possible kinds of spatial representation upon which attention might operate: a 2-D retina-centered representation, a 3-D viewer-centered representation, an environment-centered representation, and an action-centered representation. A 2-D retina-centered representation is one in which the spatial relationships between objects are defined in terms of the objects' relative positions in the 2-D retinal image. Thus, when it comes to attention, a distractor on the far side of a target (with respect to the viewer) would produce more interference than a distractor on the near side of the target, according to Tipper et al., because in the 2-D image the far object is closer to the target than the near object is. A 3-D viewer-centered representation, on the other hand, is one in which the distance of objects from the viewer is a relevant factor. If attention operates within this kind of representation, distractors on the near side of a target would potentially produce greater interference than distractors on the far side of the target. This type of representation differs from an environment-centered representation in that the orientation of the viewer with respect to the objects affects their salience. In the environment-centered representation, viewer orientation is irrelevant. Finally, the action-centered representation is one in which an object's potential for interference depends upon its relationship to a planned action path. Thus, a distractor that resides within the action path will potentially produce greater interference than one that resides beyond the path.

Tipper et al. [60] provided evidence that, during a reaching task, attention operates within an action-centered representation. They had participants reach and press target buttons that were arranged in a 3 x 3 array in the horizontal (transverse) plane. Below each button were a red and a yellow light. Illumination of the red light indicated that the corresponding button was the target; the yellow light was irrelevant to the task, but it would sometimes be illuminated simultaneously at a different location, serving as a distractor. Tipper et al. examined the cost to the total time (TT) of the reaching movement produced by the distractor, and found that TT suffered more (i.e., there was greater interference) when the distractor fell within the same row as the target or in a row between the hand start position and the target row. Furthermore, when the hand start position was moved to the opposite end of the board (i.e., to the far end of the board), the same pattern of results was found, ruling out a 3-D viewer-centered representation. Tipper et al., in discussing the mechanism underlying the action-centered interference, suggest that motor programs are activated, simultaneously, to both the target and the distractor.

A later experiment by Meegan and Tipper [65] investigated whether the pattern of interference observed by Tipper et al. [60] was due to the distractor's relationship to the response path, as Tipper et al. [60] had suggested, or to the distractor's proximity to the start position of the hand. Meegan and Tipper [65] found that proximity to the hand was a better predictor of distractor interference. This finding does not necessarily undermine the action-centered model; Meegan and Tipper [65], for instance, suggest that objects nearer to the hand might produce greater response competition than objects farther from the hand, a framework consistent with the parallel response activation proposed by Tipper et al. [60]. However, it is also possible that, because information about the location of the hand is important during action preparation [66], attention may initially be oriented to it, leading to greater interference from objects in its vicinity.

4.6. The Visual Attention Model and action-perception coupling

The Visual Attention Model (VAM), like premotor theory, posits that motor preparation and perceptual selection are coupled [61,67]. However, VAM differs from premotor theory in two major ways. For one, VAM suggests that the coupling between selection-for-action and selection-for-perception is bi-directional. In other words, selecting an object based on perceptual attributes (e.g. colour) also binds action systems to that object, and selecting an object for action (e.g. preparing to grasp an apple) also binds perceptual systems to that object. (Premotor theory only allows for action preparation to bind perceptual attention to an object.) The other way that VAM differs from premotor theory is that VAM posits an independent, higher-level, attention mechanism that binds action and perceptual processes. (Premotor theory argues against an independent attention system.) Much of the research that has been conducted within the VAM framework does not directly test VAM's predictions against those of premotor theory. As a result, the research presented in this section – research that demonstrates the coupling between action and perceptual selection – can be taken as support for either VAM or premotor theory.

Deubel and Schneider [68] provide strong evidence of the coupling between oculomotor preparation and visual attention. In one experiment participants were instructed to make a saccade to a peripheral target based on a central cue (a number specifying the location of the target). After cue presentation, but prior to saccade initiation, a discrimination target (DT) (which was a normal 'E' or a reverse 'E') appeared either at the same location as the saccade target (ST) or at a different location. The DT was present very briefly, and was masked prior to the onset of the saccade. Participants' discrimination performance was the dependent measure, and Deubel and Schneider [68] used this measure to infer the locus of attention. They found that participants' performance was considerably enhanced when the DT was at the ST position. Performance dropped off considerably when the DT was at a different position than the ST, even if by only 1 or 2 degrees of visual angle. Because all perceptual discrimination occurred prior to any movement of the eyes, these results provide evidence of covert orienting resulting from oculomotor preparation. In another experiment, Deubel and Schneider [68] showed the same effect when the ST was specified exogenously. Furthermore, in order to control for the possibility that covert orienting might be occurring independently of saccade preparation rather than being driven by it, Deubel and Schneider [68] conducted an experiment in which participants were told beforehand the upcoming location of the DT. Participants could then try to attend to the DT location while programming a saccade to a different location. Again, however, discrimination performance was best at the ST location, suggesting strong coupling between oculomotor programming and perceptual selection.

Deubel, Schneider, and Paprotta [69] extended these findings to show that reaching movements have the same impact as oculomotor programming on perceptual selection. The experiment's design was similar to that of Deubel and Schneider [68], but with manual aiming movements instead of saccades. A central cue indicated which peripheral object was the aiming target (AT), and the participant's task was to rapidly aim his/her finger to it while maintaining central fixation. The DT was always presented in the same location, so participants could attempt to attend to the DT while reaching to the AT. Despite participants' foreknowledge of the DT location, discrimination performance was best when the AT coincided with the DT, suggesting obligatory coupling between reach programming and perceptual selection. A later study by Deubel and Schneider [70], however, showed that the coupling between reaching and perceptual selection persists only for a short period of time. If movement onset was delayed by more than 300ms after the imperative stimulus, attention could be decoupled from the action target and oriented elsewhere. Eye movements, on the other hand, always bound attention to the saccade target, regardless of delay.

Baldauf, Wolf, and Deubel [71] replicated Deubel et al.'s [69] finding that manual preparation orients attention to the aiming target and extended it to show that preparing a multiple component movement can orient attention to multiple targets simultaneously. Participants executed rapid sequential aiming movements to 2 or 3 targets within a circular array of 12 stimuli. Identification of the transiently displayed DT was enhanced when its location coincided with the location of any one of the targets of the movement. Identification of the DT was poor at other locations, even a location falling directly between two target locations. This suggests that action preparation can drive multiple attention 'spotlights' in parallel.

A further example of the link between action intention and visual attention was provided by Bekkering and Neggers [72], who showed that visual target selection was influenced by whether the participant intended to grasp an object or point to it. When participants planned to *grasp* an object within a field of distractor objects, their initial eye movements, which were used as a marker of attention capture, were drawn less often to distractors of the wrong orientation than when participants intended to *point* to the target. That is, the intention to grasp may have allowed a pre-filtering of object orientation (a grasp-relevant, but not pointing-relevant, feature), thereby reducing the effect of the distractors on the initial eye movement.

4.7. Section summary

The studies discussed in this section have provided behavioural evidence that both eye and hand movement preparation produce covert orienting of attention. Furthermore, this binding of action and perception appears to be obligatory; even when participants attempt to orient elsewhere, motor preparation carries attention to the action target. So, although high-level decisions about how to interact with the world rely on perceptual representations, once the decision to act has been made, visual perception becomes yoked to action.

5. Conclusion

We set out to show that a great deal of our daily visual processing is intimately linked with the motor system. Much of that processing, in fact, proceeds without our being aware of it, and it automatically drives our actions. We began the chapter by describing some of the cortical areas that have been shown to provide direct links between incoming visual information and real-time motor output. Investigations of neurological conditions such as visual agnosia and blindsight (impaired visual awareness), optic ataxia (impaired control to peripheral targets), and hemispatial neglect (impaired attention and perceptual representation in one half of visual space) have furthered our understanding of visuomotor control, and many of the findings from these populations are consistent with the idea that visual processing in the PPC is action-related and inaccessible to conscious awareness. Behavioural studies in non-patient participants have also shown that vision-for-action can operate without any awareness on the part of the performer. For instance, masking studies reveal motor responses driven by unperceived stimuli; saccadic suppression studies show automatic responses to unperceived location changes; and motor learning studies show that awareness of a perturbation is not necessary for, and may even be detrimental to, visuomotor adaptation.

Having demonstrated that actions can sometimes access visual information that perception does not, we went on to examine ways in which our actions can also dictate what our perceptual system sees. We discussed the link between eye movements and the pick up of visual information, and we provided evidence that many of our eye movements are directly driven by our plans for manual action. Moreover, visual attention for perception was shown to be bound to the saccade and/or the reach target. At the risk of overstating our case, we propose that one think of action as a tour guide to the gallery of the visual world; it dictates what the perceptual visitors get to see, and it has access to locked rooms that perception never enters.

Author details

Brendan D. Cameron and Gordon Binsted
School of Health and Exercise Sciences, University of British Columbia Okanagan, Canada

6. References

[1] Norman J (2002) Two visual systems and two theories of perception: An attempt to reconcile the constructivist and ecological approaches. Behavioural and Brain Sciences 25: 73-144.
[2] Gibson JJ (1986) The Ecological Approach to Visual Perception. New Jersey: Lawrence Erlbaum Associates. 333p.
[3] Mishkin M, Ungerleider LG, Macko KA (1983) Object vision and spatial vision: Two cortical pathways. Trends in Neurosciences 6: 414-417.
[4] Goodale MA, Milner AD (1992) Separate visual pathways for perception and action. Trends in Neurosciences 15: 20-25.
[5] Milner AD, Goodale MA (2006) The Visual Brain in Action, 2nd edition. New York: Oxford University Press. 297p.
[6] Glover S (2004) Separate visual representations in the planning and control of action. Behavioral and Brain Sciences 27: 3-24.

[7] Goodale MA, Milner AD, Jakobson LS, Carey DP (1991) A neurological dissociation between perceiving objects and grasping them. Nature 349: 154-156.
[8] James TW, Culham J, Humphrey GK, Milner AD, Goodale MA (2003) Ventral occipital lesions impair object recognition but not object-directed grasping: an fMRI study. Brain 126: 2463-2475
[9] Aglioti S, DeSouza JFX, Goodale MA (1995) Size-contrast illusions deceive the eye but not the hand. Current Biology 5: 679-685.
[10] Haffenden AM, Goodale MA (1998) The effect of pictorial illusion on prehension and perception. Journal of Cognitive Neuroscience 10: 122-136.
[11] Westwood DA, Goodale MA (2011) Converging evidence for diverging pathways: Neuropsychology and psychophysics tell the same story. Vision Research 51: 804-811.
[12] Schenk T, Franz V, Bruno N (2011) Vision-for-perception and vision-for action: which model is compatible with the available psychophysical and neuropsychological data? Vision Research 51: 812-818.
[13] Glover S, Dixon P (2002) Dynamic effects of the Ebbinghaus illusion in grasping: Support for a planning/control model of action.
[14] Rizzolatti G, Matelli M (2003) Two different streams form the dorsal visual system: anatomy and function. Experimental Brain Research 153: 146-157.
[15] Pisella L, Binkofski F, Lasek K, Toni I, Rossetti Y (2006) No double-dissociation between optic ataxia and visual agnosia: multiple sub-streams for multiple visuo-manual integrations. Neuropsychologia 44: 2734-2748.
[16] Weiskrantz L, Warrington EK, Sanders MD, Marshall J (1974) Visual capacity in the hemianopic field following a restricted occipital ablation. Brain 97: 709-728.
[17] Weiskrantz L (1996) Blindsight revisited. Current Opinion in Neurobiology 6: 215-220.
[18] Cowey A (2010) The blindsight saga. Experimental Brain Research 200: 3-24.
[19] Poppel E, Held R, Frost D (1973) Residual visual function after brain wounds involving the central visual pathways in man. Nature 243: 295-296.
[20] Perenin MT, Rossetti Y (1996) Grasping without form discrimination in a hemianopic field. Neuroreport 7: 793-797.
[21] Whitwell RL, Striemer CL, Nicolle DA, Goodale MA (2011) Grasping the non-conscious: Preserved grip scaling to unseen objects for immediate by not delayed grasping following a unilateral lesion to primary visual cortex. Vision Research 51: 908-924.
[22] Binsted G, Brownell K, Vorontsova Z, Heath M, Saucier D (2007) Visuomotor system uses target features unavailable to conscious awareness. Proceedings of the National Academy of Sciences 104: 12669-12672.
[23] Perenin MT, Vighetto A (1988) Optic ataxia: a specific disruption in visuomotor mechanisms. I. Different aspects of the deficit in reaching for objects. Brain 111: 643-674.
[24] Pisella L, Grea H, Tilikete C, Vighetto A, Desmurget M, Rode G, Boisson D, Rossetti Y (2000) An 'automatic pilot' for the hand in human posterior parietal cortex: toward reinterpreting optic ataxia. Nature Neuroscience 3: 729-736.
[25] Rossetti Y, Pisella L, Vighetto A (2003) Optic ataxia revisited: visually guided action versus immediate visuomotor control. Experimental Brain Research 153: 171-179.

[26] Milner AD, Goodale MA (2008) Two visual systems re-viewed. Neuropsychologia 46: 774-785.

[27] Pisella L, Sergio L, Blangero A, Torchin H, Vighetto A, Rossetti Y (2009). Optic ataxia and the function of the dorsal stream: Contributions to perception and action. Neuropsychologia 47: 3033-3044.

[28] McIntosh RD, Mulroue A, Blangero A, Pisella L, Rossetti Y (2011) Correlated deficits of perception and action in optic ataxia. Neuropsychologia 49: 131-137.

[29] Harvey M, Rossit S (2011) Visuospatial neglect in action. http://dx.doi.org/10.1016/j.neuropsychologia.2011.09.030

[30] Himmelbach M, Karnath HO (2003) Goal-directed hand movements are not affected by the biased space representation in spatial neglect. Journal of Cognitive Neuroscience 15: 972-980.

[31] Himmelbach M, Karnath HO, Perenin MT (2007) Action control is not affected by spatial neglect: A comment on Coulthard et al. Neuropsychologia 45: 1979-81.

[32] Coulthard E, Parton A, Husain M (2006) Action control in visual neglect. Neuropsychologia 44, 2717-2733.

[33] Rossit S, McIntosh RD, Malhotra P, Butler SH, Muir K, Harvey M (2011) Attention in action: Evidence from on-line corrections in left visual neglect. http://dx.doi.org/10.1016/j.neuropsychologia.2011.10.004

[34] Rossit S, Fraser JA, Teasell R, Malhotra PA, Goodale MA (2011) Impaired delayed but preserved immediate grasping in a neglect patient with parieto-occipital lesions. Neuropsychologia 49: 2498-2504.

[35] Milner AD, Dijkerman HC, Pisella L, McIntosh RD, Tilikete C, Vighetto A, Rossetti Y (2001) Grasping the past: delay can improve visuomotor performance. Current Biology 23: 1896-1901.

[36] Klotz W, Neumann O (1999) Motor activation without conscious discrimination in metacontrast masking. Journal of Experimental Psychology: Human Perception and Performance 25: 976-992.

[37] Taylor JL, McCloskey DI (1990) Triggering of preprogrammed movements as reactions to masked stimuli. Journal of Neurophysiology 63: 439-446.

[38] Cressman EK, Franks IM, Enns JT, Chua R (2007) On-line control of pointing is modified by unseen visual shapes. Consciousness and Cognition 16: 265-275.

[39] Bridgeman B, Hendry D, Stark L (1975) Failure to detect displacement of the visual world due to saccadic eye movements. Vision Research 15: 719-722.

[40] Bridgeman B, Lewis S, Heit G, Nagle M (1979) Relation between cognitive and motor-oriented systems of visual position perception. Journal of Experimental Psychology: Human Perception and Performance 5: 692-700.

[41] Goodale MA, Pelisson D, Prablanc C (1986) Large adjustments in visually guided reaching do not depend on vision of the hand or perception of target displacement. Nature 320: 748-750.

[42] Pelisson D, Prablanc C, Goodale MA, Jeannerod M (1986) Visual control of reaching movements without vision of the limb. Experimental Brain Research 62: 303-311.

[43] Prablanc C, Martin O (1992) Automatic control during hand reaching at undetected two-dimensional target displacements. Journal of Neurophysiology 67: 455-469.
[44] Michel C, Pisella L, Prablanc C, Rode G, Rossetti Y (2007) Enhancing visuomotor adaptation by reducing error signals: single-step (aware) versus multiple-step (unaware) exposure to wedge prisms. Journal of Cognitive Neuroscience 19: 341-350.
[45] Magescas F, Prablanc C (2006) Automatic drive of limb motor plasticity. Journal of Cognitive Neuroscience 18: 75-83.
[46] Cameron BD, Franks IM, Inglis JT, Chua R (2011) Reach adaptation to online target error. Experimental Brain Research 209: 171-180.
[47] Magescas F, Urquizar C, Prablanc C (2009) Two modes of error processing in reaching. Experimental Brain Research 193: 337-350.
[48] Cameron BD, Franks IM, Inglis JT, Chua R (2010) Reach adaptation to explicit vs. implicit target error. Experimental Brain Research 203: 367-380.
[49] Hopp JJ, Fuchs AF (2004) The characteristics and neuronal substrate of saccadic eye movement plasticity. Progress in Neurobiology 72: 27-53.
[50] Henderson JM, Hollingworth A (1999) The role of fixation position in detecting scene changes across saccades. Psychological Science 10: 438-443.
[51] Deubel H, Schneider WX, Bridgeman B (1996) Postsaccadic target blanking prevents saccadic suppression of image displacement. Vision Research 36: 985-996.
[52] Land M, Mennie N, Rusted J (1999) The roles of vision and eye movements in the control of activities of daily living. Perception 28: 1311-1328.
[53] Johansson RS, Westling G, Backstrom A, Flanagan JR (2001) Eye-hand coordination in object manipulation. The Journal of Neuroscience 21: 6917-6932.
[54] Brouwer AM, Franz VH, Gegenfurtner KR (2009) Differences in fixations between grasping and viewing objects. Journal of Vision 9(1): 18.
[55] Neggers SFW, Bekkering H (2001) Gaze anchoring to a pointing target is present during the entire pointing movement and is driven by a non-visual signal. Journal of Neurophysiology 86: 961-970.
[56] Rensink RA, O'Regan JK, Clark JJ (1997) To see or not to see: The need for attention to perceive changes in scenes. Psychological Science 8: 368-373.
[57] Simons DJ, Chabris CF (1999) Gorillas in our midst: sustained inattentional blindness for dynamic events. Perception 28: 1059-1074.
[58] Allport A (1987) Selection for action: some behavioural and neurophysiological considerations of attention and action. In: Heuer H, Sanders AF, editors. Perspectives on Perception and Action. Hillsdale, NJ: Lawrence Erlbaum Associates. pp. 395-420.
[59] Rizzolatti G, Riggio L, Dascola I, Umilta C (1987) Reorienting attention across the horizontal and vertical meridians: evidence in favor of a premotor theory of attention. Neuropsychologia 25: 31-40.
[60] Tipper SP, Lortie C, Baylis GC (1992) Selective reaching: evidence for action-centered attention. Journal of Experimental Psychology: Human Perception and Performance 18: 891-905.

[61] Schneider WX (1995) VAM: a neuro-cognitive model for visual attention control of segmentation, object recognition, and space-based motor action. Visual Cognition 2: 331-375.
[62] Rizzolatti G, Riggio L, Sheliga BM (1994) Space and selective attention. In: Umilta C, Moscovitch M, editors. Attention and Performance XV. Cambridge, MA: MIT Press. pp. 231-265.
[63] Moore T, Fallah M (2001) Control of eye movements and spatial attention. Proceedings of the National Academy of Sciences 98: 1273-1276.
[64] Muller JR, Philiastides MG, Newsome WT (2005) Microstimulation of the superior colliculus focuses attention without moving the eyes. Proceedings of the National Academy of Sciences 102: 524-529.
[65] Meegan DV, Tipper SP (1998) Reaching into cluttered visual environments: spatial and temporal influences of distracting objects. The Quarterly Journal of Experimental Psychology 51A: 225-249.
[66] Desmurget M, Pelisson D, Rossetti Y, Prablanc C (1998) From eye to hand: planning goal-directed movements. Neuroscience and Biobehavioral Reviews 22: 761-788.
[67] Schneider WX, Deubel H (2002) Selection-for-perception and selection-for-spatial-motor-action are coupled by visual attention: A review of recent findings and new evidence from stimulus-driven saccade control. In: Hommel B, Prinz W, editors. Attention and Performance XIX. New York: Oxford University Press. pp. 609-627.
[68] Deubel H, Schneider WX (1996) Saccade target selection and object recognition: Evidence for a common attentional mechanism. Vision Research 36: 1827-1837.
[69] Deubel H, Schneider WX, Paprotta I (1998) Selective dorsal and ventral processing: Evidence for a common attentional mechanism in reaching and perception. Visual Cognition 5: 81-107.
[70] Deubel H, Schneider WX (2003) Delayed saccades, but not delayed manual aiming movements, require visual attention shifts. Annals of the New York Academy of Sciences 1004: 289-296.
[71] Baldauf D, Wolf M, Deubel H (2006) Deployment of visual attention before sequences of goal-directed hand movements. Vision Research 46: 4355-4374.
[72] Bekkering H, Neggers SFW (2002) Visual search is modulated by action intentions. Psychological Science 13: 370-374.

Chapter 7

Linking Neural Activity to Visual Perception: Separating Sensory and Attentional Contributions

Jackson E.T. Smith, Nicolas Y. Masse, Chang'an A. Zhan and Erik P. Cook

Additional information is available at the end of the chapter

http://dx.doi.org/10.5772/47270

1. Introduction

For each of the five basic senses, information about the external world begins as a physical representation in the brain. This representation exists in the structure of sensory neural activity, such as the flow of ions across neural membranes and the action potentials (or spikes) that neurons produce. At some point the brain achieves a transition – from tangible electrophysiology to something more. In other words, neural activity becomes a basic sensation that we are aware of and that we can name. For example, sensations like 'slow' or 'fast', 'far' or 'near', are some of the simplest features that we can assign to a visual stimulus and are some of the basic attributes that we can perceive.

But the transition from neural activity to perception is not simple and remains largely unknown. This process is not intractable, however, and enormous effort has been made by neuroscientists to solve it. In particular, much progress has been made to reveal how small fluctuations in cortical activity are correlated with perceptual behavior. We refer to this correlation as 'behavioral sensitivity'. New observations suggest that both bottom-up sensory mechanisms (such as neural noise) and top-down processes (such as attention) have a role to play in establishing behavioral sensitivity. How do we separate these two contributions?

Figure 1 illustrates the problem of untangling the link between a visual cortical neuron's activity and a subject's perceptual behavior. In the simplest model (Figure 1A), a visual cortical neuron contributes in a bottom-up manner to downstream networks that underlie perceptual behavior. In this case, a neuron is behaviorally sensitive because its activity is directly linked to the perception of the visual stimulus. In the alternative extreme (Figure 1B), a visual cortical neuron has no direct influence on the perceptual decision, but is

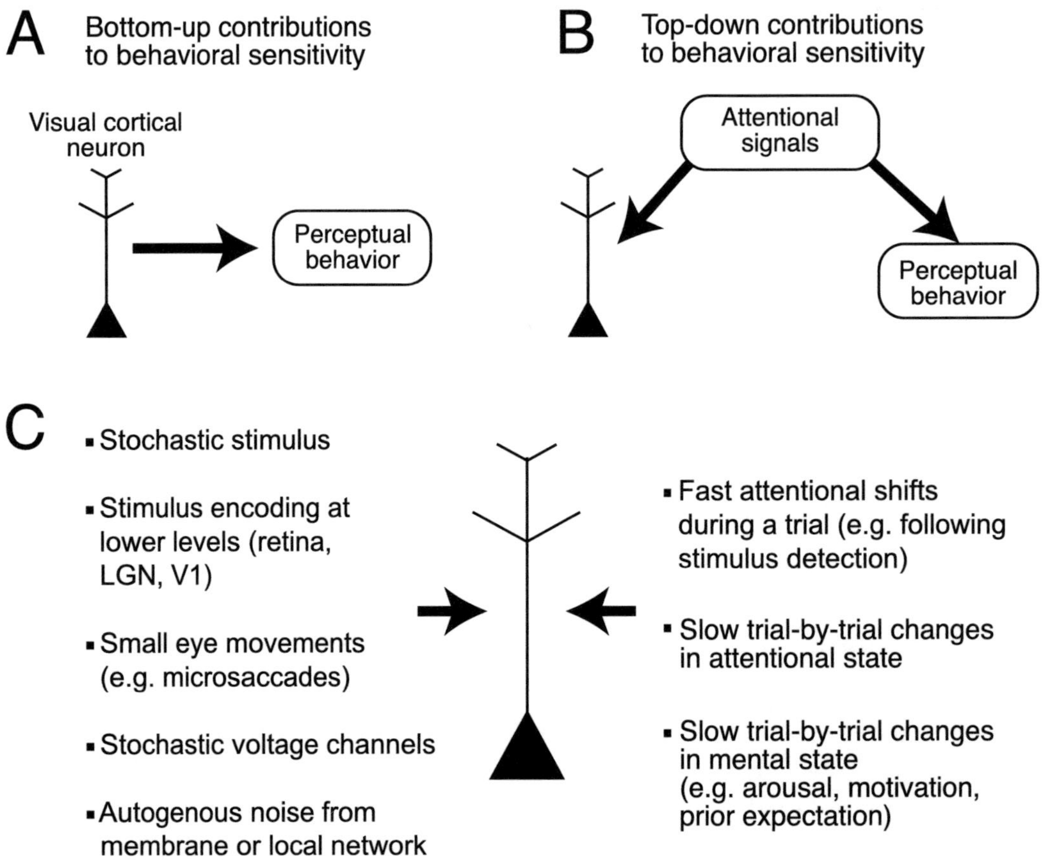

Figure 1. *Two neural mechanisms for a cortical neuron's behavioral sensitivity.* A cortical neuron exhibits behavioral sensitivity if its activity is correlated with perceptual behavior. For both mechanisms in A&B, information about the stimulus is encoded by visual cortical neurons and used to drive perceptual behavior. The arrows do not represent this flow of stimulus information; what they show are the source and destination of trial-to-trial variability. **A**, In the bottom-up mechanism, noisy sensory activity causes the variation in perceptual behavior. In this case, there is a causal link between the variability in visual cortical neurons and the variability in perceptual behavior. **B**, In the top-down mechanism, the subject's attentional state varies from trial-to-trial, causing variable perceptual behavior. However, feedback projections also allow the attentional state to affect the firing rates of visual cortical neurons. In this case, there is a non-causal link between variability in visual cortical activity and perceptual behavior. **C**, Different sources of variation that could contribute to bottom-up sensory and top-down attentional variability in cortical neurons. Note that the bottom-up and top-down hypotheses shown here are the two possible extremes. The brain may actually implement any number of hybrid models, incorporating components from both hypotheses.

modulated by top-down attentional signals that affect both its activity and the perceptual behavior. In both models a neuron can theoretically exhibit the same behavioral sensitivity, but in the top-down scenario it has no role in the perceptual process. As we will discuss, both bottom-up sensory and top-down attentional mechanisms can be at play, depending on the perceptual task. To distinguish among the many possible contributions to a neuron's behavioral sensitivity (Figure 1C), it is first important to understand the properties of behavioral sensitivity and how it is measured.

2. Area MT and visual motion perception as a model system

We can use the specialization of visual cortical neurons to begin understanding how they support visual perception. This is accomplished by comparing the activity of a neuron to the responses of an observer performing a perceptual task [1]. Neurons from the Middle Temporal area of visual cortex (MT i.e. area V5; [2]) are well suited to this purpose. In addition, the methods applied to the study of MT are generally applicable to other areas of visual cortex. MT is a part of the dorsal processing stream and it receives most of its sensory input from areas V1, V2 and V3 – while it sends output chiefly to parts of the parietal cortex [3]. In each hemisphere, area MT contains a complete topographical representation of the contralateral visual hemifield, and any one neuron receives visual information from a discrete patch of visual space, known as the neuron's receptive field (RF). MT neurons are highly selective for both the direction and speed of visual motion, and produce crisp responses to preferred stimuli that fall within their RFs [4]; they are also selective for stimulus size [5] and binocular disparity [6].

Although V1, V2, and V3 neurons can also be selective for the direction and speed of visual motion, a relatively high proportion of MT neurons have an emergent Gestalt sensitivity to the motion of objects formed from separate components. For example, when shown two superimposed sine-wave gratings that move in different directions, V1 neurons mainly respond to the motion of only one component grating or the other; however, a number of MT neurons will treat the two gratings as a single object, responding to the coherent motion of both [7, 8]. Similarly, MT neurons can detect the coherent motion of separate dots – as if the dots were painted on an invisible pane of glass that was moving – even when the coherent dots are embedded within another field of dots that move randomly and incoherently [9].

Importantly, MT has been shown to take part in the perception of coherent dot motion – as lesioning MT causes a severe deficit in a subject's ability to discriminate between opposite directions of motion [10], and microstimulating MT biases a subject to report motion in the preferred direction of the stimulation site [11]. Altogether, the robust responses and selectivity of MT neurons to visual motion, plus their involvement in motion perception, make them an excellent choice for comparison against the perceptual capabilities of a subject [1].

3. A neuron's stimulus sensitivity

The classic studies of Newsome and colleagues demonstrated the power of a careful comparison between neural activity and perceptual behavior [9, 12]. Experiments were performed to carefully measure the discrimination sensitivity of MT neurons from monkey subjects performing a two-alternative, forced-choice (2AFC), motion-discrimination task. The subjects had to report whether the coherent motion in a patch of randomly moving dots was in the preferred or null (preferred + 180°) direction of an isolated MT neuron. It was critical to match the direction, speed, and location of dot motion to the neuron's RF preferences. This ensured that the subject was responding to the same stimulus as the neuron. But more importantly: it maximized the chance that spikes recorded from the neuron were used by the subject to perform the task.

The direction of motion was randomly drawn on every trial so that the subject would have to watch the coherent dots carefully, in order to make a correct choice. However, the strength of coherent motion was also varied from trial to trial by changing the percentage of dots that moved together. This varied the difficulty of the task and therefore the subject's performance, which provided a frame of reference. The neuron's ability to discriminate the direction of coherent dot motion at any one difficulty level could be directly compared against the performance of the subject.

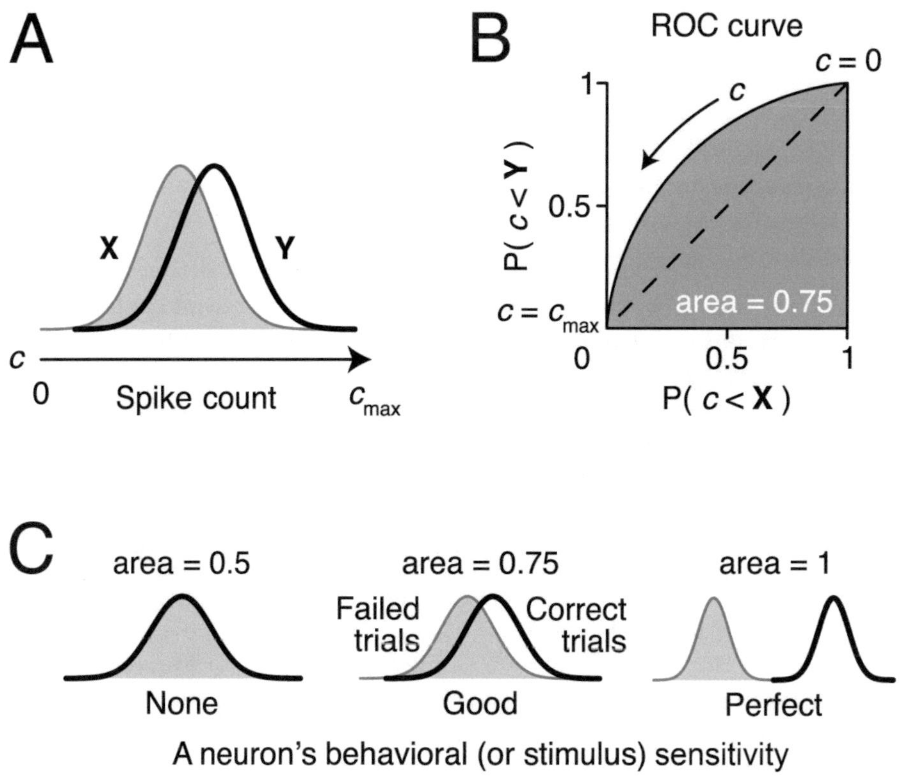

Figure 2. *Area under the receiver operating characteristic (ROC) curve.* **A**, Hypothetical example of two spike-count distributions, from trials grouped by conditions X and Y. Spike counts range between 0 and the maximum value, c_{max}. **B**, The curved line, located above the dashed 'chance' line, represents the ROC curve that is constructed from the distributions in Panel A by classifying their values with the ideal observer (see Appendix). Classification performance is tested for every possible value of the classification criterion, c, which includes all possible spike counts between 0 and c_{max}. Thus, each value of c corresponds to a point in the ROC curve; the arrow shows how increasing values of c are mapped. The grey region is the area under the ROC curve. **C**, Behavioral sensitivity (or stimulus sensitivity) are defined as the area under the ROC curve that compares a distribution of failed-trial (or noise) spike counts (grey) versus a distribution of correct-trial (or signal) spike counts (open). The area under the ROC curve quantifies the difference between the two distributions.

A receiver operating characteristic (ROC) analysis (Figure 2) was used to quantify the discrimination sensitivity of MT neurons in the 2AFC task (see Appendix). For this, two distributions of spike counts were compared against each other, the distribution of counts from trials when the coherent motion was in the neuron's preferred direction (distribution **Y** in Figure 2A) versus the distribution of counts from trials with coherent motion in the null direction (distribution **X** in Figure 2A). The resulting ROC areas (Figure 2B) described the probability that an ideal observer could tell which direction had been presented to the subject, based on the distribution of MT spike counts. This was computed separately for each level of coherent motion strength and compared directly against the subject's performance. It was found that the average MT neuron could account for the subject's discrimination sensitivity – at least under the particular conditions of the experiment [see 13].

The discrimination sensitivity of MT neurons in a 2AFC task is mirrored in experiments where the subject performs a slightly different task: motion detection. In such a task, the subject reports a change in the coherence of dot motion. The sensitivity of an MT neuron is judged by how different its firing rate is before and after the motion stimulus changes. Figure 3A shows an example motion detection task in which a monkey monitors a cloud of randomly moving dots (grey). At the start of each trial, all of the dots move independently (random dot motion) for a random duration. The subject was trained to release a lever in response to a brief (50 ms) period of coherent dot motion (motion pulse). Random dot motion resumed following the motion pulse. Trials were considered a failure if the subject did not release the lever following the coherent motion pulse. Importantly, the dots were located in the RF (dashed circle) of the MT neuron under study, and the coherent motion was always in the neuron's preferred direction and speed. Again, this maximized the chance that the recorded spikes contributed to the subject's performance.

The response of an example neuron – recorded from a monkey performing the motion detection task – is shown in Figure 3B. Each spike is represented as a black tick mark, and each row of ticks is the neuron's response on one trial. Trials are sorted vertically by whether the subject was successful (correct trials, white background) or not (failed trials, grey background). In addition, correct trials are sorted by the duration between the motion pulse and the subject's response time. All tick marks are aligned to the start of the 50 ms motion pulse (dashed line). Before the motion pulse, the neuron produced a baseline number of spikes in response to the random dot motion. Following the start of the motion pulse, however, the neuron responded with a vigorous burst of spikes. The stark contrast of the neuron's responses show that it was very sensitive to the motion pulse.

The stimulus sensitivity of this example neuron is quantified using the ROC metric (Figure 2), similar to the one used by Newsome and colleagues. First, the spikes are counted on each trial in two analysis windows (black bars); one spans the 100 ms *before* the motion pulse (b), counting spikes produced in response to the random dot motion; the other spans the 100 ms *after* the burst of spikes began, counting spikes fired in response to the motion pulse (a). The distribution of spike counts from both windows are shown in Figure 3C. The neuron's sensitivity to the motion pulse is found by comparing the distribution of spikes after the motion pulse (Figure 3C, open bars) versus the distribution of spikes before the motion pulse (Figure 3C, grey bars) using an ROC curve (refer to Figure 2). For this measure of stimulus selectivity, a value of 0.5 would indicate no difference between spike counts before and after the motion pulse, showing that a neuron's response had no information about the visual stimulus. In comparison, values of stimulus selectivity approaching 0 indicate more spikes before the motion pulse, while values approaching 1 indicate more spikes after the motion pulse. As expected, the stimulus sensitivity of this neuron is very high (0.92), meaning that this neuron conveyed reliable information about the occurrence of the motion pulse.

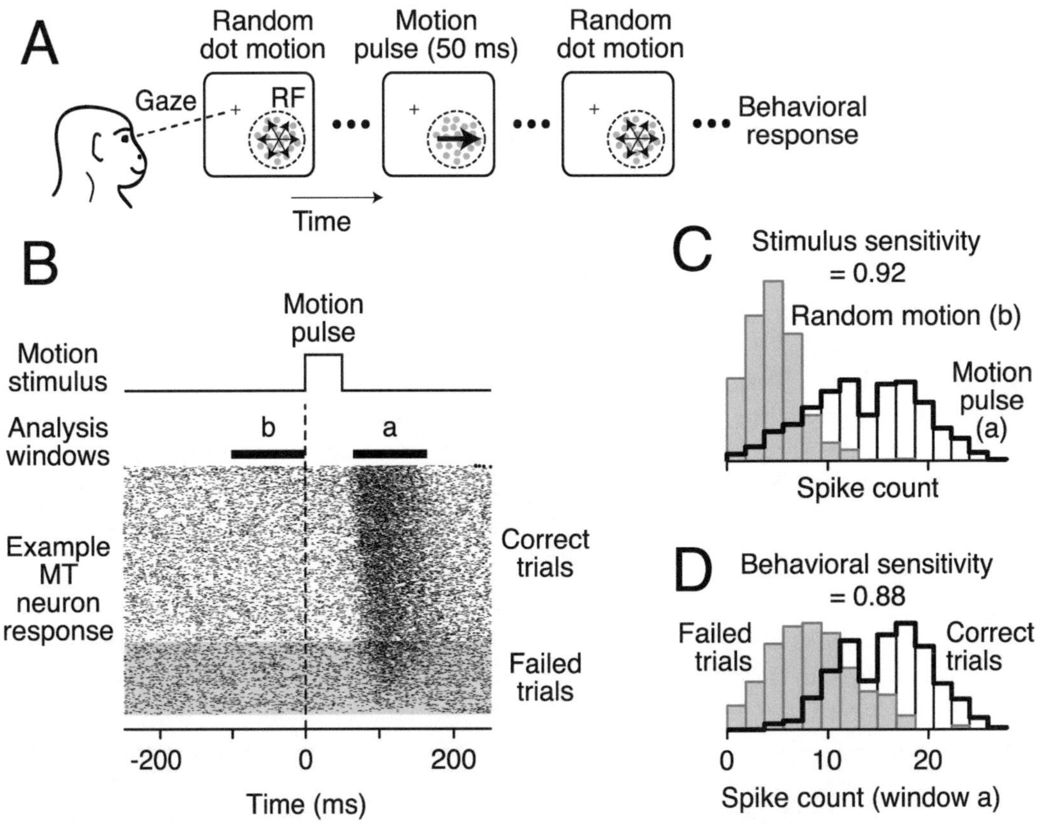

Figure 3. *Stimulus and behavioral sensitivity of an example MT neuron.* **A**, The perceptual task. A monkey directed its gaze to a fixation point (cross) and monitored a patch (grey) of randomly moving dots overlapping the neuron's receptive field (dashed circle). At a random time, the dots moved coherently for 50 ms (motion pulse) in the neuron's preferred direction and speed before reverting back to random dot motion. The trial was a success (correct trial) if the subject released a lever after the motion pulse. The trial was a failure if the subject did not respond. **B**, Raster of spike responses recorded electrophysiologically from an example MT neuron, while the animal subject performed the task in A. The analysis windows (a and b) were used to obtain the spike counts in C&D. **C**, The distribution of spike counts from before (window 'b' in panel B, grey) and after (window 'a' in panel B, open) the motion pulse used to obtain the ROC score that quantified the neuron's stimulus sensitivity. **D**, The distribution of spike counts from failed trials (grey) and correct trials (open) after the motion pulse (window 'a' in panel B) used to obtain the ROC score that quantified the neuron's behavioral sensitivity. Note that this neuron is exemplary and that few visual cortical neurons exhibit this level of behavioral sensitivity.

Whether the subject is detecting or discriminating motion, ROC analysis can be used to quantify the sensitivity of neurons to the stimulus; thus, both are referred to here as 'stimulus sensitivity'. While lesion, microstimulation, and stimulus sensitivity studies show that MT is involved in motion perception and can account for its capabilities – they do not explain how MT activity *becomes* the perception of motion. This requires the estimation of the neural link to perceptual behavior, referred to as 'behavioral sensitivity'.

4. A neuron's behavioral sensitivity

The classic studies of Newsome and colleagues highlighted the large variation in the choices made by subjects and in the number of spikes fired by MT neurons. In response to statistically identical stimuli, subjects would sometimes report the wrong direction and their neurons would sometimes fire as if the opposite direction had been shown. However, this variation presented an exciting opportunity – because the ROC curve is a versatile tool and can be used to compare any two distributions of neural activity. Celebrini and Newsome [14] performed a ground-breaking analysis: they measured the correlation between the number of spikes fired by a neuron and the choice that the subject was about to make.

They began by grouping trials based on the 'preferred' or 'null' motion discrimination report made by the subject. Then they computed the ROC curve comparing the distribution of null-trial spike counts (distribution **X** in Figure 2A) versus the distribution of preferred-trial spike counts (distribution **Y** in Figure 2A). The area under this ROC curve is the probability that the ideal observer could correctly predict which direction of motion the subject would choose, using spike counts. This kind of ROC metric was named 'choice probability' when it was later used to analyze MT neurons [15]. However, we will refer to this ROC metric, and other like it, as 'behavioral sensitivity', because it measures how much the neural response predicts perceptual behavior. It is important to keep in mind that behavioral sensitivity does not measure the correlation between spike counts and perception itself – only the perceptual report, which may not always be faithful to what was actually perceived.

Similar to stimulus sensitivity, a behavioral sensitivity of 0.5 shows that there was no difference in the number of spikes fired prior to either choice (Figure 2C, left). If more spikes were fired prior to choices coinciding with the neuron's preferred direction, then behavioral sensitivity would rise towards 1, to indicate a positive correlation (Figure 2C, middle and right). On the other hand, if more spikes were fired prior to null direction choices, then behavioral sensitivity would sink towards 0, to indicate a negative correlation. On average, MT neurons had a weak but significant, positive correlation with the subject's upcoming choice of motion direction [15]. Since then, behavioral sensitivities have been observed between MT spike counts and the subject's upcoming choice when discriminating coherent dot motion direction [16-18], speed [19, 20], disparity [21, 22], and cylindrical rotation [23-25]. Similar behavioral sensitivities have been observed between a subject's discrimination performance and spike counts from cortical areas V2 [26, 27] and MST [14, 28, 29].

When subjects are tested on their ability to detect a change in coherent dot motion (Figure 3A), the ROC curve is made by comparing the distribution of spike counts from failed trials (distribution **X** in Figure 2A) versus the distribution of spike counts from successful trials (distribution **Y** in Figure 2A). The area under this curve is the probability that the ideal observer can correctly predict the subject's detection performance, and so it was called 'detect probability' [13]. Again, we shall refer to this metric as behavioral sensitivity. A behavioral sensitivity above 0.5 indicates that the neuron fired more prior to successful detections – while behavioral sensitivity below 0.5 indicates that the neuron fired more prior to failures. Using behavioral sensitivity, correlations have been observed between MT spike counts and the subject's ability to detect a change in coherent motion strength [13, 30] and speed [31], while similar behavioral sensitivities have been observed between a subject's detection performance and spike counts from cortical areas V1 [32], V4 [33, 34], and VIP [13].

An example of how to compute behavioral sensitivity is shown for the same example MT neuron and task as before (Figure 3). This time, spike counts are only taken from the analysis window after the motion pulse (Figure 3B, bar 'a'), but they are grouped by whether the trial was correct or failed. The distributions of spike counts on correct (open, **Y** in Figure 2A) and failed (grey, **X** in Figure 2A) trials is shown in Figure 3D. As this neuron was likely to fire more spikes on correct trials, its behavioral sensitivity was very high (0.88); thus, one could reliably predict the animal's behavior from the neural responses.

5. Properties of behavioral sensitivity

The example neuron's behavioral sensitivity (shown in Figure 3) is unusually strong. In general, the average sensitivity of visual neurons to perceptual behavior is much weaker. Table 1 lists the population averages over a number of studies; for most, it was under 0.6. Nevertheless, all averages were significantly greater than chance (0.5).

A typical behavioral sensitivity distribution for an example population of MT neurons is shown in Figure 4A. These neurons were recorded from two experiments, while monkeys performed either a motion detection [35] or a speed detection task [31]. These two experiments were combined because they were both detection tasks that used short, transient stimuli (~50 ms), as illustrated in Figure 3A. The mean behavioral sensitivity was weak, but significantly greater than 0.5 (mean = 0.54, two-sided t-test, $p < 0.01$). Therefore, behavioral sensitivity in visual neurons is a robust result, even though most neurons are only weakly sensitive to the subject's upcoming behavior.

A second key observation is that neurons with high stimulus sensitivities are also highly sensitive to the subject's perceptual behavior. A tempting interpretation is that the brain can determine which neurons are best able to support the subject's performance on a task, then assign them a special role in guiding the subject's behavior. To illustrate this relationship, we plot the distribution of stimulus sensitivities for the same example population of MT neurons in Figure 4B (mean stimulus sensitivity = 0.58, two-sided t-test, $p < 0.01$). To compare stimulus and behavior sensitivities, we first normalized each metric for each animal subject using a Z-score, in order to eliminate changes in the mean from affecting our

Study	Task	Cortical Area	Behavioral Sensitivity
Liu and Newsome 2005 [19]	Speed discrimination	MT	0.52
Gu et al. 2008 [28]	Heading discrimination	MST	0.52
Sasaki and Uka 2009 [22]	Direction discrimination	MT	0.53
Cohen and Maunsell 2010 [33]	Orientation detection	V4	0.53
Cohen and Newsome 2009 [17]	Direction discrimination	MT	0.54
Britten et al. 1996 [15]	Direction discrimination	MT	0.55
Purushothaman & Bradley 2005 [16]	Direction discrimination	MT	0.55
Law and Gold 2008 [18]	Direction discrimination	MT	0.55
Price and Born 2010 [20]	Speed discrimination	MT & MST	0.55
Nienborg and Cumming 2006 [26]	Disparity discrimination	V2	0.56
Sasaki and Uka 2009 [22]	Disparity discrimination	MT	0.57
Bosking and Maunsell 2011 [30]	Coherence detection	MT	0.58
Smith, Zhan, and Cook 2011 [35]	Coherence detection	MT	0.58
Celebrini and Newsome 1994 [14]	Direction discrimination	MST	0.59
Uka and DeAngelis 2004 [21]	Disparity discrimination	MT	0.59
Herrington and Assad 2009 [31]	Speed detection	MT	0.59
Cook and Maunsell 2002 [13]	Coherence detection	MT	0.60
Palmer and Cheng 2007 [32]	Gabor detection	V1	0.61
Herrington and Assad 2009 [31]	Speed detection	LIP	0.63
Dodd et al. 2001 [23]	3D rotation discrimination	MT	0.67
Cook and Maunsell 2002 [13]	Coherence detection	VIP	0.70

Table 1. Average behavioral sensitivity across different studies.

analysis. The results of plotting the normalized stimulus sensitivity versus the normalized behavioral sensitivity is shown in Figure 4C and illustrates a significant correlation (Spearman's coefficient, $R = 0.50$, $p < 0.01$). The correlation between stimulus and behavioral sensitivity is an important property of visual neurons that is often observed [13-16, 18, 20, 21, 24, 28, 30, 35-38].

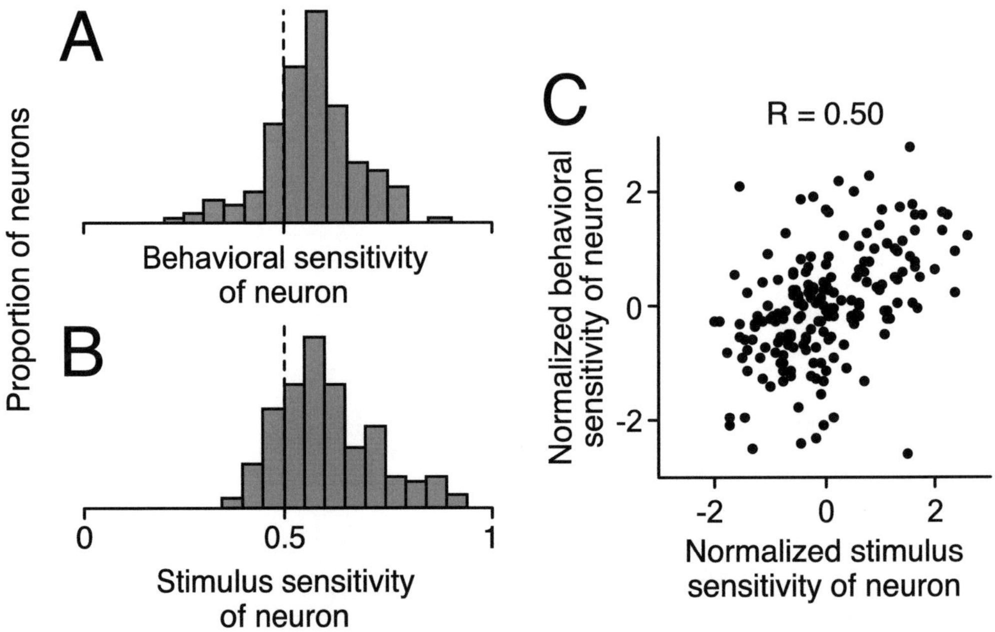

Figure 4. *Stimulus and behavioral sensitivity are correlated.* **A**, The distribution of behavioral sensitivity for an example population of MT neurons, recorded during a motion detection task similar to that in Figure 3A. **B**, The distribution of stimulus sensitivity for the same population of neurons. In A&B, the height of each histogram bin shows the relative proportion of neurons with a sensitivity that falls within the bin's range. **C**, The relationship between stimulus and behavioral sensitivity for the same population of neurons. Behavioral and stimulus sensitivity were normalized for each monkey so as not to introduce any spurious correlations when the data was combined. The Spearman's correlation coefficient is R = 0.50 ($p < 0.01$). The best-fit, linear regression line is $y = 0.46x + 0$, where x is normalized stimulus sensitivity and y is normalized behavioral sensitivity. Data are combined from two experiments using four monkeys [31, 35].

The relationship of stimulus and behavioral sensitivity has, itself, two interesting properties. First, stimulus sensitive neurons seem to become behaviorally sensitive once the subject is well trained to perform the perceptual task [18, 37]; in fact, behavioral sensitivity only appears in neurons that can support the subject's task strategy [21, 39]. Second, the correlation between stimulus and behavioral sensitivity tightens when attention is directed to the neuron's RF (Nicolas Masse, unpublished observation). Altogether, these observations suggests that the most informative neurons are recruited by the brain to drive perceptual behavior.

There is evidence that the recruitment of informative neurons is a dynamic process, and adjusts to changing task demands. For instance, when two different types of motion-disparity stimuli are presented under different task conditions, the same MT neuron may show signs of involvement in the subject's perception of one stimulus, but not another [25]. If the same task is used but the stimulus is presented through different modalities, only the MST neurons that respond in a similar manner to both modalities have strong behavioral sensitivities [28]. When the type of stimulus is consistent, behavioral sensitivity for the same MT neuron can vary as the direction of motion is dialed closer to or further from its preferred direction, in both a motion detection [30] or discrimination [16] task; a similar result holds for MST neurons during heading discrimination [29]. Lastly, when the type of stimulus is consistent but the subject performs two different perceptual tasks, behavioral sensitivity of the same MT neuron may be selective for the behavior on one task, but not the other [22]. These results suggest that the brain is constantly attempting to optimize the pool of visual neurons that it uses to drive perceptual behavior.

Several further properties of behavioral sensitivity are apparent in Table 1. Two of the studies examined neurons from different cortical areas using the same perceptual task ([13] coherence detection, MT & VIP; [31] speed detection, MT & LIP). Each study found that behavioral sensitivity was stronger in the areas further along the hierarchal processing stream (LIP and VIP). Similarly, a disparity discrimination study found behavioral sensitivity in V2 neurons but not in V1 [26]. Extensive investigation of somatosensory cortex has also shown that behavioral sensitivity grows along the hierarchal stream [40, 41]. These studies suggest that the closer a neuron is to downstream decision centers, the better its behavioral sensitivity becomes.

However, even lower level visual areas can demonstrate relatively strong behavioral sensitivity. Although V1 neurons had no sensitivity in a disparity-discrimination task [26], V1 is not thought to be directly involved in disparity perception [42]. On the other hand, V1 neurons are much better suited to supporting the perception of simpler stimuli, such as Gabor patches; accordingly, behavioral sensitivity emerges in V1 neurons when the subject detects Gabors [32]. Similarly, MT neurons are thought to participate in the perception of both motion [10, 11] and disparity [43]. When the subject discriminates a stimulus that requires the perception of both factors, MT neurons become more sensitive to the upcoming behavior [23]. Thus, the behavioral sensitivity of a neuron seems to reflect the extent to which it can support the subject's perception of a given stimulus.

A critical observation is that the strength of behavioral sensitivity is strongly contextual [reviewed by 44]. When subjects are presented with ambiguous stimuli, MT neurons maintain sensitivity to the subject's upcoming behaviour, in 2AFC motion direction [15] and cylindrical rotation [23] discrimination tasks. Ambiguous stimuli carry no meaningful signal; that is, both directions of motion or rotation are equally well represented. In this case, the subject can make no correct choice based on the stimulus and is forced to guess. Although the ambiguous motion direction stimuli are not altogether different from the ambiguous rotation stimuli, MT neurons have much stronger behavioral sensitivities when the subject attempts to discriminate the latter. The main factor accounting for this is that the subject is looking for two-dimensional, linear motion in the first case – and three-dimensional, cylindrical rotation in the second.

A second effect of context is that behavioral sensitivity can strengthen over time on the same trial, following the onset of the stimulus [13, 21, 23, 27, 28, 30] but this is not always the case [15]. An important point to note is that behavioral sensitivity may rise even while the stimulus parameters remain constant. However, some results suggest that the duration of behavioral sensitivity is confined to the time in each trial when the neuron receives useful stimulus information [15, 21, 35].

One last contextual effect was demonstrated in a recent study of V2 neurons [27]; the subject's motivation to perform a perceptual task was varied by changing the expected reward size. Smaller rewards, and therefore less motivation, were accompanied by a decrease in behavioral sensitivity.

A final property of behavioral sensitivity is that it persists when stimulus variation is removed. In both a motion direction discrimination [15] and motion detection [13] task, stimulus variation was removed by repeating the same random dot sequence on multiple trials. In conjunction with contextual effects, these results strongly suggest that behavioral sensitivity comes from mechanisms internal to the brain.

6. Bottom-up sensory versus top-down attentional contributions to behavioral sensitivity

The sensitivity of visual cortical neurons to the subject's impending perceptual behavior is a robust result. Ironically, this fundamental observation has generated some controversy. The trouble is to explain which neural mechanisms produce behavioral sensitivity. Recently, two competing theories have emerged.

The first is the bottom-up hypothesis (Figure 1A). Formulated by Newsome and colleagues [15, 36], it was built upon a foundation of earlier results from psychophysics and neurophysiology, suggesting that the value of a perceived stimulus feature is coded by the collective firing rates from a population of sensory neurons [reviewed by 1]. A population is required when the stimulus responses of individual neurons are noisy; but, by averaging together the noisy responses of a population, an accurate representation of the stimulus can be obtained and used to drive behavior. Bottom-up sources of variation (Figure 1C) may include noise in the stimulus, noisy output from earlier stages of visual processing (e.g. retina, LGN), random eye movements [45], stochastic voltage channels [46], and autogenous noise from local networks [47, 48]. The central idea is that variability in perceptual performance comes directly from the noisy cortical representations of the stimulus.

In the context of the 2AFC direction discrimination task discussed above [12], Shadlen et al. [36] built a bottom-up model using two pools of noisy MT neurons; the first pool preferred motion in one direction, and the second pool preferred motion in the opposite direction. The responses of all neurons in a pool were summed together, and the two pooled signals were used by the model to asses the direction of motion: it chose the preferred direction of whichever pooled response was stronger. Because a direct, causal connection was established between the spike counts of each MT neuron and the model's choice of direction, the model neurons had behavioral sensitivities above 0.5.

For purely bottom-up models, however, the impact of a sensory neuron on perceptual behavior should never change – nor should its behavioral sensitivity. And yet, behavioral sensitivity changes contextually depending on what the subject is looking for, how long the subject has viewed the stimulus, and the subject's motivation level. A bottom-up model can not fully account for these observations, suggesting that high-order processes are involved in the behavioral sensitivity of neurons. The alternative top-down hypothesis (Figure 1B) was formulated to explain these results – in which signals are despatched to sensory cortex from high-order areas of the brain.

In this model, the subject's attentional state varies from trial-to-trial, resulting in variable perceptual performance [see discussion of 15, 27, see review 44]; for example (Figure 1C), changes in spatial attention, prior expectation, motivation, or simply alertness can all affect the subject's chance of success. If the same processes alter the firing rates of sensory neurons, then sensory spike counts would have a non-causal correlation with the subject's performance. In other words, visual cortical neurons could exhibit behavioral sensitivity without actually affecting the perceptual behavior. Attention is a good example of a process that varies from trial to trial and affects both firing rates and perceptual performance [33, 34].

It is important to note that the bottom-up and top-down models, as described, are the two possible extremes at each end of a spectrum. For simplicity's sake, they have been discussed separately. But the brain could implement a hybrid model [e.g. 37].

7. Evidence of bottom-up and top-down sources of behavioral sensitivity

Despite almost twenty years of study, there is no clear proof that one mechanism for behavioral sensitivity is entirely correct. The bottom-up hypothesis is attractive because it ties together a number of observations parsimoniously; neurons are weakly sensitive to the subject's behavior when they are responding to an informative stimulus, when they are able to support perception of the stimulus features, and when they are able to support the subject's task strategy. Furthermore, a neuron's behavioral sensitivity scales with its sensitivity to the stimulus (Figure 4C). These properties are accounted for if the brain pools the output from a select set of informative neurons to form perceptual decisions, while ignoring output from uninformative neurons. The action of pooling offers a reason that the average behavioral sensitivity is weak: because the impact on behavior of any one neuron is diluted in the population response. However, the size of a neural pool required to form perceptions is unknown. There is some evidence that perceptual decisions are formed using only a few, highly informative neurons [38]. But the complication of correlated activity between neurons [49, 50] may require neural populations on a scale of hundreds [36].

A further attraction of the bottom-up hypothesis is that computational models with a bottom-up structure are able to emulate the subject's behavior, neural responses and neural behavioral sensitivity, for a variety of tasks [13, 35-37]. Unfortunately, bottom-up models have difficulty explaining other properties of behavioral sensitivity without resorting to complex mechanisms. Although it would seem sensible that a subject should guide visual judgements using the most informative visual cortical neurons, it is uncertain how a purely bottom-up mechanism could recruit them. A simple way would be to change the synaptic weighting downstream of sensory areas, strengthening the connections from informative neurons and weakening the connections from uninformative neurons. This technique is able to alter the mean behavioral sensitivity of a simulated neural population [37]. Unexpectedly, synaptic weight changes alone cannot account for the correlation between a neuron's stimulus and behavioral sensitivities (Figure 4C).

Correlations between the spiking activity of neurons can be the determining factor of behavioral sensitivity, especially for large pools of neurons [36]. Weak, inter-neural correlations have been observed throughout the brain [29, 49, 51-54] – with diverse implications [reviewed by 50]. Importantly, the level of correlation between neurons can inflate their behavioral sensitivities in two ways: in a bottom-up model, it reduces the independence of sensory neurons and tightens the covariance of any single one with the pooled response [36]; it can also cause neurons with no impact on perception to mimic other neurons that directly support perception [17, 55]. These effects of correlation on behavioral sensitivity increase for larger pools of neurons, while the effect of synaptic weighting decreases [36]. Thus, one cannot model the relationship between a neuron's stimulus and behavioral sensitivity (Figure 4C) with synaptic weight changes, alone. However, if the correlation between two neurons is scaled by the similarity of their RF tuning and by the similarity of their stimulus sensitivity, then selectively weighting the more informative neurons can reproduce the observed relationship between stimulus and behavioral sensitivity [37]. Although an interplay between stimulus sensitivity, behavioral sensitivity, and the correlation between neurons is predicted, very little empirical verification has been published to date [24].

Bottom-up models also fail to explain the contextual variation of behavioral sensitivity. If top-down signals are able to selectively modulate the activity of targeted sensory neurons, then the top-down hypothesis is better placed to explain contextual variation, dynamic changes in behavioral sensitivity from trial to trial, and the relationship between stimulus and behavioral sensitivity. Attention [56] can modulate the activity of select neurons as well as affect the subject's behavior; thus it is a good candidate for the source of top-down behavioral sensitivity. Trial-to-trial fluctuations in attention could equally as well have been the source of behavioral sensitivity in studies that otherwise supported a bottom-up model [15, 21, 35]. Furthermore, two recent multielectrode studies were able to estimate the level of attention on each trial, from the collective responses of many simultaneously recorded neurons [33, 34]; it was found that fluctuations in attention could account for the behavioral sensitivity of V4 neurons. Thus, a top-down mechanism is better able to account for some properties of behavioral sensitivity than a bottom-up mechanism.

8. Local field potentials and top-down mechanisms of behavioral sensitivity

Whether the behavioral sensitivity is due to top-down or bottom-up mechanisms depends entirely upon whether or not cortical neurons receive top-down signals in the first place. Specifically, attentional signals that predict the subject's upcoming performance. But how can such signals be measured and separated from bottom-up visual inputs? When microelectrodes are used to record a voltage trace from the brain, they deliver far more information than just neural spiking activity. The short, discrete, high frequency waveforms of spikes ride on top of lower frequency changes in voltage.

Cortical local field potentials (LFP) are defined as the 1-200 Hz frequency bandwidth of the electrode voltage trace, and they result from the collective activity of neurons within approximately 250μm of the electrode tip [57, 58] – roughly the same spacial scale as a cortical column [59]. Because cortical tissue has no bandpassing effect on LFPs [60] and because their measurement is robust to the choice of microelectrode [61], LFPs are a clean way of taking neural activity measurements that are comparable across studies. Neurons generate LFPs in many ways [see review 62], including sub-threshold membrane activity and local oscillatory interactions between excitatory and inhibitory neurons; but an important source of LFP fluctuations are synaptic potentials in the dendrites: in other words, LFPs indirectly measure the input received by the local population of neurons.

Different sources of LFP fluctuations that operate at different time-scales can be partially isolated from each other by analyzing LFPs in the frequency domain [63]. The stimulus response of visual cortical LFPs from 3 to 90 Hz have been found to resemble the behavior of spiking responses from earlier processing stages [64-66], while higher frequency LFPs (>80 Hz) resemble the spiking responses of local neurons [67-71] – suggesting that LFPs below 80 Hz reflect synaptic activity. Upon closer inspection, it is found that LFPs from 1 to 12 Hz carry stimulus information that is independent of the stimulus information in LFPs above 40 Hz [72, 73]; but the band from 12 to 40 Hz does not carry stimulus information at all, raising the question of what its function is.

As visual neurons receive a substantial proportion of their input recurrently [74], LFPs must capture synaptic activity that results from neuromodulatory feedback. Generally, the spectral power of gamma band (40-80 Hz) LFPs is increased when attention is directed to the recording site's RF [75-77], although it may decrease as well [78]. In area MT, this increase of gamma LFP power resembles the increase in firing rates of neurons in the same vicinity; however, beta band (12-24 Hz) LFP power from the same recordings behave differently in the face of attention – decreasing instead of increasing [79]. The decrease in low frequency LFP power is thought to result from the same attention related feedback that causes neurons to decorrelate from each other and reduce the variability of their responses [80]; this hypothesis is bolstered by the observation that the coherence of beta band LFPs from visual areas at different stages of hierarchal processing is strengthened by goal-directed attention [81, 82]. The relationship of beta band LFPs to top-down neuromodulatory signals – and their distinct response to them – make beta LFPs a good candidate measurement of the top-down input that arrives in sensory cortex.

The first demonstration that LFP spectral power is sensitive to the subject's upcoming perceptual behavior was made from recordings in MT by Liu and Newsome [83]. Their innovation was to use distributions of spectral power rather than spike counts to compute the behavioral sensitivity of LFPs – by using a ROC curve to compare the distribution of power from trials when the subject reported the preferred stimulus of the recording site versus the distribution of power from trials when the subject reported the null stimulus. As a result, LFP behavioral sensitivity was a function of LFP frequency. Liu and Newsome observed that LFPs above 50 Hz had sensitivities above 0.5, indicating more spectral power when the subject was about to choose the preferred stimulus, which was similar to the positive spike-count behavioral sensitivities of MT neurons. Lower frequency LFPs, within the realm of alpha (8-12 Hz) and beta (12-24 Hz), showed a distinct behavior: they had sensitivities less than 0.5, which indicated less spectral power when the subject was about to choose the preferred stimulus. Since top-down neuromodulatory signals can explain this result, it may be the first demonstration that correlations between neural activity and perceptual behavior come from a top-down mechanism. However, it was also found that a trial-to-trial shift of LFP spectral power from lower frequencies to high frequencies could explain this result, without top-down signals.

9. Bottom-up and top-down processes work in sequence to produce behavioral sensitivity

Studies of behavioral sensitivity have had difficulty validating either the bottom-up or top-down hypothesis. But certain aspects of their experimental designs may have led to ambiguity. For example, many key studies have used long duration stimuli of 500 ms or more [13-16, 19-23, 25, 27, 30, 83]. This is problematic when trying to distinguish between a bottom-up and top-down mechanism – because it is impossible to tell when, or even whether, the neuron is responding to the stimulus or to top-down attentional signals. Recent studies, however, have begun to dissect bottom-up from top-down processes. They suggest that both mechanisms contribute to behavioral sensitivity, one after the other (illustrated in Figure 5).

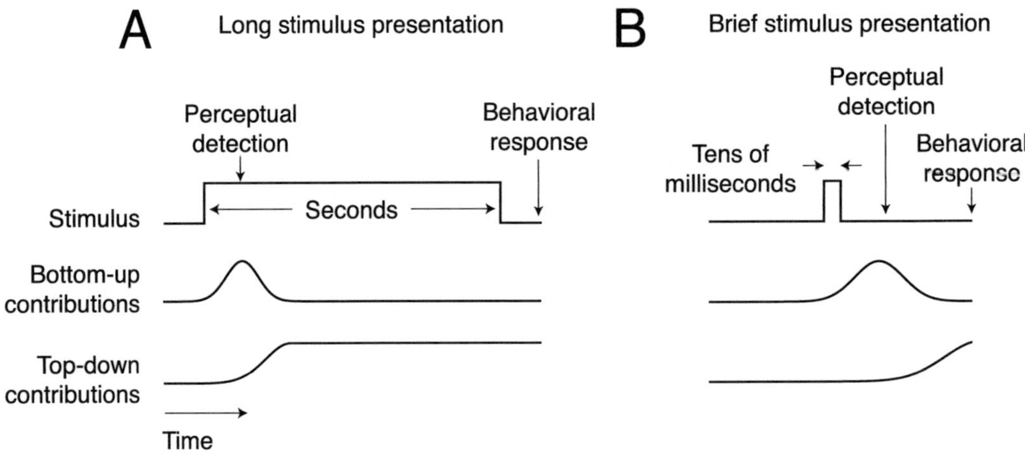

Figure 5. *Bottom-up and top-down contributions to behavioral sensitivity are sequential.* **A**, The order of perceptual events during the presentation of a long-duration stimulus, such as in [27]. The long duration stimulus allows a neuron's behavioral sensitivity to be dominated by top-down contributions. **B**, The order of perceptual events following the presentation of a brief stimulus, as in [35]. Because the subject tends to respond before top-down contributions take effect, a neuron's behavioral sensitivity is dominated by bottom-up contributions.

Nienborg and Cumming have demonstrated two contrasting processes by developing a psychophysical, reverse-correlation technique and comparing the results with the behavioral sensitivity of V2 neurons [27, 39]. Psychophysical reverse-correlation provided an estimate of the subject's strategy when performing a disparity discrimination task. More importantly, it estimated when the subject was accumulating stimulus information. They found that subjects made the most use of stimulus information early in the trial – with later information being used progressively less, even though it was equally useful. In disagreement with a bottom-up prediction, they found that behavioral sensitivity moved in the opposite direction; it was weakest at the start of the trial, and then grew for approximately 500 ms before plateauing. A similar rise in behavioral sensitivity over time has been observed in other studies [13, 17, 20, 21, 23, 28, 30]. Together, these observations suggest an early, sensory accumulation process followed by a later process that was predictive of the subject's upcoming behavior.

Rapid sensory accumulation and evaluation is necessary to explain any perceptual decision that is made before the late rise in behavioral sensitivity [84]. Accordingly, Nienborg and Cumming [27] observed behavioral sensitivity that was significantly greater than 0.5 within the first 500 ms of stimulation, when the subject made the most use of the stimulus information. But because their stimulus was long in duration and always appeared at the same time and location, it is impossible to know if the early component of behavioral sensitivity resulted from the early, sensory-accumulation process or from the late, behaviorally sensitive process (illustrated in Figure 5A).

Another recent study has looked exclusively at the behavioral sensitivity of MT neurons during early sensory accumulation, while subjects performed a motion-detection, reaction-time task [35]. This was achieved by using a very short (50 ms) motion signal that occurred at an unpredictable time and location. Unlike studies that used long stimulus presentation times, the neural sensitivity to behavior peaked approximately 100 ms after the motion signal began, during the short burst of spikes that neurons fired in response to the motion signal. Critically, both the transient neural response and the subject's perceptual report (median RT = 400 ms) occurred well before the time in other studies that a late rise in behavioral sensitivity was established. Lastly, all aspects of the behavioral sensitivity time-courses and of the subject's perceptual behavior were well accounted for by a purely bottom-up model. Together, these results suggest that sensory neurons have a bottom-up link to perceptual behavior during the early, sensory-accumulation process (illustrated in Figure 5B).

The late rise in behavioral sensitivity has parallels in other studies as well. In V1 neurons, spikes fired in response to a contour are able to distinguish whether it is the target or distractor stimulus, approximately 200–600 ms after the contour appeared [85, 86]. Similarly, the aperture problem is disentangled by MT firing rates approximately 150 ms after stimulus motion begins [8]. Of special interest is the recent evidence that stimulus information arrives in MT from outside the RF through top-down channels, approximately 400-500 ms following the onset of test stimuli in a match-to-sample task [87]. In these cases, late sensory neural activity carries information that was not originally available in the initial transient response, but likely arrives from a top-down source that has solved the problem at hand. These observations further support the idea that a top-down source of behavioral sensitivity engages sensory neurons following the initial transient response. While attention-like signals could fill the role of a top-down source following the start of the stimulus, it would have to allow for other attentional effects that are present earlier in the trial [33, 34, 52, 88].

10. Conclusion

To study the neural correlates of sensory perception in visual cortex, it is first necessary to understand how neural activity becomes selective for the upcoming perceptual behavior of a subject. This is referred to as a neuron's behavioral sensitivity. There has been debate in the literature about whether the brain links sensory neural activity to perceptual behavior using a bottom-up or top-down mechanism. New results suggest that both mechanisms are active, but in a sequential fashion. The initial, transient responses of sensory neurons have a direct, bottom-up impact upon the subject's behavior. Later responses reflect top-down signals that are linked to high-order processes, and attention fills the criteria necessary to drive top-down behavioral sensitivity. Although potentially difficult, new studies are needed to carefully distinguish and compare the contribution of both processes to the behavioral sensitivity of visual cortical neurons.

Author details

Jackson E. T. Smith and Erik P. Cook
Department of Physiology, McGill University, Montreal, Québec

Nicolas Y. Masse
Department of Neurobiology, University of Chicago, Chicago, Illinois

Chang'an A. Zhan
School of Biomedical Engineering, Southern Medical University, Guangzhou, China

Acknowledgement

The authors wish to thank John Assad and Todd Herrington for the speed-pulse data used in Figure 4. The authors also acknowledge funding support from the Canadian Institutes of Health Research, The Natural Sciences and Engineering Research Council of Canada, and The EJLB Foundation.

Appendix: Area under the receiver operating characteristic (ROC) curve

The method used to quantify the discrimination sensitivity of MT neurons in a 2AFC task [9, 12] has since become a common technique of behavioral neurophysiology, and forms the basis of all major results reported in this study. The key question is whether the neurons fired more spikes in one condition than in another. Traditional parametric methods for answering this question place restrictive assumptions on the statistics of neural activity; for example, neurons do not always resemble a Poisson process [89]. Receiver operating characteristic (ROC) curves provide an unbiased, non-parametric way of quantifying the difference between any two distributions [90] – in this case, the number of spikes fired by a neuron on one set of trials versus another. Figure 2 illustrates how a ROC curve is used to quantify the difference between two distributions of spike counts (Figure 2A).

Faced with the problem of classifying a randomly sampled spike count as being from either distribution **X** (filled) or **Y** (open), the strategy adopted by the ideal observer is to choose a criterion level of c and assign any spike count less than c to **X**, and any spike count above c to **Y**. All possible values of c between 0 and the maximum spike count (c_{max}) must be tested to find the optimal criterion that makes correct classifications the most often.

To do so, a ROC curve is built by plotting the probability that spike counts sampled from **X** are greater than c against the probability that spike counts sampled from **Y** are greater than c (Figure 2B). When $c = 0$, all spike counts are greater than c, thus the beginning point of the ROC curve is always (1,1). As c is increased (Figure 2B, arrow) the performance of the ideal observer using that criterion level is plotted. When c hits c_{max}, no spike count is greater than c and the end point of the curve is (0,0).

The area under the ROC curve (Figure 2B, grey shading) is the probability that the ideal observer will correctly classify any given spike count from either distribution, and ranges between 0 and 1 accordingly; this probability is 0.75 for distributions **X** and **Y** from Figure 2A. Therefore, when **X** and **Y** are completely distinct from each other, the ideal observer correctly classifies 100% of all spike counts (area = 1, Figure 2C, right). On the other hand, if there is no distinction between **X** and **Y**, then the ideal observer has a 50% chance of correct classification – a coin toss (area = 0.5, left). If **X** and **Y** from Figure 2A switch positions then the difference between them remains the same; this is reflected by the area under the ROC curve, which is an equal distance below 0.5 after the switch (0.25 = 0.5 - 0.25, solid curve) as it was before (0.75 = 0.5 + 0.25, dotted curve).

Abbreviations

LGN – lateral geniculate nucleus
MT i.e. V5 – middle temporal area of visual cortex
MST – medial superior temporal area of visual cortex
VIP – ventral intraparietal area of visual cortex
LIP – lateral intraparietal area of visual cortex
2AFC – two-alternative forced choice
LFP – local field potential
RF – receptive field
ROC – receiver operating characteristic
RT – reaction time

11. References

[1] Parker, A.J. and W.T. Newsome, *SENSE AND THE SINGLE NEURON: Probing the Physiology of Perception.* Annual Review of Neuroscience, 1998. 21(1): p. 227-277.

[2] Vanessen, D.C., J.H.R. Maunsell, and J.L. Bixby, *The Middle Temporal Visual Area in the Macaque - Myeloarchitecture, Connections, Functional-Properties and Topographic Organization.* Journal of Comparative Neurology, 1981. 199(3): p. 293-326.

[3] Felleman, D.J. and D.C. Van Essen, *Distributed hierarchical processing in the primate cerebral cortex.* Cereb Cortex, 1991. 1(1): p. 1-47.

[4] Maunsell, J.H. and D.C. Van Essen, *Functional properties of neurons in middle temporal visual area of the macaque monkey. I. Selectivity for stimulus direction, speed, and orientation.* J Neurophysiol, 1983. 49(5): p. 1127-47.

[5] Allman, J., F. Miezin, and E. McGuinness, *Direction- and velocity-specific responses from beyond the classical receptive field in the middle temporal visual area (MT).* Perception, 1985. 14(2): p. 105-26.

[6] DeAngelis, G.C. and W.T. Newsome, *Organization of disparity-selective neurons in macaque area MT.* J Neurosci, 1999. 19(4): p. 1398-415.

[7] Movshon, J.A. and W.T. Newsome, *Visual response properties of striate cortical neurons projecting to area MT in macaque monkeys.* J Neurosci, 1996. 16(23): p. 7733-41.

[8] Pack, C.C. and R.T. Born, *Temporal dynamics of a neural solution to the aperture problem in visual area MT of macaque brain.* Nature, 2001. 409(6823): p. 1040-2.

[9] Britten, K.H., et al., *The Analysis of Visual-Motion - a Comparison of Neuronal and Psychophysical Performance.* Journal of Neuroscience, 1992. 12(12): p. 4745-4765.

[10] Newsome, W.T. and E.B. Pare, *A selective impairment of motion perception following lesions of the middle temporal visual area (MT).* J Neurosci, 1988. 8(6): p. 2201-11.

[11] Salzman, C.D., et al., *Microstimulation in visual area MT: effects on direction discrimination performance.* J Neurosci, 1992. 12(6): p. 2331-55.

[12] Newsome, W.T., K.H. Britten, and J.A. Movshon, *Neuronal correlates of a perceptual decision.* Nature, 1989. 341(6237): p. 52-4.

[13] Cook, E.P. and J.H.R. Maunsell, *Dynamics of neuronal responses in macaque MT and VIP during motion detection.* Nature Neuroscience, 2002. 5(10): p. 985-994.

[14] Celebrini, S. and W.T. Newsome, *Neuronal and Psychophysical Sensitivity to Motion Signals in Extrastriate Area Mst of the Macaque Monkey.* Journal of Neuroscience, 1994. 14(7): p. 4109-4124.

[15] Britten, K.H., et al., *A relationship between behavioral choice and the visual responses of neurons in macaque MT.* Visual Neuroscience, 1996. 13(1): p. 87-100.

[16] Purushothaman, G. and D.C. Bradley, *Neural population code for fine perceptual decisions in area MT.* Nature Neuroscience, 2005. 8(1): p. 99-106.

[17] Cohen, M.R. and W.T. Newsome, *Estimates of the Contribution of Single Neurons to Perception Depend on Timescale and Noise Correlation.* Journal of Neuroscience, 2009. 29(20): p. 6635-6648.

[18] Law, C.T. and J.I. Gold, *Neural correlates of perceptual learning in a sensory-motor, but not a sensory, cortical area.* Nature Neuroscience, 2008. 11(4): p. 505-513.

[19] Liu, J. and W.T. Newsome, *Correlation between speed perception and neural activity in the middle temporal visual area.* J Neurosci, 2005. 25(3): p. 711-22.

[20] Price, N.S.C. and R.T. Born, *Timescales of Sensory- and Decision-Related Activity in the Middle Temporal and Medial Superior Temporal Areas.* Journal of Neuroscience, 2010. 30(42): p. 14036-14045.

[21] Uka, T. and G.C. DeAngelis, *Contribution of area MT to stereoscopic depth perception: Choice-related response modulations reflect task strategy.* Neuron, 2004. 42(2): p. 297-310.

[22] Sasaki, R. and T. Uka, *Dynamic Readout of Behaviorally Relevant Signals from Area MT during Task Switching.* Neuron, 2009. 62(1): p. 147-157.
[23] Dodd, J.V., et al., *Perceptually bistable three-dimensional figures evoke high choice probabilities in cortical area MT.* J Neurosci, 2001. 21(13): p. 4809-21.
[24] Parker, A.J., K. Krug, and B.G. Cumming, *Neuronal activity and its links with the perception of multi-stable figures.* Philosophical Transactions of the Royal Society of London Series B-Biological Sciences, 2002. 357(1424): p. 1053-1062.
[25] Krug, K., B.G. Cumming, and A.J. Parker, *Comparing perceptual signals of single V5/MT neurons in two binocular depth tasks.* Journal of Neurophysiology, 2004. 92(3): p. 1586-1596.
[26] Nienborg, H. and B.G. Cumming, *Macaque V2 neurons, but not V1 neurons, show choice-related activity.* Journal of Neuroscience, 2006. 26(37): p. 9567-9578.
[27] Nienborg, H. and B.G. Cumming, *Decision-related activity in sensory neurons reflects more than a neuron's causal effect.* Nature, 2009. 459(7243): p. 89-U93.
[28] Gu, Y., D.E. Angelaki, and G.C. Deangelis, *Neural correlates of multisensory cue integration in macaque MSTd.* Nat Neurosci, 2008. 11(10): p. 1201-10.
[29] Gu, Y., et al., *Perceptual learning reduces interneuronal correlations in macaque visual cortex.* Neuron, 2011. 71(4): p. 750-761.
[30] Bosking, W.H. and J.H. Maunsell, *Effects of stimulus direction on the correlation between behavior and single units in area MT during a motion detection task.* J Neurosci, 2011. 31(22): p. 8230-8.
[31] Herrington, T.M. and J.A. Assad, *Neural Activity in the Middle Temporal Area and Lateral Intraparietal Area during Endogenously Cued Shifts of Attention.* Journal of Neuroscience, 2009. 29(45): p. 14160-14176.
[32] Palmer, C., S.Y. Cheng, and E. Seidemann, *Linking neuronal and behavioral performance in a reaction-time visual detection task.* Journal of Neuroscience, 2007. 27(30): p. 8122-8137.
[33] Cohen, M.R. and J.H.R. Maunsell, *A Neuronal Population Measure of Attention Predicts Behavioral Performance on Individual Trials.* Journal of Neuroscience, 2010. 30(45): p. 15241-15253.
[34] Cohen, M. and J. Maunsell, *Using Neuronal Populations to Study the Mechanisms Underlying Spatial and Feature Attention.* Neuron, 2011. 70(6): p. 1192-1204.
[35] Smith, J.E., C.A. Zhan, and E.P. Cook, *The Functional Link between Area MT Neural Fluctuations and Detection of a Brief Motion Stimulus.* J Neurosci, 2011. 31(38): p. 13458-68.
[36] Shadlen, M.N., et al., *A computational analysis of the relationship between neuronal and behavioral responses to visual motion.* Journal of Neuroscience, 1996. 16(4): p. 1486-1510.
[37] Law, C.T. and J.I. Gold, *Reinforcement learning can account for associative and perceptual learning on a visual-decision task.* Nature Neuroscience, 2009. 12(5): p. 655-663.
[38] Ghose, G.M. and I.T. Harrison, *Temporal Precision of Neuronal Information in a Rapid Perceptual Judgment.* Journal of Neurophysiology, 2009. 101(3): p. 1480-1493.
[39] Nienborg, H. and B.G. Cumming, *Psychophysically measured task strategy for disparity discrimination is reflected in V2 neurons.* Nature Neuroscience, 2007. 10(12): p. 1608-1614.
[40] de Lafuente, V. and R. Romo, *Neuronal correlates of subjective sensory experience.* Nature Neuroscience, 2005. 8(12): p. 1698-1703.

[41] Hernandez, A., et al., *Decoding a Perceptual Decision Process across Cortex.* Neuron, 2010. 66(2): p. 300-314.

[42] Cumming, B.G. and A.J. Parker, *Responses of primary visual cortical neurons to binocular disparity without depth perception.* Nature, 1997. 389(6648): p. 280-3.

[43] DeAngelis, G.C., B.G. Cumming, and W.T. Newsome, *Cortical area MT and the perception of stereoscopic depth.* Nature, 1998. 394(6694): p. 677-80.

[44] Krug, K., *A common neuronal code for perceptual visual cortex? Comparing choice and processes in attentional correlates in V5/MT.* Philosophical Transactions of the Royal Society of London Series B-Biological Sciences, 2004. 359(1446): p. 929-941.

[45] Herrington, T.M., et al., *The Effect of Microsaccades on the Correlation between Neural Activity and Behavior in Middle Temporal, Ventral Intraparietal, and Lateral Intraparietal Areas.* Journal of Neuroscience, 2009. 29(18): p. 5793-5805.

[46] White, J.A., J.T. Rubinstein, and A.R. Kay, *Channel noise in neurons.* Trends in Neurosciences, 2000. 23(3): p. 131-137.

[47] Sanchez-Vives, M.V. and D.A. McCormick, *Cellular and network mechanisms of rhythmic recurrent activity in neocortex.* Nat Neurosci, 2000. 3(10): p. 1027-34.

[48] Timofeev, I., et al., *Origin of slow cortical oscillations in deafferented cortical slabs.* Cereb Cortex, 2000. 10(12): p. 1185-99.

[49] Bair, W., E. Zohary, and W.T. Newsome, *Correlated firing in macaque visual area MT: Time scales and relationship to behavior.* Journal of Neuroscience, 2001. 21(5): p. 1676-1697.

[50] Averbeck, B.B., P.E. Latham, and A. Pouget, *Neural correlations, population coding and computation.* Nature Reviews Neuroscience, 2006. 7(5): p. 358-366.

[51] Vaadia, E., et al., *Dynamics of Neuronal Interactions in Monkey Cortex in Relation to Behavioral Events.* Nature, 1995. 373(6514): p. 515-518.

[52] Cohen, M.R. and J.H.R. Maunsell, *Attention improves performance primarily by reducing interneuronal correlations.* Nat Neurosci, 2009. 12(12): p. 1594-1600.

[53] Roelfsema, P.R., V.A. Lamme, and H. Spekreijse, *Synchrony and covariation of firing rates in the primary visual cortex during contour grouping.* Nat Neurosci, 2004. 7(9): p. 982-991.

[54] Romo, R., et al., *Correlated neuronal discharges that increase coding efficiency during perceptual discrimination.* Neuron, 2003. 38(4): p. 649-657.

[55] Nienborg, H. and B. Cumming, *Correlations between the activity of sensory neurons and behavior: how much do they tell us about a neuron's causality?* Current Opinion in Neurobiology, 2010. 20(3): p. 376-381.

[56] Knudsen, E.I., *Fundamental components of attention.* Annual Review of Neuroscience, 2007. 30: p. 57-78.

[57] Katzner, S., et al., *Local Origin of Field Potentials in Visual Cortex.* Neuron, 2009. 61(1): p. 35-41.

[58] Xing, D.J., C.I. Yeh, and R.M. Shapley, *Spatial Spread of the Local Field Potential and its Laminar Variation in Visual Cortex.* Journal of Neuroscience, 2009. 29(37): p. 11540-11549.

[59] Mountcastle, V.B., *The columnar organization of the neocortex.* Brain, 1997. 120: p. 701-722.

[60] Logothetis, N.K., C. Kayser, and A. Oeltermann, *In vivo measurement of cortical impedance spectrum in monkeys: Implications for signal propagation.* Neuron, 2007. 55(5): p. 809-823.

[61] Nelson, M.J. and P. Pouget, *Do electrode properties create a problem in interpreting local field potential recordings?* J Neurophysiol, 2010. 103(5): p. 2315-7.
[62] Logothetis, N.K., *The underpinnings of the BOLD functional magnetic resonance imaging signal.* Journal of Neuroscience, 2003. 23(10): p. 3963-3971.
[63] Siegel, M., T.H. Donner, and A.K. Engel, *Spectral fingerprints of large-scale neuronal interactions.* Nat Rev Neurosci, 2012.
[64] Monosov, I.E., J.C. Trageser, and K.G. Thompson, *Measurements of simultaneously recorded spiking activity and local field potentials suggest that spatial selection emerges in the frontal eye field.* Neuron, 2008. 57(4): p. 614-625.
[65] Viswanathan, A. and R.D. Freeman, *Neurometabolic coupling in cerebral cortex reflects synaptic more than spiking activity.* Nature Neuroscience, 2007. 10(10): p. 1308-1312.
[66] Khawaja, F.A., J.M.G. Tsui, and C.C. Pack, *Pattern Motion Selectivity of Spiking Outputs and Local Field Potentials in Macaque Visual Cortex.* Journal of Neuroscience, 2009. 29(43): p. 13702-13709.
[67] Ray, S. and J.H.R. Maunsell, *Different Origins of Gamma Rhythm and High-Gamma Activity in Macaque Visual Cortex.* Plos Biology, 2011. 9(4).
[68] Ray, S., et al., *Neural Correlates of High-Gamma Oscillations (60-200 Hz) in Macaque Local Field Potentials and Their Potential Implications in Electrocorticography.* Journal of Neuroscience, 2008. 28(45): p. 11526-11536.
[69] Rasch, M.J., et al., *Inferring spike trains from local field potentials.* Journal of Neurophysiology, 2008. 99(3): p. 1461-1476.
[70] Ray, S., et al., *Effect of stimulus intensity on the spike-local field potential relationship in the secondary somatosensory cortex.* Journal of Neuroscience, 2008. 28(29): p. 7334-7343.
[71] Whittingstall, K. and N.K. Logothetis, *Frequency-band coupling in surface EEG reflects spiking activity in monkey visual cortex.* Neuron, 2009. 64(2): p. 281-9.
[72] Belitski, A., et al., *Low-frequency local field potentials and spikes in primary visual cortex convey independent visual information.* Journal of Neuroscience, 2008. 28(22): p. 5696-5709.
[73] Belitski, A., et al., *Sensory information in local field potentials and spikes from visual and auditory cortices: time scales and frequency bands.* J Comput Neurosci, 2010. 29(3): p. 533-45.
[74] Sillito, A.M., J. Cudeiro, and H.E. Jones, *Always returning: feedback and sensory processing in visual cortex and thalamus.* Trends Neurosci, 2006. 29(6): p. 307-16.
[75] Womelsdorf, T., et al., *Gamma-band synchronization in visual cortex predicts speed of change detection.* Nature, 2006. 439(7077): p. 733-736.
[76] Rotermund, D., et al., *Attention Improves Object Representation in Visual Cortical Field Potentials.* Journal of Neuroscience, 2009. 29(32): p. 10120-10130.
[77] Fries, P., et al., *Modulation of oscillatory neuronal synchronization by selective visual attention.* Science, 2001. 291: p. 1560-1563.
[78] Chalk, M., et al., *Attention Reduces Stimulus-Driven Gamma Frequency Oscillations and Spike Field Coherence in V1.* Neuron, 2010. 66(1): p. 114-125.
[79] Khayat, P.S., R. Niebergall, and J.C. Martinez-Trujillo, *Frequency-Dependent Attentional Modulation of Local Field Potential Signals in Macaque Area MT.* Journal of Neuroscience, 2010. 30(20): p. 7037-7048.

[80] Harris, K.D. and A. Thiele, *Cortical state and attention.* Nature Reviews Neuroscience, 2011. 12(9): p. 509-523.

[81] Buschman, T.J. and E.K. Miller, *Top-down versus bottom-up control of attention in the prefrontal and posterior parietal cortices.* Science, 2007. 315(5820): p. 1860-1862.

[82] Saalmann, Y.B., I.N. Pigarev, and T.R. Vidyasagar, *Neural mechanisms of visual attention: How top-down feedback highlights relevant locations.* Science, 2007. 316(5831): p. 1612-1615.

[83] Liu, J. and W.T. Newsome, *Local field potential in cortical area MT: Stimulus tuning and behavioral correlations.* Journal of Neuroscience, 2006. 26(30): p. 7779-7790.

[84] Stanford, T.R., et al., *Perceptual decision making in less than 30 milliseconds.* Nat Neurosci, 2010. 13(3): p. 379-85.

[85] Roelfsema, P.R., V.A.F. Lamme, and H. Spekreijse, *Object-based attention in the primary visual cortex of the macaque monkey.* Nature, 1998. 395(6700): p. 376-381.

[86] Moro, S.I., et al., *Neuronal Activity in the Visual Cortex Reveals the Temporal Order of Cognitive Operations.* Journal of Neuroscience, 2010. 30(48): p. 16293-16303.

[87] Lui, L.L. and T. Pasternak, *Representation of comparison signals in cortical area MT during a delayed direction discrimination task.* Journal of Neurophysiology, 2011. 106(3): p. 1260-1273.

[88] Mitchell, J.F., K.A. Sundberg, and J.H. Reynolds, *Spatial Attention Decorrelates Intrinsic Activity Fluctuations in Macaque Area V4.* Neuron, 2009. 63(6): p. 879-888.

[89] Kara, P., P. Reinagel, and R.C. Reid, *Low response variability in simultaneously recorded retinal, thalamic, and cortical neurons.* Neuron, 2000. 27(3): p. 635-646.

[90] Swets, J.A., *Measuring the accuracy of diagnostic systems.* Science, 1988. 240(4857): p. 1285-93.

[91] Buschman, T.J. and E.K. Miller, *Serial, Covert Shifts of Attention during Visual Search Are Reflected by the Frontal Eye Fields and Correlated with Population Oscillations.* Neuron, 2009. 63(3): p. 386-396.

[92] Pillow, J.W., et al., *Spatio-temporal correlations and visual signalling in a complete neuronal population.* Nature, 2008. 454(7207): p. 995-U37.

[93] Williams, Z.M., et al., *Parietal activity and the perceived direction of ambiguous apparent motion.* Nature Neuroscience, 2003. 6(6): p. 616-623.

Chapter 8

Bio-Inspired Architecture for Clustering into Natural and Non-Natural Facial Expressions

Claudio Castellanos Sánchez, Manuel Hernández Hernández
and Pedro Luis Sánchez Orellana

Additional information is available at the end of the chapter

http://dx.doi.org/10.5772/48508

1. Introduction

Over the past years there has been an increasing surge of interest in automated facial expression analysis but there are several situations where the analysis of the expressions cannot be successfully done with the different classical approaches due to the variations in the environmental conditions (like illumination changes).

A way to face these variations in the environmental conditions is by looking at the existing systems that efficiently locate, extract and analyse the face information. An example of these systems is the brain of the human being.

According to several researchers [2, 27, 36], emotion processing is done in the amygdala, an area located within medial temporal lobes in the brain. Experiments carried out by [35] demonstrated that face recognition process can be achieved with the simple facial features (eyebrows and eyes vs eyebrows) of threatening and friendly faces. These experiments confirm that emotion processing involves other areas like the visual cortex, e.g. V1 [32]. Later, [17] demonstrated that fast, automatic, and parallel processing of unattended emotional faces provide important insights into the specific and dissociated neural pathways in emotion and face perception.

Although, there are different areas involved in the analysis of facial expressions in the brain of the human being, there is no consensus about how this process is done.

Clues from the psychological point of view, like that proposed by Ekman and Friesen [9], point out the importance of the symmetry in this process and the facial asymmetry (with left part of the face stronger than that of right part) is apparent only with deliberate and non-spontaneous (non-natural) expressions. According to this work, the symmetrical expressions show a true or natural emotion. Nevertheless, the asymmetrical expressions show a false or non-natural emotion.

In this research, we take advantage of psychological point of view to interpret our results issued by symmetrical and asymmetrical face measures when we model the visual areas of brain of the human being. Furthermore, we are inspired by early visual areas for processing the visual stream. Then, the interaction between neurons of visual cortex lead us to introduce our proposed architecture based on the detection of asymmetrical facial expressions and their clustering into natural/non-natural expressions.

In this chapter, we will present an architecture composed of five stages in order to cluster into natural/non-natural facial expressions in a sequence of images.

The first stage process a sequence of images for eyes and mouth corners detection inspired by the sensibility of cone-cells in the eyes. With these corners we build an anthropometrical grid of six vertical bands.

The second stage is a bio-inspired treatment through three steps:

- Contrast and orientation detection inspired in the simple neurons in V1 (primary visual cortex) that are modelled by Gabor-like filters.
- Integration and smoothing contours due to the performance of complex neurons in V1.
- The coherence and integration activity of neurons in MT (middle temporal area) inspire us to detect the motion through a temporal interaction of our consecutive complex neurons.

The third stage computes the ratio between the quantity of active neurons and the maximum quantity of neurons in each of six bands built in the first stage. A process inspired in the visual stream integration in IT (infero-temporal area).

The fourth stage compares each symmetrical band with an empirical threshold κ obtained in our experiments.

The end stage clusters in natural/non-natural expressions. This stage uses the results of the fourth stage with a bio-inspired neural network model.

In the following sections, we will present an overview of the state of the art in research of facial expressions. In addition, we present our proposed architecture to analyse the asymmetrical responses of the faces from a sequence of images. We also mention the experiments, discuss the results and finally comment on the future work.

2. State of the art

The analysis of facial expressions constitute a critical and complex part of our non-verbal social interactions. Therefore, over the past years there has been an increasing surge of interest to create tools that allow to analyse the facial expression automatically. This analysis is a complex task; on one hand facial expression structure of human beings are different from one another. On the other hand, faces are analysed from sequences of images captured in different environments with variations of lighting, pose and scale changes that difficult the extraction of their structure. Traditionally, the analysis of facial expressions has been focused on identify emotions; however, both deformation and face information can be originated by other factors (like verbal communication or fatigue) rather than emotions. The emotions can be evaluated from two main perspectives: psychological, physiological and neurophysiological points of view versus computational point of view.

2.1. Psychological and physiological perspective

From the psychological and physiological perspective, the emotions can be analysed considering the symmetry of the expressions. According to Ekman and Friesen [9] through the analysis of symmetry it can be evaluated the veracity (naturalness) of an emotion. In the brain, the information about emotions is processed in the amygdala [2, 27, 36], an area located within medial temporal lobes in the brain. By using fMRI some researchers [1, 13, 32] have discovered that in this area the processing is modulated by the significance of faces, particularly with fearful expressions, also with others like gaze direction. Visual search paradigms have provided evidence the enhanced capture of attention by threatening faces. Experiments carried out by [35] demonstrated that the recognition process can be achieved with simple facial features (expressions of eyebrows and eyes together vs only eyebrows) of threatening and friendly faces. These experiments confirm that emotion processing involves other areas like the visual cortex, e.g. V1 [32].

2.2. Neurophysiological perspective

According to neurophysiological studies [15, 16], the task of facial expression recognition also occurs in some regions in the visual cortex (ventral and dorsal pathways). The neurons in these areas respond mainly to gesticulations and identity. In the case of gesticulations, the neurons in the superior temporal sulcus involve the dynamics of the face. In the case of identity, the neurons in the inferior temporal gyrus imply the analysis of invariant facial features. In both cases the processing is modulated by attentional mechanisms [37]. Later, [17] demonstrated that fast, automatic, and parallel processing of unattended emotional faces, provides important insights into the specific and dissociated neural pathways in emotion and face perception.

In the figure 1 we show the main pathways of processing visual stream in the cortex of the human being. The dorsal pathways analyse the motion and localisation of information, while ventral pathways analyse information about form and colour. Both pathways have the same source, V1. The visual cortex is the last specialised layer of evolution in mammals; the limbic system (not shown in the figure) is the first and primitive layer in the mammals where the amygdala is situated in the temporal lobes. Then, it is covered by visual cortex.

2.3. Computational perspective

From the computational point of view, facial expression recognition implies the classification of facial motion and facial structure deformation into abstract representations completely based on visual information. To address this analysis it is necessary to perform two main tasks: face detection and facial feature extraction. In the first one, techniques have been developed to deal with the extraction and normalization of the face considering variations in the pose [10, 28] and illumination [3, 12]. However, according to [11] the main effort has been focused to feature facial extraction where techniques like appearance-based models [6, 18, 19] work with significant variations in the acquired face images without normalization.

Basically, the facial feature extraction has been approached by two main streams [11, 23]: facial deformation extraction models and facial motion extraction models. Motion extraction approaches focus on facial changes produced by facial expressions, whereas deformation-based methods contrast the visual information against face models to extract features produced by expressions and not by age deformation like wrinkles. The main

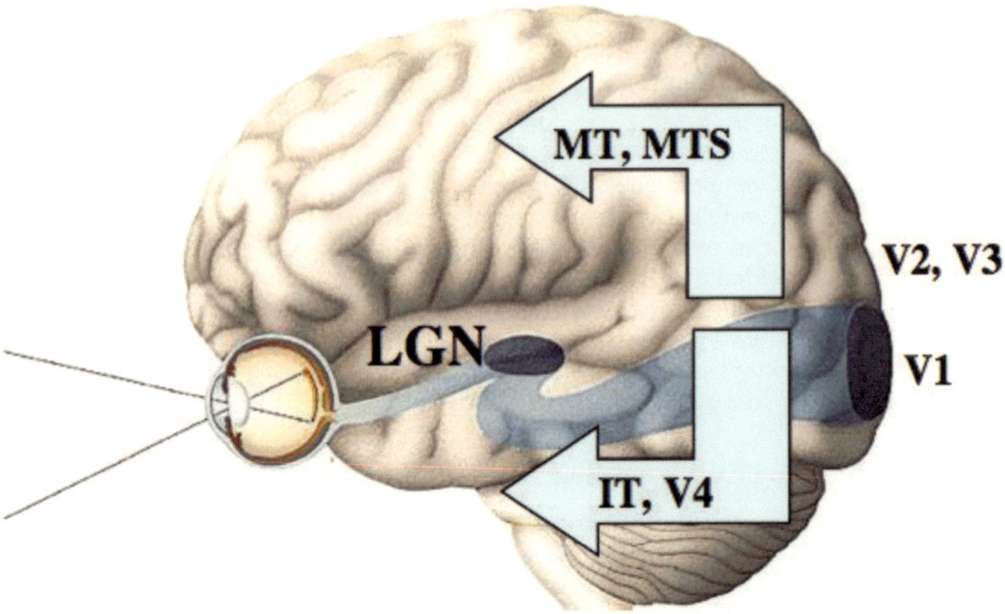

Figure 1. The visual pathway. The information comes in from the retina, next it is integrated in LGN, treated in V1, and finally processed in two different pathways : dorsal (MT, MTS, etc.) and ventral (V4, IT, etc.). The amygdala are almond-shaped groups of nuclei located deep within the medial temporal lobes and perform a primary role in the processing and memory of emotional reactions.

difference between these two methods is that deformation-based methods can be applied to single images as well as image sequences, and motion methods need a sequence of images. In both cases the facial features may be processed holistically (the faces are analysed as a whole) or locally (focusing on features from specific areas). In the case of deformation methods, the extraction of features relies on shape and texture changes through a period of time. On one hand the Holistic approaches either use the whole face [7, 25] or partial information about regions in the face like mouth or eyes [14, 21, 31]. For the motion extraction methods, the features are extracted by analysing motion vectors: holistically [8, 29], and locally [26, 34, 39] obtained.

3. Proposed bio-inspired architecture

A general diagram of the proposed methodology is shown in the figure 2. In the beginning, a sequence of images or video is captured in RGB format. Next, a processing based on green and red colours is realized to detect eyes and mouth corners. In this stage, we generate a grid of 6×5 based on coordinates of eyes and mouth corners. In this chapter, we only chose the six vertical bands for our experiments, the other combinations for analysis of the antropomorphical grid are subjects our future analysis.

Our bio-inspired treatment obtain the simple and complex neuron responses following the function of basic neurons of visual primary cortex (V1). Next, a temporal integration in complex neuron responses simulates the neurons in middle temporal cortex (MT).

Then, we extract the active neurons for each vertical band and compute their ratio of active quantity neurons. Next, each vertical band is compared to their symmetrical band.

Finally, we detect the asymmetries for each pair of vertical bands and cluster it in three classes applying the self-organizing maps (SOM).

In the next subsections we give a brief explanation of the steps of our approach where we assume that the face has been located correctly.

3.1. Description of input image sequences

In our proposed approach, the images of each sequence are in RGB colour, because we use the colour during the pre-processing to detect eyes and mouth corners. The process is described below. We suggest sampling capture to 25 frames per second and 1024×768 pixels. High sampling and high resolution is desirable.

3.2. Pre-processing

In this stage we realize three steps which are (1) the eyes and mouth detection, (2) we build the grid and finally we utilize only six regions, the six vertical bands (6-RVB) to analyse it (with left side of the stronger than right one). These steps will be briefly explained in the following paragraphs.

In the first step, let $I = \{I_1, I_2, I_3, \ldots I_t\}$ be an image face sequence where the eyes and mouth corners are correctly detected using red and green band colours as the sensibility of cones cells in our eyes. We work on the rectangle that contains the face; next, we define the point corresponding to the center of the face (x_c and y_c) and two parameters (width and height) for the size of the face. We use these anthropometric measures in the order to define three regions of interest that probably contain the mouth and eyes (left and right). For each region we find the corresponding coordinates of detected corners in both eyes and mouth and these coordinates are used in the next step.

In the second step, we use the coordinates of eyes and mouth corners to build an antropomorphical grid on the face. With the processing we can obtain twenty-five small regions, we also split the central part in two regions such as can see in the figure 2 obtaining thirty small regions (the step anthropometrical segmentation using black line doted).

Finally in this stage, we use only six symmetrical columns ($R_1, R_2, R_3, R_4, R_5, R_6$) of proposed grid to analyse expressions in the face.

3.3. Bio-inspired treatment

The facial expressions carry much more information that cannot be extracted from traditional facial expression analysis. So we propose, from the bio-inspired point of view, a methodology to analyse the symmetry of facial expressions. The objective with this is to achieve both a perspective, according to brain mechanisms, of the interpretation of facial motion relevance and a methodology that takes advantage of the tolerance to illumination change of the brain mechanisms. This can be divided into three main processing steps:

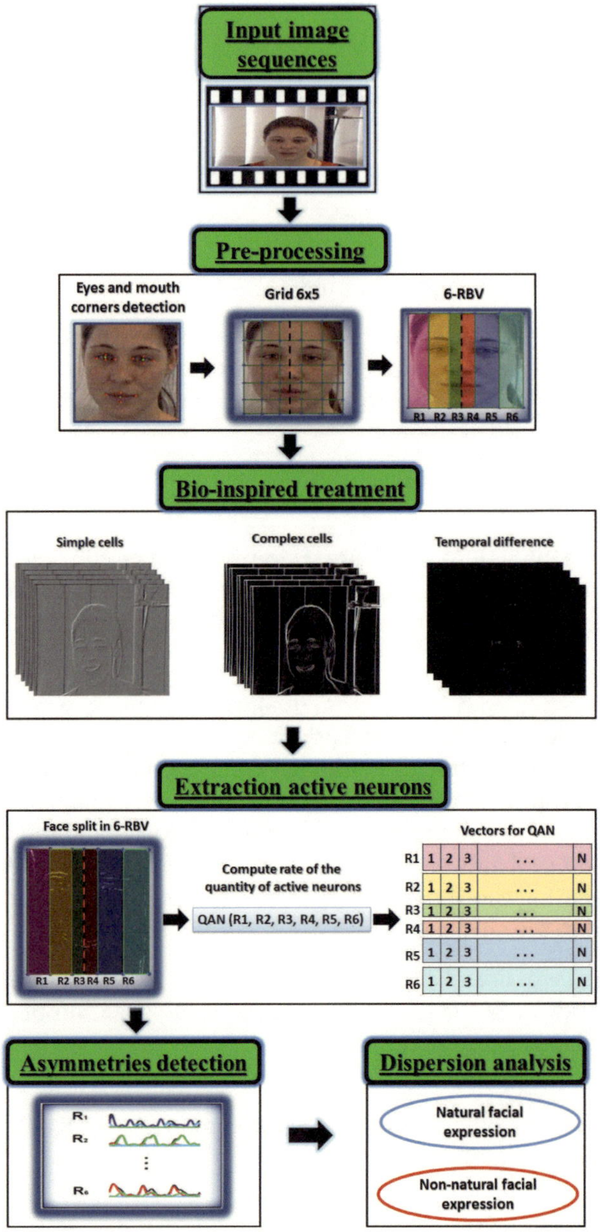

Figure 2. General architecture of bio-inspired proposed model. After video acquisition, a pre-processing generates an anthropometrical grid. Next, a treatment inspired in V1 determines the active neurons. Then, we compare two symmetrical regions: hears, eyes and nose to extract the vector composed of ratio of quantity active neurons. Finally, the asymmetries detection are evaluated with SOM to cluster into natural or non-natural facial expressions.

- Inspiring in simple neurons of V1 (primary visual cortex) and modelled by Gabor-like filters, we extract the simple active neurons in eight different orientations and two different phases.

- Two simple neurons with different phase are merged to generate a complex neuron.
- A temporal integration between two consecutive complex neurons models MT neurons (Middle temporal area). The neurons with a major response to a threshold are considered as active neurons.

In the first proposed step, considering the processing done by the visual cortex, the first neurons that receive the stimuli from the eyes are the simple cells. Physiological evidence [5, 38] affirms that neuronal populations in the primary visual cortex (V1) of mammals exhibit contrast normalization. Neurons that respond strongly to simple visual stimuli, such as sinusoidal gratings, respond less well to the same stimuli when they are presented as part of a more complex stimulus which also excites other, neighbouring neurons. The behaviour of these neurons show a preference to specific orientations, which can be modelled computationally by the oriented Gabor-like filters [4, 22]:

$$S_{\theta,\varphi}(x,y,t) = \sum_{t=0}^{t} I(x,y,t) * G_{\theta}(\hat{x},\hat{y},\varphi) \tag{1}$$

where $S_{\theta}(x,y,t)$ are simple cells which is the result of the convolution between a pool of Gabor functions ($G_{\theta}(\hat{x},\hat{y})$), in our case with 8 orientation and 2 phases, and the image t of the image sequences, ($\hat{x}$, $\hat{y}$) are the rotational components and (x,y) a position of the image. The Gabor function $G_{\theta}(\hat{x},\hat{y})$ is defined as:

$$G_{\theta}(\hat{x},\hat{y},\varphi) = exp\left(-\frac{\hat{x}^2+\gamma^2\hat{y}^2}{2\sigma^2}\right) cos\left(2\pi\frac{\hat{x}}{\lambda}+\varphi\right) \tag{2}$$

where $\hat{x} = x\cos\theta + y\sin\theta$, $\hat{y} = -x\sin\theta + y\cos\theta$, λ is the length-width, θ represent the orientation, φ the phase, σ the standard deviation and γ represent the relation of aspect.

In the second step, the responses of two diffent phases of simple cells $S_{\theta}(x,y,t)$ are then integrated in the complex cells by using a non-linear model that allows to merge the responses. Then, the complex cells responses are estimated by

$$C_{\theta}(x,y,t) = \sqrt{S_{\theta,\frac{\pi}{2}}(x,y,t)^2 + S_{\theta,-\frac{\pi}{2}}(x,y,t)^2} \tag{3}$$

where $C_{\theta}(x,y,t)$ represent complex cells responses, $\frac{\pi}{2}$ and $-\frac{\pi}{2}$ are the symmetric and anti-symmetric phases, respectively. Then, the eight orientations are integrated of the complex cells responses $C_{\theta}(x,y,t)$ for obtain one matrix of the map active neurons complex $C(x,y,t)$ for the image t.

Finally the third step, the neurons in the human brain are connected to MT neurons allowing a temporal processing that is defined as the temporal integration between $C(x,y,t)$ and $C(x,y,t-1)$ obtaining the map of active complex neurons by

$$D(x,y,t) = C(x,y,t) - C(x,y,t-1) \tag{4}$$

where $D(x,y,t)$ is the result of active complex neurons in the image t, $C(x,y,t)$ and $C(x,y,t-1)$ are the current image and the previous image, respectively. We use the information $D(x,y,t)$ to compute the number of active neurons.

3.4. Extraction of active neurons

In this stage, we realize the extraction of active complex neurons of the active map complex neurons ($D(x, y, t)$). For this, we use the six vertical bands and the map of active neurons. The 6-RVB overlapping in the map of active neurons. So, we compute the quantity of active neurons (QAN) for each region ($R_1, R_2, R_3, R_4, R_5, R_6$) and find the region with the maximum quantity of active neurons (QAN). The QAN is the number of active complex neurons in a region of the image.

So, we obtain six vectors of the quantity of active neurons (QAN): one for the QAN obtained and one for QAN expected for a region. The last one is the total possible QAN in a region. The first one computes only the active present neurons such that the ratio is always between 0 and 1. This information is used to compare two symmetric regions to detect temporal asymmetries.

3.5. Asymmetry detection

Next stage, we detect the asymmetries for each region (6-RVB) of the map of active complex neurons. To obtain or detect asymmetries in each image during two seconds using 6-RVB we follow the next steps:

- First step, we compute the difference between the symmetric regions. For example, the difference between region R_1 and R_6, that are the extreme regions.
- Then, compute average and standard deviation for each difference of the regions.
- So, we calculate a threshold (a minimum and a maximum) using the average and standard deviation.
- Then, we detect the asymmetries for each difference of regions in the image sequences, using the "rule": for each difference of regions, we verify that the difference is outside the threshold (i.e., minor to minimum and major to maximum). We count each outsider in the sequence, *Out*.
- Finally, we compute the *Out* for each pair of regions in the images sequence.

The detected asymmetries (*Out*) in the facial expression during the image sequences are weighed for each pair of symmetrical regions (R_1 with R_6, R_2 with R_5 and R_3 with R_4). For each database, we proposed an empirical threshold κ that we apply to all image sequence in the same database. This κ considers various aspects as the sampling frequency (we used two seconds in our experiments), the personal conditions, head motion and luminance-capture conditions.

3.6. Clustering in natural/non-natural expressions

For each different database we obtain a κ adapted to number of images in each sequence. So, we used the equation 5 for cluster the facial expressions in the natural/non-natural expressions:

$$C_{\kappa} = \frac{C_A}{C_E} \frac{2F}{T\kappa} \tag{5}$$

where $\frac{C_A}{C_E}$ is the ratio of quantity of active neurons (QAN) in a region, T is the total number of images in a typical sequence in the database to compute κ, F is the capture frequency for the sequences in this database and the κ index. With C_κ values we cluster in natural expression and non-natural expression.

These values are sending to SOM 1D that performs 5000 epochs, with a $\eta = 1.000$ to $\eta = 0.0001$ and they were analysed statistically.

4. Experimental results

We take six columns of proposed face grid. The symmetrical regions are: R1 with R6 (ears), R2 with R5 (eyes) and R3 with R4 (nose).

The tests for our approach took only the colour sequence of images for the CK+ database while for FG-Net and LTI-HIT we take all sequences of images. The last database was split per question in each interview (sequence of images).

Figure 3 shows a sequence of image of CK+ database for a non-natural expression. There are 11 asymmetries in both ears and nose regions, and 9 asymmetries in eyes region, the weighted sum is $10 = 11 * 0.3 + 11 * 0.2 + 9 * 0.5$. But this ratio is higher than fixed threshold $\kappa = 7$, then this sequence is non natural. We tested all the experiments for two seconds independently of sampling frequency (see table 1). We fix κ according table 1 for test our all available databases. In our experiments this threshold tolerates the generated asymmetries by illumination, environment, and personal conditions.

We test the databases Cohn-Kanade (CK+) (only colour images) [20], FG-Net [33], and LTI-HIT as shown in the table 2. We confirm that FG-Net is the most natural database. Our classification error was of 12% in average.

4.1. Description of databases

We used three databases to test our proposed approach: FG-Net, CK+, and LTI-HIT.

4.1.1. Cohn-Kanade (CK+) database

In 2000 and 2010, The Institute of Electrical & Electronics Engineers at Grenoble, France, created the CK and CK+, respectively (the same CK database but 107 new sequences of which 33 are in color), consists of 123 persons with 7 different expressions per person: anger, contempt, disgust, fear, happy, sadness and surprise. The image sequences vary in duration (i.e. 10 to 60 frames) and incorporate the onset of a neutral frame at the moment of peak formation of the facial expressions. This database was captured to 30 frames per second with a resolution 640×480. The final frame of each image sequence was coded using FACS (Facial Action Coding System) which describes person's expression in terms of action units (AUs) [20]. Participants were instructed by an experimenter to perform a series of 23 facial displays including single action units and specified emotion like expressions of joy, surprise, anger, disgust, fear, and sadness. Each display began and ended in a neutral face.

4.1.2. FG-Net database

In 2006, Facial Expressions and Emotions from the Munich Technical University created the FG-Net database. This is an image database containing face images showing a number of persons performing six different basic emotions defined by Ekman & Friesen: anger, fear,

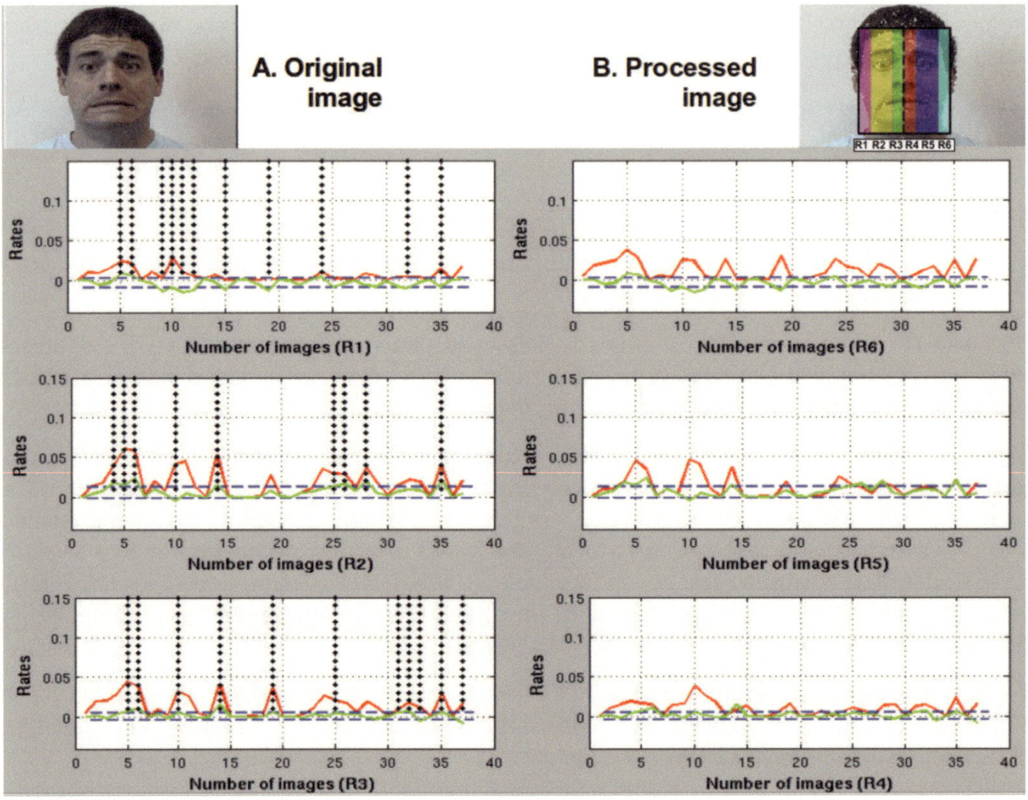

Figure 3. Asymmetry in vertical regions for a sequence of images in CK+. Horizontal red (black) line represents the data; horizontal green (gray) line, the difference between symmetrical regions; the separation between horizontal dashed lines is the symmetrical tolerance, and vertical dotted lines show the asymmetry (we show it only in the left graphics).

surprise, disgust, sadness and happiness. They also add the neutral expression for each person. This database consists of 19 persons with 21 sequences for each person, then it contains 399 different sequences. The sequences of images were captured to 25 frames per second with a resolution of 640 × 480 pixels [33]. This database allows to observe people react as natural as possible. As a consequence, it was tried to wake real emotions by playing video clips or still images after a short introductory phase instead of telling the person to play a role. This is in contrast to the asymmetry of luminance of the face, which includes not only asymmetry introduced by lighting, but also asymmetry introduced by the face itself.

4.1.3. LTI-HIT database

Finally, in 2010, the Children's Hospital of Tamaulipas created the LTI-HIT database. This database is taken from interviews that consists of 52 persons (11 men and 41 women) out of them 5 persons were put into one type of environment and 47 in the other. Each interview has between 27 and 33 different questions. The participants were between 18 and 66 years old. Each sequence of images were captured to 30 frames per second with resolution of 720 × 480 pixels and duration of 1.6 to 2.5 minutes per interviews. The interviews were made in natural conditions.

The tests for our approach took only the colour sequence of images for the CK+ database while for FG-Net and LTI-HIT we take all sequences images. The last database was split per question.

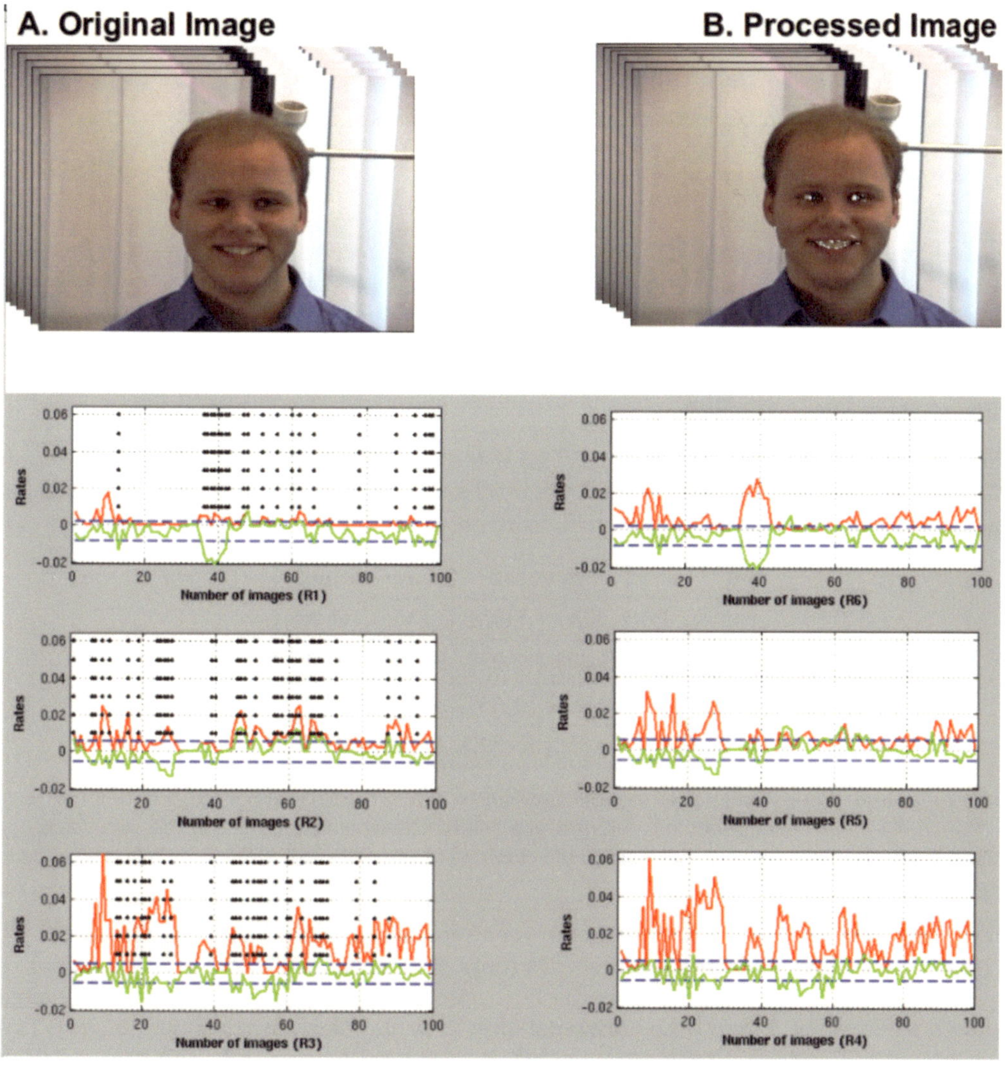

Figure 4. Results for face asymmetry detection in a sequence of images for FGNet. In this case, the boy is suspect to deceitful clues.

4.2. Remarks

The three databases are very different in its acquisition, illumination and manipulation of capture conditions. For weight these databases, we propose the κ index according to table 1.

In natural conditions, facial changes on the left side are only about 2% greater than overall right-side changes [30]. We establish a level of 1 to 5 for the personal conditions (hair-style,

Database (DB)	PC	HM	LC	κ index
CK+	3	1	2	6
FG-Net	3	3	3	9
LTI-HIT	3	4	4	11

Table 1. κ index is the value for each of the three databases. PC, personal conditions (facial expression); HM, head movement, and LC, luminance conditions. Each feature is between 0 to 5.

skin colour and tolerable static face asymmetry), and, in average, we choose a level 3 to model all personal conditions (PC) for our available databases.

The head motion (HM) is very different too between these three databases. In CK+ all persons are very controlled and the original sequences were cut to show only the evident expression. Again, the FG-Net sequences show activities before and after an evident expression. Finally, the LTI-HIT sequences were not prepared for the major expression. It shows the natural reactions of the interviewed persons. Then, we assign to HM variable the values 1, 3 and 4 to each database, respectively.

The luminance and capture conditions (LC) is too different. CK+ was created in a studio, FG-Net in a controlled environment and LTI-HIT in an uncontrolled environment. Then, we assign to LC variable 2, 3 and 4 to each database, respectively.

	Natural		Non-natural	
DB	DA	SOM	DA	SOM
CK+	42.42%	27.27%	33.33%	63.64%
FG-Net	33.60%	56.65%	39.68%	29.63%
LTI-HIT	34.55%	35.37%	38.70%	52.51%

Table 2. Natural/non-natural percentages according to κ index. The quantity of active neurons is manipulated into two manipulations: statistical analysis of active neurons (DA) and self-organizing maps (SOM). The percentages correspond to the obtained results with $12\% \pm 8\%$ error with two expert responses.

The figure 4 shows another example of test for a sequence of images in FGNet database. The vertical dotted lines show the asymmetries (only shown the left side). The horizontal red lines are the ratios of quantity, while the horizontal green lines are the difference between symmetrical regions. Finally, the horizontal blue lines are tolerable threshold obtained from this sequence of images. In this case, the boy is suspected to deceitful clues because all the graphics show a higher value (22, 33 and 28 for each pair of vertical band) and the weighed sum is $29.3 = 22 * 0.2 + 33 * 0.5 + 28 * 0.3$ that is higher than $\kappa = 18.0$ index.

The table 2 resume the obtained ratios for natural/non-natural facial expressions with statistical analysis and SOM. If we see SOM percentages, these percentages show FG-Net as greater in natural facial expressions than the other two databases, CK+ also has greater percentage followed by LTI-HIT with non-natural facial expressions.

For statistical analysis we have the opposed results. This difference is due to concentration of values and the dispersion. With a simple statistical analysis, all responses are separated based

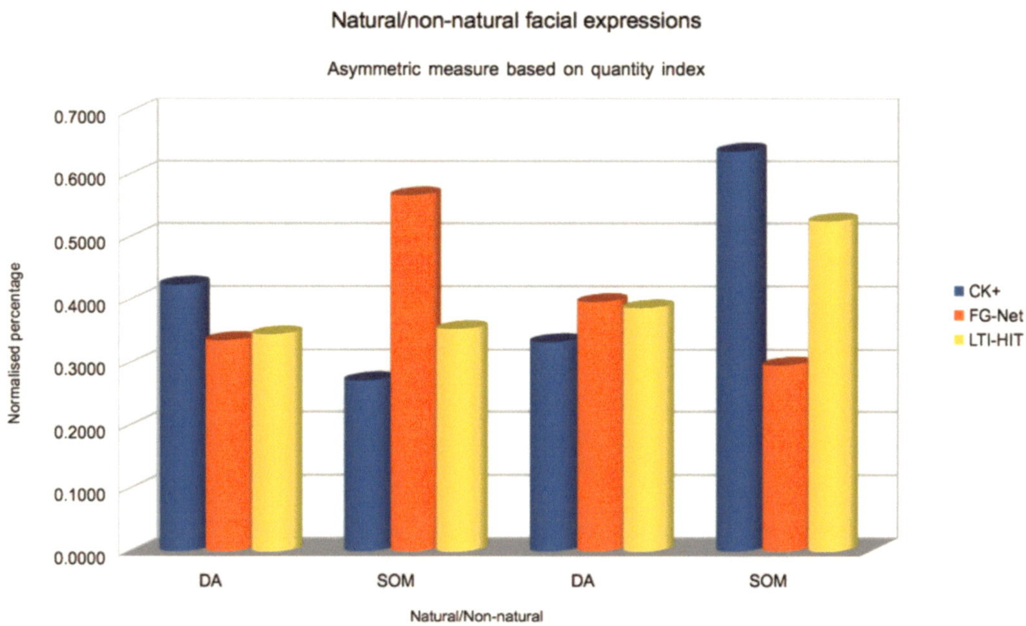

Figure 5. Asymmetry based on the quantity index. The first DA and SOM blocks correspond to Natural facial expressions. The last two DA and SOM correspond to Non-Natural facial expression.

on average and standard deviation, while the SOM application shows the centroids guided by the density and dispersion.

5. Conclusion

We have shown a bio-inspired approach to processing facial gesture for clustering into natural and non-natural facial expressions. It takes advantage of early primary visual areas in the brains of human beings for feature-extraction. Futhermore, it simulates the integration and discrimination of the superior visual areas considering the symmetrical and asymmetrical measures within the respective time span. This process ends in a bio-inspired neural network for clustering into natural and non-natural facial expressions.

The asymmetry between symmetrical regions of the face analysed during two seconds allows us to classify in: natural or non-natural facial expression. The quantity of asymmetries and its relations with different symmetrical regions is applied as a new biometric measure [24] (the precision of measurement is necessary). But we apply it for classification of natural or non natural expressions (the precision is not necessary).

In our bio-inspired proposed architecture, after face detection, an anthropomorphical grid is proposed. For each region, we obtain the ratio of quantity of active neurons (QAN) obtained from the modelled simple and complex neurons by our Gabor-like filters.

This proposed model can work for any database. Furthermore, the database FG-Net and Cohn-Kanade were tested. More than 63% of CK+ video sequences contain asymmetries. This database was built with simulation expressions (non natural expressions) and we confirm that our results are modelled correctly regarding the capture, illumination and personal conditions.

The different conditions of each database do not allow a simple characterization. We proposed an experimental index to model these conditions (e.g. personal conditions, head motion and luminance-capture), κ. In future, we will determine this index automatically for each database and, more precisely, for each sequence of images into database.

Using the index κ we have shown that our approach is independent of each database. This independence was tested in our experiments.

The preliminary steps of our approach show the feasibility to detect suspected persons in nervous or altered situations. Here is the beginning of our methodology to detect deceitful clues in facial expressions.

Author details

Claudio Castellanos Sánchez
Laboratory of Information Technology, Cinvestav-Tamaulipas and División de Estudios de Posgrado e Investigación, Instituto Tecnológico de Ciudad Victoria, Mexico

Manuel Hernández Hernández
Departamento de Ingeniería en Sistemas Computacionales, Instituto Tecnológico Superior de Tantoyuca, Mexico

Pedro Luis Sánchez Orellana
División de Estudios de Posgrado e Investigación, Instituto Tecnológico de Ciudad Victoria, Mexico

6. References

[1] Adolphs, R., Tranel, D. & Damasio, A. R. [Sep-1998]. The human amygdala in social judgment., *Nature* 393(6684): 470–474.

[2] Adolphs, R., Tranel, D., Damasio, H. & Damasio, A. R. [1995]. Fear and the human amygdala, *The Journal of Neuroscience* 15(9): 5879–5891.

[3] Belhumeur, P. N., Hespanha, J. & Kriegman, D. J. [1997]. Eigenfaces vs. Fisherfaces: Recognition Using Class Specific Linear Projection, *IEEE Transactions on Pattern Analysis and Machine Intelligence* 19(7): 711–720.

[4] Castellanos-Sánchez, C. [2005]. *Neuromimetic connectionist model for embedded visual perception of motion*, PhD thesis, Université Henri Poincaré (Nancy I), Nancy, France. Bibliothèque des Sciences et Techniques.

[5] Clatworthy, P., Chirimuuta, M., Lauritzen, J. & Tolhurst, D. [2003]. Coding of the contrasts in natural images by populations of neurons in primary visual cortex (v1), *Vision Research* 43(18): 1983 – 2001.

[6] del Solar, J. R. & Quinteros, J. [2008]. Illumination compensation and normalization in eigenspace-based face recognition: A comparative study of different pre-processing approaches, *Pattern Recognition Letters* 29(14): 1966 – 1979.

[7] Devi, B. J., Veeranjaneyulu, N. & Kishore, K. [2010]. A novel face recognition system based on combining eigenfaces with fisher faces using wavelets, *Procedia Computer Science* 2(0): 44 – 51.

[8] Dornaika, F., Lazkano, E. & Sierra, B. [2011]. Improving dynamic facial expression recognition with feature subset selection, *Pattern Recognition Letters* 32(5): 740 – 748.

[9] Ekman, P. [1980]. Asymmetry in facial expression, *Science* 209(4458): 833–834.

[10] Essa, I. A. & Pentland, A. P. [1997]. Coding, analysis, interpretation, and recognition of facial expressions, *IEEE Trans. Pattern Anal. Mach. Intell.* 19: 757–763.

[11] Fasel, B. & Luettin, J. [2003]. Automatic facial expression analysis: a survey, *Pattern Recognition* 36(1): 259 – 275.

[12] Fellenz, W., Taylor, J., Tsapatsoulis, N. & Kollias, S. [1999]. Comparing template-based, feature-based and supervised classification of facial expressions from static images, *Proceedings of Circuits, Systems, Communications and Computers* pp. 5331–5336.

[13] Gosselin, F., Spezio, M. L., Tranel, D. & Adolphs, R. [2011]. Asymmetrical use of eye information from faces following unilateral amygdala damage, *Social Cognitive and Affective Neuroscience* 6(3): 330–337.

[14] Gu, W., Xiang, C., Venkatesh, Y., Huang, D. & Lin, H. [2012]. Facial expression recognition using radial encoding of local gabor features and classifier synthesis, *Pattern Recognition* 45(1): 80 – 91.

[15] Hasselmo, M. E., Rolls, E. T. & Baylis, G. C. [1989]. The role of expression and identity in the face-selective responses of neurons in the temporal visual cortex of the monkey, *Behavioural Brain Research* 32(3): 203 – 218.

[16] Haxby, J. V., Hoffman, E. A. & Gobbini, M. I. [2000]. The distributed human neural system for face perception., *Trends in cognitive sciences* 4(6): 223–233.

[17] Hung, Y., Smith, M. L., Bayle, D. J., Mills, T., Cheyne, D. & Taylor, M. J. [2010]. Unattended emotional faces elicit early lateralized amygdala-frontal and fusiform activations, *NeuroImage* 50(2): 727 – 733.

[18] Kim, H.-C., Kim, D., Bang, S.-Y. & Lee, S.-Y. [2004]. Face recognition using the second-order mixture-of-eigenfaces method, *Pattern Recognition* 37(2): 337 – 349.

[19] Lanitis, A., Taylor, C. J. & Cootes, T. F. [1997]. Automatic interpretation and coding of face images using flexible models, *IEEE Trans. Pattern Anal. Mach. Intell.* 19: 743–756.

[20] Lucey, P., Cohn, J., Kanade, T., Saragih, J., Ambadar, Z. & Matthews, I. [2010]. The extended cohn-kanade dataset (ck+): A complete dataset for action unit and emotion-specified expression, *Computer Vision and Pattern Recognition Workshops (CVPRW), 2010 IEEE Computer Society Conference on*, pp. 94–101.

[21] Maalej, A., Amor, B. B., Daoudi, M., Srivastava, A. & Berretti, S. [2011]. Shape analysis of local facial patches for 3d facial expression recognition, *Pattern Recognition* 44(8): 1581 – 1589.

[22] Marcelja, S. [1980]. Mathematical description of the reponses of simple cortical cells, *Journal of the Optical Society of America A* 70(11): 1297–1300.

[23] Mitra, S. & Acharya, T. [2007]. Gesture recognition: A survey, *IEEE Transactions on Systems, Man and Cybernetics - Part C* 37(3): 311–324.

[24] Mitra, S. & Savvides, M. [2005]. Analyzing asymmetry biometric in the frequency domain for face recognition, *IEEE ICASSP* II: 953–956.

[25] Nair, B. M., Foytik, J., Tompkins, R., Diskin, Y., Aspiras, T. & Asari, V. [2011]. Multi-pose face recognition and tracking system, *Procedia Computer Science* 6(0): 381 – 386.

[26] Park, S. & Kim, D. [2009]. Subtle facial expression recognition using motion magnification, *Pattern Recognition Letters* 30(7): 708 – 716.

[27] Phillips, M. L., Young, A. W., Senior, C., Brammer, M., Andrews, C., Calder, A. J., Bullmore, E. T., Perrett, D. I., Rowland, D., Williams, S. C. R., Gray, J. A. & David, A. S.

[1997]. Aspecific neural substrate for perceiving facial expressions of disgust, *Nature* 389(6650): 174 – 194.

[28] Rowley, H. A., Baluja, S. & Kanade, T. [1998]. Neural network-based face detection, *IEEE Trans. Pattern Anal. Mach. Intell.* 20: 23–38.

[29] Sánchez, A., Ruiz, J., Moreno, A., Montemayor, A., Hernández, J. & Pantrigo, J. [2011]. Differential optical flow applied to automatic facial expression recognition, *Neurocomputing* 74(8): 1272 – 1282. Selected Papers from the 3rd International Work-Conference on the Interplay between Natural and Artificial Computation (IWINAC 2009).

[30] Schmidt, K. L., Liu, Y. & Coh, J. F. [2006]. The role of structural facial asymmetry in in asymmetry peak facial expressions, *Literality* 11(6): 540–561.

[31] Venkatesh, Y., Kassim, A. A. & Murthy, O. R. [2009]. A novel approach to classification of facial expressions from 3d-mesh datasets using modified pca, *Pattern Recognition Letters* 30(12): 1128 – 1137.

[32] Vuilleumier, P. & Pourtois, G. [2007]. Distributed and interactive brain mechanisms during emotion face perception: Evidence from functional neuroimaging, *Neuropsychologia* 45(1): 174 – 194.

[33] Wallhoff, F. [2006]. Facial expressions and emotion database. URL: *http://www.mmk.ei.tum.de/~waf/fgnet/feedtum.html*

[34] Wang, T.-H. & Lien, J.-J. J. [2009]. Facial expression recognition system based on rigid and non-rigid motion separation and 3d pose estimation, *Pattern Recognition* 42(5): 962 – 977.

[35] Weymar, M., Law, A., Ohman, A. & Hamm, A. O. [2011]. The face is more than its parts: Brain dynamics of enhanced spatial attention to schematic threat, *NeuroImage* 58(3): 946 – 954.

[36] Whalen, P. J., Rauch, S. L., Etcoff, N. L., McInerney, S. C., Lee, M. B. & Jenike, M. A. [January-1998]. Masked presentations of emotional facial expressions modulate amygdala activity without explicit knowledge., *The Journal of Neuroscience* 18(1): 411–418.

[37] Williams, M. A., McGlone, F., Abbott, D. F. & Mattingley, J. B. [2005]. Differential amygdala responses to happy and fearful facial expressions depend on selective attention, *NeuroImage* 24(2): 417 – 425.

[38] Willmore, B. D., Bulstrode, H. & Tolhurst, D. J. [2012]. Contrast normalization contributes to a biologically-plausible model of receptive-field development in primary visual cortex (v1), *Vision Research* 54(0): 49 – 60.

[39] Xiang, T., Leung, M. & Cho, S. [2008]. Expression recognition using fuzzy spatio-temporal modeling, *Pattern Recognition* 41(1): 204 – 216.

Chapter 9

Vision as a Fundamentally Statistical Machine

Zhiyong Yang

Additional information is available at the end of the chapter

http://dx.doi.org/10.5772/50165

1. Introduction

As a vital driving force of systems neuroscience, visual neuroscience had its conceptual framework established more than 40 years ago based on Hubel and Wiesel's groundbreaking work on the receptive-field properties of visual neurons (Hubel & Wiesel, 1977). This framework was subsequently strengthened by David Marr's influential book (Marr, 2010). In this paradigm, visual neurons are conceived to perform bottom-up, image-based processing to build a series of symbolic representations of visual stimuli. This paradigm, however, is deeply misleading since the generative sources in the three-dimensional (3**D**) physical world of any stimulus, to which visual animals must respond successfully, cannot be determined by image-based processing (due to the inverse optics problem). This is perhaps the reason why "Now, thirty years later, the main problems that occupied Marr remain fundamental open problems in the study of perception" (Marr, 2010), as assessed by two prominent vision scientists and Marr's close associates.

During the last 30 years, dramatic progress in computing hardware, digital imaging, statistical modeling, and visual neuroscience has promoted researchers to re-examine the computations and representations (see above) for natural vision examined in Marr's book. A range of new ideas have been proposed, many of which are summarized in books (Knill & Richards, 1996; Rao et al., 2002; Purves & Lotto, 2003; Doya et al., 2007; Trommershauser et al., 2011) and reviews (Simoncelli & Olshausen, 2001; Yuille & Kersten, 2006; Geisler, 2008; Friston, 2010). The unified theme is that vision and visual system structure and function must be understood in statistical terms. How this feat can be achieved, however, is not clear at all.

Since humans and other visual animals must respond successfully to visual stimuli whose generative sources cannot be determined in any direct way, the visual system can only generate percepts according to the probability distributions (**PDs**) of visual variables underlying the stimuli. The information pertinent to the generation of these PDs, namely, the statistics of natural visual environments, must have been incorporated into the visual circuitry by successful behavior in the world over evolutionary and developmental time.

During the last two decades, this statistical concept of vision has been successful in explaining aspects of vision that would be difficult to understand otherwise (see references cited above). In this chapter, I will describe several recent studies that relate the statistics of 2D and 3D natural visual scenes to visual percepts of brightness, saliency, and 3D space.

In the second section of this chapter, I will discuss how the PDs of luminance in specific contexts in natural scenes, referred to as the context-mediated PDs in natural scenes, predict brightness, the perception elicited by the luminance of a visual target. Our results show that brightness generated on this statistical basis accounts for a range of observations, whose causes have been debated for a long time without consensus. In the third section, I will present a simple, elegant model of the context- mediated PDs in natural scenes and a measure of visual saliency derived from these PDs. Our results show that this measure of visual saliency is a good predictor of human gaze in free-viewing both static and dynamic natural scenes. In the fourth section, I will present the statistics of 3D natural scenes and their relationship to human visual space. Our results show that human visual space is not a direct mapping of the 3D physical space but rather generated probabilistically. Finally, I will discuss the implications of these and other results for our understanding of the response properties of visual neurons, the intricate visual circuitries, the large-scale cortical organizations, the operational dynamics of the visual system, and natural vision.

2. The statistical structure of natural light patterns determines perceived light intensity

2.1. Introduction

In this section, I present evidence that the context-mediated PDs of luminance in natural scenes predict brightness, the perception elicited by the luminance of a visual target. A central puzzle in understanding how such percepts are generated by the visual system is that brightness does not correspond in any simple way to luminance. Thus, the same amount of light arising from a given region in a scene can elicit dramatically different brightness percepts when presented in different contexts (Fig. 1) (Kingdom, 2011). For example, in Fig.1 (a), the central square (T) in the left panel appears brighter than the same target in the right panel. This is the standard simultaneous brightness contrast effect.

A variety of explanations have been suggested since the basis for such phenomena was first debated by Helmholtz, Hering, Mach, and others (Gichrist et al., 1999; Purves et al., 2004; Kingdom, 2011). Although lateral inhibition in the early visual processing has often been proposed to account for these "illusions", this mechanism cannot explain instances in which similar overall contexts produce different brightness effects (compare Fig. 1 (a) with Figs. 1 (b) and (e); see also Fig. 1 (c)). This failure has led to several more recent suggestions, including complex filtering (Blakeslee & McCourt, 2004), the idea that brightness depends on detecting edges and junctions that promote the grouping of various luminances into interpretable spatial arrangements (Adelson, 2000; Anderson & Winawer, 2005), and the proposal that brightness is "re-synthesized" from 3D scene properties "inferred" from the stimulus (Wishart et al., 1997).

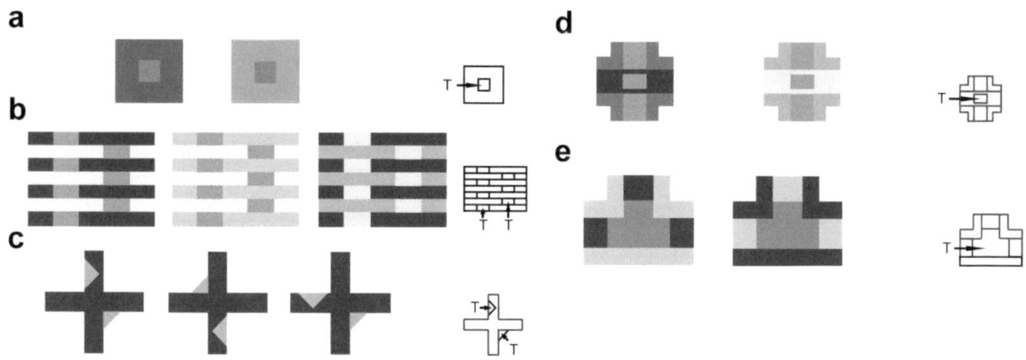

(a), Standard simultaneous brightness contrast effect. The central square in the dark surround (left panel) appears brighter than the equiluminant square in the light surround (right panel). (b), White's illusion. Although the gray rectangles in the left panel are all equiluminant, the ones surrounded by the generally lighter context on the left appear brighter than those surrounded by the generally darker context on the right. When, however, the luminance of the target rectangles is the lowest (middle panel) or highest (right panel) value in the stimulus, the targets in the generally lighter context (on the left in the middle and right panels) appear less brighter than ones in the generally darker context (called the "inverted White's effect"). (c), Wertheimer-Benary illusion. The triangle embedded in the arm of the black cross appears brighter than the one that abuts the corner of the cross. The slightly different brightness of the equiluminant triangles is maintained whether the presentation is upside down (middle panel), or reflected along the diagonal (right panel). (d), The intertwined cross illusion. The target on the left appears substantially brighter than the equiluminant target on the right. (e), The inverted T-illusion. The inverted T-shape on the left appears somewhat brighter than the equiluminant target on the right (modified from Yang & Purves, 2004).

Figure 1. The influence of spatial patterns of luminance on the apparent brightness of a target (the targets [T] in each stimulus are equiluminant, and are indicated in the insets on the right).

2.2. Context-mediated PDs of luminance in natural scenes

To examine whether the statistics of natural light patterns predict the perceptual phenomena shown in Fig. 1, we obtained the relevant PDs of luminance in natural scenes by sampling a database of natural scenes (van Hateren & van der Schaaf, 1998) with target-surround configurations that had the same local geometry as the stimuli in Fig. 1. As a first step, these configurations were superimposed on the images to find light patterns in which the luminance values of both the surround and target regions were approximately homogeneous; for those configurations in which the surround comprised more than one region of the same luminance (see Fig. 1), we also required that the relevant sampled regions meet this criterion. The sampling configurations were moved in steps of one pixel to screen the full image. The mean luminance values of the target and the surrounding regions in the samples were then calculated, and their occurrences tallied.

2.3. Brightness signifies context-mediated PDs of luminance in natural scenes

Natural environments comprise objects of different sizes at various distances that are related to each other and the observer in a variety of ways (Yang & Purves, 2003a,b). When the light arising from objects is projected onto an image plane, these complex relationships are transformed into 2D patterns of light intensity with highly structured statistics. Thus, the PD of the luminance of, say, the central target in a standard simultaneous brightness contrast stimulus (Fig. 2 (a)) depends on the surrounding luminance values (Fig. 2 (b)).

Fig. 2 (c) illustrates the supposition that, for any context, the visual system generates the brightness of a target according to the value of its luminance in the probability distribution function (PDF, the integral of PD) of the possible target luminance experienced in that context (Yang & Purves, 2004). This value is referred to subsequently as the percentile of the target luminance among all possible luminance values that co-occur with the contextual luminance pattern in the natural environment. In formal terms, this supposition means that the visual system generates brightness percepts according to the relationship Brightness=$A\Phi(P)+A_0$, where A and A_0 are constants, and $\Phi(P)$ is a monotonically increasing function of the PDF, P.

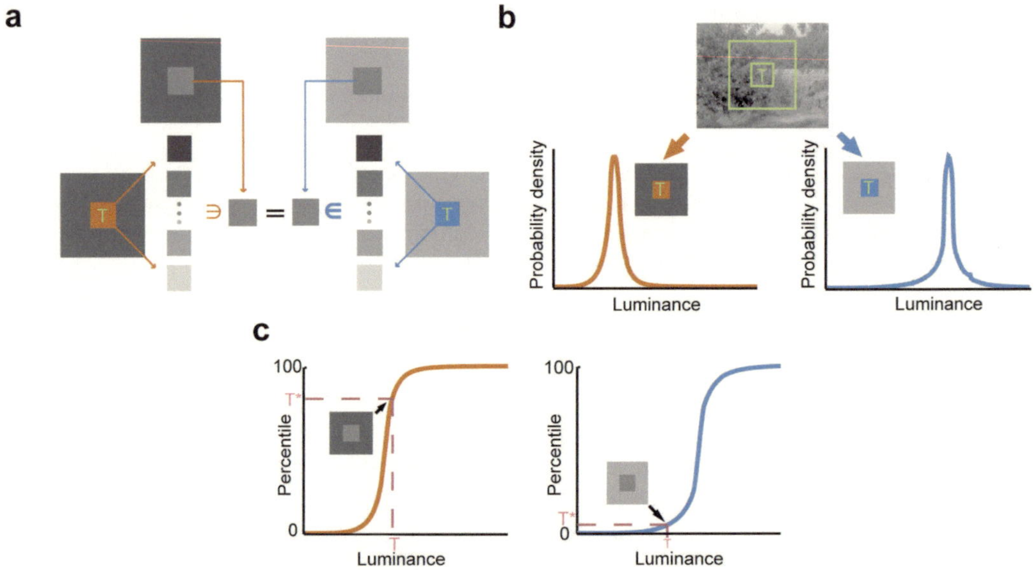

(a), The brightness elicited by a given target luminance in any context depends on the frequency of occurrence of that luminance relative to all the possible target luminance values experienced in that context in natural environments. This concept is illustrated here using the standard simultaneous brightness contrast stimulus in Fig. 1 (a). The series of squares with different luminance values indicate all the possible occurrences of luminance in the target (T) in the two different contexts; the symbol ∊ indicates the relationship of a particular occurrence of luminance to the all possible occurrences of target luminance values experienced in the two contexts in natural environments. (b), This statistical relationship can be derived from the PD of target luminance values co-occurring with the luminance values and pattern of the two contexts of interest. The red and blue curves indicate the PDs of the luminance of the targets in (a), obtained by sampling the natural image database. The size of the sampling configuration was 1°x1°. (c), The brightness elicited by the luminance of the targets in (a) is based on the percentile of that luminance in the PDFs for the two different contexts, which are indicated by the icons (modified from Yang & Purves, 2004).

Figure 2. Brightness percepts signify context-mediated PDs of luminance in natural scenes.

By definition, then, the percentile of target luminance for the lowest luminance value within any contextual light pattern is 0% and corresponds to the perception of maximum darkness; the percentile for the highest luminance within any contextual pattern is 100% and corresponds to the maximum perceivable brightness. In any given context, a higher luminance will always have a higher percentile, and will always elicit a perception of greater brightness compared to any luminance that has a lower percentile. Since the relation Brightness=$A\Phi(P)+A_0$ is not based on a particular luminance within the context in question, but rather on the entire PD of possible luminance values experienced in that context, the context-dependent relationship between brightness and luminance is highly nonlinear (see Fig. 2 (c)). In consequence, the same physical difference between two luminance values will often signify different percentile differences, and thus perceived differences in brightness. Furthermore, because the percentiles change more rapidly as the target luminance approaches the luminance of the surround one would expect greater changes of brightness, an expectation that corresponds to the well known "crispening" effect in perception.

Finally, because the same value of target luminance will often correspond to different percentiles in the PDFs of target luminance in different contexts, two targets having the same luminance can elicit different brightness percepts, the higher percentile always corresponding to a brighter percept. Thus, in the standard simultaneous brightness contrast stimulus in Fig. 1 (a), the target (T) in the left panel in Fig. 2 (a) appears brighter than the equiluminant target in the right panel.

2.4. White's illusion

White's illusion (Fig. 1 (b)) presents a particular challenge for any explanation of brightness (White, 1979). The equiluminant rectangular areas surrounded by predominantly more luminant regions in the stimulus (on the left in the left panel of Fig. 1 (b); see also the area in the red frame in Fig. 3 (a) appear brighter than areas of identical luminance surrounded by less luminant regions (on the right in the left panel of Fig. 1 (b); see also the area in the blue frame in Fig. 3 (a). The especially perplexing characteristic of this percept is that the effect is opposite that elicited by standard simultaneous brightness contrast stimuli (Fig. 1 (a)). Even more puzzling, the effect reverses when the luminance of the rectangular targets is either the lowest or highest value in the stimulus (middle and right panels in Fig. 1 (b).

The explanation for White's illusion provided by the statistical framework outlined above is shown in Fig. 3. When presented separately, as in Fig. 3 (a), the components of White's stimulus elicit much the same effect as in the usual presentation. By sampling the images of natural visual environments using configurations based on these components (Fig. 3 (b)), we obtained the PDFs of the luminance of a rectangular target (T) embedded in the two different configurations of surrounding luminance in White's stimulus. As shown in Fig. 3 (c), when the target in the intermediate range of luminance values (i.e., in between the luminance values at the two crossover points) abuts two dark rectangles laterally (left panel in Fig. 3 (b)), the percentile of the target luminance (red line) is higher than the percentile when the target abuts the two light rectangles (right panel in Fig. 3(b); blue line in Fig. 3 (c)). If, as we suppose, the percentile in the PDF of target luminance within any specific context determines the brightness perceived, the target with an intermediate luminance on the left in Fig. 3 (b) should appear brighter than the equiluminant target on the right. Finally, when all the luminance values in the stimulus are limited to a very narrow range (e.g., from 0 to 100 cd/m^2 or from 1000 to 1100 cd/m^2), when the sampling configurations are orientated vertically, or when the aspect ratio of the sampling configurations is changed (e.g., from 1:2 to 1:5), the PDFs derived from the database are not much different. These further results are consistent with the observations that White's stimulus elicits the similar effect when presented at a wide range of overall luminance levels, in a vertical orientation, or with different aspect ratios.

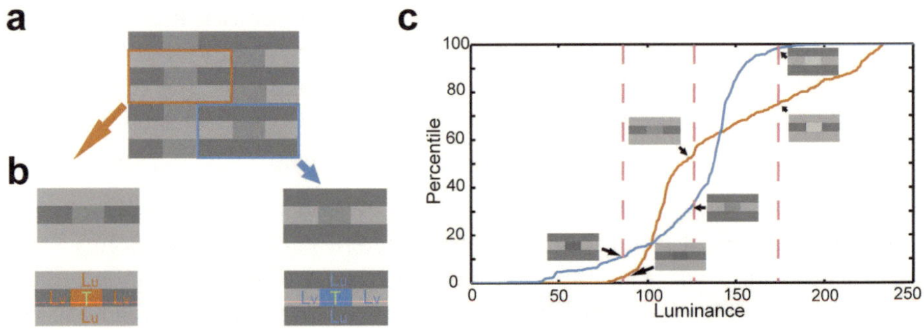

(a), The usual presentation of White's illusion; boxed areas indicate the basic components of the stimulus, which when separated elicit about the same effect as the usual presentation. (b), The sampling configurations used to obtain the PDFs of target luminance (the red and blue rectangles), given a pattern of surrounds with luminance values L_u and L_v (size of the sampling configuration in this example was 0.6°[H]×0.3°[V] and the unit of luminance was cd/m²). (c), The PDFs of the luminance of the targets in these contexts (red curve: L_u=145, L_v=105; blue curve: L_u=105, L_v=145). For the middle luminance values lying within the two crossover points (at ~105 and 145), the red curve is above the blue curve; as a result, the luminance configurations in (b) generate White's illusion (as indicated by the insets). For other luminance values of the target, the blue curve is above the red curve; as a result, the luminance configurations in (b) generate the inverted White's effect (modified from Yang & Purves, 2004).

Figure 3. Statistical explanation of White's illusion.

An aspect of White's illusion that has been particularly difficult to explain is the so-called "inverted White's effect": when the target luminance is either the lowest or the highest value in the stimulus, the effect is actually opposite the usual percept (see the middle and right panels in Fig. 1 (b)). The explanation for this further anomaly is also evident in Fig. 3 (c). When the target luminance is the lowest value in the presentation (see insets), the blue curve is above the red curve. As a result, a relatively dark target surrounded by more light area should now appear darker, as it does (see also the middle panel of Fig. 1 (b)). By the same token, when the target luminance is the highest value in the stimulus (see insets), the blue curve is also above the red curve. Accordingly, the relatively light target surrounded by more dark area should appear brighter, as it does (see also the right panel of Fig. 1 (b)). Thus the statistical structure of natural light patterns predicts not only White's illusion, but the inverted White's effect as well. Notice further that the two crossover points of the blue and red curves shift to the right when the contextual luminances increase, and to the left when they decrease; thus the inverted effect will be apparent, although altered in magnitude, for any luminance values of the surrounding areas.

2.5. The Wertheimer-Benary illusion

In the Wertheimer-Benary illusion (Fig. 1(c)), the equiluminant gray triangles appear differently bright, the triangle embedded in the arm of the cross looking slightly brighter than the triangle in the corner of the cross.

The explanation of the Wertheimer-Benary illusion provided by the statistical framework outlined above is shown in Fig. 4. By sampling the images of natural environments using configurations based on the components of the stimulus (Fig. 4 (b)), we obtained the PDFs of target luminance in these contexts. As shown in Fig. 4 (c), when the triangular patch is embedded in a dark bar with its base facing a lighter area, the percentile of the luminance of the triangular patch (red line) is higher than the percentile when the triangular patch abuts a dark corner with its base facing a similar light background (blue line). Accordingly, the same gray patch should appear brighter in the former context than in the latter, as is the case. The PDFs obtained after changing the triangles to rectangles, rotating the configurations in Fig. 4 (b) by 180°, or reflecting the configurations along the diagonal of the cross (cf. middle and right panels in Fig. 1 (c)) were much the same as those shown in Fig. 4 (c). These several observations accord with the fact that the Wertheimer-Benary effect is little changed by such manipulations.

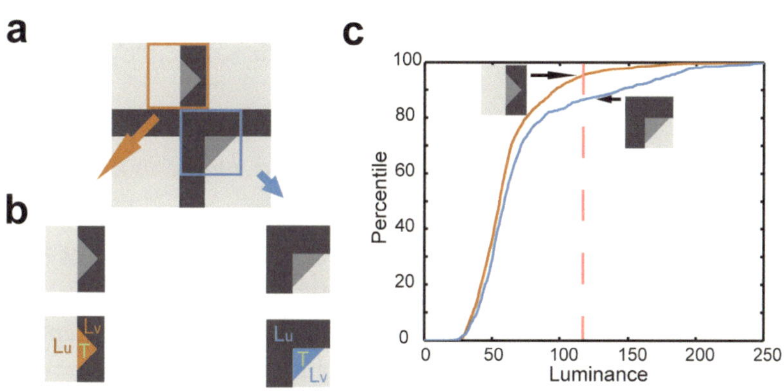

(a), The usual presentation of the Wertheimer-Benary stimulus. The separated components of the stimulus (boxed areas) elicit about the same effect as the usual presentation. (b), Configurations used to sample the database (size=0.4°×0.4°). (c), The PDFs of target luminance, given the surrounding luminances in (b) (The unit of luminance was cd/m^2). The red curve corresponds to the condition shown in the left panel in (b) (L_u=205, L_v=45), and the blue curve to the condition shown in the right panel in (b) (L_u=45, L_v=205) (modified from Yang & Purves, 2004).

Figure 4. Statistical explanation of the Wertheimer-Benary illusion.

The context-mediated PDs of luminance in natural scenes predict equally well other brightness phenomena shown in Fig. 1 (Yang & Purves, 2004).

2.6. Discussion

2.6.1. The statistical nature of perception

I showed that brightness percepts do not encode luminance as such, but rather the statistical relationship between the luminance in an area within a particular contextual light pattern and all possible occurrences of luminance in the context that have been experienced by humans in natural environments during evolution. The statistical basis for this aspect of visual perception is quite different from traditional approaches to rationalizing brightness. In the "relational approach" (Gichrist et al., 1999), an idea that evolved from the late 19th C.

debate between Helmholtz, Hering, and others, brightness percepts are "recovered" by the visual system from explicitly coded luminance contrasts and gradients. Another idea is that brightness depends on intermediate-level visual processes that detect edges, gradients and junctions, which are then grouped into specific spatial layouts (Adelson, 2000; Anderson & Winawer, 2005). Finally, the brightness elicited by a given luminance has been also considered as being "re-synthesized" by processing at several levels of the visual system that is based on inferences about the possible arrangements of surfaces in 3D, their material properties and their illumination (Wishart et al., 1997).

The common deficiency of these several ways of thinking about brightness is their failure to relate the statistics of light patterns experienced in the course of evolution to what the corresponding brightness percepts need to signify (namely, the relationship of a particular occurrence of luminance to all possible occurrences of luminance in a given context). Since light patterns on the retina are the only information the visual system receives, basing brightness percepts on the statistics of natural light patterns allows visual animals to deal optimally with all possible natural occurrences of luminance, employing the full range of perceivable brightness to represent the physical world.

2.6.2. Neural instantiation of context-mediated PDs of luminance in natural scenes

What sort of neural mechanisms, then, could incorporate these statistics of natural light patterns and relate them to brightness percepts? Although the answer is not known, the present results suggest that the circuitry at all levels of the visual system instantiates the statistical structures of light patterns in natural environments. In this conception, the center-surround organization of the receptive fields of retinal ganglion cells provides the initial basis for representing the necessary statistics. A further speculation would be that neural circuitry at the level of visual cortex is organized to instantiate the statistics of luminance patterns with arbitrary target and context shapes and sizes. As a result, the neuronal response at each location would signify the percentile of the target luminance in the PDF pertinent to a given context.

3. Visual saliency emerging from context-mediated PDs in natural scenes

3.1. Introduction

In this section, I present a simple model of the context-mediated PDs in natural scenes and derive a measure of visual saliency from these PDs. Visual saliency is the perceptual quality that makes some items in visual scenes stand out from their immediate contexts (Itti & Koch, 2001). Visual saliency plays important roles in natural vision in that saliency can direct eye movements and facilitate object detection and scene understanding. We developed a model of the context-mediated PDs in natural scenes using a modified algorithm for independent component analysis (**ICA**) (Hyvarinen, 1999) and demonstrated that visual saliency based on the context-mediated PDs in natural scenes is a good predictor of human gaze in free-viewing both static and dynamic natural scenes (Xu et al., 2010).

3.2. Context-mediated PDs in natural scenes and visual saliency

A visual feature is a random variable and co-occurs at certain probabilities with other visual features in natural scenes. We call these the context-mediated PDs in natural scenes. Here, a context refers to the natural scene patch that co-occurs with a visual target in question in space and/or time domains. We proposed to represent the context-mediated PDs in natural scenes using independent components (**ICs**) of natural scenes. There are two reasons for this. First, it has been argued extensively that the early visual cortex represents incoming stimuli in an efficient manner (Simoncelli & Olshausen, 2001). Second, the filters of the ICs of natural scenes are very much like the receptive fields of simple cells in V1 (van Hateren & van der Schaaf, 1998).

To model the context-mediated PDs in static natural scenes, we used a center-surround configuration in which the scene patch within the circular center serves as the target and the scene patch in the annular surround as the context (Xu et al., 2010). We sampled a large number of scene patches from the McGill calibrated color image database of natural scenes (Olmos & Kingdom, 2004). Thus, each sample is a pair of a patch in center (X_c) and a patch in the surrounding area (X_s) (Fig. 5 (a)). We developed a model of natural scenes in this configuration (Eq. (1)). In Eq. (1), A_s, A_c, and A_{sc} are ICs. This model allows us to calculate the ICs for the context first and then the other ICs of natural scenes.

$$\begin{bmatrix} X_s \\ X_c \end{bmatrix} = \begin{bmatrix} A_s & 0 \\ A_{sc} & A_c \end{bmatrix} \begin{bmatrix} U_s \\ U_{sc} \end{bmatrix} \tag{1}$$

ICA filters (i.e., W_s, W_{sc}, W_c) can be obtained as follows

$$\begin{bmatrix} U_s \\ U_{sc} \end{bmatrix} = \begin{bmatrix} W_s & 0 \\ W_{sc} & W_c \end{bmatrix} \begin{bmatrix} X_s \\ X_c \end{bmatrix} \tag{2}$$

Therefore, we obtained three sets of ICs. First, the columns of A_s are the ICs for X_s. Second, the columns of A_{sc} are the ICs for X_c that are paired with the ICs for X_s. Finally, the columns of A_c are the ICs for X_c that are not paired with any ICs for X_s.

Fig. 5 (b) shows paired chromatic ICs for X_c and X_s. Fig. 5 (c) shows paired achromatic ICs for X_c and X_s. The chromatic ICs for the surround have red-green (L-M) or blue-yellow [S-(LM)] opponency. The chromatic paired ICs for the center are extensions of the ICs for the surround. Fig. 5 (d) shows the ICs for X_c, including chromatic and achromatic ICs, that are not paired with any ICs for X_s. Fig. 5 (e) shows examples of the ICs for the center computed alone.

To obtain the context-mediated PDs in dynamic natural scenes, we used sequences of image patches in which the current frame severed as the target and the three preceding frames as the context. We sampled a large number of sequences of image patches (~ 490,000) from a video database (Itti & Baldi, 2009) and performed the ICA according to Eq. (1). Fig. 6 (a) shows the paired chromatic spatiotemporal ICs. Fig. 6 (b) shows the paired achromatic spatiotemporal ICs. Fig. 6 (c) shows the unpaired ICs for the current frame, which are oriented bars and have red-green or blue-yellow opponency.

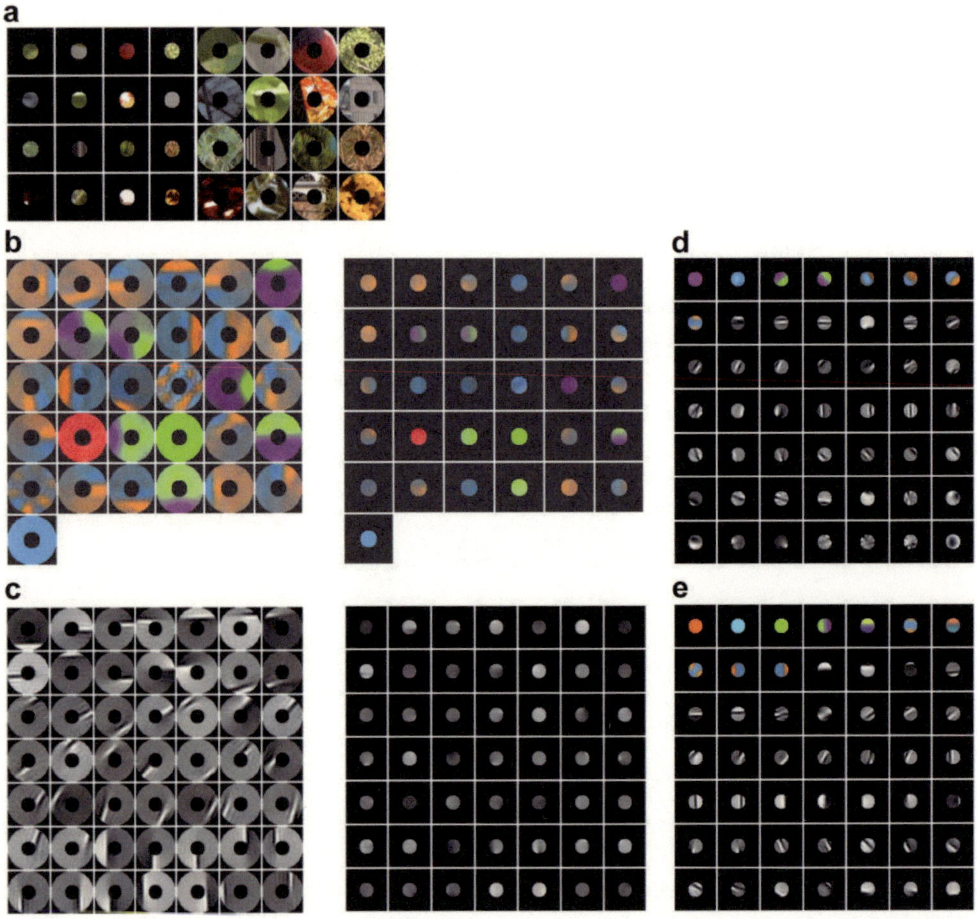

(a), Samples of patches of natural scenes. Each central patch in the left panel is paired with a surrounding patch in the right panel in the same raster order. (b), Examples of paired chromatic center and surround ICs. ICs in the panels are paired in the same raster order. (c), Examples of paired achromatic center and surround ICs. (d), Examples of unpaired center ICs. (e), Examples of the ICs for the center computed alone (modified from Xu et al., 2010).

Figure 5. ICs of color images of natural scenes.

The context-mediated PDs of natural scenes, i.e., the conditional PDs, $P(X_c \mid X_s)$, can be derived using the Bayesian formula as follows

$$P(X_c \mid X_s) = \frac{P(X_c, X_s)}{P(X_s)} \propto \frac{P(U_s)P(U_{sc})}{P(U_s)} = \prod_i P(u_{sc}^i) \tag{3}$$

where u_{sc}^i is the amplitude of the ith unpaired IC for X_c. Therefore, the context-mediated PDs depend only on the unpaired ICs for X_c. We modeled $P(u_{sc}^i)$ as generalized Gaussian PDs.

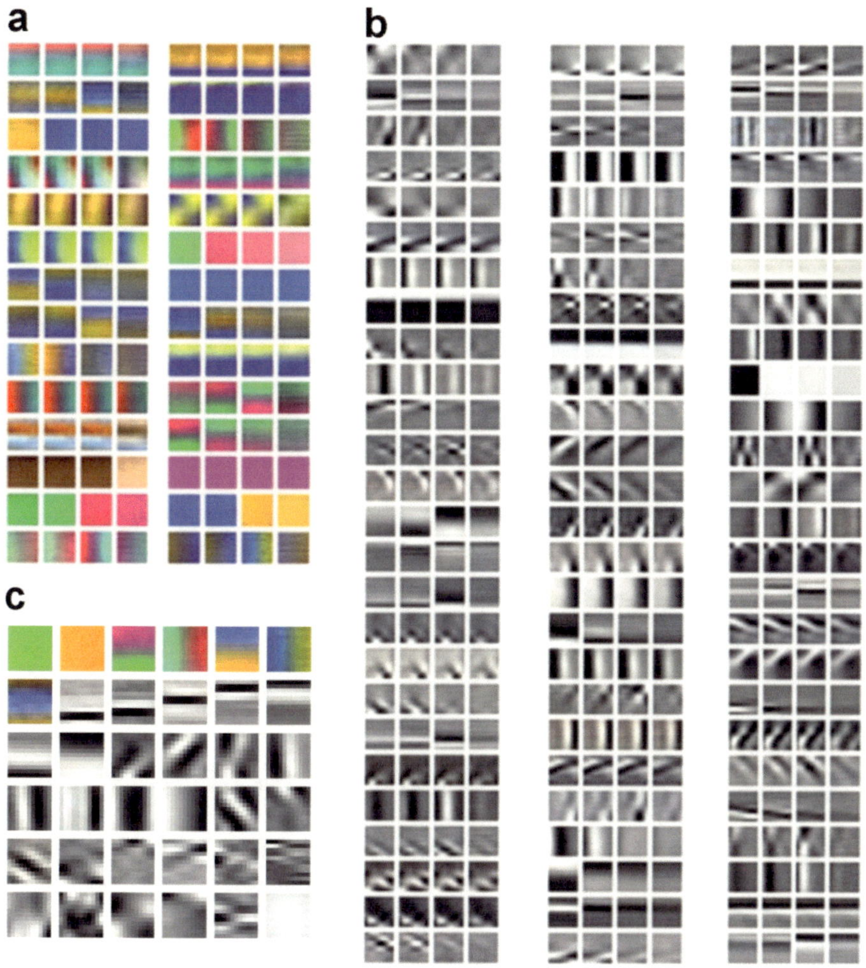

(a), Selected 28 red/green or blue/yellow paired ICs. (b), Selected 78 paired bright/dark ICs. (c), Examples of unpaired target ICs (modified from Xu et al., 2010).

Figure 6. ICs of natural moving scenes.

We proposed a measure of visual saliency as

$$S = \ln P_{\max}(X_c \mid X_s) - \ln P(X_c \mid X_s) \tag{4}$$

Substituting Eq. (3) into Eq. (4), we have

$$S = \sum_i \ln P_{\max}(u_{sc}^i) - \sum_i \ln P(u_{sc}^i) \tag{5}$$

where $P_{\max}(X_c \mid X_s)$ is the maximum probability of a target, X_c, that co-occurs with a context, X_s, in natural scenes. Thus, if the probability of the occurrence of a target is low relative to that of the most likely occurrence in the context in natural scenes, the target is salient within the context (Fig. 7).

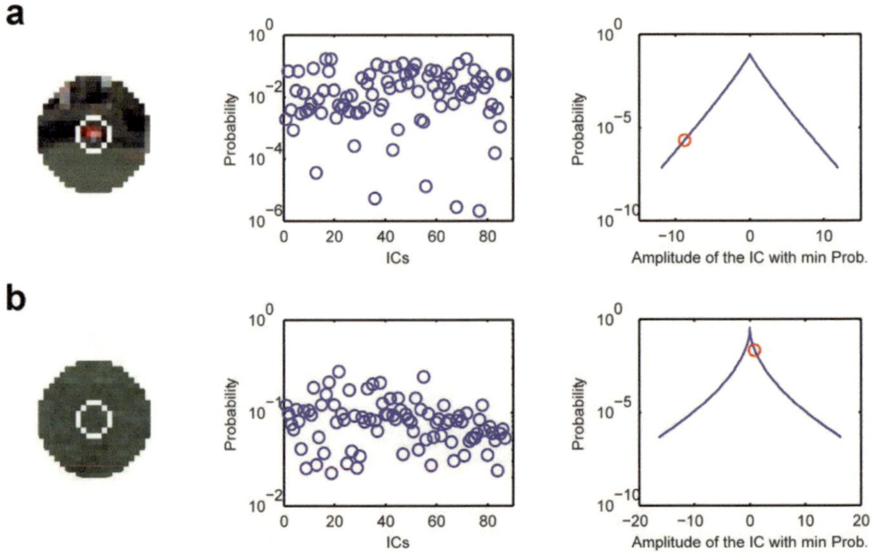

(a), An image patch with an salient feature at the center (left), the probabilities of the ICs (middle), and the PD of the IC that has the smallest probability (right). (b), An image patch with an non-salient feature at the center (left), the probabilities of the ICs (middle), and the PD of the IC that has the smallest probability (right). In (a) and (b), the red circles indicate the probability of the amplitude of the IC of the features in the centers (modified from Xu et al., 2010).

Figure 7. Visual saliency based on the context-mediated PDs in natural scenes.

3.3. Visual saliency and human gaze in free-viewing static natural scenes

Human gaze in free-viewing natural scenes is probably driven by visual saliency in natural scenes. To test this hypothesis, we used a dataset of human gaze collected from 20 human subjects in free-viewing 120 images (Bruce & Tsotsos, 2009). Fig. 8 shows the saliency maps based on the context-mediated PDs in natural scenes and the density maps of human gaze for six scenes. The saliency maps based on the information maximization (**AIM**) model are also shown (Bruce & Tsotsos, 2009). Evidently, the salient features and objects in these scenes predicted by the saliency maps accord with human observations and the saliency maps predicted by our model qualitatively matched the density maps of human gaze.

To quantitatively examine how well this model of visual saliency predicts human fixation, we used the receiver operating characteristic (**ROC**) metric and the Kullback–Leibler (**KL**) divergence. The ROC metric measures the area under the ROC curve. To calculate this metric, we used visual saliency as a feature to classify the locations where the saliency measures are greater than a threshold as fixations and the rest as nonfixated locations. By varying the threshold, we obtained an ROC curve and calculated the area under the curve, which indicates how well the saliency maps predict human gaze.

To avoid a central tendency in human gaze, we used the ROC measure described in (Tatler et al., 2005). We compared the saliency measures at the attended locations to the saliency measures in that scene at the locations that are attended in different scenes in the dataset, called shuffled fixations. The average area under the ROC curve is 0.6803, which means the saliency measures at fixations are significantly higher than the saliency measures at shuffled fixations. Similarly, we measured the KL divergence between two histograms of saliency measures: the histogram of saliency measures at the fixated locations in a test scene and the histogram of saliency measures at the same locations in a different scene randomly selected from the dataset (Zhang et al., 2008).

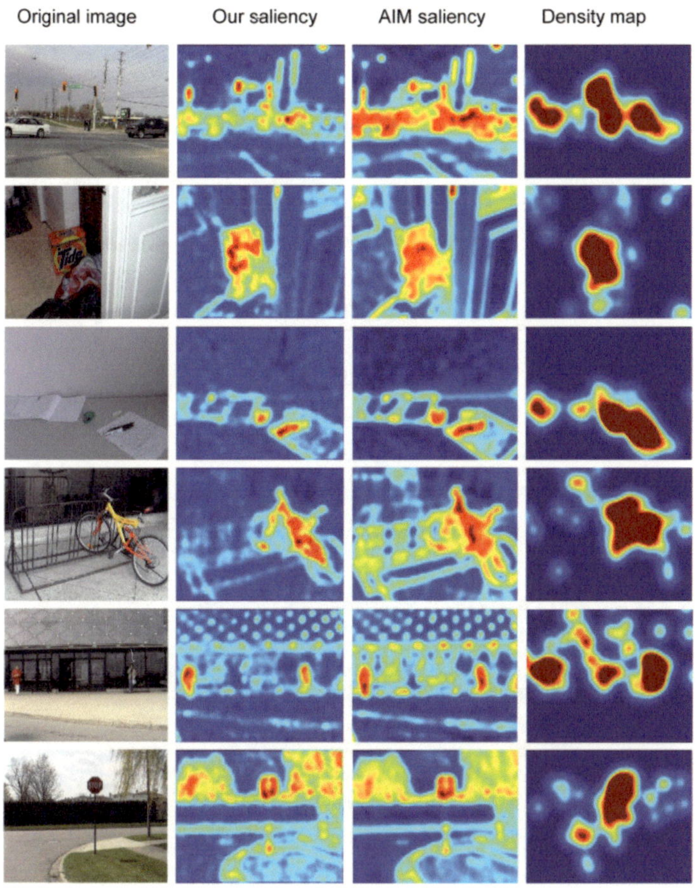

First column: input scenes. Second column, saliency maps produced by our model. Third column: saliency maps given by the AIM model. Fourth column: density maps of human fixation. Saliency is coded in color-scale (red/blue: high/low saliency) (modified from Xu et al., 2010).

Figure 8. Examples of saliency maps of natural scenes.

Our model of visual saliency is a good predictor of human gaze in free-viewing static natural scenes, outperforming all other models that we tested. As shown in Table 1 (Xu et al., 2010), our model has an average KL divergence of 0.3016 and the average ROC measure is 0.6803. The average KL divergence and ROC measure for the AIM model are 0.2879 and 0.6799 respectively, which were calculated using the code provided by the authors. The results for other models in Table 1 were given in (Zhang et al., 2008).

Model	KL (SE)	ROC (SE)
Bruce et al. (2009)	0.2879(0.0048)	0.6799(0.0024)
Itti et al. (1998)	0.1130(0.0011)	0.6146(0.0008)
Gao et al. (2009)	0.1535(0.0016)	0.6395(0.0007)
Zhang et al.: DOG (2008)	0.1723(0.0012)	0.6570(0.0007)
Zhang et al.: ICA (2008)	0.2097(0.0016)	0.6682(0.0008)
Our model	0.3016(0.0051)	0.6803(0.0027)

Table 1. ROC metric and KL-divergence for saliency maps of static natural scenes (SE: standard error).

3.4. Visual saliency and human gaze in free-viewing natural movies

We used a database of human gaze collected from 8 subjects in free-viewing 50 videos, including indoor scenes, outdoor scenes, television clips, and video games (Itti & Baldi, 2009). Fig. 9 shows the saliency maps for selected frames in 6 videos. The 3 contextual video frames and the target frame are shown to the left and the saliency maps to the right. As predicted by the saliency maps, the moving objects in these videos appear to be salient (e.g., the character in the game video, the falling water drop, the soccer player and the ball, the moving car and the walking policeman, and the jogger and the football player). These predictions accord well with human observations.

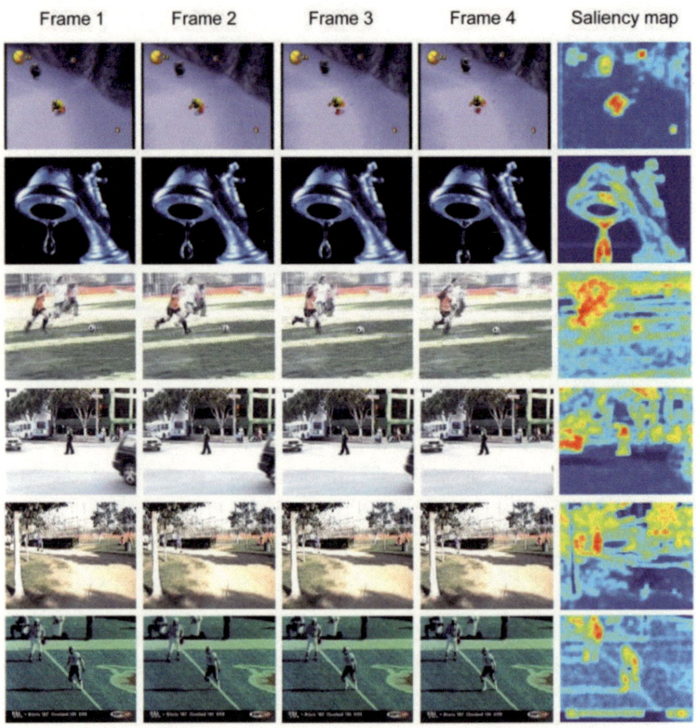

Figure 9. Saliency maps of dynamic natural scenes. Examples of contextual frames (3 left columns) and target frames (4th column) in 6 video clips and saliency maps (rightmost column) (modified from Xu et al., 2010).

We calculated the KL-divergence for this dataset as described above. Humans tend to gaze at visual features that have high saliency, as shown by the KL divergence measures in Table 2 (Xu et al., 2010). The KL-divergence measure for our model is 0.3153, which is higher than the saliency metric (0.205) (Itti et al., 1998) and the surprise metric 0.241 (Itti & Baldi, 2009), but slightly lower than the AIM model (0.328) (Bruce & Tsotsos, 2009).

3.5. Discussion

3.5.1. Distinctions from other models of visual saliency

Our model of visual saliency is different from all other models. There are four classes of models of visual saliency. The first class of models do not use PDs in natural scenes but involve complex image-based computation that includes feature extraction, feature pooling, and normalization (Itti et al., 1998). The second class of models make use of PDs computed from the current scene the subject is seeing (Bruce & Tsotsos, 2009). The third class of models are based on PDs in natural scenes that are not dependent on specific contexts (Zhang et al., 2008). Finally, there is a biologically inspired neural network model (Zhaoping & May, 2007). Our model is unique in that: 1) the PDs are computed from an ensemble of natural scenes that presumably approximate the statistics human experienced during evolution and development; and 2) the PDs are dependent on specific contexts in natural scenes.

Model	**KL (SE)**
Bruce et al. (2009)	0.328(0.009)
Itti et al. (2009)	0.241(0.006)
Zhang et al. (2009)	0.181
Itti et al. (1998)	0.205(0.006)
Our model	0.315(0.003)

Table 2. KL-divergence for saliency maps of dynamic natural scenes (SE: standard error).

3.5.2. Neurons as estimators of context-mediated PDs in natural scenes

These results support the notion that neurons in the early visual cortex act as estimators of the context-mediated PDs in natural scenes. This way, any single neuron relates an occurrence of any visual variable to the underlying PD in natural scenes. These PDs are related to all possible stimuli in natural scenes experienced by the visual animals over evolutionary and developmental time.

This hypothesis is distinct from the conventional view of neurons as feature detectors, the efficient coding hypothesis (Simoncelli & Olshausen, 2001), predictive coding (Rao & Ballard, 1999), the proposal that neurons encode logarithmic likelihood functions (Rao, 2004), and several recent V1 neuronal models that involve complex spatial-tempo structures but don't function as estimators of PDs in natural scenes (Rust et al., 2005; Chen at al., 2007).

Since the response of any single neuron encodes and decodes the PD of the visual variable in natural scenes, this concept is also different from probabilistic population codes where populations of neurons automatically encode PDs due to varying tuning among neurons and noise (Ma et al., 2005).

4. Statistics of 3D natural scenes and visual space

4.1. Introduction

In the last two sections, I presented evidence that aspects of human natural vision are generated on the basis of the PDs of visual variables in 2D natural scenes. However, the most fundamental task of vision is to generate visual percepts and visually guided behaviors in the 3D physical world. In this section, I present PDs in 3D natural scenes and relate them to the characteristics of human visual space.

Visual space is characterized by perceived geometrical properties such as distance, linearity, and parallelism. An appealing intuition is that these properties are the result of a direct transformation of the Euclidean characteristics of physical space (Hershenson, 1998; Loomis et al., 1996; Gillam, 1996). This assumption is, however, inconsistent with a variety of puzzling and often subtle discrepancies between the predicted consequences of any direct mapping of physical space and what people actually see. A number of examples in perceived distance, the simplest aspect of visual space, show that the apparent distance of objects bears no simple relation to their physical distance from the observer (Loomis et al., 1996; Gillam, 1996) (Fig. 10). Although a variety of explanations have been proposed, there has been little or no agreement about the basis of this phenomenology.

We tested the hypothesis that these anomalies of perceived distance are all manifestations of a probabilistic strategy for generating visual percepts in response to inevitably ambiguous visual stimuli (Knill & Richards, 1996; Purves & Lotto, 2003; Trommershauser et al., 2011). A straightforward way of examining this idea in the case of visual space is to analyze the statistical relationship between geometrical features (e.g., points, lines and surfaces) in the image plane and the corresponding physical geometry in representative visual scenes. Accordingly, we used a database of natural scene geometry acquired with a laser range scanner to test whether the otherwise puzzling phenomenology of perceived distance can be explained in statistical terms (Fig. 11).

4.2. A probabilistic concept of visual space

The challenge in generating perceptions of distance (and spatial relationships more generally) is the inevitable ambiguity of visual stimuli. When any point in space is projected onto the retina, the corresponding point in projection could have been generated by an infinite number of different locations in the physical world. In consequence, the relationship between any projected image and its source is inherently ambiguous. Nevertheless, the PD of the distances of un-occluded object surfaces from the observer must have a potentially informative statistical structure. Given this inevitable ambiguity, it seems likely that highly evolved visual systems would have taken advantage of this probabilistic information in generating perceptions of physical space.

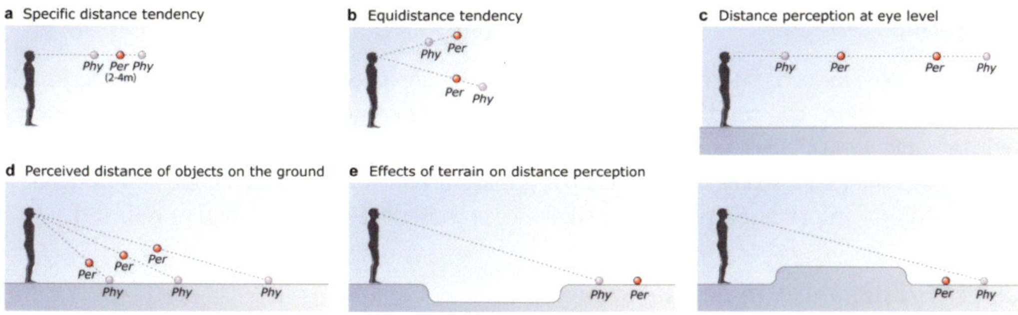

(a), Specific distance tendency. When a simple object is presented in an otherwise dark environment, observers usually judge it to be at a distance of 2-4m, regardless of its actual distance. In these diagrams, which are not to scale, 'Phy' indicates the physical position of the object and 'Per' the perceived position. (b), Equidistance tendency. Under these same conditions, an object is usually judged to be at about the same distance from the observer as neighboring objects, even when their physical distances differ. (c), Perceived distance of objects at eye-level. The distances of nearby objects presented at eye-level tend to be overestimated, whereas the distances of further objects tend to be underestimated. (d), Perceived distance of objects on the ground. An object on the ground a few meters away tends to appear closer and slightly elevated with respect to its physical position. Moreover, the perceived location becomes increasingly elevated and relatively closer to the observer as the angle of the line of sight approaches the horizontal plane at eye-level. (e), Effects of terrain on distance perception. Under more realistic conditions, the distance of an object on a uniform ground-plane a few meters away from the observer is usually accurately perceived. When, however, the terrain is disrupted by a dip, the same object appears to be further away; conversely, when the ground-plane is disrupted by a hump, the object tends to appear closer than it is (modified from Yang & Purves, 2003a).

Figure 10. Anomalies in perceived distance.

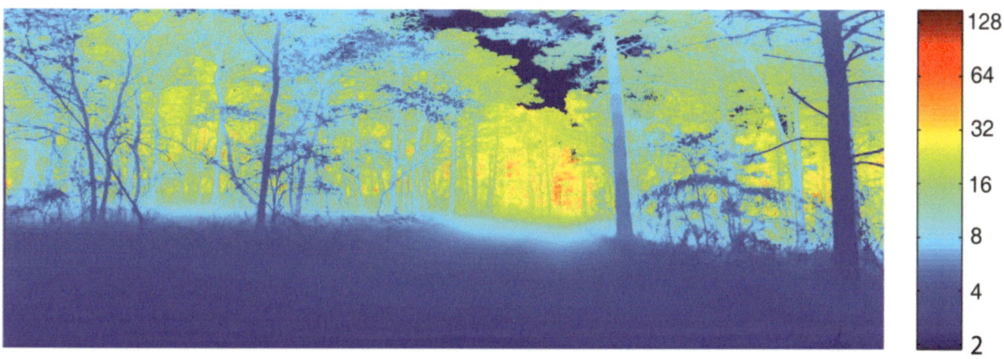

The distance (in meters) of each pixel is indicated by color coding. Black areas are regions where the laser beam did not return a value.

Figure 11. A range image acquired by laser range scanning.

This probabilistic strategy can be formalized in terms of Bayesian inference (Knill & Richards, 1996; Trommershauser et al., 2011). In this framework, the PD of the physical sources underlying a visual stimulus, P(S|I) can be expressed as

$$P(S|I)=P(I|S)P(S)/P(I) \quad (6)$$

where S represents the parameters of physical scene geometry and I the visual image. P(S) is the PD of scene geometry in typical visual environments (the prior), P(I|S) the PD of stimulus I generated by the scene geometry S (the likelihood function), and P(I) a normalization constant.

If visual space is indeed determined by the PD of 3D scene geometry underlying visual stimuli, then, under reduced-cue conditions, the prior PD of distances to the observer in typical viewing environments should bias perceived distances. By the same token, the PD of the distances between locations in a scene should bias the apparent relative distances among them. Finally, when additional information pertinent to distance is present, these biases will be reduced.

4.3. PDs of distances in natural scenes

The information at each pixel in the range image database is the distance, elevation, and azimuth of the corresponding location in the physical scene relative to the laser scanner (Fig. 11). These data were used to compute the PD of distances from the center of the scanner to locations in the physical scenes in the database.

The first of several statistical features apparent in the analysis is that the PD of the radial distances from the scanner to physical locations in the scenes has a maximum at about 3 m, declining approximately exponentially over greater distances (Fig. 12 (a)). This PD is scale-invariant, meaning that any scaled version of the geometry of a set of natural scenes will, in statistical terms, be much the same (Lee et al., 2001). A simple model of natural 3D scenes generates a scaling-invariant PD of object distances nearly identical to that obtained from natural scenes (see legend of Fig. 12).

A second statistical feature of the analysis concerns how different physical locations in natural scenes are typically related to each other with respect to distance from the observer. The PD of the differences in the distance from the observer to any two physical locations is highly skewed, having a maximum near zero and a long tail (Fig. 12 (b)). Even for physical separations as large as 30°, the most probable difference between the distances from the image plane of two locations is minimal.

A third statistical feature is that the PD of horizontal distances from the scanner to physical locations changes relatively little with height in the scene (the height of the center of scanner was always 1.65m above the ground, thus approximating eye-level of an average adult) (Fig. 12 (c)). The PD of physical distances at eye-level has a maximum at about 4.7 m and decays gradually as the distances increase. The PDs of the horizontal distances of physical locations at different heights above and below eye-level also tend to have a maximum at about 3m, and are similar in shape.

4.4. Perceived distances in impoverished settings

How, then, do these scale-invariant PDs of distances from the image plane in natural scenes account for the anomalies of visual space summarized in Fig. 10?

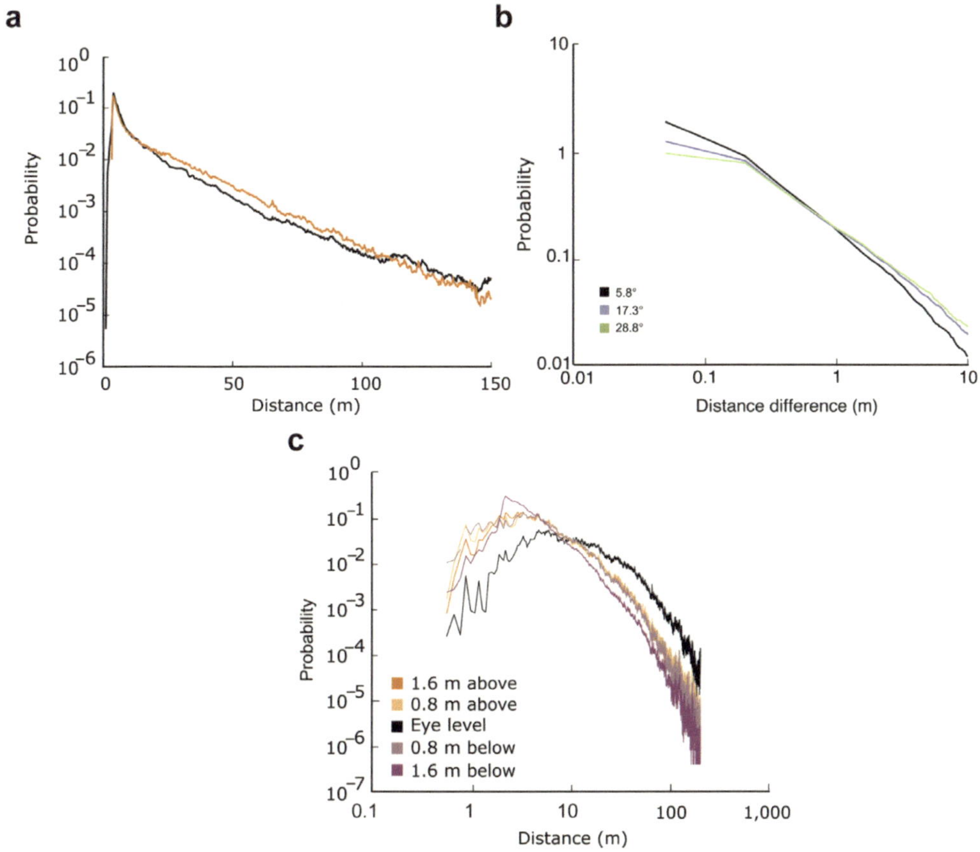

(a), The scale-invariant PD of the distances from the center of the laser scanner to all the physical locations in the database (black line). The red line represents the PD of distances derived from a simple model in which 1000 planar rectangular surfaces were uniformly placed at distances from 2.5-300 m, from 150 m left to 150 m right, and from the ground to 25 m above the ground (which was 1.65m below the image center). The sizes of these uniformly distributed surfaces ranged from 0.2-18 m. Five hundred 512×512 images of this model made by a pinhole camera method showed statistical behavior similar to that derived from the range image database for a wide variety of specific values, although with different slopes and modes. The model also generated statistical behavior similar to that shown in (b) and (c) (not shown). (b), PDs of the differences in the physical distances of two locations separated by three different angles in the horizontal plane. (c), PDs of the horizontal distances of physical locations at different heights with respect to eye-level (modified from Yang & Purves, 2003a).

Figure 12. PDs of the physical distances from the image plane of points in the range images of natural scenes.

When little or no other information is available in a scene, observers tend to perceive objects at a distance of 2-4m (Owens et al., 1976). In the absence of any distance cues, the likelihood function in Eq. (6) is flat; the apparent distance of a point in physical space should therefore accord with the PD of the distances of all points in typical visual scenes (see Eq. (6)). As indicated in Fig. 12 (a), this distribution has a maximum probability at about 3 m. The agreement between this PD of distances in natural scenes and the relevant psychophysical evidence is thus consistent with a probabilistic explanation of the 'specific distance tendency'.

The similar apparent distance of an object to the apparent distances of its near neighbors in the retinal image (the 'equidistance tendency' (Owens et al., 1976)) also accords with the PD of the distances of locations in the natural scenes. In the absence of additional information about differences in the distances of two nearby locations, the likelihood function is again more or less flat. As a result, the PD of the differences of the physical distances from the image plane to any two locations in natural scenes should strongly bias the perceived difference in their distances. Since this distribution between two locations with relatively small angular separations (the black line in Fig. 12 (b)) has a maximum near zero, any two neighboring objects should be perceived to be at about the same distance from the observer. However, at larger angular separations (the green line in Fig. 12 (b)) the probability associated with small absolute differences in the distance to the two points is lower than the corresponding probabilities for smaller separations, and the distribution relatively flatter. Accordingly, the tendency to see neighboring points at the same distance from the observer would be expected to decrease somewhat as a function of increasing angular separation. Finally, when more specific information about the distance difference is present, this tendency should decrease. Each of these several tendencies has been observed in psychophysical studies of the 'equidistance tendency'.

4.5. Perceived distances in more complex circumstances

The following explanations for the phenomena illustrated in Figs. 10 (c) and (d) are somewhat more complex since, in contrast to the 'specific distance' and 'equidistance' tendencies, the relevant psychophysical observations were made under conditions that entailed some degree of contextual visual information. Thus, the relevant likelihood functions are no longer flat. Since their form is not known, we used a Gaussian to approximate the likelihood function in the following analyses.

The PD of physical distances at eye-level (the black line in Fig. 12 (c)) accounts for the perceptual anomalies in response to stimuli generated by near and far objects presented at this height (see Fig. 10 (c)). As shown in Fig. 13 (a), the distance that should be perceived on this basis is approximately a linear function of physical distance, with near distances being overestimated and far distances underestimated; the physical distance at which overestimation changes to underestimation is about 5-6 m. The effect of these statistics accords both qualitatively and quantitatively with the distances reported under these experimental conditions (Philbeck & Loomis, 1997).

To examine whether the perceptual observations summarized in Fig. 10 (d) can also be explained in these terms, we computed the PD of physical distances of points at different elevation angles of the laser beam relative to the horizontal plane at eye-level (Fig. 14). As shown in Fig. 14 (a), the PD of distances is more dispersed when the line of sight is directed above rather than below eye-level. The distribution shifts toward nearer distances with increasing absolute elevation angle, a tendency that is more pronounced below than above eye-level. A more detailed examination of the distribution within 30 m shows a single salient ridge below eye-level (indicated in red), extending from ~3 m near the ground to ~10 m at an elevation of -10°(Fig. 14 (b)). The distances of the average physical locations at different elevation angles of the scanning beam form a gentle curve. Below eye-level, the height of this curve is relatively near the ground for closer distances, but increases slowly as the horizontal distance from the observer increases. If the portion of the curve at heights below eye-level in Fig. 14 (c) is taken as an index of the average ground, it is apparent that the average ground is neither a horizontal plane nor a plane with constant slant, but a curved surface that is increasingly inclined toward the observer as a function of horizontal distance.

These characteristics of distance as a function of the elevation of the line of sight can thus account for the otherwise puzzling perceptual effects shown in Fig. 10 (d). The perceived location of an object on the ground without much additional information varies according to the declination of the line of sight, the object appearing closer and higher than it really is as a function of this angle. The apparent location of an object predicted by the PDs in Fig. 14 is increasingly higher and closer to the observer as the declination of the line of sight decreases, in agreement with the relevant psychophysical data (Ooi et al., 2001) (Fig. 13 (b)).

Other characteristics of visual space shown in Fig. 10 can be explained in the same way (Yang & Purves, 2003a).

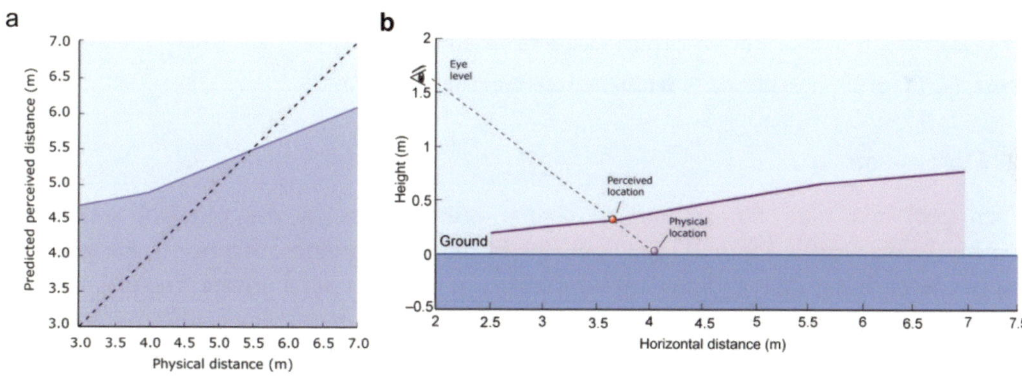

(a), The perceived distances predicted from the PD of physical distances measured at eye-level. The solid line represents the local mass mean of the PD obtained by multiplying the PD in Fig. 12 (c) (black line) by a Gaussian likelihood function of distances with a standard deviation of 1.4 m. The dashed line represents the equivalence of perceived and physical distances for comparison. (b), The perceived distances of objects on the ground in the absence of other information predicted from the PD in Fig. 14 (a). The likelihood function at an angular declination α was a Gaussian function, i.e., ~ $\exp(-(\alpha-\alpha_0)^2/2\Sigma^2)$ ($\alpha_0=\sin^{-1}(H/R)$, $\Sigma=8°$, R is radial distance, and H=1.65m). The prior was the distribution of distance at angular declinations within [α-8°, α+8°]. The ground in the diagram is a horizontal plane 1.65m below eye-level (icon). The predicted perceptual locations of objects on the ground are indicated by the solid line (modified from Yang & Purves, 2003a).

Figure 13. The perceived distances predicted for objects located at eye-level and objects on the ground.

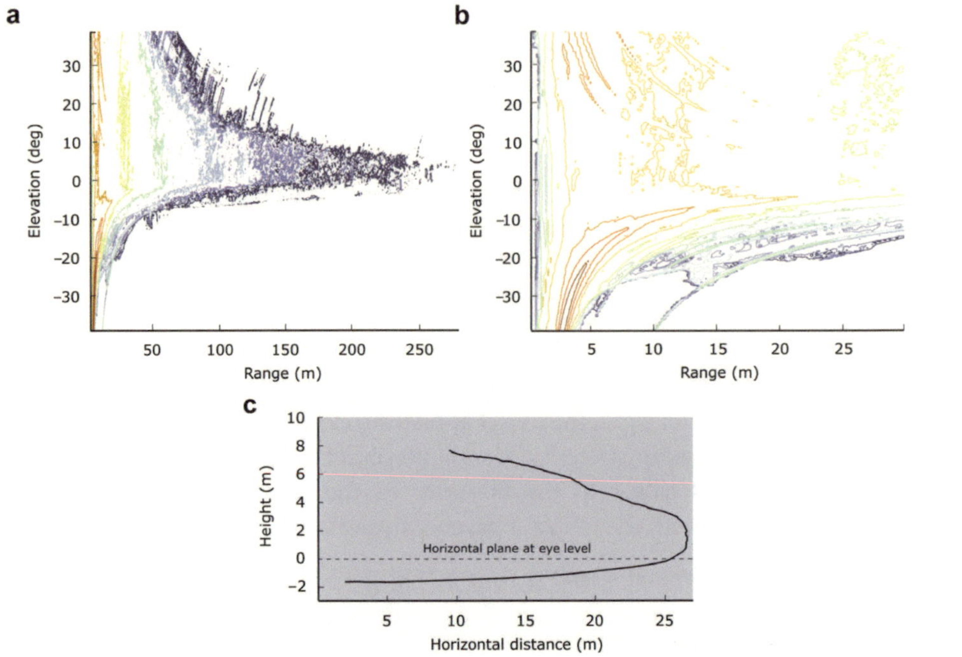

(a), Contour plot of the logarithm of the PD of distances at elevation angles indicated by color coding. Red indicates a probability value of ~10^{-2} and blue ~$10^{-5.5}$. (b), Blowup of (a) showing the PD of distances within 30 m in greater detail. In this case, red indicates a probability value of ~$10^{-1.5}$. (c), The average distance as a function of elevation angle, based on the data in (a). The vertical axis is the height relative to eye level; the horizontal axis is the horizontal distance from the image plane. The curve below eye-level, if modeled as a piece-wise plane, would have a slant of about 1.5° from 3-15 m, and about 5° from 15-24 m (modified from Yang & Purves, 2003a).

Figure 14. PD of physical distances at different elevation angles.

4.6. Discussion

When projected onto the retina, 3D spatial relationships in the physical world are necessarily transformed into 2D relationships in the image plane. As a result, the physical sources underlying any geometrical configuration in the retinal image are uncertain: a multitude of different scene geometries could underlie any particular configuration in the image. This uncertain link between retinal stimuli and physical sources presents a biological dilemma, since an observer's fate depends on visually guided behavior that accords with real-world physical sources.

Given this quandary, we set out to explore the hypothesis that the uncertain relationship of images and sources is addressed by a probabilistic strategy, using the phenomenology of visual space to test this idea. If physical and perceptual space are indeed related in this way, then the characteristics of human visual space should accord with the PDs of 3D natural scene geometry. Observers would be expected to perceive objects in positions substantially and systematically different from their physical locations when countervailing empirical information is not available, or at locations predicted by the altered PDs of the possible sources of the stimulus in question when other contextual information is available. Using a database of range images, we showed that the phenomena illustrated in Fig. 10 can all be rationalized in this framework.

If visual space is indeed generated by a probabilistic strategy, then explaining the relevant perceptual phenomenology will inevitably require knowledge of the statistical properties of natural visual environments with respect to observers. Visual space generated probabilistically will necessarily be a space in which perceived distances are not a simple mapping of physical distances; on the contrary, apparent distance will always be determined by the way all the available information at that moment affects the PD of the gamut of the possible sources of any physical point in the scene.

5. Conclusion

These and many other studies present a strong case supporting the concept that vision works as a fundamentally statistical machine. In this concept, even the simplest visual percept has a statistical basis, i.e., it is related to a certain statistics in the natural environments that supports routinely successful visually guided behavior. The statistics of natural visual environments must have been incorporated into the visual circuitry by successful behavior in the world over evolutionary and developmental time.

There are a range of statistics in the natural environments. These include the statistics of 2D and 3D natural scenes in both space and time domains. As discussed here and elsewhere (Geisler, 2008), these statistics are related to a range of aspects of human natural vision. Since natural environments consist of objects of various physical properties that are arranged in 3D space and move in a variety of ways, the statistics of natural objects, activities, and events, though not discussed here, are critical for our understanding of human object recognition and activity and event understanding (Yuille & Kersten, 2006; Doya et al., 2007; Friston, 2010).

What could be the neural mechanisms underlying this fundamentally statistical machine? A broad hypothesis is that the response properties of visual neurons and their connections, the organization of visual cortex, the patterns of activity elicited by visual stimuli, and visual perception are all determined by the PDs of visual stimuli. In this conception, neurons do not detect or encode features, but by virtue of their activity levels, act as estimators of the PDs of the variables underlying any given stimulus. From this perspective, the function of visual cortical circuitry is to propagate, combine, and transform these PDs. The iterated structure of the primary visual cortex in primates may thus be organized in the way it is in order to generate PDs pertinent to simpler aspects of visual stimuli. By the same token, the extrastriate visual cortical areas may serve to generate PDs pertinent to more complex aspects of visual stimuli by propagating, combining, and transforming the PDs elaborated in the V1 area. The activity patterns elicited by any visual stimulus would, in this conception, be determined by the joint PDs of the variables underlying visual stimuli, which, in turn, determine what people actually see.

This statistical concept of vision and visual system structure and function is radically different from the conventional view, where visual neurons are conceived to perform bottom-up, image-based processing (e.g., computing zero-crossing, luminance and texture gradients, stereoscopic and motion correspondence, and grouping) to build a series of symbolic representations of visual stimuli (e.g., primal sketch, 2½) sketch, and 3D representation) (Marr, 2010). Since the statistics of natural scenes, which are, as argued above, fundamental to the generation of natural vision and visually guided behaviors, are not contained in any current stimulus the visual animal is seeing, any image-based feature extraction/representation construction in the current stimulus *per se* will not generate percepts that allow routinely successful behaviors. The results presented here and many others support this statistical concept of vision and visual system structure and function and several recent reviews also point to this new concept (Knill & Richards, 1996; Rao et al., 2002; Purves & Lotto, 2003; Doya et al., 2007; Trommershauser et al., 2011; Simoncelli & Olshausen, 2001; Yuille & Kersten, 2006; Geisler, 2008; Friston, 2010), but much is left to the next generation of neuroscientists.

Author details

Zhiyong Yang
Brain and Behavior Discovery Institute and Department of Ophthalmology,
Georgia Health Sciences University, USA

6. References

Adelson, E. H. (2000). Lightness and perception and lightness illusion. In: *The New Cognitive Neuroscience (2nd Ed)*, M. Gazzaiga, (Ed.), pp. 339-351, MIT Press, ISBN 0262071959, Cambridge, MA, USA.

Anderson, B. L. & Winawer, J. (2005). Image segmentation and lightness perception. *Nature*, Vol. 434, pp. 79-83.

Blakeslee, B. & McCourt, M. E. (2004). A unified theory of brightness contrast and assimilation incorporating oriented multiscale spatial filtering and contrast normalization. *Vision Research*, Vol. 44, No. 21, pp. 2483-2503.

Bruce, N. D. & Tsotsos, J. K. (2009). Saliency, attention, and visual search: an information theoretic approach. *Journal of Vision*, Vol. 9, No. 5, pp. 1-24.

Chen, X.; Han, F.; Poo, M. M. & Dan, Y. (2007). Excitatory and suppressive receptive field subunits in awake monkey primary visual cortex (V1). *Proc. Natl. Acad. Sci. USA*, Vol. 104, No. 48, pp. 19120-19125.

Doya, K.; Ishii, S.; Pouget, A. & Rao, R. P. N. (Eds.). (2007). *Bayesian Brain, Probabilistic Approaches to Neural Coding*. MIT Press, ISBN 0-262-04238-X, Cambridge, MA, USA.

Friston, K. (2010). The free-energy principle: a unified brain theory? *Nature Reviews Neuroscience*, Vol. 11, p. 127-138..

Gao, D.; Han, S. & Vasconcelos, N. (2009). Discriminant saliency, the detection of suspicious coincidences, and applications to visual recognition. *IEEE Transactions on Pattern Analysis and Machine Intelligence*, Vol. 31, No. 6, pp. 989-1005.

Geisler, W. S. (2008). Visual perception and the statistical properties of natural scenes. *Annu. Rev. Psychol.* Vol. 59, pp. 167-192.

Gichrist, A. et al. (1999). An anchoring theory of lightness perception. *Psychological Review*, Vol. 106, No. 4, pp. 795-834.

Gillam, B. (1995). The perception of spatial layout from static optical information. In: *Perception of space and motion, W.* Epstein & S. Rogers, (Eds.), pp. 23-67, Academic Press, Inc., ISBN 978-0122405303, San Diego, CA, USA.

Hershenson, M. (1998). *Visual space perception: A Primer.* MIT Press, ISBN 978-0262581677, Cambridge, MA, USA.

Hubel, D. H. & Wiesel, T. N. (1977). Functional architecture of macaque monkey visual cortex. *Proc. R. Soc. Lond. B*, Vol. 198, No. 1130, pp 1-59.

Hyvarinen, A. (1999). Fast and robust fixed-point algorithms for independent component analysis. *IEEE Trans Neural Netw*, Vol. 10, No. 3, pp. 626-634

Itti, L. & Baldi, P. (2009). Bayesian surprise attracts human attention. *Vision Research*, Vol. 49, pp. 1295-1306.

Itti, L. & Koch, C. (2001). Computational modelling of visual attention. *Nature Reviews Neuroscience*, Vol. 2, No. 3, pp. 194-203.

Itti, L.; Koch, C. & Niebur, E. (1998). A model of saliency-based visual attention for rapid scene analysis. *IEEE Transactions on Pattern Analysis and Machine Intelligence*, Vol. 20, No. 11, pp. 1254-1259.

Kingdom, F. A. A. (2011). Lightness, brightness and transparency: A quarter century of new ideas, captivating demonstrations and unrelenting controversy. *Vision Research*, Vol. 51, No. 7, pp. 652-673.

Knill, D. C. & Richards, W. (Eds.). (1996). *Perception as Bayesian Inference.* Cambridge Univ. Press, ISNB 052146109X, New York, USA.

Lee, A. B.; Mumford, D. & Huang, J. (2001). Occlusion models for natural images: A statistical study of a scale-invariant dead leaves model. *International Journal of Computer Vision*, Vol. 41, No. 1-2, pp. 35-59.

Loomis, J. M.; Da Silva, J. A.; Philbeck, J. W. & Fukusima, S. S. (1996). Visual perception of location and distance. *Current Directions in Psychological Science*, Vol. 5, No. 3, pp. 72-77.

Ma, W. J.; Beck, J. M.; Latham, P. E. & Pouget, A. (2006). Bayesian inference with probabilistic population codes. *Nature Neuroscience*, Vol. 9, pp. 1432-1438.

Marr, D. (2010). *Vision: A Computational Investigation into the Human Representation and Processing of Visual Information* (reprinted from 1982 edition). MIT Press, ISBN 978-0-262-51462-0, Cambridge, MA, USA.

Olmos, A. & Kingdom, F. A. A. (2004). A biologically inspired algorithm for the recovery of shading and reflectance images. *Perception*, Vol. 33, No. 12, pp. 1463 - 1473.

Ooi, T. L.; Wu, B. & He, Z. J. (2001). Distance determined by the angular declination below the horizon. *Nature*, Vol. 414, pp. 197-200.

Owens, D. A. & Leibowitz, H. W. (1976). Oculomotor adjustments in darkness and the specific distance tendency. *Attention, Perception, & Psychophysics*, Vol. 20, No. 1, pp. 2-9.

Philbeck, J. W. & Loomis, J. M. (1997). Comparison of two indicators of perceived egocentric distance under full-cue and reduced-cue conditions. *J. Exp. Psychol. Hum. Percept. Perform.*, Vol. 23, No. 1, pp. 72-85.

Purves, D.; Williams, S. M.; Nundy, S. & Lotto, R. B. (2004). Perceiving the Intensity of Light. *Psychological Review*, Vol. 111, No. 1, pp. 142-158.

Purves, D. & Lotto, R. B. (2003). *Why We See What We Do, AN EMPIRICAL THEORY OF VISION*. Sinauer Associates, Inc., ISBN 0-87893-752-8, Sunderland, MA, USA.

Rao, R. P. (2004). Bayesian computation in recurrent neural circuits. *Neural Computation*, Vol. 16, No. 1, pp. 1-38.

Rao, R. P. N. & Ballard, D. H. (1999). Predictive coding in the visual cortex: a functional interpretation of some extra-classical receptive-field effects. *Nature neuroscience*, Vol. 2, pp. 79-87.

Rao, R. P. N.; Olshausen, B. A. & Lewicki, M. S. (Eds.). (2002). *PROBABILISTIC MODELS OF THE BRAIN, Perception and Neural Function*. MIT Press, ISBN 0-262-18224-6, Cambridge, MA, USA.

Rust, N. C.; Schwartz, O.; Movshon, J. A. & Simoncelli, E. P. (2005). Spatiotemporal elements of macaque v1 receptive fields. *Neuron*, Vol. 46, No. 6, pp. 945-956.

Simoncelli, E. P. & Olshausen, B. A. (2001). Natural image statistics and neural representation. *Ann. Rev. Neurosci.* Vol. 24, pp. 1193-1216.

Tatler, B. W.; Baddeley, R. J. & Gilchrist, I. D. (2005). Visual correlates of fixation selection: effects of scale and time. *Vision Research*, Vol. 45, No. 5, pp. 643-659.

Trommershauser, J.; Kording, K. & Landy, M. L. (Eds.). (2011). *Sensory Cue Integration*. Oxford Univ. Press, ISBN 978-0-19-538724-7, New York, USA.

van Hateren, J. H. & van der Schaaf, A. (1998). Independent component filters of natural images compared with simple cells in primary visual cortex. *Proc. Biol. Sci.*, Vol. 265, No. 1394, pp. 359–366.

White, M. (1979). A new effect of pattern on perceived lightness. *Perception*, Vol. 8, No. 4, pp. 413-416.

Wishart, K. A.; Frisby, J. P. & Buckley, D. (1997). The role of 3-D surface slope in a lightness/brightness effect. *Vision Research*, Vol. 37, No. 4, pp. 467-473.

Xu, J.; Yang, Z. & Tsien, J. (2010). Emergence of Visual Saliency from Natural Scenes via Context-mediated Probability Distributions Coding. *PLoS ONE*, 5(12):e15796. doi:10.1371/journal.pone.0015796.

Yang, Z. & Purves, D. (2003a). A statistical explanation of visual space. *Nat. Neurosci.*, Vol. 6, No. 6, pp. 632-640.

Yang, Z. & Purves, D. (2003b). Image/source statistics of surfaces in natural scenes. *Network: Computation in Neural Systems*, Vol. 14, No. 3, pp. 371-390.

Yang, Z. & Purves, D. (2004). The statistical structure of natural light patterns determines perceived light intensity. *Proc. Natl. Acad. Sci. USA*, Vol. 101, No. 23, pp. 8745-8750.

Yuille, A. & Kersten, D. (2006). A Vision as Bayesian inference: analysis by synthesis? *Trends Cogn. Sci.*, Vol. 10, No. 7, pp. 301-308.

Zhang, L.; Tong, M. H. & Cottrell, G. W. (2009). SUNDAy: Saliency using natural statistics for dynamic analysis of scenes. *Proceedings of the 31st Annual Conference of the Cognitive Science Society*. Amsterdam, Netherlands, August, 2009.

Zhang, L.; Tong, M. H.; Marks, T. K.; Shan, H. & Cottrell, G. W. (2008). SUN: A Bayesian framework for saliency using natural statistics. *Journal of Vision*, Vol. 0, No. 1, pp. 1-20.

Zhaoping, L. & May, K. A. (2007). Psychophysical tests of the hypothesis of a bottom-up saliency map in primary visual cortex. *PLoS Comput. Biol. 3(4)*: e62. doi:10.1371/journal.pcbi.0030062.

Chapter 10

Models of Information Processing in the Visual Cortex

Vincent de Ladurantaye, Jean Rouat and Jacques Vanden-Abeele

Additional information is available at the end of the chapter

http://dx.doi.org/10.5772/50616

1. Introduction

In the most general meaning of the word, a model is a way of representing something of interest. If we ask a biologist to model the visual system, he will probably talk about neurons, dendrites and synapses. On the other hand, if we ask a mathematician to model the visual system, he will probably talk about variables, probabilities and differential equations.

There are an almost infinite number of ways to model any given system, and this is particularly true if we are interested in something as complex as the human brain, including the visual cortex. It is impossible to review every type of model present in the literature. This chapter does not, by any means, claim to be an accurate review of all the models of vision published so far. Instead, we try to regroup the different types of models into small categories, to give the reader a good overview of what is possible to achieve in terms of modeling biological vision. Each section of the chapter concentrates on one of these categories, begins with an outline of the general properties and goals of the global model category, and then explores different implementation methods (i.e. specific models).

1.1. Why models?

There are many reasons why one might want to elaborate and use a model. Different kinds of models achieve different goals, however they all serve a common purpose: a tool to learn and better understand our world. Models are used as a simplification of reality. Many models only represent a specific aspect of a complex system and make arbitrary assumptions about the rest of the system which may be unrelated, judged negligible or simply unknown. A good example is the fact that current neurobiological models of the brain mainly focus on modeling neurons, neglecting interneurons and glial cells. Current models ignore glial cells, probably because they are not fully understood. Some models might purposefully ignore some parts of a system to isolate a specific structure and/or function that we want to understand.

Because of the extreme complexity of the cortex, simplification is unavoidable and even productive. Modeling is an efficient approach for simplifying reality as a way to gain a better understanding of the system in question. In fact, one should strive to design the simplest possible model that could be complexified if necessary.

For a more philosophical discussion on the role of models in science, the work by Frigg and Hartmann [15] can be recommended. They describe two fundamental functions of models. First, models can represent a selected part of the world, and second, models can represent a theory. The two notions are not mutually exclusive, but they provide a good distinction between more practical models trying to reproduce a certain system, and more theoretical models constrained to a certain set of laws. As we don't have yet an established theory as how the brain works, this chapter focuses on the former.

Moreover, models can also be categorized into models of data and models of phenomena. This is an important distinction because they consist of two drastically different approaches to the same problem that, in our case, is understanding the visual cortex. Models of data try to reproduce data we observe in the brain, and models of phenomena try to reproduce the "miracle" of the visual cortex, which is vision. This chapter emphasizes practical models and the functioning of the visual cortex from an information-processing point of view.

1.2. Modeling the visual cortex

As established in previous section, we concentrate more on models of phenomena to understand how the visual system works, instead of models of data that are trying to be biologically accurate. We do so, because science is yet to provide a full understanding of the brain, thus it is not possible to propose accurate overall models of data.

The chapter rather gives an overview of different kinds of models of vision present in the literature, whether they are biologically accurate or not. Modeling with artificial neural networks is not the only way. There are many other models based on mathematical representations, statistics, physics principles that can represent behaviors observed in the visual system. Any model able to represent some aspects of the vision process can provide valuable insights as to how the visual cortex really works.

Because of the complexity, there exists no model in the literature that can represent visual cortex as a whole. For the sake of simplicity, when designing a model, only specific functions of the visual system are usually considered . Of course, there are models more encompassing than others with more functionalities. However, most of them deal with only one of the two main visual functions, that is, localization or recognition. Ironically, this fits the often used ventral vs. dorsal stream model of the visual cortex, where the ventral stream explains the "what?" and the dorsal steam the "where?". This chapter is thus divided into three main sections:

1. A short section concerning models trying to be biologically accurate.
2. A section concerning models associated with the dorsal pathway, which deals with movement and localization.
3. A section on models related to the ventral pathway, which mainly deals with object recognition.

Before doing so, we first discuss the point that the visual cortex is embedded in a huge neural network, interacting and cooperating with other cortical and sensorial areas.

2. Visual cortex: integrated into a cooperative network

2.1. Integration into a collaborative network

Even if the organization of the brain is considered to be specific to the task, the various modalities seem to use the same independent processing mechanism [57]. Specialization of the cortices appears with the stimulation through specific sensory pathways. The visual cortex is interconnected with other sensory modalities and is therefore multisensorial [6]. For example, the visual cortex is also involved in the perception of tactile orientations as observed by Zangaladze et al. [68] and other authors. Many models of interactions between the visual cortex and other modalities are presented in the literature. For example, the recent work by Ohshiro et al. [43] in which a model of multisensory neural layer is proposed. From an engineering perspective, new applications that integrate multisensory perception can be designed. Wysoski et al. [64] give an example of a multimedia application in which models of audition and vision are combined through an implementation of a network of spiking neurons for the identification of 35 persons.

Figure 1 is our sketchy representation summarizing our integrated and general view of how functional multimodal information processing is done in the cortex. By no means, are we attempting to reproduce the biological characteristics of the cortex in relation to this figure. Emphasis is put on the main streams of information processing in relation with the visual cortex. We symbolize the cortical polysensoriality with a dedicated neural cortical layer, while there is no physiological agreement on the existence of such dedicated layer. In this section, interpretation of the functioning of the visual cortex is based on information and signal processing techniques to facilitate model designs without taking into account all physiological complexities.

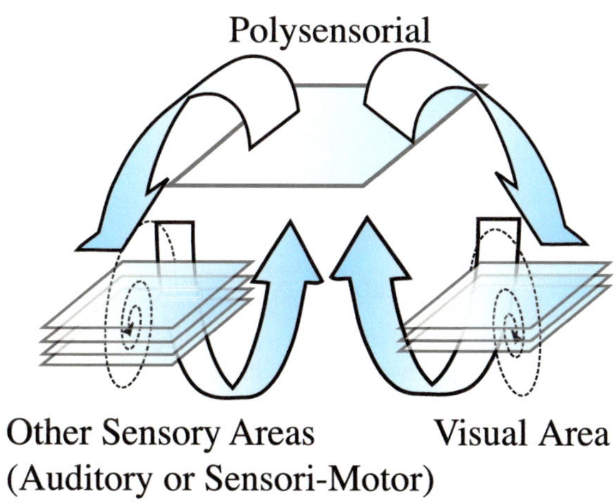

Figure 1. Functional view of the information processing going on in the cortex and between various sensorial areas of the cortex. Layers at bottom illustrate the hierarchical structure of feature extraction, corresponding to visual, auditory, somato-sensorial, sensori-motor, etc. The upper layer represents the multisensorial areas of the cortex. Large arrows represent the feedforward flow of information going from the sensorial areas to the polysensorial "layer" and feedbacks from the upper layer to the sensorial (and hierarchical feature) layers. Dotted arrows represent the iterative process of feature extraction which is occuring inside the sensory layers.

According to the common view, we represent sensing areas of the cortex in figure 1 as a hierarchy of layers and the "polysensorial" layer represents the connectivity between cortical areas. We known that connectivities between audition, vision and the motor system at lower levels of the senses exist (e.g. in the colliculus [6]), but these interactions are not discussed in this chapter.

Even if the perspective presented here is very schematic, it is still of interest for research and a better understanding of the cortex. Next subsections introduce models of feature-extraction through the visual sensory layers.

2.2. Hierarchical and sparse low level feature extractions

Low level features and characteristics are hypothesized to be hierarchically obtained through a succession of feedforward and feedback loops. This process is commonly modeled as a cascade of layers made of filters that mimic the receptive fields of neurons. Each layer output is subject to nonlinear transformations. Layers are interconnected into hierarchical structures that can be feedforward or include feedbacks as illustrated at the bottom of figure 1. We introduce here two types of models based on signal processing techniques or on artificial neural networks.

2.2.1. Signal processing models

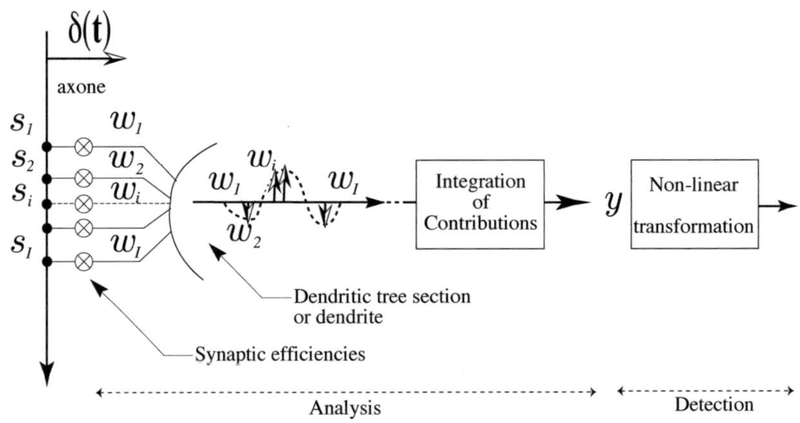

Figure 2. Illustration of the receptive field of a neuron representing an elementary analysis function and the nonlinear output being associated to a decision function. In this illustration, a hypothetic presynaptic axon is sketched and it synapses with I contacts on a postsynaptic neuron.

In these approaches, neurons are assumed to be made of two simple modules: analysis and then detection. The analysis is modeled as a filter which characterizes to some extent the receptive field of a neuron. Detection is modeled as a threshold or a nonlinear function. When the input to the neuron matches its receptive field, the detection module has a strong response.

There is an intense research work going on the automatic finding and generation of receptive fields to be used in computational models or artificial vision models and systems. Signal processing methods estimating the receptive fields of models are briefly summarized here.

These models assume that any stimulus $\mathbf{s}(t)$ (denoted as a vector) to a neuron is transformed by this neuron into a new representation by projection on an elementary function $\mathbf{w}(t)$

(also denoted as vector). Each elementary function $\mathbf{w}(t)$ (or "basis function", in the signal processing jargon) represents the receptive field of a particular neuron (or group of neurons). The result of the projection of $\mathbf{s}(t)$ on the specific basis function $\mathbf{w}(t)$ is a scalar number $y(t)$ that is added to the transmembrane potential of the neuron. It corresponds to the contribution of the stimulus input $\mathbf{s}(t)$ to the neuron-activity. It is summarized below in mathematical terms.

$$y(t) = \mathbf{w}(t).\mathbf{s}(t)$$

or

$$y(t) = \sum_{i=1}^{I} w_i(t) s_i(t) \tag{1}$$

with

$$\mathbf{w}(t) = \begin{bmatrix} w_1(t) \\ w_2(t) \\ . \\ . \\ w_I(t) \end{bmatrix} \text{ and } \mathbf{s}(t) = \begin{bmatrix} s_1(t) \\ s_2(t) \\ . \\ . \\ s_I(t) \end{bmatrix}$$

I is the dimension of the stimulus and receptive field (assuming that the neuron has I synapses). w_i is the efficiency at time t of synapse i from the neuron. In other words, at time t, $y(t)$ (equation 1) is the degree of similarity between the input stimulus $\mathbf{s}(t)$ and the receptive field $\mathbf{w}(t)$ of the neuron. In signal processing jargon, $y(t)$ is the basis coefficient.

To some extent, a set of I neurons can be assimilated into a bank of I finite impulse response filters (FIR) which impulse response is equal to a set of I receptive fields $\mathbf{w}$. Depending on the number of neurons, the characteristics of the receptive field functions $\mathbf{w}$, and the constraints on the coefficients y, the analysis operation performed by a set of neurons can be equivalent to an independent component analysis (ICA) decomposition [27], a wavelet decomposition [33], or an overcomplete and sparse decomposition [39, 56].

- ICA [24, 27] constraints the output coefficients $y_i(t)$ to be independent for a set of dependent input receptive fields $\mathbf{w}$. Therefore, a layer of postsynaptic neurons can uncouple the features coming from a presynaptic layer in which receptive fields are dependent. This is particularly efficient for hierarchical analysis systems. Applications in image processing commonly use ICA to find basis functions to decompose images into features [26].
- Wavelet decomposition [34] of signals is a well established field in signal processing. A layer of neurons can approximate a wavelet decomposition as long as the receptive fields $\mathbf{w}$ respect some mathematical constraints such as limited support, bounded energy, and constraints on the Fourier transform of the receptive fields [17].
- Sparsity in the activity of neurons in the visual cortex can also be taken into account with equation 1. Sparsity in the activity means that very few neurons are active, that is only a few y_i are sufficiently high to generate a response in the neuron. $\mathbf{w}$ is called the dictionary on which the presynaptic signals are projected on. To be sparse, the size of the dictionary should be sufficient, that is, the number of neurons is sufficiently high so that the basis is overcomplete.

Equation 1 is a simple model of a layer of neurons (at least for the receptive fields). Bank of neurons can be combined into hierarchical layers of filters that follow equation 1. Different combinations are possible. Depending on the architecture and on the connectivity, different hierarchical structures can be obtained.

We introduce in the following subsection 3 types of such structures.

2.2.2. Hierarchical neural network structures

Previous signal processing modules can be combined into hierarchical structures of neural networks. We list below some of the known models.

- Convolutional neural networks like the one proposed by Lecun et al. [30] have a mostly feedforward architecture;
- Deep learning machines [22] are layered neural networks that can be trained layer by layer. Theses layers are placed in a hierarchy to solve complex problems like image or speech recognition. First layers extract features and last layers perform a kind of classification by filtering the activity of the incoming layers. Feedbacks are established between layers.
- An example of a Bayesian neural network is given by Hawkins et al. [16, 20]. The connectivity between neurons inside a layer reflects partially the architecture of the cortex. Neurons are nodes of a statistical graphical model and feedbacks between layers are also established.

2.3. Summary

Simple models of the visual cortex have been presented. The present section has opened the way to a more integrated view in which peripheral and other senses interact with the visual cortex.

3. Biological models

This section reviews some models trying to reproduce as accurately as possible the biological visual system. The ultimate goal of those researches is having models able to represent the data we observe in the brain.

One of the earliest models is the Hodgkin & Huxley neuron model [23]. It is popular in the field of computational neuroscience and uses 4 differential equations to represent a biologically realistic neuron. Such models are important as they are one of the corner stones to the simulators that are used for a better understanding of the visual system. They can help us understand more precisely the different cortical mechanisms. Nowadays, computer simulations are very important in neuroscience and to the understanding of the visual cortex. Hundreds of computational models (along with their reference papers) are available to the computational neuroscientist. Many different models can be downloaded from the modelDB database [21]. Compartment, channel, spiking, continuous or discrete models cover a wide range of simulators and are available in different languages and simulators.

One of the biggest challenge when implementing biologically accurate models of the visual cortex is the amount of calculations required for the simulations. Even with massively parallel computer architectures, we cannot effectively rival the level of parallelism and computing power of the brain. As such, works claiming to represent the visual cortex in a biologically accurate fashion have to cut corners by modeling only isolated sections of the cortex and sometimes also by simplifying the neuron model.

The section presents biologically accurate models, that is, models trying to fit the data observed in the brain. And then, some models are reviewed that are not exactly biologically accurate, but that are striving to reproduce biology.

3.1. Biologically accurate models

Since the primary visual cortex is the most studied and best understood, most models try to reproduce parts of the early visual system. In the work of McLaughlin et al. [36], a small local patch (1 mm^2) of V1 is reproduced. They use a relatively complex, and thus accurate, neuron model. The work focuses upon orientation preference and selectivity, and upon the spatial distribution of neuronal responses across the cortical layer. Furthermore, they discuss how large-scale scientific computation can provide significant understanding about the possible cortical mechanisms.

Similarly, Basalyga and Wennekers [4] are able to model a simplified version of the visual pathway of a cat's eye using three connected subsystems: the retina, the Thalamus and V1. They model a patch of about 1.9 mm^2 of cortical surface using a Hodgkin-Huxley neuron model. They are able to reproduce the orientation preference and direction selectivity of cortical cells.

While biologically accurate neuron models are closer to reality, they are also computationally very expensive. By using a simpler, "integrate-and-fire" neuron model, Rangan et al. [47] are able to model a patch of 25 mm^2. They focus on reproducing V1 orientation preference maps with hypercolumns in a pinwheel organization. Models such as these give insights into the neuronal dynamics in V1.

3.2. Biologically realist models

Not all models are trying to directly reproduce biology. Most vision models use a more functional approach, trying to mimic the architecture and the behavior instead of the exact dynamics. Many distinct visual areas have been identified in the cerebral cortex, and functional organization of these areas has been proposed [62]. Such models do not generally use large-scale simulations, but are still trying to reproduce the biological architecture. As such, they are able to model a much larger part of the visual cortex.

A good example of such a model is based on the Adaptive Resonance Theory (ART) proposed by Grossberg. More specifically, the LAMINART model [19]. This model is a relatively complex system that is based on bottom-up, top-down and lateral interactions. The model integrates a "what" and a "where" stream, and as such, offers a very complete model of the visual cortex.

Another interesting work is a computational model of the human visual cortex based on the simulation of arrays of cortical columns [1]. The model suggests an architecture by which the brain can transform the external world into internal interpretable events. Furthermore, they argue that the model could be a good start for reverse engineering the brain. Modern super-computers have enough computational capacity to simulate enough cortical columns to achieve such a goal. However, the problem resides in the communication between the cortical columns. Communication between processing units in super-computer is a major bottleneck. There is also the question of how the model should connect those cortical columns between them. How many must communicate with each other? How much information do they communicate? Nevertheless, reverse engineering of the brain is an objective that is becoming more and more realistic.

4. Visual localization and planning

In this section we present models that are related to the "where?" pathway of the visual cortex, that is, models having to do with movement and localization. However, another important function of our visual system is to anticipate trajectories of moving objects. In computer vision, this is commonly called target tracking. Many of these algorithms are based on probabilistic approaches which we will present in the first part of this section. In the second part, we will discuss the importance of vision in motion control, which uses the concepts of localization and planning to control actions.

4.1. Movement detection and prediction

Movement detection is a crucial element of our visual system. Moving objects attract more attention than stationary objects. Optical flow models implement the capture of movement in a sequence of images. Such models compute the local displacement gradient for each pixel in a sequence of images. The result is a series of gradient fields such as illustrated in figure 3. These methods can be used for a multitude of applications such as detecting motion, segmenting moving objects and analyzing stereo disparity to extract 3D information out of 2 cameras. Further information about optical flow models can be found in the work of Fleet and Weiss [14].

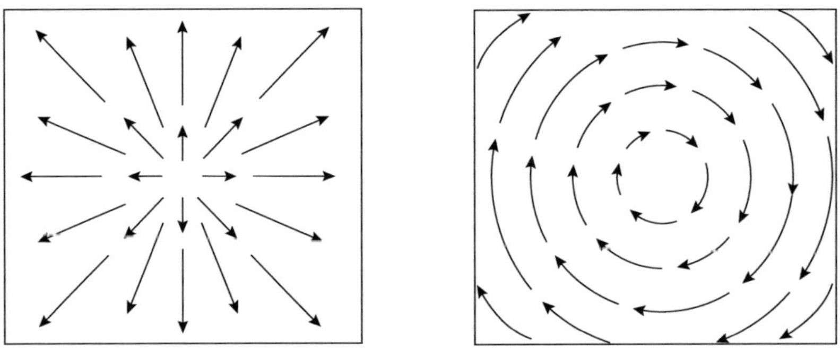

Figure 3. Example of optical flow gradient. In the left figure, a scene of forward movement is illustrated, thus, gradients are growing from the center toward the edges. In the right figure, the scene is rotating, thus forming a rotational pattern. In both scenes, the center of the image is moving slower than the rest, thus the arrows are shorter.

Optical flow models can detect movement, however, they are unable to achieve tracking in a reliable fashion because they lack anticipating behavior. The human brain is very good at predicting short term events. In fact, it is believed that the brain anticipates almost everything in our environment [20]. Indeed, brain activity is greater when we encounter an unanticipated event [2]. When we see a moving object, we automatically anticipate its trajectory. To do so, our brain unconsciously estimates the object speed and direction, and "runs" these number in a "mental physic model", which is acquired through experience". This anticipation allows us to perform actions such as catching a ball, by placing our hands in the predicted trajectory estimated by our brain.

Models that use such anticipation principle have applications in target tracking. Most of these models are based on a method known as Recursive Bayesian Estimation. To put things simply, the algorithm consists of a loop that constantly tracks the movement of the target based on its current position and speed. The loop estimates and corrects the previous estimation using new data acquired from the moving object. Similar principles can also apply to visual control tasks. A quick overview of the mathematical framework can be found in the work of Diard et al. [10].

One of the most popular implementation of recursive Bayesian estimation is the Kalman filter. Many applications have used this algorithm to achieve target tracking. The model proposed by Bai [3] is a good example that achieves tracking of not only the target position in space, but also its size and rotation. Many different methods can be used for tracking. For instance, an approach based on a low pass filter has been shown to give better precision than traditional Kalman filters [7]. For tracking targets with more unreliable movement patterns, particle filters can be used [8]. These approaches are not making predefined assumptions about the target, and are thus more polyvalent, but generally slower. However, optimization techniques such as the one proposed by Zhou et al. [69] can be used for faster processing.

4.2. Visual control

The predictive behavior mentioned previously is used by the visual system for planning and controlling many of our actions. This section is divided in two parts. The first section present studies discussing the importance of vision in visual control models. The second section presents different models using visual stimuli for controlling actions such as pointing, grasping and locomotion.

4.2.1. Importance of vision in motion control

A study from Kawato [29] analyses the internal models for trajectory planning and motor control. It is suggested that humans or animals use the combination of a kinematic and dynamic model for trajectory planning and control. To catch a ball, one must anticipate the trajectory of the ball and position the hand and orient adequately the palm. Fajen and Cramer [13] study the positioning of the hand in function of distance, the angle and the speed. They discuss the implications for predictive models of catching based on visual perception. However, the targeted object is not the only thing tracked by our visual system. The movement of the hand itself needs to be anticipated. Saunders and Knill [53] study the visual feedback to control movements of the hand. Alternatively, Tucker and Ellis [59] are interested in the cortical area of visuomotor integration. They discuss on the fact that motor involvement impacts visual representations. They set up 5 experiments in which they study the impact of grasping and touching objects on the speed of visual perception.

The use of vision for motion control is thus a very complex process using both feedforward and feedback visual information to achieve movement.

4.2.2. Visual control models

Now that we know vision plays an important role in movement, we present some models using vision to achieve motion control. Fagg and Arbib [12] developed the FARS model for grasping. They study the interaction between anterior intra-parietal and premotor areas. They also make predictions on neural activity patterns at population and single unit levels.

Moving on to models with more concrete applications, Yoshimi and Allen [65] propose an integrated view with a robotic application. They describe a real-time computer vision system with a gripper. A closed feedback loop control is used between the vision system and the gripper. Visual primitives are used to assist in the grasping and manipulation. Böhme and Heinke [5] implement the Selective Attention for Action model (SAAM) by taking into account the physical properties of the hand including anatomy. Their model is based on the fact that visual attention is guided by physical characteristics of objects (like the handle of a cup). Mehta and Schaal [37] study the visuomotor control of an unstable dynamic system (the balancing of a pole on a finger) with Smith predictors, Kalman filters, tapped-delay lines, and delay-uncompensated control. After validation with human participants, they exclude these models and propose the existence of a forward model in the sensory preprocessing loop.

5. Object recognition

5.1. Overview

In this section, we present models that are related to the ventral pathway of the visual cortex, that is, models that have to do with form and object recognition. For many years, object recognition has been one of the most challenging problems in the field of artificial intelligence. However, for humans, this task is something so simple that we do it unconsciously within a fraction of a second. For this reason, the visual cortex has been used as an inspiration in many artificial vision systems.

There are many ways to categorize the different object recognition models present in the literature. For the purpose of this chapter, we will discern two main categories: spiking and non-spiking models. The principal differences between those two approaches are that spiking models use bio-inspired spiking mechanism like STDP, synchrony and oscillations while non-spiking approaches tend to use statistical methods to achieve brain-like behavior. Spiking models are less popular in the literature because they tend to be computationally more expensive. However, they offer models that are more biologically plausible, and in specific cases more robust.

5.2. Non-spiking models

Since there are so many non spiking visual models in the literature, we further divide this section into three parts. We first review bottom-up models, which are strictly feed forward. We then review models incorporating top-down components, that is, models using feedback from previous or learned data to influence the input. We then take a quick look at models based on modeling visual attention.

5.2.1. Bottom-up models

One of the earliest models of the visual cortex originated in the work of Hubel and Wiesel[25]. They described a hierarchical organization of the primary visual cortex where the lower level cells were responsive to visual patterns containing bars (edges-like). These "simple cells", as they called them, are selective to bars of specific orientation, location and phase. Higher up

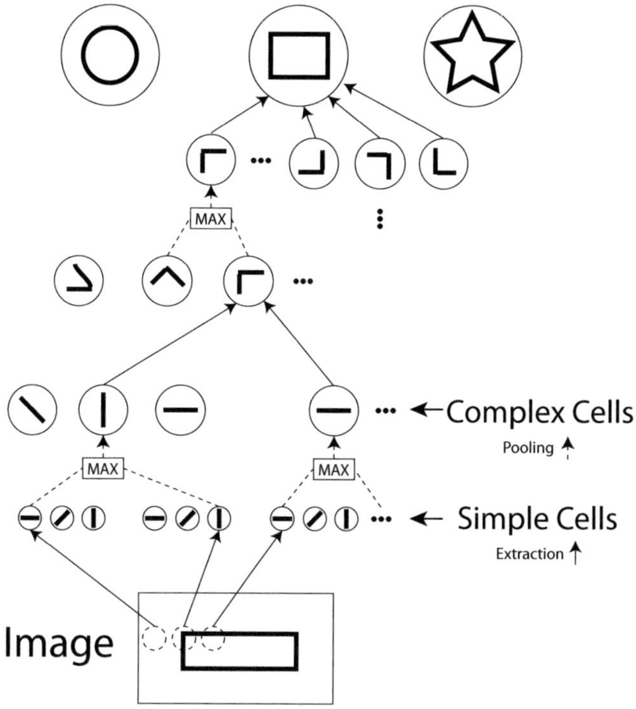

Figure 4. Example of a hierarchical model [51], consisting of multiple layers organized hierarchically. Each level in the hierarchy is composed of a layer of simple cells followed by a layer of complex cells. The simple cells are doing an extraction operation, combining features of the lower level to form more complex features. Complex cells are doing a pooling operation, selecting only the strongest (MAX) features for passage to the next level.

in the hierarchy, they found what they called "complex cells", which are insensitive to phase and location in the visual field, but are still sensitive to oriented bars. This is explained in their model by the complex cells having a larger receptive field than simple cells, thus integrating outputs of many simple cells.

5.2.1.1. Hierarchical models

Inspired by the hierarchical model of Hubel and Wiesel, convolutional neural networks were proposed. Good examples of such networks are LeNet-5[30] and HMAX[54]. As illustrated in figure 4, a typical hierarchical model is composed of multiple layers of simple and complex cells. As we go up in the hierarchy, lower level features are combined into more and more complex patterns.

Simple cells achieve feature extraction while complex cells realize a pooling operation. Feature extraction is done using the convolution between the input and the features, hence the name "convolutional neural networks". The pooling operation can be achieved in many different ways, but the most popular is the one used in the HMAX model, that is, the MAX operation. The MAX operation selects the highest input on its receptive field, and thus only allows the strongest features to be propagated to the next level of the hierarchy.

5.2.1.2. Learning feature extractors

The biggest problem with convolutional networks is to find a way to learn good features to extract at each level. In our visual cortex, visual stimuli are perceived from birth and visual features are learned in function of what we see in our everyday life. In the primary visual cortex, these features happen to be, as discussed earlier, edge extractors. Interestingly enough, using natural image statistics, mathematical algorithms are able to reproduce this result. Figure 5 shows some of the features learned with different algorithms. Moreover, we can see that it is possible to learn these features in a topographical organization, just like cortical maps.

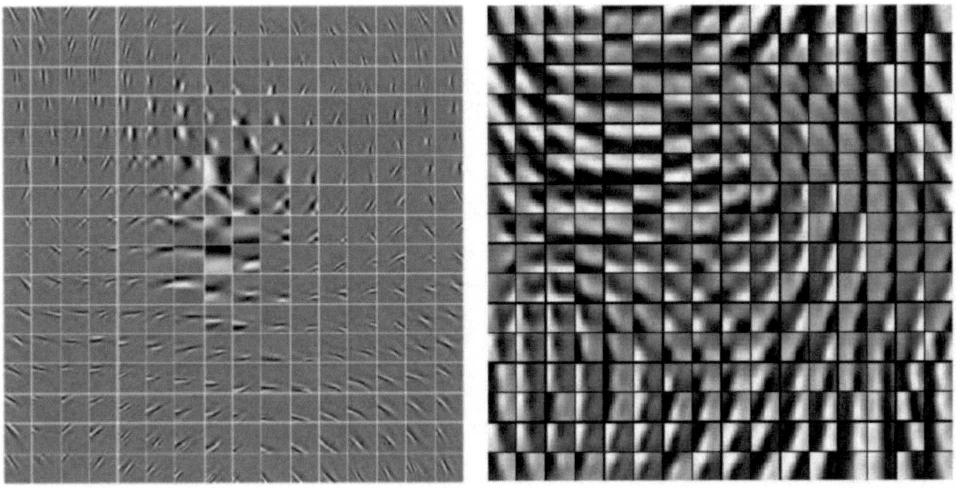

Figure 5. Visual features learned using image statistics. The features on the right are obtained using TICA (Topographic Independent Component Analysis) [26] and the left features are obtained using the IPSD algorithm [28]. In both cases, the features are learned in a pinwheel fashion, using unsupervised learning.

However, those features are only first level features, and learning good features for higher levels is a great challenge. Networks composed of multiple layers are typically referred to as "Deep Belief Networks". Hinton et al. [22] were the first to be able to effectively learn multi-level features using his RBM (Restricted Boltzman Machine) approach. This learning method has later been extended to deep convolutional networks [48]. An approach combining RBM and a convolutional approach has also been proposed [31].

However, deep belief networks are not the only way to learn feature extractors. The SIFT features [32] are a very popular and for a long time have been considered state of the art. More recently, it has also been shown that the concepts behind SIFT features are biologically plausible [40].

5.2.2. Top-down models

As mentioned earlier in the planning section, the brain is very good at anticipating our environment. While this is obvious for applications such as target tracking, this behavior is also applied to object recognition. When we see an object, a top-down process based partly on the context and the shape of the object helps the recognition process. This section presents some of the models trying to reproduce this prediction process.

One of the fist models to include a top-down process involving prediction was an hierarchical neural network incorporating a Kalman Filter [49]. An improved version of this model has since been proposed [41], where sparse coding is used as a pretreatment. Another model using top-down prediction to influence inputs is Grossberg's ART model (Adaptive Resonance Theory)[18]. If complementarity is detected between ascendant (bottom-up) and descendent (top-down) data, the network will enter a resonance state, amplifying complementary data. Hawkins has proposed the HTM model (Hierarchical Temporal Memory) [20] [16], which is based on a hierarchical Bayesian network.

Another category of top-down models are the ones learning a compositional representation of objects. They learn object structures by combining objects parts, and can then use this representation in a top-down fashion to help recognition or fill in missing elements. One such approach is known as hierarchical recursive composition [70]. This method is able to form segments of objects and combine them in a hierarchical representation that can be used to segment and recognize objects. Another approach using a compositional method is based on a Bayesian network [45]. They demonstrate the power of their system by showing their ability to construct an image of an object using only their top-down process.

5.2.3. Visual attention models

Visual attention models try to reproduce the saccadic behavior of the eyes by analyzing specific regions of the image in sequence, instead of perceiving the whole image simultaneously. One of the first models of pattern recognition using the concept of visual attention has been proposed by Olshausen [44]. The visual attention process is driven by the interaction between a top-down process (memory) and bottom-up data coming from the input. In this section, we quickly review some of the most recent models for both bottom-up and top-down guidance of the visual glaze.

Bottom-up visual attention models mostly rely on visual saliency maps. Such maps use algorithms trying to reproduce the visual saliency properties observed in the biological visual cortex. Examples of such maps are given in figure . Many algorithms for computing such maps have been proposed. For a recent review of the most popular of these algorithms, refer to the work of Toet [58].

5.3. Spiking and synchronisation models

All the neural models presented until now in this section are using simpler neuron models that do not have a time component. They give a numerical value as output, that can be interpreted as a strong firing rate if the value is strong, or weak otherwise. However, they do not generate spikes as biological neurons do. By modeling spikes, we can model a phenomenon such as synchronization, oscillation and Hebbian learning.

5.3.1. Spiking models

This section presents general models using spiking neurons in a way that is not using synchrony or oscillation. Many models have been proposed to achieve spike-timing-

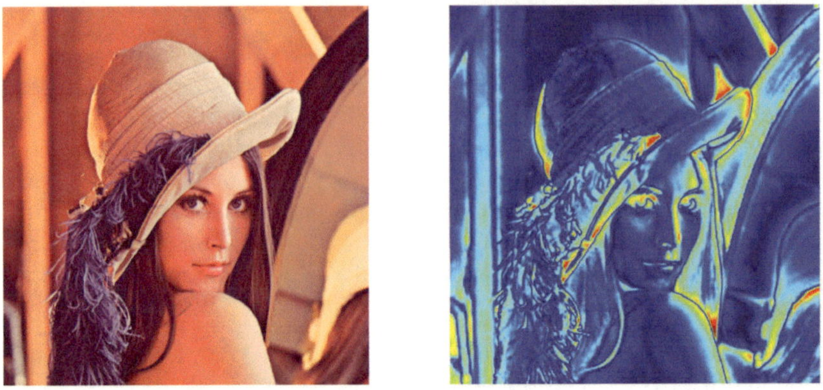

Figure 6. Example of saliency map. Using a JET color map, regions in red are considred to be more visualy salient. The saliency was computed using the FastSUN algorithm [42].

dependent plasticity (STDP). Thorpe and Masquelier have proposed an implementation of HMAX using spiking neurons [35]. They show that such hierarchical models can be implemented and trained using STDP.

Another concept that can be implemented using spiking neurons is rank-order coding (ROC). In ROC, the activation order of neurons transports information. Neurons firing first represent more important information than neurons firing at a later time after presentation of stimuli. A recognition model based on this principle is the SpikeNet network [9].

Many spiking models are now proposed to achieve different vision tasks. For instance, a vision system achieving image recognition using spiking neurons [55] has been shown to be robust to rotation and occlusion.

5.3.2. Synchrony models

Most of the vision models based on synchrony and oscillations are based on the binding problem and the binding-by-synchrony hypothesis. In this section, we first give a quick overview of what is the binding problem and we then describes some of the models implementing it.

5.3.2.1. The binding problem

A fundamental dilemma in the brain, or in any recognition system, is the combinational problem. When a signal is perceived, it is broken down into a multitude of features, which then need to be recombined to achieve recognition. This has been defined by Malsburg [61] as the "Binding Problem".

One solution proposed to solve the binding problem is the binding-by-synchrony hypothesis. According to Milner [38] and van der Malsburg [61], groups of neurons in the brain can be bound by synchrony when these groups belong to a same external entity. The validity of this hypothesis is however highly debated in the literature. The binding problem itself is highly controversial [50]. In fact, no real evidence has yet been found regarding the synchronization

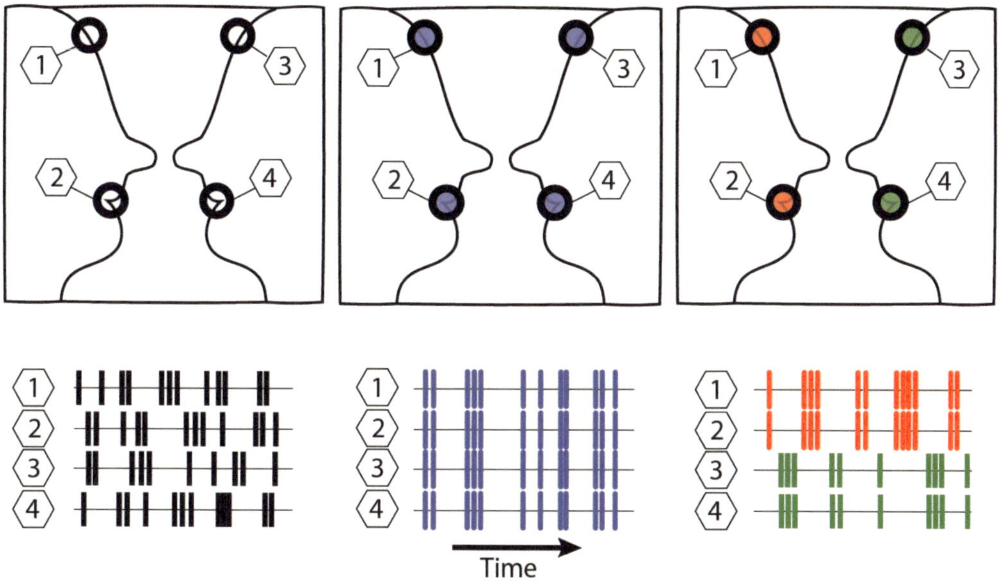

Figure 7. The binding problem [11]. In the leftmost column, we have an image from which 4 features are responding. Each feature is represented by a neuron spiking through time in the lower part of the figure. The binding problem consists in grouping these features together to recognize objects. The binding-by-synchrony offers a solution to this problem by using rhythmic oscillations. Features belonging to a same object will oscillate in synchrony, as shown in the middle column, where all the features combine to form a vase. In the rightmost column, with the same 4 features responding, 2 distinct groups of oscillation occur, thus forming 2 faces looking at each other.

of groups of neurons encoding an extended object [60]. Most studies however agree that synchrony and oscillation plays a role in the functioning of the visual cortex. Mechanisms such as binding-by-synchrony and temporal binding could very well be occurring in higher areas of the brain which are harder to study and understand [60].

5.3.2.2. Binding-by-synchrony models

One of the most popular models based on temporal binding is the LEGION network[63]. It was first developed to provide a neurocomputational foundation to the temporal binding theory. There are many applications for legion in scene analysis, particularly for image segmentation[67]. Pichevar and Rouat then proposed the ODLM network [46], which extends the LEGION model. ODLM is able to perform binding and matching in signal processing applications that are insensitive to affine transforms. Therefore, patterns can be recognized independently of their size, position and rotations. They have shown how binding can be used to segment and/or compare images based on pixel-values, and also to achieve sound source separation.

Slotine and his group have also proposed a model based on synchronization [66] that achieves visual grouping of orientation features. However, they do not use real images, but only orientation features. The only binding model that reproduces the vision process from real images is the Maplet model [52] from Malsburg's lab. Their model is computationally quite intensive, but is able to achieve face recognition.

6. Conclusion

This chapter presented different types of models of the visual cortex. We first discussed the idea that the visual cortex is in fact only a part of a more complex system, cooperating with other sensorial areas. However, because models are mainly used for simplifying reality, we then focused on vision specific models. We first presented models closely related to biology, with models directly trying to reproduce biological data, and others trying to reproduce the global architecture of the visual cortex. We then presented models related to movement detection and planning. Anticipation being an important mechanism in the brain we presented models using vision for planning and controlling movements. Finally, we glanced through vision models related to form and object recognition. We looked at feedforward and top-down models, as well as models based on neural synchrony and oscillations. Since all these models are very different, there is no consensus on how the visual cortex should be modeled. Also, all models do not have the same goals. The best possible model for a given situation is the simplest model that allows reaching the targeted goals.

We have only given a small overview of all the models of vision reported in the literature. This chapter was only intended to have a quick peek into the world of visual cortex models. We also have to keep in mind that our current understanding of the brain is far from complete. What we are doing right now is akin to trying to understand the mechanics of the ocean by studying one drop of water at a time. Considering the rapid evolution of knowledge about the brain, it is quite possible that some of the currently available models may become obsolete. But this is the basic characteristic of any scientific endeavor.

Author details

Vincent de Ladurantaye, Jean Rouat and Jacques Vanden-Abeele
NECOTIS, Université de Sherbrooke, Québec, Canada

7. References

[1] Albus, J. [2008]. A computational model of the human visual cortex, *Proceedings of the SPIE - The International Society for Optical Engineering*, Vol. 6943, pp. 69430 – 1.

[2] Alink, A., Schwiedrzik, C. M., Kohler, A., Singer, W. & Muckli, L. [2010]. Stimulus predictability reduces responses in primary visual cortex., *The Journal of neuroscience : the official journal of the Society for Neuroscience* 30(8): 2960–2966.

[3] Bai, K.-J. [2010]. A new object tracking algorithm based on mean shift in 4-d state space and on-line feature selection, *Information and Computing (ICIC), 2010 Third International Conference on*, Vol. 1, pp. 39 –42.

[4] Basalyga, G. & Wennekers, T. [2009]. Large-scale computational model of cat primary visual cortex, *BMC Neuroscience* 10: 358.

[5] Böhme, C. & Heinke, D. [2009]. Modeling visual affordances: The selective attention for action model (saam), *Connectionist Models of Behaviour and Cognition II Proceedings of the 11th Neural Computation and Psychology Workshop* (April): 39–50.

[6] Calvert, G., Spence, C. & Stein, B. E. [2004]. *The handbook of multisensory processes*, MIT Press.

[7] Chen, K., Li, D. & Jhun, C. G. [2010]. Video motion predictive tracking quality: Kalman filter vs. lowpass filter, *2010 International Conference on Multimedia Technology (ICMT)*, pp. 1–4.

[8] Czyz, J. [2006]. Object detection in video via particle filters, *Proceedings - International Conference on Pattern Recognition*, Vol. 1, Hong Kong, China, pp. 820 – 823.

[9] Delorme, A. & Thorpe, S. [2001]. Face identification using one spike per neuron: resistance to image degradations, *Neural Networks* 14(6-7): 795 – 803.

[10] Diard, J., Bessière, P. & Mazer, E. [2003]. A survey of probabilistic models, using the bayesian programming methodology as a unifying framework, *In The Second International Conference on Computational Intelligence, Robotics and Autonomous Systems (CIRAS 2003)*.

[11] Engel, A. K., Fries, P. & Singer, W. [2001]. Dynamic predictions: oscillations and synchrony in top-down processing., *Nature Reviews Neuroscience* 2(10): 704–716.

[12] Fagg, A. & Arbib, M. [1998]. Modeling parietal-premotor interactions in primate control of grasping., *Neural Networks* 11: 1277 – 1303.

[13] Fajen, B. & Cramer, C. [2007]. Visual control of hand position and orientation during one-handed catching, *Journal of Vision* 7(9): 165–165.

[14] Fleet, D. & Weiss, Y. [2005]. *Optical Flow Estimation*, Vol. 19, Springer, pp. 1–10.

[15] Frigg, R. & Hartmann, S. [2012]. Models in science, *in* E. N. Zalta (ed.), *The Stanford Encyclopedia of Philosophy*, spring 2012 edn.

[16] George, D. & Hawkins, J. [2005]. A hierarchical bayesian model of invariant pattern recognition in the visual cortex, *In Proceedings of the International Joint Conference on Neural Networks. IEEE*, pp. 1812–1817.

[17] Goupillaud, P., Grossmann, A. & Morlet, J. [1984]. Cycle-Octave and related transforms in seismic signal analysis, *Geoexploration* 23: 85–102.

[18] Grossberg, S. [1999]. The link between brain learning, attention, and consciousness, *Consciousness and Cognition* 8(1): 1 – 44.

[19] Grossberg, S., for Adaptive Systems, B. U. C., of Cognitive, B. U. D. & Systems, N. [2006]. *Towards a Unified Theory of Neocortex: Laminar Cortical Circuits for Vision and Cognition*, Technical report CAS/CNS, Boston University, Center for Adaptive Systems and Department of Cognitive and Neural Systems.

[20] Hawkins, J. & Blakeslee, S. [2004]. *On Intelligence*, Times Books.

[21] Hines, M., Morse, T., Migliore, M., Carnevale, N. & Shepherd, G. [2004]. Modeldb: A database to support computational neuroscience, *Journal of Computational Neuroscience* 17(1): 7–11.

[22] Hinton, G. E., Osindero, S. & Teh, Y.-W. [2006]. A fast learning algorithm for deep belief nets, *Neural Comp.* 18(7): 1527–1554.

[23] Hodgkin & Huxley [1952]. A quantitative description of membrane current and its application to conduction and excitation in nerve, *The Journal of Physiology* 117(4): 500–544.

[24] Hoyer, P. O. & Hyvärinen, A. [2000]. Independent component analysis applied to feature extraction from colour and stereo images, *Network: Computation in Neural Systems* 11(3): 191–210.

[25] Hubel, D. H. & Wiesel, T. N. [1965]. Receptive fields and functional architecture in two nonstriate visual areas (18 and 19) of the cat, *J Neurophysiol* 28(2): 229–289.

[26] Hyvärinen, A., Hurri, J. & Hoyer, P. [2009]. *Natural Image Statistics: A Probabilistic Approach to Early Computational Vision.*, Springer.

[27] Hyvärinen, Karhunen & Oja [2001]. *Independent Component Analysis*, Wiley.

[28] Kavukcuoglu, K., Ranzato, M., Fergus, R. & LeCun, Y. [2009]. Learning invariant features through topographic filter maps, *Proc. International Conference on Computer Vision and Pattern Recognition (CVPR'09)*, IEEE.

[29] Kawato, M. [1999]. Internal models for motor control and trajectory planning., *Current Opinion in Neurobiology* 9: 718–727.

[30] Lecun, Y., Bottou, L., Bengio, Y. & Haffner, P. [1998]. Gradient-based learning applied to document recognition, *Proceedings of the IEEE*, Vol. 86, pp. 2278–2324.

[31] Lee, H., Grosse, R., Ranganath, R. & Ng, A. Y. [2009]. Convolutional deep belief networks for scalable unsupervised learning of hierarchical representations, *Proceedings of the Twenth-Sixth International Conference on Machine Learning* .

[32] Lowe, D. G. [2004]. Distinctive image features from scale-invariant keypoints, *International Journal of Computer Vision* 60: 91–110.

[33] Mallat, S. [1996]. Wavelets for a vision, *Proceedings of the IEEE* 84(4): 604–614.

[34] Mallat, S. [1997]. *A wavelet tour of signal processing*, ACADEMIC PRESS.

[35] Masquelier, T. & Thorpe, S. J. [2007]. Unsupervised learning of visual features through spike timing dependent plasticity, *PLoS Computational Biology* 3(2): e31.

[36] McLaughlin, D., Shapley, R. & Shelley, M. [2003]. Large-scale modeling of the primary visual cortex: influence of cortical architecture upon neuronal response., *Journal Of Physiology Paris* 97(2-3): 237–252.

[37] Mehta, B. & Schaal, S. [2002]. Forward models in visuomotor control, *Journal of Neurophysiology* 88(2): 942–953.

[38] Milner, P. [1974]. A model for visual shape recognition, *Psychological Review* 81: 521–535.

[39] Molotchnikoff, S. & Rouat, J. [2012]. Brain at work: Time, sparseness and superposition principles, *Frontiers in Bioscience* 17(1): 583–606.

[40] Muralidharan, K. & Vasconcelos, N. [2010]. A biologically plausible network for the computation of orientation dominance, *in* J. Lafferty, C. K. I. Williams, J. Shawe-Taylor, R. Zemel & A. Culotta (eds), *NIPS*, pp. 1723–1731.

[41] Murray, J. F. & Kreutz-Delgado, K. [2007]. Visual Recognition and Inference Using Dynamic Overcomplete Sparse Learning, *Neural Comp.* 19(9): 2301–2352.

[42] Nicholas J. Butko, Lingyun Zhang, G. W. C. & Movellan, J. R. [2008]. Visual salience model for robot cameras, *Proceedings of the 2008 IEEE International Conference on Robotics and Automation (ICRA)*, p. 2398Ű2403.

[43] Ohshiro, T., Angelaki, D. E. & DeAngelis, G. C. [2011]. A normalization model of multisensory integration, *Nat Neurosci* 14(6): 775–782.

[44] Olshausen, B., Anderson, C. & Essen, D. V. [1993]. A neurobiological model of visual attention and invariant pattern recognition based on dynamic routing of information, *J.Neurosci.* 13(11): 4700–4719.

[45] Ommer, B. & Buhmann, J. [2010]. Learning the compositional nature of visual object categories for recognition, *IEEE Trans. Pattern Anal. Mach. Intell.* 32: 501–516.

[46] Pichevar, R., Rouat, J. & Tai, L. [2006]. The oscillatory dynamic link matcher for spiking-neuron-based pattern recognition, *Neurocomputing* 69(16-18): 1837–1849.

[47] Rangan, A., Tao, L., Kovacic, G. & Cai, D. [2009]. Multiscale modeling of the primary visual cortex, *Engineering in Medicine and Biology Magazine, IEEE* 28(3): 19–24.
[48] Ranzato, M., Poultney, C., Chopra, S. & Lecun, Y. [2006]. Efficient learning of sparse representations with an energy-based model, *Advances in Neural Information Processing Systems (NIPS)*.
[49] Rao, R. P. N. & Ballard, D. H. [1997]. Dynamic Model of Visual Recognition Predicts Neural Response Properties in the Visual Cortex, *Neural Computation* 9(4): 721–763.
[50] Riesenhuber, M. & Poggio, T. [1999a]. Are cortical models really bound by the "binding problem"?, *Neuron* 24(1).
[51] Riesenhuber, M. & Poggio, T. [1999b]. Hierarchical models of object recognition in cortex, *Nature neuroscience* 2(11): 1019–1025.
[52] Sato, Y. D., Jitsev, J. & Malsburg, C. [2008]. A visual object recognition system invariant to scale and rotation, *Proceedings of the 18th international conference on Artificial Neural Networks, Part I*, Springer-Verlag, pp. 991–1000.
[53] Saunders, J. & Knill, D. [2004]. Visual feedback control of hand movements, *The Journal of Neuroscience* 24(13): 3223–3234.
[54] Serre, T., Wolf, L., Bileschi, S., Riesenhuber, M. & Poggio, T. [2007]. Robust object recognition with cortex-like mechanisms, *Pattern Analysis and Machine Intelligence, IEEE Transactions on* 29(3): 411–426.
[55] Shin, J.-H., Smith, D., Swiercz, W., Staley, K., Rickard, J., Montero, J., Kurgan, L. & Cios, K. [2010]. Recognition of partially occluded and rotated images with a network of spiking neurons, *Neural Networks, IEEE Transactions on* 21(11): 1697 –1709.
[56] Starck, J.-L., Murtagh, F. & Fadili, J. M. [2010]. *Sparse Image and Signal Processing: Wavelets, Curvelets, Morphological Diversity*, Cambridge University Press.
[57] Striem-Amit, E., Dakwar, O., Reich, L. & Amedi, A. [2011]. The large-scale organization of "visual" streams emerges without visual experience, *Cerebral Cortex* .
[58] Toet, A. [2011]. Computational versus Psychophysical Image Saliency: A Comparative Evaluation Study, *IEEE Transactions on Pattern Analysis and Machine Intelligence* 99(PrePrints).
[59] Tucker, M. & Ellis, R. [2001]. The potentiation of grasp types during visual object categorization, *Visual Cognition* 8(6): 769–800.
[60] Uhlhaas, P., Pipa, G., Lima, B., Melloni, L., Neuenschwander, S., Nikolic, D. & Singer, W. [2009]. Neural synchrony in cortical networks: history, concept and current status, *Frontiers in Integrative Neuroscience* 3(00017).
[61] v. d. Malsburg, C. [1981]. The correlation theory of brain function, *Technical Report Internal Report 81-2*, Max-Planck Institute for Biophysical Chemistry.
[62] Van Essen, D. C. & Maunsell, J. H. [1983]. Hierarchical organization and functional streams in the visual cortex, *Trends in Neurosciences* 6(0): 370–375.
[63] Wang, D. & Terman, D. [1995]. Locally excitatory globally inhibitory oscillator networks., *IEEE Transactions on Neural Networks* 6(1): 283–286.
[64] Wysoski, S. G., Benuskova, L. & Kasabov, N. [2010]. Evolving spiking neural networks for audiovisual information processing, *Neural Networks* 23(7): 819–835.
[65] Yoshimi, B. & Allen, P. [1998]. The confluence of vision and control, *in* D. Kriegman, G. Hager & A. Morse (eds), *Lecture Notes in Control and Information Sciences*, Vol. 237, Springer Berlin / Heidelberg, pp. 195–209.

[66] Yu, G. & Slotine, J. [2009]. Visual grouping by oscillator networks, *I.E.E.E. Transactions on Neural Networks* 49: 4528–4538.

[67] Yuan, J., Wang, D., Wu, B., Yan, L. & Li, R. [2009]. Legion-based automatic road extraction from satellite imagery, *IEEE Transactions on Geoscience and Remote Sensing* 49: 4528–4538.

[68] Zangaladze, A., Epstein, C. M., Grafton, S. T. & Sathian, K. [1999]. Involvement of visual cortex in tactile discrimination of orientation, *Nature* 401(6753): 587–590.

[69] Zhou, H., Zhang, X., Li, H. & Li, J. [2010]. Video object tracking based on swarm optimized particle filter, *Industrial Mechatronics and Automation (ICIMA), 2010 2nd International Conference on*, Vol. 2, pp. 702–706.

[70] Zhu, L. L., Lin, C., Huang, H., Chen, Y. & Yuille, A. L. [2008]. Unsupervised structure learning: Hierarchical recursive composition, suspicious coincidence and competitive exclusion, *ECCV (2)*, Vol. 5303 of *Lecture Notes in Computer Science*, Springer, pp. 759–773.

Chapter 11

Neurovascular and Neurometabolic Uncoupling in the Visual Cortex

Ai-Ling Lin, Jia-Hong Gao and Peter T. Fox

Additional information is available at the end of the chapter

http://dx.doi.org/10.5772/51074

1. Introduction

The quest to understand the functional organization of the brain by assessing changes in brain circulation has occupied scientists for more than a century. Significant increases in cerebral blood flow (CBF) accompany brain activity. The direct relationship between CBF and brain activity has been known since 1881(1). For more than a century, neuroscientists have assumed that increased metabolic demands in response to brain activation drive the elevation of CBF. Researchers could not investigate the hypothesis further until the 1980s, with the development of positron emission tomography (PET), a noninvasive imaging method to measure hemodynamic and metabolic changes in response to task-induced brain activation. Using PET and visual stimulation, Fox and colleagues (2) found that CBF increases were linearly coupled with neuronal activity as expected; however, changes in the cerebral metabolic rate of oxygen ($CMRO_2$) were significantly lower than that of CBF. The CBF–$CMRO_2$ "uncoupling" phenomenon therefore contradicts the early hypothesis.

The "uncoupling" discovery not only reshaped our understanding of the flow–metabolism interaction in response to brain activation but also led to the discovery of blood oxygenation level–dependent (BOLD) functional magnetic resonance imaging (fMRI) in the 1990s (3, 4). Further, the discovery evoked heated debate on physiological interpretations—for example, whether oxidative metabolism or glycolysis meets the energy demand during brain activation, and whether oxygen demand or some other mechanism mediates increases in CBF. In this chapter, we review the historical events that led to using PET to discover the neurovascular and neurometabolic "uncoupling"; the invention of BOLD fMRI techniques; and the development of physiological hypotheses to resolve the "uncoupling" mystery in the visual cortex.

2. Neurovascular and neurometabolic uncoupling in the visual cortex

2.1. Brain Activity vs. Cerebral Blood Flow

Italian physiologist Angelo Mosso first observed the relationship between CBF and neuronal activity in the late nineteenth century (1). Mosso invented an apparatus to simultaneously compare human intracranial pressure changes measured through a traumatic skull injury with pressure changes in the forearm or foot (Figure 1). Using this approach, he investigated particular cerebral hemodynamic patterns during emotional and cognitive experiences. His most famous report was the case of Michele Bertino, a 37-year-old farmer who had a large fracture to the skull (1). The fractured bone pieces were removed and the cerebral mass was exposed through a 2-cm bone breach in the right frontal region. Mosso recorded changes in brain volume related to CBF through a button fixed to the wooden cupola with a sheet of gutta-percha resting on Bertino's exposed dura mater and connected to a screw on the recording drum (Figure 2A).

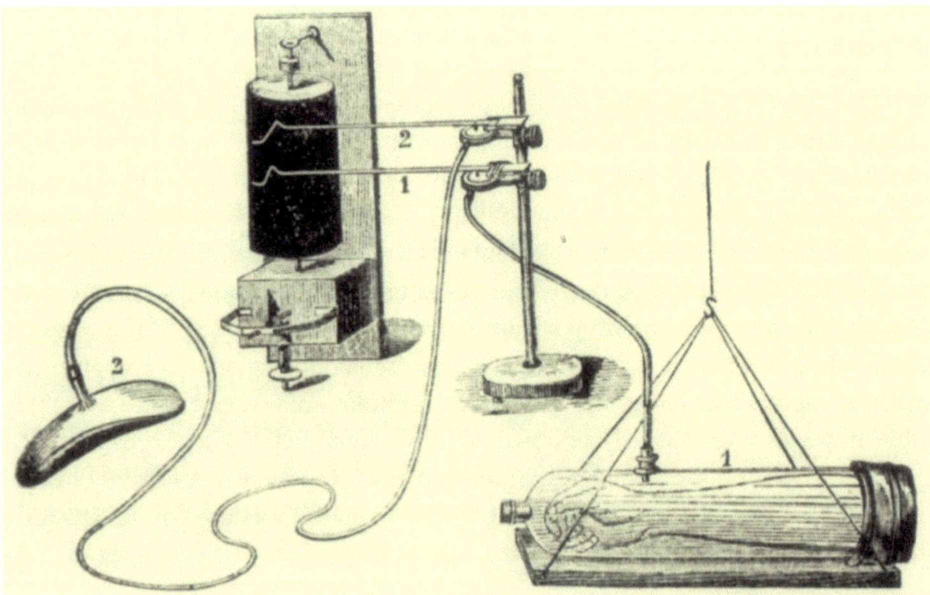

Figure 1. Mosso's devices for recording the blood volumes in arm and brain. 1, Forearm pulsation recording; 2, brain pulsation recording. Source: (5).

When the blood volume in the brain changed, the pulsation of the brain increased, increasing the pressure on the button and on the screw, thus compressing the air inside the drum. Changes in air compression were transmitted to a second recording drum and then written on a rotating cylinder. When Mosso asked Bertino to multiply 8×12, the pulsations of the brain increased within a few seconds after the request—but pulsations in the forearm did not. Similarly, when Mosso asked whether the chiming of the local church bell reminded Bertino that he had forgotten his midday prayers, Bertino said yes, and his brain pulsated again (Figure 2B).

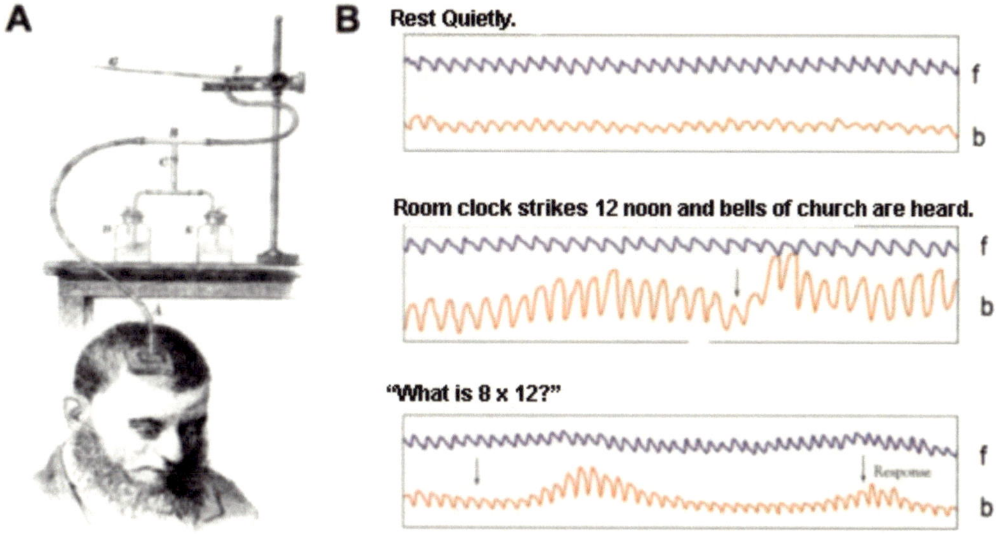

Figure 2. **(A)** The apparatus Mosso used to record Bertino's brain pulsations. **(B)** Mosso's recordings, taken from the forearm (f) and the brain (b), show stronger brain pulsations after events (marked by the arrows) that stimulated brain activity. Source: (1).

These studies suggested that measuring CBF might be an important way to assess brain function during mental activity. Roy and Sherrington, two distinguished British physiologists, further characterized the relationship between brain function and CBF (6). They attributed task-induced vasodilation to an increased demand for cerebral metabolism in response to neuronal activity. They stated, "the chemical products of cerebral metabolism contained in the lymph which bathes the walls of the arterioles of the brain can cause variations of the caliber of the cerebral vessels: that in this re-action the brain possesses an intrinsic mechanism by which its vascular supply can be varied locally in correspondence with local variations of functional activity". This statement implies that cerebral functional activity, energy metabolism, and blood flow are closely related. Researchers have interpreted the Roy–Sherrington principle to mean that CBF changes reflect a tight coupling between cellular energy requirements and vascular delivery of glucose and oxygen.

Over the past century, the visual cortex has made significant contributions to the evolving investigations of the Roy–Sherrington principle. The first report of the close relationship between CBF and neuronal activation in the visual cortex was in 1928 by Dr. John Fulton, of the neurosurgery clinic at the Peter Bent Brigham Hospital in Boston (7). Fulton's patient had suffered a gradual loss of vision due to a collection of congenitally abnormal blood vessels serving his visual cortex. Unlike the smooth, silent blood flow in normal blood vessels, the blood flow through these abnormal vessels was turbulent and created a brief rushing sound with each heartbeat. The patient could hear this sound, as could his physicians when they listened with their stethoscope through a defect in the skull (Figure 3A). The sound increased whenever the patient opened his eyes and especially when he read a newspaper (Figure 3B).

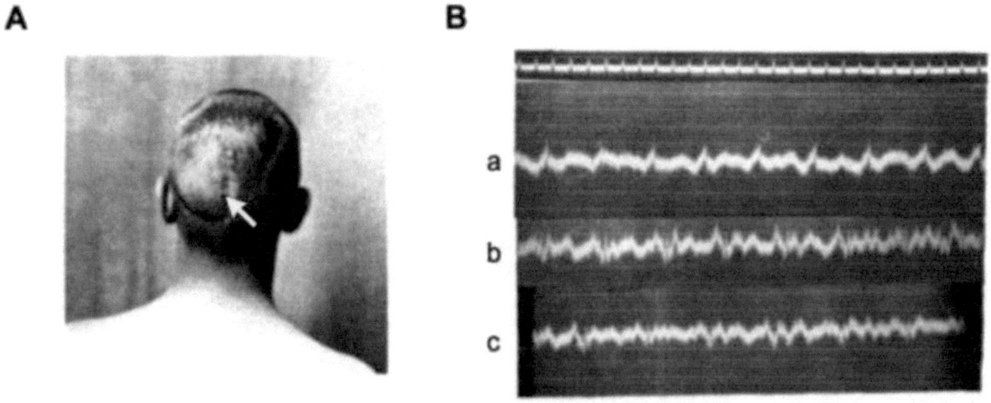

Figure 3. **(A)** Patient 3 weeks after operation, showing the region explored. The arrow indicates the point of maximum intensity of the bruit. This overlies the region of greatest vascularity of the angioma. **(B)** Typical electrophonograms of bruit **(a)**, after 10 minutes' rest in a darkened room; **(b)**, after 2 minutes' reading of small print illuminated by a single 40-watt tungsten bulb at 5 feet; **(c)**, 3 minutes later, after 2.5 minutes' rest in a darkened room. Time above: 0–2 sec. Source: (7).

The correlation between CBF changes in a specific sensory system (visual system) during mental activity (reading) was remarkable. However, the full importance of this work was not appreciated until the development of accurate techniques to measure CBF and brain metabolism in laboratory animals and in humans.

The development of positron emission tomography (PET) in the 1960s further advanced the field of research. PET is a nuclear medicine imaging technique that produces a three-dimensional, in vivo image of functional processes in the body. Using ^{15}O-labeled water (i.e., $H_2{}^{15}O$; half-life = 123 sec) as a freely diffusible tracer, PET can measure CBF in less than 1 min. With these techniques, Fox and Raichle (8) revisited the task-induced neurovascular coupling in the human visual cortex in vivo. They measured CBF changes with a visual system that delivered full-field flashes of fixed wavelength, luminance, and duration over frequencies from 1 to 60 Hz (Figure 4A). For the first time, noninvasive neuroimaging showed localized CBF changes in the human visual cortex in response to neuronal activation (Figure 4, B to D). Knowing that the time for full recovery of the visual-evoked potential was approximately 125 msec and that $H_2{}^{15}O$ PET measurements integrated over 40 sec, Fox and colleagues reasoned that the CBF response should be linear at least up to a repetition rate of 8 Hz (i.e., 1/0.125 sec; the stimulation is not effective for stimulus frequency >8 Hz). The findings were in excellent agreement with their hypothesis: CBF rose linearly with stimulus rate (r = 0.886; p < 0.0005), peaking at 7.8 Hz (Figure 5, A and B). Response locations also were tightly grouped. The rate–response function soon was replicated and extended by using a reversing checkerboard, constant-luminance stimulus (9). The pioneer works by Fox and colleagues were significant in two aspects: they were the first studies to show CBF in response to visual stimulation in conscious adult humans, and they confirmed that CBF is linear coupled with neuronal activity till it reaches the maximal visual-evoked potential.

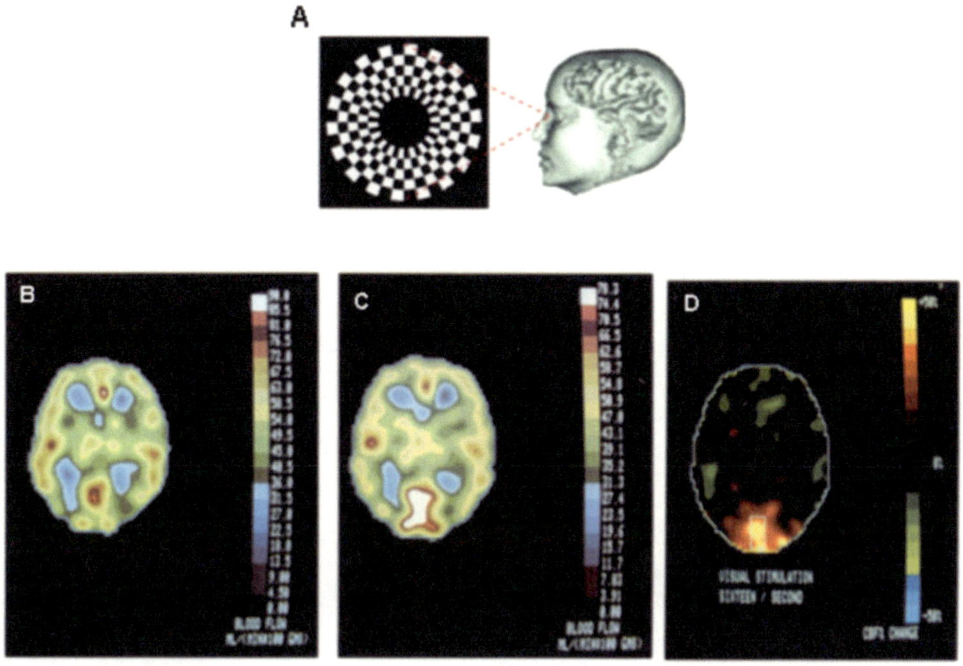

Figure 4. (A) Checkerboard stimulation. **(B)** CBF image during the initial unstimulated state. **(C)** CBF image during 16-Hz photic stimulation. **(D)** CBF image of panel C (16 Hz) versus panel B (unstimulated). The position and configuration of the regional CBF response elicited by repetitive patterned-flash stimuli are illustrated. Source: (8).

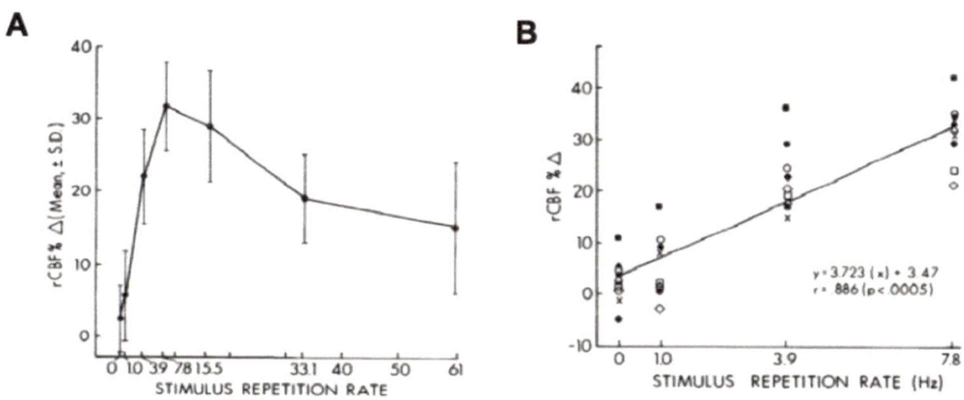

Figure 5. (A) Photic stimulation caused a selective regional CBF (rCBF) increase in the striate cortex up to a maximum response at 7.8 Hz. The rCBF declined with frequency increases beyond 7.8 Hz but remained above the unstimulated state. Each point and error bar represent the mean ± SD at each stimulus frequency. rCBF response is expressed as the percent change from the initial unstimulated scan. **(B)** Striate cortex percent change in rCBF from the initial unstimulated state, varied as a linear function of stimulus frequency between 0 and 7.8 Hz. The function of the linear regression is given and the regression line plotted. Source: (8).

2.2. Discovery of the neurovascular and neurometabolic uncoupling

With these powerful tools in hand, Fox and colleagues took a further step to test the Roy–Sherrington principle, that is, to determine whether increased metabolic demands (i.e., glucose and oxygen consumption) in response to neuronal activity drove the task-evoked CBF changes. At first, researchers rationally assumed that cerebral metabolic rate of glucose (CMR_{Glc}) and oxygen ($CMRO_2$) would increase proportionally with the increased CBF and neuronal activity because neurons account for most of the energy consumption during brain activation through ATP generated by oxidative phosphorylation of glucose. In addition to CBF, they measured CMR_{Glc} by using ^{18}F-labeled 2-fluoro-2-deoxy-D-glucose (^{18}FDG) and $CMRO_2$ by using ^{15}O-labeled oxygen ($^{15}O_2$). Again, using visual stimulation as a paradigm, Fox and colleagues used PET to simultaneously measure the task-induced changes in CBF, CMR_{Glc}, and $CMRO_2$ in the activated human cortex. As expected, task performance reliably elicited large, highly focal increases in CBF (2) and CMR_{Glc} (2, 10) (Figure 6A). The observed increases in CBF and CMR_{Glc} were similar in magnitude, typically 30%–50%.

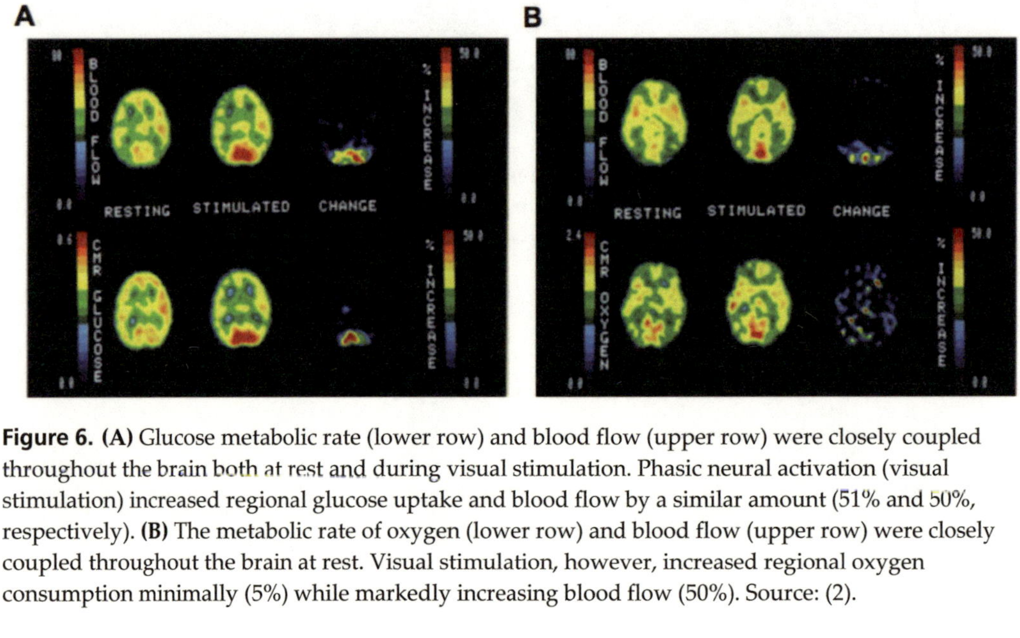

Figure 6. (A) Glucose metabolic rate (lower row) and blood flow (upper row) were closely coupled throughout the brain both at rest and during visual stimulation. Phasic neural activation (visual stimulation) increased regional glucose uptake and blood flow by a similar amount (51% and 50%, respectively). **(B)** The metabolic rate of oxygen (lower row) and blood flow (upper row) were closely coupled throughout the brain at rest. Visual stimulation, however, increased regional oxygen consumption minimally (5%) while markedly increasing blood flow (50%). Source: (2).

However, to their surprise, Fox and colleagues (2) observed that task-induced increases in $CMRO_2$ (5%) were much lower than those in CBF or CMR_{Glc} (Figure 6B). The $CMRO_2$ shortfall during focal neuronal activation, in fact, caused a local oxygen surplus, with the oxygen extraction fraction falling from a resting value of ~40% to a task-state value of ~20%. These findings contradicted the Roy–Sherrington hypothesis.

Because either oxidative or nonoxidative (i.e., lactate producing) pathways can metabolize glucose and because the increase of $CMRO_2$ was minimal, Fox and colleagues suggested that (i) glucose is predominately metabolized by anaerobic glycolysis; (ii) the energy demand associated with neuronal activation is small (as opposed to resting-state demand), and glycolysis alone may provide the energy needed for the transient changes in brain activity; and (iii) factors other than oxidative metabolism and total energy demand must regulate CBF response.

Using ¹H nuclear magnetic resonance spectroscopy (MRS), a method that exploits the magnetic properties of metabolites, Prichard and colleagues observed that tissue lactate concentration [Lac] significantly increases during visual stimulation (Figure 7, A and B). The observation confirmed that the stimulus-evoked increase in glucose consumption observed with PET is at least partially nonoxidative (11, 12).

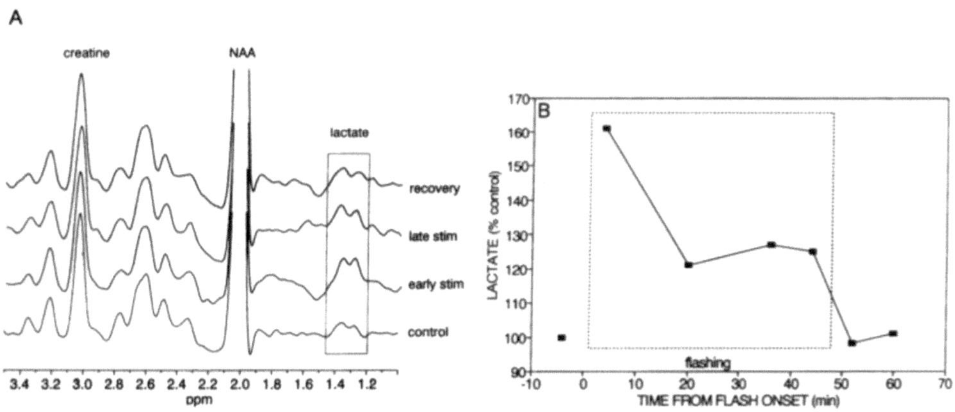

Figure 7. **(A)** ¹H spectra from 13 cc of human visual cortex before, during, and after photic stimulation (stim) by red dot grids flashing at 16 Hz in front of each eye. The frequency axis is in ppm and was set from the prominent resonance of *N*-acetylaspartate (NAA) at 2.02 ppm. The shaded area highlights the lactate methyl proton resonance at 1.33 ppm, with its characteristic 7-Hz splitting. The creatine resonance at 3.04 ppm is the total signal from methyl protons of phosphocreatine and creatine. **(B)** Time course of the experiment illustrated in panel A, with intensities of the lactate resonance plotted as a percentage of its control intensity. Source: (11).

Later studies further identified that CBF–$CMRO_2$ uncoupling also depended on rate and duration (13, 14). Using graded visual stimulation, Vafaee and Gjedde (13) found that the percent fractional changes (%Δ) in CBF peaked at 8 Hz, similar to the finding of Fox and colleagues, whereas %Δ$CMRO_2$ reached a maximum at 4 Hz (Figure 8). With prolonged visual stimulation (25 min), Mintun and colleagues (14) found that after 1 min of stimulation, $CMRO_2$ increased only 4.7% compared with baseline and CBF increased 40.7% (Figure 9, A and B). However, after 25 min of stimulation, the increase in $CMRO_2$ compared with baseline was 15.0%, having tripled from that measured at 1 min (Figure 9B). CBF decreased to 37.1% after 1 min of visual stimulation and then returned almost to baseline values after 25 min of activation (Figure 9A). These two studies further supported the Fox group's argument that factors other than oxidative metabolism regulate CBF response.

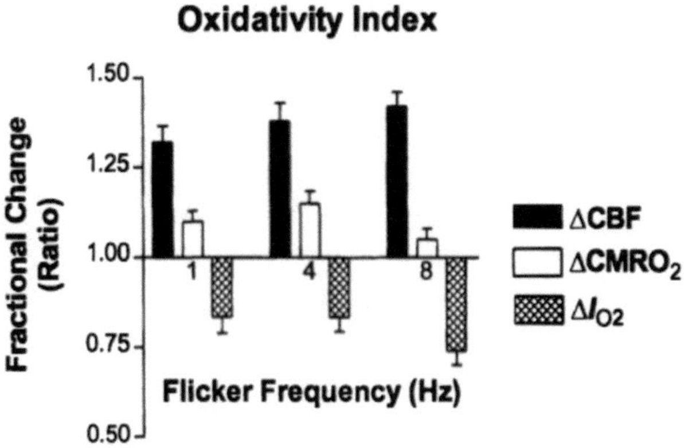

Figure 8. Percent changes of CBF, $CMRO_2$, and $CMRO_2$:CBF ratio index (I_{O2}) in the primary visual cortex as a function of checkerboard contrast reversal rate. Note maximum I_{O2} change at 8 Hz. Source: (13).

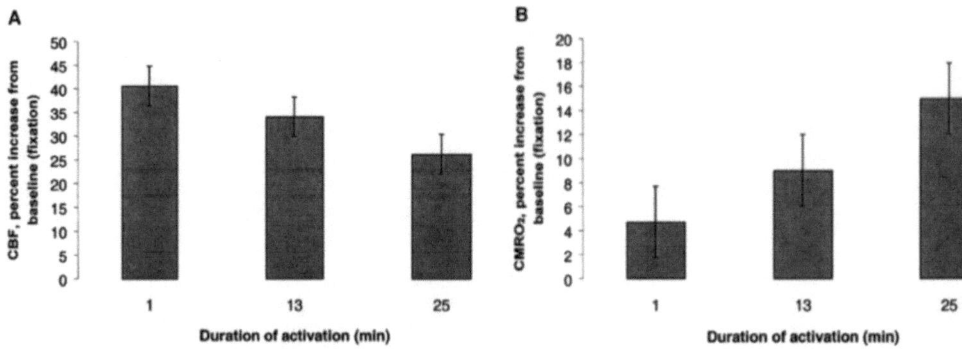

Figure 9. Effects of continuous visual stimulation on rCBF **(A)** and $CMRO_2$ **(B)**. Data shown represent the mean percent change from baseline (fixation) in seven subjects. CBF increased significantly early after the onset of visual stimulation and then had a nonsignificant tendency to decrease. Initial increase in $CMRO_2$ was small (4.7%); however, it tripled during continued stimulation and reached significant levels (15%, $p < 0.01$) at 25 min. Source: (14).

2.3. Discovery of functional magnetic resonance imaging

The CBF–$CMRO_2$ uncoupling phenomenon led to the discovery of functional magnetic resonance imaging (fMRI), known as the blood oxygenation level–dependent (BOLD) contrast, by Ogawa and others (3, 4). The physical effect is based on the magnetic property difference between deoxyhemoglobin (dHb; i.e., hemoglobin not bound with oxygen) and oxyhemoglobin (Hb; i.e., hemoglobin that binds with oxygen). Magnetic fields can weakly repel Hb, which is diamagnetic, whereas they can attract dHb, which is paramagnetic (which makes the magnetic field less uniform and thus decreases MR signal). The dramatic increases in CBF, relative to $CMRO_2$, bring in excess Hb (relative to dHb) to the venous blood, which causes measurable changes in the MRI signal (BOLD contrast).

In 1992, Kwong et al. used the BOLD contrast to study activation in the human visual cortex (15). During stimulation, they detected local increases in signal intensity in the medial-posterior regions of the occipital lobes along the calcarine fissures (Figure 10A). Their results independently confirm PET observations that little or no increase in tissue oxygen consumption accompanies activation-induced changes in blood flow and volume (2). They also observed rate-dependent increases of BOLD signal, peaking at 8 Hz, consistent with the PET observations for CBF (8) (Figure 10B).

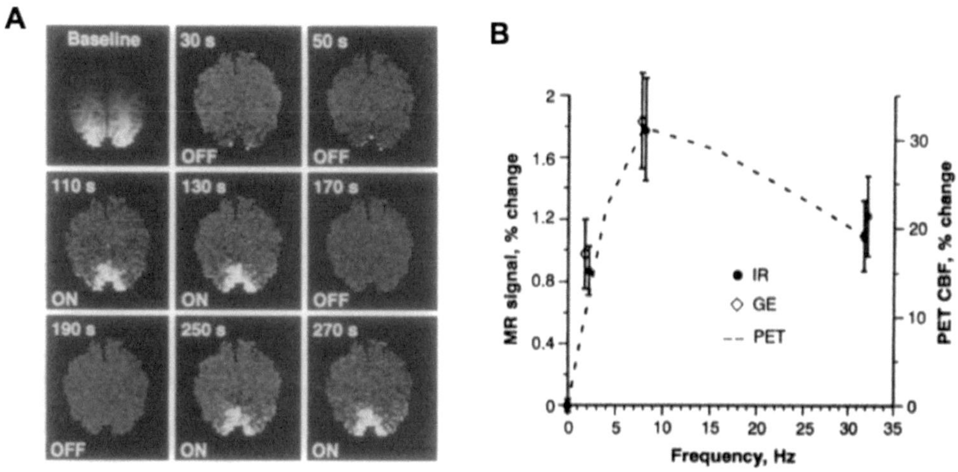

Figure 10. (A) Noninvasive, real-time MRI mapping of V1 activation during visual stimulation. A baseline image acquired during darkness (upper left) was subtracted from subsequent images. Eight of these subtraction images are displayed, chosen when the image intensities reached a steady-state signal level, during darkness (OFF) and during 8-Hz photic stimulation (ON). **(B)** BOLD signal as a function of the frequency of light stimulus (0 Hz = darkness). Signal response is expressed as percent change from baseline unstimulated level. The largest observed response occurred at 8 Hz. For comparison with data from Fox and colleagues, CBF percent changes obtained by PET with the same stimulation paradigm at 0, 1, 4, 8, 16, and 32 Hz are superimposed on the MR data. Source: (15).

Using BOLD signal, Davis and colleagues developed mathematical modeling to determine task-induced changes in $CMRO_2$. By combining with MRI-based CBF measurement using arterial spin labeling techniques (16), researchers can compute relative $CMRO_2$ changes ($rCMRO_2$) by measuring evoked-induced changes in BOLD and CBF and basal BOLD relaxation rate (*M* value) (Eq. [1]). Consistent with the PET-based measurement, $CMRO_2$ changes (16%) were much smaller than CBF changes (45%) during visual stimulation (17).

$$\mathrm{rCMRO}_2(t) = CBF(t)^{1-\alpha/\beta}\left(1-\frac{BOLD(t)-1}{M}\right)^{1/\beta} \tag{1}$$

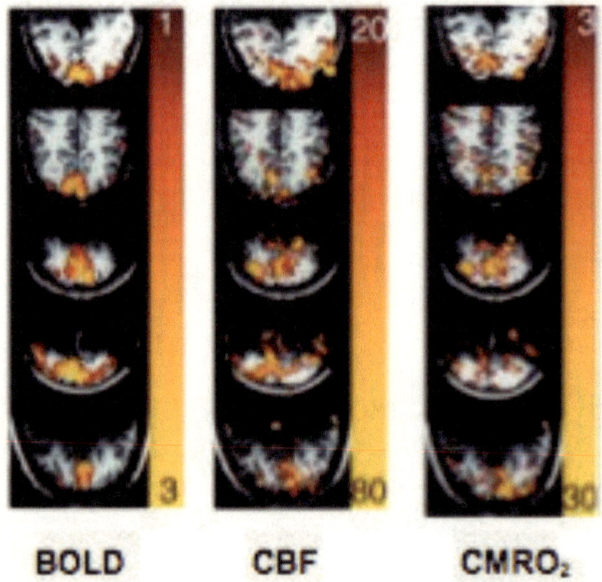

Figure 11. The left column shows BOLD task activation responses as color overlays: colors represent signal increases from 1% (red) to 3% (yellow). The center column shows CBF task activation increasing from 20% to 80%. The rightmost column shows $rCMRO_2$ for each subject, from 3% to 30%. All subjects show a confluent patch of increased $rCMRO_2$ in the visual cortex, averaging from 13% to 19%. Some peaks reach up to 30% increase in metabolism, corresponding to peaks of blood flow up to 70%. Source: (17).

Taken together, the PET and fMRI results showed that the increases in CBF and $CMRO_2$ during visual stimulation are uncoupled, summarized as follows (18): Compared with viewing a blank screen, visual stimulation produces marked changes in activity in visual areas of the brain, as shown in the PET images (from small increase, blue, to major increase, red; Figure 12). Increases in both blood flow and glucose use in the visual cortex could be observed, without similar increases in oxygen use. As a result, local oxygen availability increases because of the increased supply of oxygen from flowing blood that exceeds the increased local demand for oxygen, which forms the fMRI BOLD contrast.

2.4. Bioenergetics in the Visual Cortex

Despite the agreement across imaging modalities in the observation of CBF–$CMRO_2$ uncoupling, the physiological interpretation for this phenomenon has been controversial. Two major debates were whether oxidative metabolism regulates CBF and whether oxidative metabolism or nonoxidative glycolysis meets the energy demands for neuronal activity.

In contrast to the suggestion of Fox and colleagues that oxygen demand did not regulate CBF increases and that glycolysis can meet the neuronal energy requirements, others argued

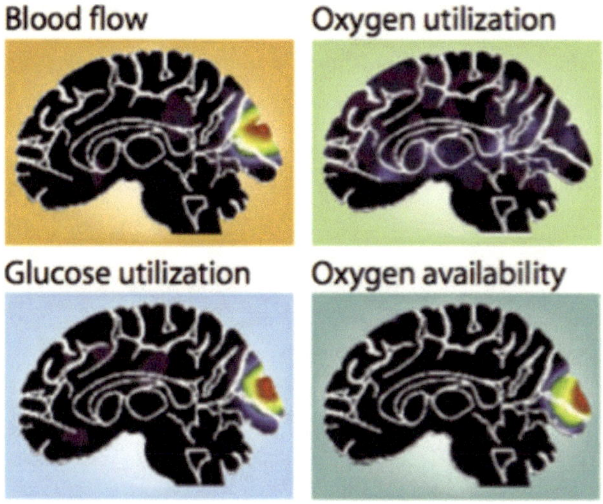

Figure 12. Visual stimulation produces marked changes in activity in visual areas of the brain. Blood flow, glucose utilization, and oxygen availability significantly increase, but the change of the oxygen utilization is minimal. Source: (18).

that significant increases of CBF were needed to facilitate oxygen delivery and that predominately oxidative metabolism should meet energy demands (19). To clarify whether oxidative metabolism or glycolysis regulates CBF and energy demands, Lin and colleagues (20) performed a concurrent fMRI and ^{1}H MRS study using graded visual stimulation (4, 8, and 16 Hz). They used fMRI to determine %ΔCBF and %$\Delta CMRO_2$ and used ^{1}H MRS to determine %Δ[Lac].

Findings for %ΔCBF, %$\Delta CMRO_2$, and %Δ[Lac] varied with frequency, with %ΔCBF and %Δ[Lac] peaking at 8 Hz, whereas %$\Delta CMRO_2$ reached a maximum at 4 Hz (Figure 13, A and B). The magnitudes of %ΔCBF (57.1%–65.1%) and %Δ[Lac] (31.3%–50.0%) were much larger than that of %$\Delta CMRO_2$ (12.2%–17.0%). As a result, %ΔCBF was tightly coupled with lactate production rate (Figure 14A) but negatively correlated with %$\Delta CMRO_2$ (Figure 14B).

ATP production (J_{ATP}) was calculated, using a stoichiometric equation, from the determined %$\Delta CMRO_2$ and lactate production rate. J_{ATP} was not significantly different among the three stimulus frequencies, and the increment was smaller (12%–17%) than the baseline (Rest) state. Further, oxidative metabolism predominately contributed to J_{ATP} and linearly correlated with %$\Delta CMRO_2$ (Figure 14C and Figure 15).

Taken together, the major findings from the study were as follows: (i) Increases in oxygen metabolism and energy demand of task-induced neuronal activation were small (12%–17%); (ii) oxidative (indexed by $CMRO_2$) and nonoxidative (indexed by lactate production) metabolism coexisted during visual stimulation; and (iii) CBF increase was much larger (52%–65%) than the increase in energy demand and highly correlated with lactate production, but not with $CMRO_2$. In response to the two main debated questions mentioned above, Lin et al's observations supported that (i) anaerobic glycolysis, rather than oxygen demand, drives CBF response to neuronal activity, and (ii) energy demand is predominately met through the oxidative metabolic pathway even though the $CMRO_2$ increases are much lower than those of [Lac] (19, 21, 22).

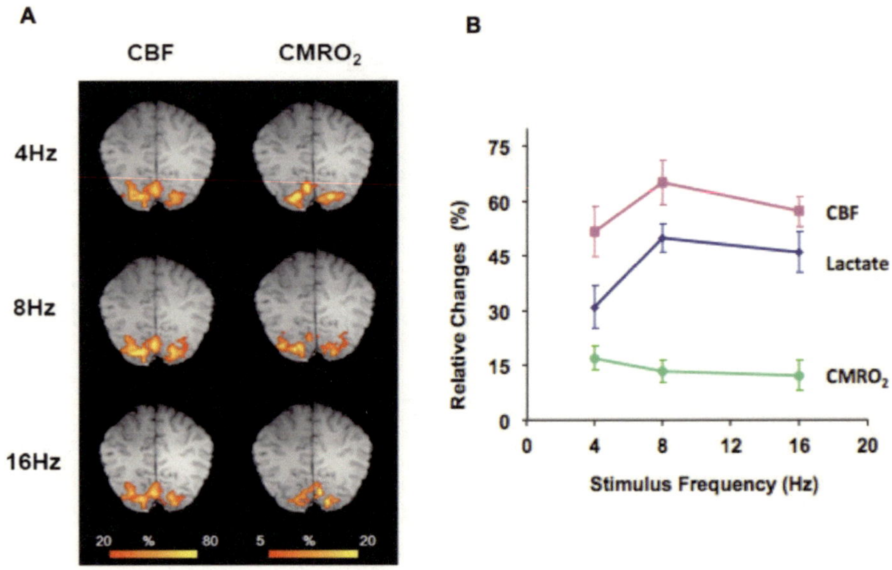

Figure 13. **(A)** Location and magnitude of $\%\Delta CBF$ and $\%\Delta CMRO_2$ in the primary visual cortex during 4-, 8-, and 16-Hz visual stimulation. **(B)** Magnitude of $\%\Delta CBF$, $\%\Delta[Lac]$, and $\%\Delta CMRO_2$ in the primary visual cortex during 4-, 8-, and 16-Hz visual stimulation. Source: (20).

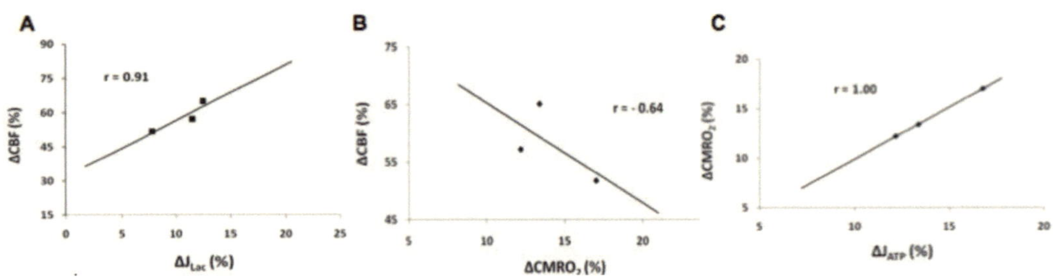

Figure 14. **(A)** CBF–lactate coupling. Significant correlation existed between $\%\Delta CBF$ and $\%\Delta J_{Lac}$ at the three visual stimulation rates ($r = 0.91$; $p < 0.001$). **(B)** CBF–$CMRO_2$ coupling. Negative correlation existed between $\%\Delta CBF$ and $\%\Delta CMRO_2$ at the three visual stimulation rates ($r = -0.64$; $p = 0.024$). **(C)** $CMRO_2$–ATP coupling. Significant correlation existed between $\%\Delta CMRO_2$ and $\%\Delta J_{ATP}$ at the three visual stimulation rates ($r = 1.00$; $p < 0.001$). Source: (20).

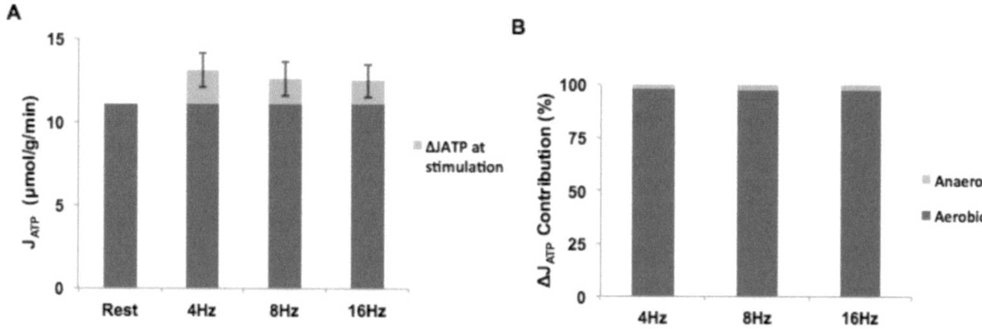

Figure 15. **(A)** J_{ATP} at rest and the three levels of visual stimulation. The J_{ATP} values during activation are independent of stimulus rate. The increments at activation are smaller (1.4–2.0 μmol/g/min) than the rest value (11.1 μmol/g/min). **(B)** Aerobic and anaerobic relative contributions (%) to ΔJ_{ATP}. The ΔJ_{ATP} at the three stimulation rates is due predominately to aerobic metabolism (~98%, including both neuronal and astrocytic contributions). Source: (20).

2.5. Astrocyte–Neuron Lactate Shuttle (ANLS) Model

The collective evidence from the functional imaging literature (PET, fMRI, and MRS) has forced the development of alternatives to the Roy–Sherrington hypothesis. Of these, the astrocyte–neuron lactate shuttle (ANLS) model (Figure 16) is the most conceptually evolved and widely accepted (23, 24). The ANLS model posits a cooperation between neurons and astrocytes in meeting the activation-induced needs both for energy production and for neurotransmitter production. Upon neuronal firing, both neurons and astrocytes take up glucose. Astrocytes take up most of the glucose, and neurons take up the rest. Though the level of glucose metabolism in neurons is low, the process is entirely aerobic to support neurotransmission (25, 26). The level of astrocytic glucose consumption, however, is high but much less energetically efficient because it is predominately anaerobic. Astrocytic glycolysis (2 ATP) is used to support Na^+/K^+ ion pumping and glutamate (Glu)–glutamine (Gln) conversion. Lactate generated by astrocytic glycolysis is eventually transported to neurons as fuel, but with some loss into the circulation, which increases hyperemia (26, 27). The ANLS hypothesis implies that (i) oxygen demand does not drive increases in CMR_{Glc}, which serve other purposes such as astrocyte-mediated neurotransmitter recycling; (ii) task-induced oxygen demand is small; and (iii) factors other than oxidative metabolism regulate CBF increases.

The three findings that Lin and colleagues reported, described above, were in good agreement with the ANLS hypothesis. The first finding (small $CMRO_2$ increase) was in line with the ANLS implication that the energy demands of acute, transient increases in neuronal activity are small (~15% increase in $CMRO_2$; at most, 30%). Oxidative metabolism should increase as neuronal activation continues because neurons eventually take up astrocytic lactate into the tricarboxylic acid cycle as a fuel substrate. In support of this formulation, prolonged visual stimulation (>20 min) can induce gradually rising levels of $CMRO_2$ and gradually decreasing CMR_{Glc}, J_{Lac}, and CBF under high-frequency stimulation

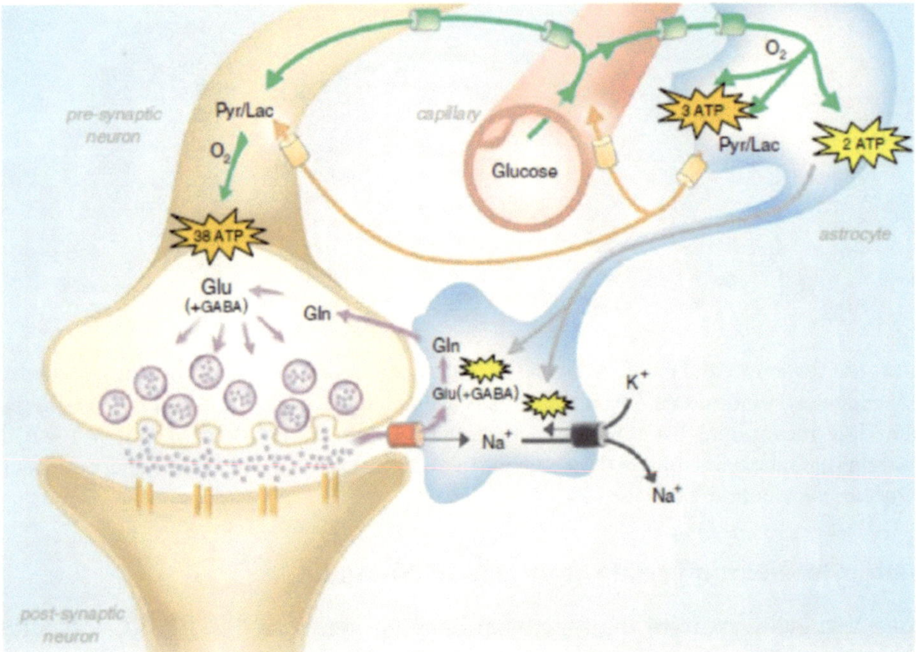

Figure 16. The Astrocyte-neuron lactate shuttle (ANLS) model. Glucose (green arrows) is delivered via the capillaries to both neurons (beige) and astrocytes (blue). In neurons, glucose consumption is predominately oxidative, generating 38 ATP at a glucose oxidation rate of 1.00 μmol/g/min. In astrocytes, glucose consumption is both oxidative and nonoxidative, generating 3 ATP oxidatively and 2 ATP nonoxidatively (at a glucose oxidation rate of 1.00 μmol/g/min). The energy from nonoxidative metabolism is used to convert glutamate to glutamine, the predominant excitatory neurotransmitter. Neurons take up the lactate that glycolysis generates to fuel further glucose oxidation. A small amount of lactate will efflux to the capillaries and thus increase cerebral blood flow (CBF). Source: (26).

(e.g., 8 Hz) (11, 14, 28-30). Consequently, %ΔCBF and %ΔCMRO$_2$ were recoupled as stimulation continued (14, 28), as mentioned in section 2.2.

The second finding supported the ANLS hypothesis construct of two metabolic pathways (oxidative and nonoxidative) that coexist, are dissociable, and serve different purposes in maintaining neuronal functions during visual stimulation. Oxidative metabolism is predominantly neuronal and supports ATP production for the release of neurotransmitters, whereas nonoxidative metabolism occurs mainly in astrocytes and supports Glu–Gln recycling and lactogenesis-mediated hyperemia.

The third finding was consistent with the ANLS prediction that some lactate produced by anaerobic glycolysis in astrocytes is effluxed into the circulation. The increased lactate:pyruvate and NADH:NAD$^+$ ratios in blood then activate the nitric oxide signaling pathway, to increase local CBF (27, 29, 31). However, astrocyte-mediated glycolytic metabolism may not be the sole mechanism to elicit this CBF response. Local CBF increase also has been proposed via Ca^{2+}, K^+, and adenosine signaling pathways (29, 32, 33).

Although findings from (20) support current neurophysiological hypotheses, such as the ANLS hypothesis, theories of neurovascular and neurometabolic mechanisms continue to evolve (34). Some aspects of the ANLS hypothesis remain controversial. For example, whether the lactate transferred to neurons as a fuel substrate is from astrocytic or neuronal activity (30), and whether lactate is the preferential substrate of neurons for neurotransmission-related energy needs are still under debate. (See review in (35)). Finally, whether J_{ATP} is constant during continuous stimulation, as this study assumes, remains open. Further investigations are needed to resolve these issues.

In summary, the ANLS model offers a more explicit and comprehensive explanation of the interplay of neuronal activation, metabolism, and hemodynamics that is based on the discovery of the CBF–$CMRO_2$ uncoupling phenomenon.

3. Conclusion

Over the past century, the visual cortex has played a significant role in revealing the fundamental relationship among brain activity, metabolism, and hemodynamics. The development of PET imaging facilitated the investigations and led to the discovery of flow–metabolism uncoupling, the development of fMRI BOLD techniques, and the evolution of the physiological interpretation. These revolutionized changes enable us to better understand the metabolic physiology of brain activity, giving us the bases to predict metabolic physiology in neurological disorders, including stroke or Alzheimer's disease.

Author details

Ai-Ling Lin and Peter T. Fox
Research Imaging Institute, University of Texas Health Science Center, San Antonio, TX, USA

Jia-Hong Gao
Brain Research Imaging Center, University of Chicago, Chicago, IL, USA

4. References

[1] Mosso A. *Ueber den Kreislauf des Blutes im menschlichen Gehirn*. Leipzig: Verlag von Veit. 1881.

[2] Fox PT, Raichle ME, Mintun MA, Dence C. Nonoxidative glucose consumption during focal physiologic neural activity. Science. 1988;241(4864):462-4. Epub 1988/07/22.

[3] Ogawa S, Menon RS, Tank DW, Kim SG, Merkle H, Ellermann JM, et al. Functional brain mapping by blood oxygenation level-dependent contrast magnetic resonance imaging. A comparison of signal characteristics with a biophysical model. Biophys J. 1993;64(3):803-12. Epub 1993/03/01.

[4] Ogawa S, Tank DW, Menon R, Ellermann JM, Kim SG, Merkle H, et al. Intrinsic signal changes accompanying sensory stimulation: functional brain mapping with magnetic resonance imaging. Proc Natl Acad Sci U S A. 1992;89(13):5951-5. Epub 1992/07/01.

[5] Patrizi ML. Primi esperimenti intorno all'influenza della musica sulla circolazione del sangue nel cervello dell'uomo. Rivista Musicale Italiana. 1896;3:275-94.
[6] Roy CS, Sherrington CS. On the Regulation of the Blood-supply of the Brain. J Physiol. 1890;11(1-2):85-158 17. Epub 1890/01/01.
[7] Fulton JF. Observation upon the vascularity of the human occipital lobe during visual activity. Brain. 1928;51:310-20.
[8] Fox PT, Raichle ME. Stimulus rate dependence of regional cerebral blood flow in human striate cortex, demonstrated by positron emission tomography. J Neurophysiol. 1984;51(5):1109-20. Epub 1984/05/01.
[9] Fox PT, Raichle ME. Stimulus rate determines regional brain blood flow in striate cortex. Ann Neurol. 1985;17(3):303-5. Epub 1985/03/01.
[10] Phelps ME, Mazziotta JC. Positron emission tomography: human brain function and biochemistry. Science. 1985;228(4701):799-809. Epub 1985/05/17.
[11] Prichard J, Rothman D, Novotny E, Petroff O, Kuwabara T, Avison M, et al. Lactate rise detected by 1H NMR in human visual cortex during physiologic stimulation. Proc Natl Acad Sci U S A. 1991;88(13):5829-31. Epub 1991/07/01.
[12] Frahm J, Kruger G, Merboldt KD, Kleinschmidt A. Dynamic uncoupling and recoupling of perfusion and oxidative metabolism during focal brain activation in man. Magn Reson Med. 1996;35(2):143-8. Epub 1996/02/01.
[13] Vafaee MS, Gjedde A. Model of blood-brain transfer of oxygen explains nonlinear flow-metabolism coupling during stimulation of visual cortex. J Cereb Blood Flow Metab. 2000;20(4):747-54. Epub 2000/04/25.
[14] Mintun MA, Vlassenko AG, Shulman GL, Snyder AZ. Time-related increase of oxygen utilization in continuously activated human visual cortex. Neuroimage. 2002;16(2):531-7. Epub 2002/05/29.
[15] Kwong KK, Belliveau JW, Chesler DA, Goldberg IE, Weisskoff RM, Poncelet BP, et al. Dynamic magnetic resonance imaging of human brain activity during primary sensory stimulation. Proc Natl Acad Sci U S A. 1992;89(12):5675-9. Epub 1992/06/15.
[16] Detre JA, Leigh JS, Williams DS, Koretsky AP. Perfusion imaging. Magn Reson Med. 1992;23(1):37-45. Epub 1992/01/01.
[17] Davis TL, Kwong KK, Weisskoff RM, Rosen BR. Calibrated functional MRI: mapping the dynamics of oxidative metabolism. Proc Natl Acad Sci U S A. 1998;95(4):1834-9. Epub 1998/03/21.
[18] Gusnard DA, Raichle ME. Searching for a baseline: functional imaging and the resting human brain. Nat Rev Neurosci. 2001;2(10):685-94. Epub 2001/10/05.
[19] Hoge RD, Atkinson J, Gill B, Crelier GR, Marrett S, Pike GB. Linear coupling between cerebral blood flow and oxygen consumption in activated human cortex. Proc Natl Acad Sci U S A. 1999;96(16):9403-8. Epub 1999/08/04.
[20] Lin AL, Fox PT, Hardies J, Duong TQ, Gao JH. Nonlinear coupling between cerebral blood flow, oxygen consumption, and ATP production in human visual cortex. Proc Natl Acad Sci U S A. 2010;107(18):8446-51. Epub 2010/04/21.

[21] Chen W, Zhu XH, Gruetter R, Seaquist ER, Adriany G, Ugurbil K. Study of tricarboxylic acid cycle flux changes in human visual cortex during hemifield visual stimulation using (1)H-[(13)C] MRS and fMRI. Magn Reson Med. 2001;45(3):349-55. Epub 2001/03/10.

[22] Kim SG, Rostrup E, Larsson HB, Ogawa S, Paulson OB. Determination of relative CMRO2 from CBF and BOLD changes: significant increase of oxygen consumption rate during visual stimulation. Magn Reson Med. 1999;41(6):1152-61. Epub 1999/06/17.

[23] Pellerin L, Magistretti PJ. Glutamate uptake into astrocytes stimulates aerobic glycolysis: a mechanism coupling neuronal activity to glucose utilization. Proc Natl Acad Sci U S A. 1994;91(22):10625-9. Epub 1994/10/25.

[24] Belanger M, Allaman I, Magistretti PJ. Brain energy metabolism: focus on astrocyte-neuron metabolic cooperation. Cell Metab. 2011;14(6):724-38. Epub 2011/12/14.

[25] Brand MD. The efficiency and plasticity of mitochondrial energy transduction. Biochem Soc Trans. 2005;33(Pt 5):897-904. Epub 2005/10/26.

[26] Hyder F, Patel AB, Gjedde A, Rothman DL, Behar KL, Shulman RG. Neuronal-glial glucose oxidation and glutamatergic-GABAergic function. J Cereb Blood Flow Metab. 2006;26(7):865-77. Epub 2006/01/13.

[27] Mintun MA, Vlassenko AG, Rundle MM, Raichle ME. Increased lactate/pyruvate ratio augments blood flow in physiologically activated human brain. Proc Natl Acad Sci U S A. 2004;101(2):659-64. Epub 2004/01/06.

[28] Lin AL, Fox PT, Yang Y, Lu H, Tan LH, Gao JH. Time-dependent correlation of cerebral blood flow with oxygen metabolism in activated human visual cortex as measured by fMRI. NeuroImage. 2009;44(1):16-22. Epub 2008/09/23.

[29] Vlassenko AG, Rundle MM, Raichle ME, Mintun MA. Regulation of blood flow in activated human brain by cytosolic NADH/NAD+ ratio. Proc Natl Acad Sci U S A. 2006;103(6):1964-9. Epub 2006/02/01.

[30] Gjedde A, Marrett S. Glycolysis in neurons, not astrocytes, delays oxidative metabolism of human visual cortex during sustained checkerboard stimulation in vivo. J Cereb Blood Flow Metab. 2001;21(12):1384-92. Epub 2001/12/12.

[31] Mangia S, Tkac I, Gruetter R, Van de Moortele PF, Maraviglia B, Ugurbil K. Sustained neuronal activation raises oxidative metabolism to a new steady-state level: evidence from 1H NMR spectroscopy in the human visual cortex. J Cereb Blood Flow Metab. 2007;27(5):1055-63. Epub 2006/10/13.

[32] Takano T, Tian GF, Peng W, Lou N, Libionka W, Han X, et al. Astrocyte-mediated control of cerebral blood flow. Nat Neurosci. 2006;9(2):260-7. Epub 2006/01/03.

[33] Haddy FJ, Vanhoutte PM, Feletou M. Role of potassium in regulating blood flow and blood pressure. Am J Physiol Regul Integr Comp Physiol. 2006;290(3):R546-52. Epub 2006/02/10.

[34] Attwell D, Buchan AM, Charpak S, Lauritzen M, Macvicar BA, Newman EA. Glial and neuronal control of brain blood flow. Nature. 2010;468(7321):232-43. Epub 2010/11/12.

[35] Mangia S, Giove F, Tkac I, Logothetis NK, Henry PG, Olman CA, et al. Metabolic and hemodynamic events after changes in neuronal activity: current hypotheses, theoretical predictions and in vivo NMR experimental findings. J Cereb Blood Flow Metab. 2009;29(3):441-63. Epub 2008/11/13.

Chapter 12

Experience Mediated Development of the Visual Cortex Vascularization

Enrike G. Argandoña, Harkaitz Bengoetxea, Naiara Ortuzar, Susana Bulnes, Irantzu Rico-Barrio and José Vicente Lafuente

Additional information is available at the end of the chapter

http://dx.doi.org/10.5772/48749

1. Introduction

The vascular system of every organ is composed of an afferent arterial system that ensures metabolic support, and an efferent venous drainage system that evacuates the substances produced by the organ as well as the catabolites that are generated. Both systems communicate via a terminal network in which the arterial capillaries anastomose with the venous ones. Vascular organisation depends on the structure and function of each organ, thus there is not a general vascular system, but an organ-specific one. The large blood vessels supplying the brain are the carotid and vertebral arteries, which then branch to form the network of pial arteries covering the surface of the brain. In the cerebral cortex, the pial vessels branch into smaller arteries, which enter the brain tissue itself and are called the penetrating arterioles. These arterioles branch into secondary and tertiary arterioles, until they reach the smallest vessel supplying the brain tissue, the capillary, which is only wide enough for one red blood cell to pass through it at a time. The capillaries then feed into the venules and veins, which carry the blood away [1].

Brain vascularisation is especially important due to brain metabolic peculiarities. Although the brain represents only 2% of the body weight and vascularisation is only 1% of brain size, it receives 20% of the cardiac output, 20% of total body oxygen consumption, and 25% of total body glucose utilization [2, 3]. As the brain lacks a glucose storage system, most of it has to be supported by a constant blood supply. Within the brain vascularisation, the vascularisation of the cerebral cortex has differential features compared not only to other body regions, but also to other brain areas. The two main differential features are the Blood Brain Barrier function and the dense capillary network.

2. Blood brain barrier

The endothelium of the CNS vessels is a structure specialised in the maintenance of the homeostasis of the internal environment of the brain parenchyma. This function is crucial in the CNS, as its function requires a strict regulation of the neuronal environment, which is extremely sensitive to ionic and/or metabolic changes. In fact, most of the substances freely available in blood from daily food intake that are constantly metabolised and excreted, are potentially neurotoxic [4]. This function is known as the Blood Brain Barrier, and was first described in 1885 by Paul Ehrlich, who found that soluble dyes injected into the system stained all organs but the brain and the spinal cord [5].

The Blood Brain Barrier is the set of mechanisms (physical and metabolic) that regulate the passage of compounds from blood to brain, allowing the regulation of the internal environment of the CNS with independence of fluctuations in blood composition. These mechanisms include, among others, the enzymatic systems that transform some compounds during their passage through the endothelium, as well as the specific transporters of some substances, such as glucose or aminoacids. Bigger molecules, such as insulin, use exocytosis systems mediated by receptors. Some of these enzymatic mechanisms have been used to quantify vascular distribution, e.g., butyryl cholinesterase histochemistry [6], alkaline phosphatase histochemistry [7], LEA lectin histochemistry [8-10] and immunohistochemistry against antigens such as glucose transporter-1 (GluT-1) [11], PECAM [12], RECA-1 [13] and the endothelial barrier antigen (EBA) [11, 14-18].

Among the cellular components of the BBB, we could mention the following:

a. Endothelial cells. The cortical endothelium is formed by a layer of endothelial cells with a higher mitochondrial component, almost complete absence of pinocytic activity, absence of fenestrations and presence of interendothelial junctions [19, 20].
b. Pericytes. Joined to the abluminal membrane of the endothelium, pericytes are included in the same basal membrane as the endothelium. The pericyte is a cell of heterogeneous origin that is related to macrophages, muscle cells, etc. Despite the fact that they have been largely neglected, recent studies show that they play a relevant role in angiogenesis and in the BBB function, by, among other mechanisms, inhibiting apoptosis of endothelial cells. Apart from their vascular role, recent studies have demonstrated a crucial role of pericytes in the formation of the glial scars produced after brain injuries, thus linking the maintenance of the Blood Brain Barrier with scarring and tissue repair, a role that has long been attributed to astrocytes [21].
c. Astrocytes. These play a relevant role in the dual nature of the BBB, physical and metabolic. On the one hand, their prolongations ensheathing the endothelial wall (astrocytic endfeet) are closely related to the basal membrane. Astrocytes induce several metabolic BBB properties, such as the enzymatic activity of the capillary wall, the uptake of glucose and the establishment of tight junctions. In general, astrocytes play a key role in the induction, expression and maintenance of the BBB. Although astrocytes are implicated in flow regulation and microvascular permeability by elevating calcium

levels in endothelial intervention, they are less involved than expected in the structural properties of the BBB [4].

d. Extracellular matrix. Apart from the afore-mentioned cells and neurons, that also regulate blood flow to cope with energy requirements and that even regulate vascular permeability, the extracellular matrix plays a key role in the interaction with vascular permeability, even regulating the expression of proteins that constitute the TJ of the BBB. On the other hand, the ECM has to be digested in order to allow angiogenesis, thus liberating non-soluble VEGF. This function is performed by the matrix metalloproteases [22].

Due to the cellular heterogeneity that constitutes the BBB, all the elements can be described as a neurogliovascular unit, where all elements are interrelated, as can be seen in pathological processes such as Alzheimer's, Parkinson's or stroke, where all elements are implicated [4, 23].

Among the structural elements of the BBB, tight junctions play a crucial role in the control of the paracellular diffusion of blood compounds to brain parenchyma. Tight Junctions coexist with other junction structures, such as belt desmosomes and gap junctions; nevertheless, tight junctions are still the main ones [23].

The proteins that constitute the tight junctions share a common cytoplasmatic location, and are linked to the actin cytoskeleton (ZO-1 and 2, cingulin, AF-6 and 7H6). The transmembrane proteins are JAM-1, occludin and claudin [24]. Actin plays an even greater role than TJ proteins in the maintenance of BBB integrity [22].

Although the development of cortical vascularisation is closely related to the development of the cortical function, in previous work we have demonstrated that despite the effects of sensorial deprivation on the development of the vascularisation of the visual cortex, the maturation of the BBB is not related to the functional maturation of the cortex, as neither visual deprivation nor environmental enrichment induced changes in the maturation of early and late markers of barrier maturation [14]. As most of the barrier structural and functional markers are fully developed prior to the beginning of the critical period, experience-mediated modifications do not appear to influence barrier maturation.

3. Capillary network

On the other hand, 90% of the cortical vascularisation is constituted by a fine capillary network that spreads all over the cortex and whose density is related to local neuronal activity. This network was described by Galen, who called it *rete mirabile* [25, 26]. Estimations suggest that the human brain contains up to 100 billion vessels, suggesting a ratio of one vessel per neuron [3]. In prior work, we have demonstrated that this relationship is maintained in the visual cortex despite deprivation of visual inputs. Indeed, both the number of vessels per neuron and the vascular surface per neuron maintain similar values when comparing normal and visually deprived rats [27]. In contrast, visual environmental enrichment does increase the ratio of vessels per neuron in response to the increased demand [28, 29].

The vascular system of the rat cerebral cortex is organised from the penetrating vessels perpendicular to the surface, emanating from the leptomeningeal vascular system. These vascular trunks branch, forming the capillary network that is the essential nutritional sector of the cortex, although metabolic exchange also takes place in the microcirculation sectors preceding the capillary network in small calibre arterioles [6].

When determining the three types of intracerebral vessels, although the vessel size is not a firm criterion for differentiating between capillary venules and arterioles, in general it can be established that the arterioles are vessels of 10 to 100 microns gauge. Arterioles with a caliber between 50 and 100 microns are called large arterioles, and arterioles smaller than 50 microns are called terminals. The capillaries are vessels under 10 microns, while venules are vessels of about 30 microns in diameter.

The main differences between these two types of vessel are in the structure of the wall:

- Arterioles lack a complete internal elastic membrane despite having a middle layer consisting of three layers of smooth muscle. A distinctive feature of the arteriolar wall structure is the adventitia, much thinner in cerebral arterioles than in the arterioles of the rest of the body, becoming discontinuous in some points, thus allowing the exchange of nutrients.
- Venules lack a distinct muscular middle layer. In its place is a layer of periendotelial cells. Periendotelial cells are a cell type that does not correspond clearly to smooth muscle cells or to pericytes, and that play a phagocytic function. The endothelium is structurally similar to the capillary structure.
- The capillary wall thickness is 4 to 10 times lower than the arteriolar wall thickness. The capillary wall has no muscle layer and is in close relationship with glia, physically structuring the blood brain barrier.

The study of the vascular system of the cerebral cortex requires the establishment of the topographical relationships between neurons, and blood vessels must provide a sufficient supply. Vascular density is closely related to local metabolic activity and oxygen consumption of different cortical regions. In areas with increased activity, characterised by an increase in mitochondrial volume density and increased local consumption of glucose, there was an increase in capillary density [2].

The differences in capillary density between different areas are mainly due to neuronal density and activity, and more specifically due to synaptic density. Being structurally similar, the differences will be based solely on the degree of activity. Furthermore, the development of the vascular bed is the result and runs parallel to the development of the cortex. Thus, in animal species in which the cerebral cortex is not fully mature at birth, there is little cortical vascularisation, and as the cortex matures, it develops its vascular architecture. This does not happen in lower species that are born relatively mature in which we see a vascular network similar to the adult animal brain. Similarly, phylogenetically older regions such as the entorhinal cortex have a more primitive vascular structure [30].

4. Development of the vascularisation of the visual cortex

The development of new blood vessels can occur via two mechanisms: vasculogenesis and angiogenesis. Vasculogenesis is the development of new vessels from differentiated endothelial cells in situ. Angiogenesis is the development of capillaries from preexisting vessels and is the way that cerebral vessels develop. Angiogenesis is a process that coordinates the precise timing and location of all the cells belonging to the NeuroGlioVascular unit to form a hierarchical vascular network with CNS specifications, including BBB function, reciprocal interactions between neurons, glia and pericytes and a vascular niche for neural stem cells [31]. The angiogenic process starts when one endothelial cell, in response to the VEGF secreted following local hypoxia, differentiates into a tip cell that advances according to the VEGF signal. The adjacent endothelial cells are destined to become stalk cells that follow the tip cell, providing a lumenized endothelial cell chain. The signal to inhibit tip cell differentiation and to become stalk cell is mediated by the Notch pathway [32, 33]. This process is functionally similar to axon growth cones [34, 35].

The development of intracortical vascularisation starts at 12 days post coitum with radially penetrating stem vessels following the pattern of neural tube growth, and is completed when these vessels form new cortical branches terminating in different cellular layers with 'en bouquet' [36] terminations. This is the vascular pattern of the mature neocortex.

The first draft of brain vessels is formed starting from where the aortic arches approach the ventral neural tube to form a primary vascular plexus. Vessels from the primary plexus reach the vesicles developing in the telencephalic basolateral surface, and vascular buds penetrate perpendicularly to the walls of the hemisphere [3, 37]. The development of the cerebral vasculature is divided into two stages, one extracerebral and the other intracerebral.

a. Extracerebral vascularisation (leptomeningeal)

The arterial and venous vessels that cover the entire cerebral cortex are formed from undifferentiated capillary plexus. This perineural vascular system ends when the development of intracerebral vascularisation finishes. At first, the density of leptomeningeal arteries decreases, and then the veins, which indicates that the venous system reaches its final pattern after the arterial [36].

b. Intracerebral vascularisation

The vascularisation of the cerebral cortex begins with the development of vascular trunks penetrating radially, perpendicular to the cortical surface. The development of these early intracerebral vessels begins in the early days of embryonic development and is completed during postnatal life [38].

The first vascular sprouts penetrate the cortex before the development of the cortical plate, so that the first vessels reach the ventricular zone perpendicularly opposite the leptomeningeal plexus. The earliest vessels that arise during development penetrate the cortical plate throughout its depth. This is reflected in the vascular structure of the adult cortex, where we can distinguish the radial trunks originated at first and going through all cortical layers without collateral branches. During development of the cortex, the vascular leptomeningeal system issues new branches that penetrate the cortical plate, covering a territory that corresponds to their age so that the first vessels supply the deeper layers and the later ones supply the outermost layers. In the rat, from the second week of postnatal life there is no new perpendicular growth that enters the cortex from the leptomeningeal vascular system. The volume and surface area of the cortex continue to increase, so the vessel density decreases in proportion, penetrating perpendicularly to the cortical surface.

The cerebral cortex, in addition to thickening, undergoes a three-dimensional growth process accompanied by vascular arborization involving penetrating vessels. As was the case with the increase in thickness, the most ancient vessels provide greater horizontal branches due to the fact that older vessels occupy a larger area.

After maturation of the capillary network there is no budding of new vascular branches, indicating that the process of budding of new vascular branches ends when the vascular wall has fully developed. During the first phase of vascular development, a basic pattern is provided to suit the needs of each cortical area, showing specific regional differences in relation to the further development of different areas. During the second phase of vascularisation, a large increase in the vascular bed density occurs which corresponds to a large increase of the capillary surface closely associated with increased metabolic demands of the tissue. Between 8 and 20 days of postnatal life the microvascular endothelial cells proliferate rapidly. It is during this period that virtually all vascular branches form. The mitotic activity of endothelial cells drops sharply during the third week of postnatal life, as can be verified by tritiated thymidine incorporation into endothelial cells [36].

The third phase of vascular development is the elongation of existing branches. Originally, successive vascular branches are established, and then the vessels grow in length to cover the whole territory they serve. This elongation stage of pre-existing capillaries extends from day 20 until adulthood. This is the physiological pattern of development. In animals kept under normal conditions the definitive pattern of vascularisation culminates in the third week of postnatal life. Subsequent changes in transient local metabolic demands are supplied by local flow changes, but there are special circumstances that occur in which definitive increases in metabolic demand are offset by extending or adapting the normal pattern of development, as happens in adaptation to altitude hypoxia [39].

The development of the vascularisation of the visual cortex has one main specificity in rats, as the first phases of cortical development occur prior to eye opening, and thus are not experience-mediated. So, the experience-mediated vascular development happens during the so-called critical period. Sensory modifications during the early critical period result in substantial plasticity and are a crucial factor in establishing the mature circuitry [hooks]. This time window of postnatal life is specific for each brain area, and is experience-mediated. The critical period in the rat visual system is located between the 3rd and 5th postnatal weeks with a peak at the 4th [40]. Previously, we have shown that vascular density is closely related to neuronal activity, and by increasing and decreasing visual experience, we have found that the peak of VEGF expression is also at the 4th postnatal week [41], corresponding to the activity peak.

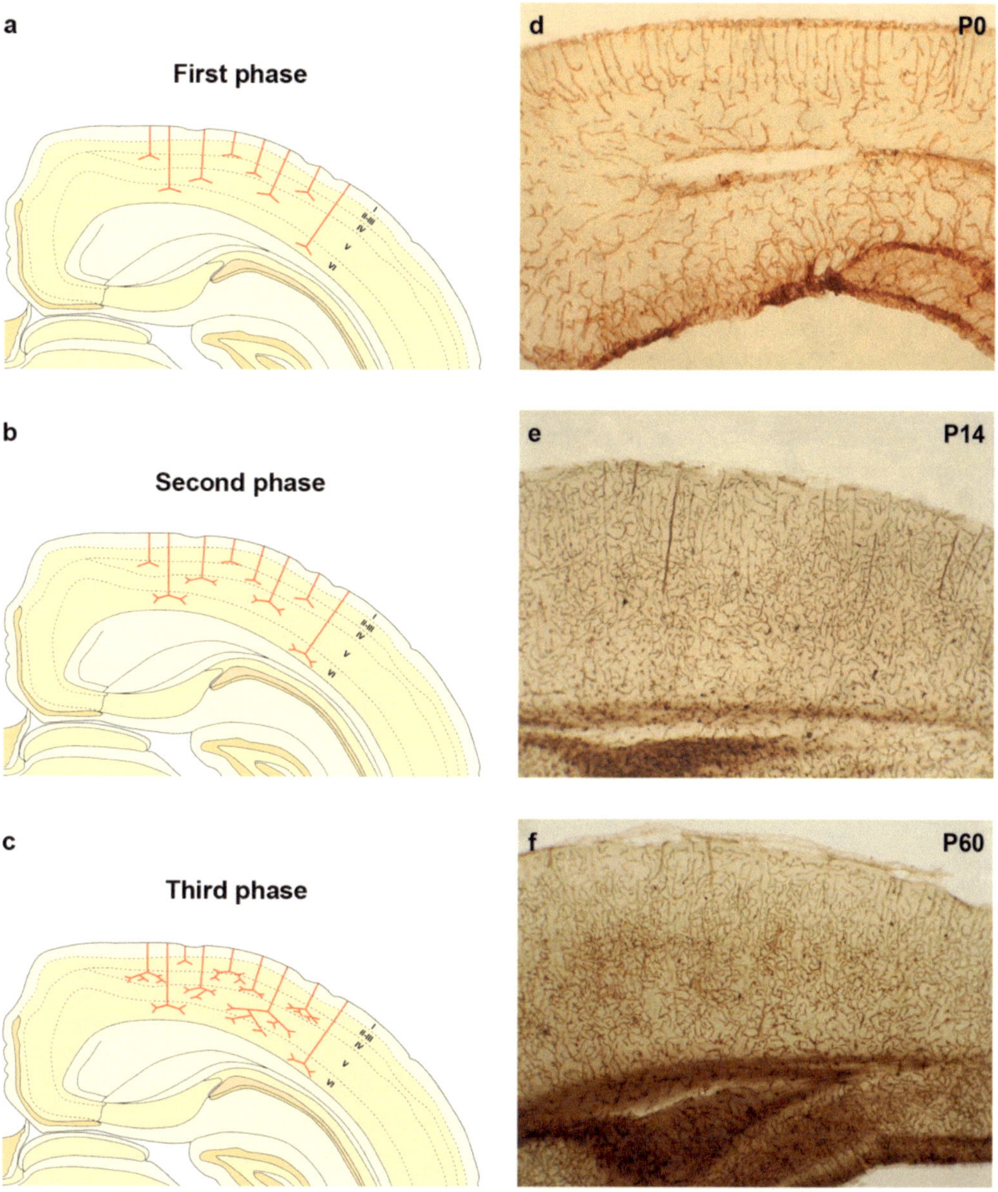

Figure 1. Schematic representation and histochemical sections of the development of the vascularisation of the visual cortex: a) first phase where vascular sprouts penetrate the cortex; b) during the second phase an increase in the vascular bed occurs; c) in the third phase the vessels grow in length and cover the whole territory they serve; d,e,f) show visual cortex vascularisation by butyrylcholinesterase histochemistry during these phases at P0 (first phase), P14 (second phase) and P60 (third phase), when the rats reach adulthood.

Thus, during the first two weeks of postnatal development, most of the vessels are the perpendicularly penetrating vessels, and this terminates at the end of the second postnatal week, just at the opening of the eyes. At this point, the adult pattern starts, characterised by a dense capillary network that is thicker in the most active areas, such as layer IV [6, 30]. The influence of experience can be demonstrated in visually-deprived dark-reared rats, that have an immature vascular pattern characterised by a higher prevalence of perpendicularly penetrant trunks and a much sparser vascular network. In contrast, environmental enrichment induces just the opposite, a faster development of the mature pattern and a higher vascular density [14]. These changes occur in parallel to the development of the rest of the elements of the neurogliovascular unit, and we have demonstrated that the development of the astroglial population in layer IV of the visual cortex mirrors the vascular behaviour [42, 43]. In a similar way, vascular density is also higher in layer IV of the auditory cortex and lower in layer I [30]. On the other hand, we have recently described upregulated neuropeptides in the visual system, and as some of them have also strong angiogenic properties, and as neuropeptides are among the main regulators of the critical period in the visual cortex along with angioglioneurins, this finding is also consistent with the common patterns for neural and vascular development [44].

There is a direct relationship between vascular density and metabolic activity. This is evidenced by the correlation between vascular density and mitochondria. Local capillary density, local utilization of glucose and local cerebral blood flow [45, 46] have also been found to be correlated. The relationship between the increase in neural activity and the increase in perfusion to supply this requirement is the so-called neurovascular coupling, that is the basis of modern neuroimaging techniques and that has been recently described as neurogenic instead of metabolic [47].

5. Angioglioneurins

Neovascularisation is mediated by a variety of cytokines, including Vascular Endothelial Growth Factor (VEGF). VEGF is a hypoxia-inducible secreted homodimeric glycoprotein of 45,000 daltons that plays a major role in developmental [48-51] and pathological angiogenesis [52-57]. Five major isoforms of human VEGF exist, of which VEGF165 is the predominant one in most mammals. However, VEGF164 is shorter by one amino acid in rodents. VEGF isoforms are differentially expressed in disease, suggesting differences between pathological entities in the mechanisms of VEGF up-regulation as well as in their employment of distinct isoforms for neovascularisation [58]. The main receptors for the Vascular Endothelial Growth Factor (VEGF) family are the feline sarcoma virus-like tyrosine kinase receptor (Flt-1 or VEGFR-1) and the fetal liver kinase receptor (Flk-1) or VEGFR-2, also known as KDR [49, 51, 59, 60].

VEGFR-2 plays a critical role in some permeability-enhancing effects of VEGF [54]. In pathological conditions, VEGFR-2 mediates an antiapoptotic effect via Phosphoinositide 3-kinase (PI3K)-dependent signalling pathways which promote the survival of endothelial cells induced by VEGF [61-63] and is related to the blood-brain barrier (BBB) opening in brain injury [54, 64, 65]. A neuroprotective role for VEGF via VEGFR-2 has also been described [59, 66-68], which occurs via the PI3k/Akt and the mitogen-activated protein kinase/ERK kinase/extracellular signal-regulated protein kinase (MEK/ERK) pathways [69, 70].

But despite VEGF being the main angiogenic molecule, there are others that also play a multicellular role. Molecules that affect both neural and vascular cell processes have recently been termed angioneurins [71]. Angioneurins include molecules first described as vascular growth factors, such as Vascular Endothelial Growth Factor (VEGF), molecules first described as neurotrophins such as Brain-Derived Neurotrophic Factor (BDNF), and other factors such as Insulin-Like Growth Factor-1 (IGF-I) or Erythropoietin (EPO). Independently of their origin, all angioneurins share a common action on vascular and neuronal function. As most of these molecules also have effects on the third component of the neurogliovascular unit, the glia, we propose the term angioglioneurins to describe them [39, 72].

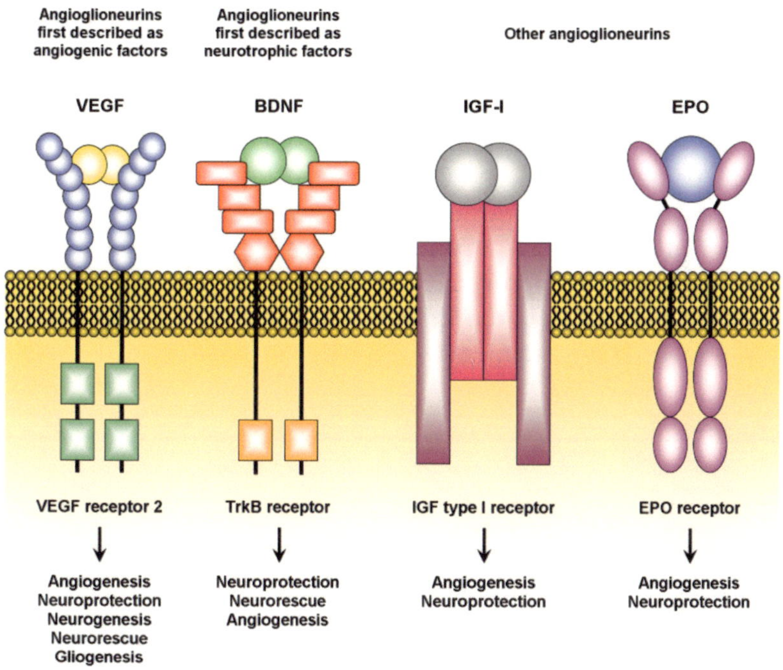

Figure 2. Schematic representation of referred angioglioneurins and their receptors. Some angioglioneurins were originally discovered through their angiogenic effects and then later found to also have neuroprotective activity (for example, vascular endothelial growth factor (VEGF)); some neurotrophic factors were originally discovered through their neuronal effects and then later found to also have angiogenic activity (for example, brain derived neurotrophic factor (BDNF)); others are more pleiotropic but still have relevant neurovascular activities, being involved in both angiogenesis and neuroprotection (for example, insulin-like growth factor 1 (IGF1) and erythropoietin (EPO)) (modified from Zacchigna et al., Nat Rev Neurosci; 9(3):169-81. Review).

6. Conclusions

The brain is highly vascularised, containing a very intricate network of capillaries (nearly every brain cell is located within 20 μm of a capillary). The endothelial cells that form the brain capillaries are sealed together by tight junctions, and have no fenestrations and very low pinocytosis. This combination of features creates the BBB, which is both a physical and enzymatic barrier.

Angiogenesis is one of the main adaptive mechanisms of brain microcirculation to changing needs of the CNS, as happens in the development of the visual cortex under the influence of visual activity, mainly during the critical period.

The nervous system needs a stable internal environment, which is created by the Blood Brain Barrier (BBB). The BBB function is related to structural and functional features of the vascular endothelium. Both the development of angioarchitecture and the functional maturation of the BBB occur postnatally and are regulated by tissue microenvironment and external environment. The development of the vascular tree, the acquisition of functional competence by the BBB and the induction and modulation of neoangiogenesis are closely dependent on the changes in metabolic demand induced by functional modifications (increases or decreases of stimuli).

The vascular network plays a crucial role in development and function of the CNS. It adapts to specific changes of metabolic demand and local flow modifications. However, if these changes become permanent, the supply is ensured by neoangiogenesis. Angiogenic, neurotrophic and neuroprotective factors participate in the development and maintenance of vascular, astroglial and neuronal structures, suggesting that the neurogliovascular unit preserves brain integrity. The improvement of the neurogliovascular unit by mechanisms such as the direct administration or the indirect stimulation of secretion of angioglioneurins could be an efficient strategy in brain diseases.

Author details

Enrike G. Argandoña
Department of Medicine, Unit of Anatomy, University of Fribourg, Fribourg, Switzerland

Harkaitz Bengoetxea, Naiara Ortuzar, Susana Bulnes,
Irantzu Rico-Barrio and José Vicente Lafuente
Laboratory of Experimental Neuroscience LaNCE, Department of Neuroscience,
Faculty of Medicine and Odontology, University of the Basque Country (UPV/EHU),
Sarriena Auzoa, Leioa, Spain

7. References

[1] MacVicar BA, Salter MW (2006) Neuroscience: controlled capillaries. Nature. 443(7112):642-643.

[2] Belanger M, Allaman I, Magistretti PJ (2011) Brain energy metabolism: focus on astrocyte-neuron metabolic cooperation. Cell Metab. 14(6):724-738.
[3] Quaegebeur A, Lange C, Carmeliet P (2011) The neurovascular link in health and disease: molecular mechanisms and therapeutic implications. Neuron. 71(3):406-424.
[4] Neuwelt EA, Bauer B, Fahlke C, Fricker G, Iadecola C, Janigro D, et al. (2011) Engaging neuroscience to advance translational research in brain barrier biology. Nat Rev Neurosci. 12(3):169-182.
[5] Ehrlich P (1885) Das sauerstoff-bedurfnis des organismus. Eine farbenanalytische studie Hirschwald, Berlin.
[6] Argandona EG, Lafuente JV (1996) Effects of dark-rearing on the vascularization of the developmental rat visual cortex. Brain Res. 732(1-2):43-51.
[7] Fonta C, Imbert M (2002) Vascularization in the primate visual cortex during development. Cereb Cortex. 12(2):199-211.
[8] Ezaki T, Baluk P, Thurston G, La Barbara A, Woo C, McDonald DM (2001) Time course of endothelial cell proliferation and microvascular remodeling in chronic inflammation. Am J Pathol. 158(6):2043-2055.
[9] Mazzetti S, Librizzi L, Frigerio S, de Curtis M, Vitellaro-Zuccarello L (2004) Molecular anatomy of the cerebral microvessels in the isolated guinea-pig brain. Brain Res. 999(1):81-90.
[10] Thurston G, Murphy TJ, Baluk P, Lindsey JR, McDonald DM (1998) Angiogenesis in mice with chronic airway inflammation: strain-dependent differences. Am J Pathol. 153(4):1099-1112.
[11] Krum JM (1996) Effect of astroglial degeneration on neonatal blood-brain barrier marker expression. Exp Neurol. 142(1):29-35.
[12] Ogunshola OO, Stewart WB, Mihalcik V, Solli T, Madri JA, Ment LR (2000) Neuronal VEGF expression correlates with angiogenesis in postnatal developing rat brain. Brain Res Dev Brain Res. 119(1):139-153.
[13] Palmer TD, Willhoite AR, Gage FH (2000) Vascular niche for adult hippocampal neurogenesis. J Comp Neurol. 425(4):479-494.
[14] Argandona EG, Bengoetxea H, Lafuente JV (2005) Lack of experience-mediated differences in the immunohistochemical expression of blood-brain barrier markers (EBA and GluT-1) during the postnatal development of the rat visual cortex. Brain Res Dev Brain Res. 156(2):158-166.
[15] Cassella JP, Lawrenson JG, Allt G, Firth JA (1996) Ontogeny of four blood-brain barrier markers: an immunocytochemical comparison of pial and cerebral cortical microvessels. J Anat. 189 (Pt 2):407-415.
[16] Lin B, Ginsberg MD (2000) Quantitative assessment of the normal cerebral microvasculature by endothelial barrier antigen (EBA) immunohistochemistry: application to focal cerebral ischemia. Brain Res. 865(2):237-244.
[17] Norsted E, Gomuc B, Meister B (2008) Protein components of the blood-brain barrier (BBB) in the mediobasal hypothalamus. J Chem Neuroanat. 36(2):107-121.
[18] Orte C, Lawrenson JG, Finn TM, Reid AR, Allt G (1999) A comparison of blood-brain barrier and blood-nerve barrier endothelial cell markers. Anat Embryol (Berl). 199(6):509-517.

[19] Gomez-Gonzalez B, Escobar A (2009) Altered functional development of the blood-brain barrier after early life stress in the rat. Brain Res Bull. 79(6):376-387.

[20] Gomez-Gonzalez B, Larios HM, Escobar A (2011) Increased transvascular transport of WGA-peroxidase after chronic perinatal stress in the hippocampal microvasculature of the rat. Int J Dev Neurosci. 29(8):839-846.

[21] Goritz C, Dias DO, Tomilin N, Barbacid M, Shupliakov O, Frisen J (2011) A pericyte origin of spinal cord scar tissue. Science. 333(6039):238-242.

[22] Hawkins BT, Davis TP (2005) The blood-brain barrier/neurovascular unit in health and disease. Pharmacol Rev. 57(2):173-185.

[23] Abbott NJ, Ronnback L, Hansson E (2006) Astrocyte-endothelial interactions at the blood-brain barrier. Nat Rev Neurosci. 7(1):41-53.

[24] Liebner S, Cavallaro U, Dejana E (2006) The multiple languages of endothelial cell-to-cell communication. Arterioscler Thromb Vasc Biol. 26(7):1431-1438.

[25] Prioreschi P (1996) Galenicae Quaestiones Disputatae Duae: rete mirabile and pulmonary circulation. Vesalius. 2(2):67-78.

[26] Viale G (2006) The rete mirabile of the cranial base: a millenary legend. Neurosurgery. 58(6):1198-1208; discussion 1198-1208.

[27] Argandona EG, Lafuente JV (2000) Influence of visual experience deprivation on the postnatal development of the microvascular bed in layer IV of the rat visual cortex. Brain Res. 855(1):137-142.

[28] Beauquis J, Roig P, De Nicola AF, Saravia F (2010) Short-term environmental enrichment enhances adult neurogenesis, vascular network and dendritic complexity in the hippocampus of type 1 diabetic mice. PLoS One. 5(11):e13993.

[29] Black JE, Sirevaag AM, Greenough WT (1987) Complex experience promotes capillary formation in young rat visual cortex. Neurosci Lett. 83(3):351-355.

[30] Michaloudi H, Grivas I, Batzios C, Chiotelli M, Papadopoulos GC (2005) Areal and laminar variations in the vascularity of the visual, auditory, and entorhinal cortices of the developing rat brain. Brain Res Dev Brain Res. 155(1):60-70.

[31] Mancuso MR, Kuhnert F, Kuo CJ (2008) Developmental angiogenesis of the central nervous system. Lymphat Res Biol. 6(3-4):173-180.

[32] Carmeliet P, Jain RK (2011) Principles and mechanisms of vessel normalization for cancer and other angiogenic diseases. Nat Rev Drug Discov. 10(6):417-427.

[33] Carmeliet P, Jain RK (2011) Molecular mechanisms and clinical applications of angiogenesis. Nature. 473(7347):298-307.

[34] Gerhardt H, Golding M, Fruttiger M, Ruhrberg C, Lundkvist A, Abramsson A, et al. (2003) VEGF guides angiogenic sprouting utilizing endothelial tip cell filopodia. J Cell Biol. 161(6):1163-1177.

[35] Tam SJ, Watts RJ (2010) Connecting vascular and nervous system development: angiogenesis and the blood-brain barrier. Annu Rev Neurosci. 33:379-408.

[36] Bar T (1980) The vascular system of the cerebral cortex. Adv Anat Embryol Cell Biol. 59:I-VI,1-62.

[37] Marin-Padilla M, Knopman DS (2011) Developmental aspects of the intracerebral microvasculature and perivascular spaces: insights into brain response to late-life diseases. J Neuropathol Exp Neurol. 70(12):1060-1069.

[38] Risau W (1997) Mechanisms of angiogenesis. Nature. 386(6626):671-674.

[39] Argandona EG, Bengoetxea H, Ortuzar N, Bulnes S, Rico-Barrio I, Lafuente JV (2012) Vascular endothelial growth factor: adaptive changes in the neuroglialvascular unit. Curr Neurovasc Res. 9(1):72-81.
[40] Fagiolini M, Pizzorusso T, Berardi N, Domenici L, Maffei L (1994) Functional postnatal development of the rat primary visual cortex and the role of visual experience: dark rearing and monocular deprivation. Vision Res. 34(6):709-720.
[41] Bengoetxea H, Argandona EG, Lafuente JV (2008) Effects of visual experience on vascular endothelial growth factor expression during the postnatal development of the rat visual cortex. Cereb Cortex. 18(7):1630-1639.
[42] Argandona EG, Bengoetxea H, Lafuente JV (2009) Physical exercise is required for environmental enrichment to offset the quantitative effects of dark-rearing on the S-100beta astrocytic density in the rat visual cortex. J Anat. 215(2):132-140.
[43] Argandoña EG, Rossi ML, Lafuente JV (2003) Visual deprivation effects on the s100beta positive astrocytic population in the developing rat visual cortex: a quantitative study. Brain Res Dev Brain Res. 141(1-2):63-69.
[44] Ranc V, Petruzziello F, Kretz R, Argandoña EG, Zhang X, Rainer G (2012) Broad characterization of endogenous peptides in the tree shrew visual system. J Proteomics.
[45] Busija DW (1994) Cerebral circulation of the fetus and newborn. RD Bevan, JA Bevan (Eds), The Human Brain Circulation, Humana Press, Totowa, NJ.259–270.
[46] Toga AW (1987) The metabolic consequence of visual deprivation in the rat. Brain Res. 465(1-2):209-217.
[47] Kennerley AJ, Harris S, Bruyns-Haylett M, Boorman L, Zheng Y, Jones M, et al. (2012) Early and late stimulus-evoked cortical hemodynamic responses provide insight into the neurogenic nature of neurovascular coupling. J Cereb Blood Flow Metab. 32(3):468-480.
[48] Ferrara N, Bunting S (1996) Vascular endothelial growth factor, a specific regulator of angiogenesis. Curr Opin Nephrol Hypertens. 5(1):35-44.
[49] Ferrara N, Davis-Smyth T (1997) The biology of vascular endothelial growth factor. Endocr Rev. 18(1):4-25.
[50] Ferrara N, Gerber HP (2001) The role of vascular endothelial growth factor in angiogenesis. Acta Haematol. 106(4):148-156.
[51] Ferrara N, Gerber HP, LeCouter J (2003) The biology of VEGF and its receptors. Nat Med. 9(6):669-676.
[52] Dvorak HF (2000) VPF/VEGF and the angiogenic response. Semin Perinatol. 24(1):75-78.
[53] Greenberg DA, Jin K (2005) From angiogenesis to neuropathology. Nature. 438(7070):954-959.
[54] Lafuente JV, Argandoña EG, Mitre B (2006) VEGFR-2 expression in brain injury: its distribution related to brain-blood barrier markers. J Neural Transm. 113(4):487-496.
[55] Marti HJ, Bernaudin M, Bellail A, Schoch H, Euler M, Petit E, et al. (2000) Hypoxia-induced vascular endothelial growth factor expression precedes neovascularization after cerebral ischemia. Am J Pathol. 156(3):965-976.
[56] Plate KH, Breier G, Weich HA, Risau W (1992) Vascular endothelial growth factor is a potential tumour angiogenesis factor in human gliomas in vivo. Nature. 359(6398):845-848.

[57] Ruiz de Almodovar C, Lambrechts D, Mazzone M, Carmeliet P (2009) Role and therapeutic potential of VEGF in the nervous system. Physiol Rev. 89(2):607-648.

[58] Nishikawa R, Cheng SY, Nagashima R, Huang HJ, Cavenee WK, Matsutani M (1998) Expression of vascular endothelial growth factor in human brain tumors. Acta Neuropathol. 96(5):453-462.

[59] Moser KV, Humpel C (2005) Vascular endothelial growth factor counteracts NMDA-induced cell death of adult cholinergic neurons in rat basal nucleus of Meynert. Brain Res Bull. 65(2):125-131.

[60] Robinson CJ, Stringer SE (2001) The splice variants of vascular endothelial growth factor (VEGF) and their receptors. J Cell Sci. 114(Pt 5):853-865.

[61] Geretti E, Shimizu A, Klagsbrun M (2008) Neuropilin structure governs VEGF and semaphorin binding and regulates angiogenesis. Angiogenesis. 11(1):31-39.

[62] Jin K, Mao XO, Batteur SP, McEachron E, Leahy A, Greenberg DA (2001) Caspase-3 and the regulation of hypoxic neuronal death by vascular endothelial growth factor. Neuroscience. 108(2):351-358.

[63] Jin KL, Mao XO, Greenberg DA (2000) Vascular endothelial growth factor: direct neuroprotective effect in in vitro ischemia. Proc Natl Acad Sci U S A. 97(18):10242-10247.

[64] Fischer S, Wobben M, Marti HH, Renz D, Schaper W (2002) Hypoxia-induced hyperpermeability in brain microvessel endothelial cells involves VEGF-mediated changes in the expression of zonula occludens-1. Microvasc Res. 63(1):70-80.

[65] Ortuzar N, Argandoña EG, Bengoetxea H, Leis O, Bulnes S, Lafuente JV (2010) Effects of VEGF administration or neutralization on the BBB of developing rat brain. Acta Neurochir Suppl. 106:55-59.

[66] Oosthuyse B, Moons L, Storkebaum E, Beck H, Nuyens D, Brusselmans K, et al. (2001) Deletion of the hypoxia-response element in the vascular endothelial growth factor promoter causes motor neuron degeneration. Nat Genet. 28(2):131-138.

[67] Ortuzar N, Argandoña EG, Bengoetxea H, Lafuente JV (2011) Combination of intracortically administered VEGF and environmental enrichment enhances brain protection in developing rats. J Neural Transm. 118(1):135-144.

[68] Storkebaum E, Lambrechts D, Carmeliet P (2004) VEGF: once regarded as a specific angiogenic factor, now implicated in neuroprotection. Bioessays. 26(9):943-954.

[69] Kaya D, Gursoy-Ozdemir Y, Yemisci M, Tuncer N, Aktan S, Dalkara T (2005) VEGF protects brain against focal ischemia without increasing blood--brain permeability when administered intracerebroventricularly. J Cereb Blood Flow Metab. 25(9):1111-1118.

[70] Wick A, Wick W, Waltenberger J, Weller M, Dichgans J, Schulz JB (2002) Neuroprotection by hypoxic preconditioning requires sequential activation of vascular endothelial growth factor receptor and Akt. J Neurosci. 22(15):6401-6407.

[71] Zacchigna S, Lambrechts D, Carmeliet P (2008) Neurovascular signalling defects in neurodegeneration. Nat Rev Neurosci. 9(3):169-181.

[72] Lafuente JV, Ortuzar N, Bengoetxea H, Bulnes S, Argandoña EG (2012) Vascular Endothelial Growth Factor and Other Angioglioneurins: Key Molecules in Brain Development and Restoration. International Review of Neurobiology. 102.

Chapter 13

Insights into Visual Cortex Plasticity: Interaction Between Genes and Sensory Experience

José Fernando Maya-Vetencourt and Matteo Caleo

Additional information is available at the end of the chapter

http://dx.doi.org/10.5772/50721

1. Introduction

The central nervous system architecture is highly dynamic and continuously modified by sensory experience through processes of neuronal plasticity. Interactions with the external world, mediated by sensory input, update and modify the structural and functional architecture of the nervous system, particularly during short-term sensitive periods in early life (critical period (CP) for brain plasticity) during which experience drives the consolidation of synaptic circuitries (Katz & Shatz 1996; Berardi et al., 2000; Levelt & Hubener 2012). However, experience-dependent reorganization of neuronal circuitries continues in adult life, at least to some extent.

The visual cortex (VC) is a classical model to examine the influence of sensory experience on brain structure and function. Early electrophysiological studies demonstrated that occlusion of one eye (monocular deprivation, MD) during the CP leads to an ocular dominance (OD) shift of visual cortical neurons, i.e., a decrease in the number of cells responding to the deprived eye that is accompanied by an increment of cells driven by the open eye (Wiesel & Hubel 1963; Hubel & Wiesel 1970; Frenkel & Bear 2004). In addition, the deprived eye becomes amblyopic: its spatial acuity and contrast sensitivity are markedly impaired. At structural level, unilateral eyelid suture causes a reduction in the arborisation of geniculocortical terminals that serve the deprived eye, which parallels an increased spread of terminals serving the open eye (Antonini & Stryker 1993). Because MD does not cause amblyopia in adult life this is a typical example of a CP. These findings highlight the notion that sensory experience is critical for normal development of the nervous system.

The importance of sensory experience in development of the human brain is well exemplified by cases of strabismic or anisometric children that underwent no clinical treatment during early development. In either pathological condition proper visual experience is altered, causing a marked impairment of normal visual functions (amblyopia) that is irreversible if not treated before 8 years of age (Holmes & Clarke 2006; Friedman et al., 2009; Maurer & Hensch 2012). A similar phenomenon is described by clinical observations of children born with congenital cataracts, a pathological condition in which the lens of the eye becomes milky and therefore no longer permits images to form on the retina (Lloyd et al., 2007; Milazzo et al., 2011). The recovery of normal visual functions after long-term sensory deprivation has long been a subject of study with the prospect of finding therapies for human amblyopia. Although amblyopia can be prevented by different strategies that restore the formation of proper retinal images or by eye patching in early life, such treatments are normally ineffective in adulthood. These observations indicate that proper sensory experience during early stages of development is necessary for normal visual perception and also point towards the enhancement of neuronal plasticity as a strategy for brain repair in adult life.

2. Sensory experience triggers the maturation of inhibitory circuitries that control the time-course of the CP

Among the different factors that regulate the CP for VC plasticity, inhibitory processes seem to play a critical role. Visual experience seems to signal the time-course of the CP by promoting the transfer of the protein Otx2 from the retina to the VC, where Otx2 gradually promotes the maturation of parvalbumin-positive GABAergic interneurons (Sugiyama et al., 2008). An initial threshold of inhibition then triggers the CP in which neural networks are highly susceptible to sensory experience (Hensch et al., 1998; Fagiolini & Hensch 2000), while a second inhibitory threshold signals the end of this phase of enhanced plasticity (Huang et al., 1999). A direct demonstration that GABAergic inhibition is a crucial brake limiting VC plasticity derives from the recent observation that a pharmacological reduction of inhibitory transmission effectively restores OD plasticity in adulthood (Harauzov et al., 2010). This is consistent with the fact that experimental paradigms such as dark exposure (He et al., 2006), environmental enrichment (Baroncelli et al., 2010; Sale et al., 2010), food restriction (Spolidoro et al., 2011), long-term fluoxetine (FLX) administration (Maya-Vetencourt et al., 2008; Chen et al., 2011; Maya-Vetencourt et al., 2011), and exogenous IGF-I administration (Maya-Vetencourt et al., 2012), all promote plasticity late in life by reducing the intracortical inhibitory/excitatory (I/E) ratio. This has prompted the search for endogenous factors with the potential to enhance plasticity in adult life by modulating the intracortical I/E balance.

3. Long-distance projection systems regulate plasticity in the visual system

The major modulatory systems in the brain (i.e., noradrenaline, dopamine, histamine, acetylcholine, serotonin) regulate complex functions of the central nervous system such as cognition, behaviour, and neuronal plasticity. Experience-dependent modifications of cortical circuitries are not determined solely by local correlations of electrical activity but are also influenced by attentional mechanisms (Singer 1995). Sensory signals, for instance, promote marked modifications of neural circuitries only when animals attend to the sensory input and use this information for the control of behaviour (Singer 1990, 1995). Early studies performed in cats demonstrated that changes of visual cortical circuitries in response to experience during early life, are lessened when noradrenergic (Kasamatsu & Pettigrew 1979; Bear & Singer 1986), cholinergic (Gu & Singer 1993) and serotonergic (Gu & Singer 1995; Wang et al., 1997) projections to the cortex are inactivated. Moreover, there is evidence that these neuromodulatory systems mediate forms of plasticity in the adult visual system of cats (Pettigrew & Kasamatsu 1978; Kasamatsu et al., 1979; Kasamatsu et al., 1985; Imamura & Kasamatsu 1991; Mataga et al., 1992) and rodents (Maya-Vetencourt et al., 2008; Baroncelli et al., 2010; Maya-Vetencourt et al., 2011).

Advances in the understanding of mechanisms by which neuromodulatory systems modulate experience-dependent plasticity derive from *in vitro* studies of synaptic plasticity. There is ample evidence that noradrenaline, acetylcholine and serotonin modulate two different forms of activity-dependent synaptic modifications: long-term potentiation (LTP) and long-term depression (LTD) (Kirkwood 2000). In the visual system, LTP and LTD can be induced by different patterns of electrical stimulation. Brief and strong episodes of high frequency stimulation promote LTP while prolonged low-frequency stimulation yields LTD. In the rodent VC, upon administration of noradrenaline and acetylcholine, weaker tetanic stimulation is required to induce LTP and shorter episodes of low frequency stimulation are needed to drive LTD (Brocher et al., 1992; Kirkwood et al., 1999). Likewise, serotonin facilitates the induction of both LTP and LTD in layer IV of the kitten VC (Kojic et al., 1997). Taken together, these findings are consistent with a role for neuromodulatory systems as enabling factors for visual cortical plasticity and indicate that activation of noradrenergic, cholinergic, and serotonergic receptors lowers the threshold of activity required for the induction of LTP and LTD. Intracellular mechanisms whereby neuromodulatory systems facilitate these forms of synaptic plasticity have been subject of extensive study. In the VC, the induction of LTP and LTD requires the activation of N-methyl-D-aspartate (NMDA) receptors together with a postsynaptic rise in intracellular calcium. The available evidence is consistent with a model in which the magnitude and duration of the calcium signal determines the magnitude of the synaptic modification (Bear 1996). Brief and large calcium influxes induce LTP, whereas smaller and prolonged calcium increases yield LTD. Of note, receptors of these three major neuromodulatory systems are able to activate the IP3 second messenger pathway, which can induce calcium release from intracellular stores and therefore modulate plasticity.

Because the intracortical inhibitory/excitatory (I/E) ratio is critical for the induction of neuronal plasticity in the visual system (Jiang et al., 2005; Sale et al., 2010), the neuromodulators-mediated fine-tuning of the I/E balance may also play a critical role for the induction of experience-dependent plasticity. In line with this, the enhanced action of serotonin and/or acetylcholine decreases the intracortical I/E balance in the rodent visual system (Amar et al., 2010; Moreau et al., 2010).

4. Non-visual components of the environment alter visual system development

In addition to MD, another classical paradigm used to assess the impact of experience in the functional maturation of the visual system is dark rearing (i.e., rearing animals in total darkness from birth). When dark-reared animals are brought back into the light, they turn out to be blind or, at least, display marked impairments of normal visual functions (Fagiolini et al., 1994). Total absence of visual experience delays the functional maturation of the striate cortex; an event that seems to be mediated by a down-regulation of BDNF expression (Castren et al., 1992), which results in a retarded maturation of GABAergic circuitries (Morales et al., 2002). The spatial resolution of visual cortical neurons is, in fact, reduced in dark-reared animals, this phenomenon being accompanied by longer latencies of responses to visual stimuli (Blakemore & Price 1987; Fagiolini et al., 1994). Moreover, visual cortical neurons have larger receptive field sizes and show alterations in the density of dendritic spines, which are shorter and fewer in dark-reared animals as compared to normally reared counterparts (Wallace & Bear 2004). Noteworthy, rearing animals in complete darkness extents the critical period far beyond its normal limits (Hensch 2005).

Although early studies of the visual system showed that sensory experience after eye opening is necessary for the functional maturation of the VC (Wiesel & Hubel 1963, 1963; Hubel & Wiesel 1970; LeVay et al., 1980), the notion that non-visual components of the environment can influence the structural and functional development of the visual system has been increasingly appreciated in the last few years. Experiments in dark-reared transgenic mice overexpressing BDNF, revealed a remarkable and unexpected finding: visual cortical neurons in these animals responded normally to visual stimuli, indicating that transgenic animals could see well despite the lack of visual experience during the CP (Gianfranceschi et al., 2003). This result was the first demonstration of a gene that could substitute for functional aspects caused by experience in the nervous system. These observations are in consonance with the fact that environmental enrichment, an experimental condition characterized by an increased exploratory behavior and sensory-motor stimulation, which increases BDNF signaling and enhances GABAergic inhibition during early stages of development, prevents the effects of dark rearing in the visual system (Bartoletti et al., 2004). Of note, environmental enrichment in normally reared animals accelerates the functional development of the VC, this phenomenon being accompanied by alterations in the expression of BDNF and GABA synthesizing enzymes well before eye opening (Cancedda et al., 2004). These findings further suggest that environmental influences on visual system development may be, at least in part, independent of visual experience.

5. Inter-hemispheric projections control visual cortical maturation and plasticity

Recent studies in the rodent VC have demonstrated a key role for inter-hemispheric, transcallosal projections in processes of visual cortical development and plasticity. In rodents, as in other mammals, callosal terminals are particularly concentrated in the area of primary VC mapping the central part of the visual field (Mizuno et al., 2007), thus contributing to binding together the two representations of the visual hemifields in the two hemispheres. A crucial role for callosal input activity in the functional maturation of the VC was indicated by experiments in which activity was unilaterally blocked in the striate cortex during the CP. Transient blockade of synaptic activity arrested maturation of visual acuity not only in the treated, but also in the contralateral hemisphere (Caleo et al., 2007). The CP for plasticity was also extended in both hemispheres (Caleo et al., 2007). These findings indicate that maturation of the blocked cortex is superimposable to that of the opposite side. Since the contralateral hemisphere maintains normal vision through the retinogeniculate pathway and only lacks callosal input, these data point towards a fundamental role for callosal linkages in regulating the process of cortical maturation. Similar conclusions have been drawn from experiments in knockout mice with reduced callosal connectivity; when tested as adults, these animals display a reduced visual acuity and a persistent OD plasticity (Pinto et al., 2009). The notion that inter-hemispheric callosal projections play a key role in the maturation of visual functions is exemplified by experimental observations in cats and humans. Early sections of the callosum in kittens, indeed, cause a reduction in the behavioural measure of visual acuity (Elberger 1984). Consistently, patients with hemianopia show impairments in figure detection tasks also in the intact hemifield, suggesting that these deficits may be caused by the loss of inter-hemispheric interactions (Paramei & Sabel 2008).

Other studies have indicated a role for the callosum in determining both normal binocularity and the shift of OD that follows a period of monocular eyelid suture in juvenile rats. In rodents, retinogeniculate afferent input to the cortex from the contralateral eye is much stronger than that from the ipsilateral eye. Indeed, over 95% of retinal fibers decussate at the chiasm. However, cells mapping the central part of the visual field are highly binocular, and experiments support the view that callosal afferents contribute to this binocularity by providing input from the ipsilateral eye. In particular, acute inactivation of transcallosal input activity in rats shifts OD towards the contralateral eye (Diao et al., 1983), due to a loss of ipsilateral eye responses (Restani et al., 2009). In a complementary experiment, binocularity was recorded before and after acute inactivation of thalamocortical input to isolate visual responses driven exclusively by callosal afferents in young rats (Cerri et al., 2010). After blockade of the ipsilateral thalamus, cortical neurons display a dramatic loss of contralateral eye driven responses, while ipsilateral eye driven responses are reduced to a less extent (Cerri et al., 2010). These experiments indicate that in rats, a substantial fraction of the influence of the ipsilateral eye on cortical responses arrives via callosal connections from the opposite hemisphere, where it is the dominant eye.

Not only normal binocularity, but also the shift of OD that follows MD appears to depend on the function of callosal fibers. In particular, acute inactivation of transcallosal input activity restores binocularity after MD in juvenile rats (Restani et al., 2009). This recovery of binocularity following callosal silencing is due to an unexpected and selective increase in the strength of the deprived eye. Thus, acute removal of callosal influence following MD unmasks deprived eye inputs. These data highlight the notion that callosal afferents act primarily to inhibit closed eye inputs during visual deprivation (Restani et al., 2009).

6. Structural plasticity in the visual system

Experience-dependent functional modifications in the visual system are accompanied by a structural remodeling of synaptic connectivity, in terms of growth and loss of dendritic spines. Dendritic spines in pyramidal neurons are markedly sensitive to experience as indicated by the observation that total lack of visual experience in early life induces modifications in spine morphology and density, both of which are partially reversible by light exposure (Wallace & Bear 2004). This is consistent with the observation that monocular deprivation in early life alters the motility, turnover, number and morphology of dendritic spines in the VC (Majewska & Sur 2003; Mataga et al., 2004; Hofer et al., 2009; Tropea et al., 2010).

Structural plasticity *in vivo* studies, using two-photon imaging, indicate that dendritic spine dynamics is high during early postnatal life but decreases thereafter, in parallel to the time-course of CP plasticity over development (Fu & Zuo 2011). This suggests that, despite the absence of large-scale remodeling of dendrites, the reorganization of cortical connections in terms of growth and loss of dendritic spines may be the structural substrate for experience-dependent plasticity. Notably, chronic imaging experiments have recently demonstrated that changes in VC responsiveness after monocular deprivation during the CP correlate with structural modifications in terms of dendritic spines across the binocular VC; these two features being reversed when the deprived eye was reopened. After brief periods of MD, spine turnover increased significantly, with a larger percentage of spines being lost rather than gained, whereas after a 24-hours period of recovery (visual experience) the baseline number of dendritic spines was gained again (Yu et al., 2011). Interestingly, increasing the density and dynamics of spines by intracortical infusion of the bacterial toxin CNF1, restores a degree of plasticity in the mature cortex that is similar to that observed during early postnatal life (Cerri et al., 2011).

It is worth mentioning that new synapses formation may increase memory storage capacity of the brain and that new dendritic spines may serve as structural traces for earlier memories, enabling the brain for faster adaptations to similar future experiences (Hofer et al., 2009; Xu et al., 2009). Recent experiments carried out using the MD paradigm seem to confirm this notion. Modifications of dendritic spines caused by a first experience of unilateral eyelid suture persist even after restoration of binocular vision and may therefore be involved in the enhancement of plasticity observed after a second episode of visual deprivation (Hofer et al., 2009).

The imaging studies mentioned above raise the question of whether structural modifications of dendritic spines represent functional changes of synaptic transmission. Electrophysiological experiments in hippocampal slice cultures indicate that AMPA- and NMDA-type glutamate receptor currents of newborn spines resemble that of mature synaptic contacts (Zito et al., 2009). Interestingly, it has been recently demonstrated that dendritic spine dynamics regulate the stability of synaptic plasticity. The relationship between Calcium influx and spine size actually determines the long-term synaptic stability and synaptic strength distribution, at least in synapses of hippocampal CA3-CA1 pyramidal neurons (O'Donnell et al., 2011).

7. Epigenetics of visual cortex plasticity

Plasticity is achieved by a complex interplay of environmental influences and physiological mechanisms that ultimately set in motion intracellular signal transduction pathways directly regulating gene expression. Processes of chromatin remodeling that modulate gene transcription are, in fact, conserved mechanisms by which the mammalian's nervous system accomplishes adaptive behavioral responses upon environmental demands. In rodents, for instance, maternal care seems to influence behavioral and endocrine responses to stress in the offspring by modifying chromatin susceptibility to transcription (Francis et al., 1999).

The reorganization of cortical circuitries during early development requires the activation of sensory transduction pathways, which eventually mediate the expression of genes that act as downstream effectors of plastic phenomena. Studies performed in cats and rodents during the CP indicate that electrical activity and experience-dependent expression of neurotrophins cooperate to set in motion different protein kinases: extracellular-signal-regulated kinase (ERK1/2) (Di Cristo et al., 2001), cAMP-dependent protein kinase (PKA) (Beaver et al., 2001), and calclium/calmodulin-dependent protein kinase II (CaMKII) (Taha et al., 2002). The activation of these intracellular signal transduction pathways promotes the up-regulation of transcription factors that, in turn, mediate gene expression. A very well known activity-dependent mechanism is the activation of the transcription factor CREB, which triggers the expression of genes under control of the cAMP-response element (CRE) promoter, thus allowing phenomena of plasticity to occur (Pham et al., 1999). These findings are in consonance with the recent observation that visual experience during development promotes modifications of chromatin structure that are permissive for transcription, whereas a developmental down-regulation of histone post-translational modifications regulates the closure of the CP in the mouse visual system (Putignano et al., 2007).

In line with this notion, previous studies have demonstrated that the process of plasticity reactivation in the adult visual system is a multifactorial event that comprises the action of different cellular and molecular mechanisms, working in parallel or in series, the sum of which results in the activation of intracellular signal transduction pathways regulating the expression of plasticity genes (Putignano et al., 2007; Maya-Vetencourt et al., 2008; Bavelier et al., 2010; Morishita et al., 2010; Silingardi et al., 2010; Maya-Vetencourt et al., 2011; Maya-Vetencourt et al., 2012). Experimental paradigms based upon the manipulation of environmental stimulation levels, genetic manipulations, and pharmacological treatments in rodents have revealed that a complex interplay between the enhanced action of long-distance projection systems (e.g., serotonergic and cholinergic transmission) and IGF-I signaling seems to modulate the intracortical inhibitory/excitatory balance in favour of excitation (Amar et al., 2010; Moreau et al., 2010; Maya-Vetencourt et al., 2012), which, in turn, set in motion cellular and molecular events that eventually mediate the expression of genes associated with functional modifications in the adult visual system. The reinstatement of adult VC plasticity caused by serotonergic transmission, for instance, is mediated by 5-HT1A receptors signaling and accompanied by a transitory increment of BDNF expression. This is paralleled by an enhanced histone acetylation status at the activity-dependently regulated BDNF promoter regions and by a decreased expression of histone deacetylase enzymes (HDACs) (Maya-Vetencourt et al., 2011). In keeping with this, long-term treatment with HDACs inhibitors (e.g., Trichostatin-A, Valproic Acid and Sodium Butyrate) not only reinstates OD plasticity in adulthood (Putignano et al., 2007; Maya-Vetencourt et al., 2011) but also promotes full recovery of visual functions in adult amblyopic animals (Silingardi et al., 2010).

8. Cross-modal plasticity: Adaptive reorganization of neural networks

Sensory deprivation in one modality during early stages of development can have marked effects on the development of the remaining modalities. This phenomenon is known as cross-modal plasticity and is particularly epitomized by cases of congenital blindness or deafness from birth. In such instances, processes of cross-modal plasticity strengthen other sensory systems to compensate for the lack of vision or hearing.

Although clinical studies of deaf and blind humans have clearly demonstrated increased functional capabilities and compensatory expansion in the remaining sensory modalities (Bavelier & Neville 2002), the neurological bases for these plastic phenomena remain poorly understood. It has been reported that congenitally blind subjects show better sound localization abilities as compared to sighted individuals (Roder et al., 1999) and display better two-point tactile discrimination skills as well (Bavelier & Neville 2002). Moreover, studies that combine Braille reading and functional brain imaging revealed that early blind individuals show a strong activation of the primary VC during the Braille reading task (Sadato et al., 1996). Remarkably, the inactivation of the VC by means of transcranial electrical stimulation in blind people during Braille reading not only distorts tactile perceptions of blind subjects but also induces errors in Braille reading. These findings indicate that the VC seems to be recruited to process somatosensory information after congenital blindness (Cohen et al., 1997). Recent experimental evidence also suggests that congenital blindness enables visual circuitries to contribute to language processing (Bedny et al., 2011).

The question of whether there is a CP for cross-modal plasticity has also been addressed by examining the activation of visual cortical areas by Braille reading in early and late-onset blind individuals (blindness after 14 years of age). It has been reported that VC responsiveness to somatosensory stimuli is higher in congenitally blind and early-onset subjects as compared to the late-onset blind group (Cohen et al., 1999). These data indicate that there is a CP for the visual system to be recruited to a role in the processing of somatosensory information, which does not extend beyond 14 years of age in humans.

Phenomena of cross-modal plasticity have also been observed in the brain of deaf subjects. Functional magnetic resonance imaging studies have demonstrated that early deaf individuals use the primary auditory cortex alongside the visual system when they observe sign language (Lambertz et al., 2005). Although there is no hearing component to sign language, the auditory cortex is instead used to assist with visual and language processing. The effects of cochlear implants also provide another strategy to assess cross-modal plasticity in the deaf. Early deaf individuals, but not late-onset deaf subjects, actually display impairments in their ability to process language using a cochlear implant in adult life as the auditory cortex has been reshaped to deal with visual information and therefore it cannot deal as well with the new sensory input that the implant provides (Doucet et al., 2006).

There is evidence for potent cross-modal plastic interactions even during normal development. A recent series of experiments have demonstrated that enhancement of somatosensory stimulation in terms of body massage, affects development of another sensory modality, the visual system (Guzzetta et al., 2009). It has been reported that an enriched environment accelerates the structural and functional development of the rodent VC (Cancedda et al., 2004) and that enriching the environment in terms of tactile stimulation (body massage with a soft toothbrush) in rat pups effectively mimics the effects of enrichment on visual system development (Guzzetta et al., 2009). The massage protocol in the offspring of rats accelerated the maturation of visual functions and increased circulating levels of insulin-like growth factor 1 (IGF-I), whereas antagonizing IGF-I signaling by systemic injections of an IGF-I receptor antagonist prevented the effects of massage (Guzzetta et al., 2009). In keeping with this, enriching the environment in terms of body massage in human preterm infants accelerates the maturation of the visual system as indicated by an enhanced development of spatial acuity and, as in the offspring of rats, this phenomenon is accompanied by high IGF-I levels (Guzzetta et al., 2009). Taken together, these findings indicate that processes of cross-modal plasticity may be involved in the effects caused by environmental enrichment in VC development and portray the well-characterized visual system as a model to investigate the functional integration of two or more sensory modalities.

9. Achieving the recovery of sensory functions after long-term sensory deprivation

The recovery of normal visual functions after long-term sensory deprivation has long been a subject of study with the prospect of finding therapies for human amblyopia. In this context, perceptual learning has long been used to improve spatial acuity in adult amblyopic patients (Levi & Li 2009). Systematic training of patients with unilateral amblyopia (secondary to strabismus and anisometropia) in simple visual tasks revealed a 2-fold increase of contrast sensitivity and improved performance in letter-recognition tests (Polat et al., 2004). Likewise, Snellen acuities in anisometric amblyopes improved after intensive training in a Vernier acuity task. Moreover, video game playing appears to promote a significant rescue of visual functions in adult amblyopic patients. Playing video games for a short period of time using the amblyopic eye actually improves visual functions such as spatial acuity and stereopsis (Li et al., 2011). The improvement of performance seen in perceptual learning is proportional to the number of trials taken, although performance eventually reaches an asymptote with no further progress (Huang et al., 2008). Unfortunately, the extent to which acuity improvements occur is limited by the task specificity of perceptual learning (Crist et al., 1997). In most instances of perceptual learning, attention to the trained stimulus is necessary for improvements of vision to occur (Ahissar & Hochstein 1993). This observation is particularly important as it epitomizes the role of diffuse projection systems in the physiological state of arousal, which regulates mechanisms of attention and information processing that may contribute to functional changes of neural circuitries in the adult brain. Such notion points toward the possibility to pharmacologically enhance plasticity as a strategy for brain repair, which could facilitate restructuring of mature circuitries impaired by damage or disease.

10. Conclusion

The ability of the brain to change functionally in response to experience is most active during early stages of development but it decreases later in life when major alterations in neuronal network structures no longer take place in response to experience. For decades it has been believed that the plastic potential of the adult nervous system is insufficient to allow the recovery of lost sensory functions following long-term deprivation. Therefore, treatments for human amblyopia were generally not undertaken in older children and adults. However, novel experimental data obtained in animal models have demonstrated the effectiveness of different pharmacological treatments and experimental paradigms based upon manipulation of environmental input levels in restoring plasticity to the adult nervous system. In light of these findings, one can speculate that the beneficial effects exerted by these treatments could be exploited for clinical application. Since deterioration in functional plasticity contributes to the pathogenesis of several brain diseases, environmental enrichment (Baroncelli et al., 2010), food restriction (Spolidoro et al., 2011), brief dark exposure (He et al., 2006), long-term fluoxetine treatment (Maya-Vetencourt et al., 2008; Chen et al., 2011; Maya-Vetencourt et al., 2011) and exogenous IGF-I administration (Maya-Vetencourt et al., 2012), all of which reactivate adult brain plasticity, arise as potential therapeutic strategies for pathological conditions, such as human amblyopia, in which reorganization of neural circuitries would be beneficial in adult life. These therapeutic approaches bear some similarity to the interventions that have proved successful in promoting recovery from other pathological conditions such as stroke (Maurer & Hensch 2012). Fluoxetine treatment, indeed, enhances the effects of rehabilitation in the recovery from motor deficits after ischaemic stroke in humans (Chollet et al., 2011).

Author details

José Fernando Maya-Vetencourt *

Scuola Normale Superiore, Pisa, Italy

* Corresponding Author

Matteo Caleo
CNR Neuroscience Institute, Pisa, Italy

Acknowledgement

J.F.M.V. is supported by a research fellowship provided by the Scuola Normale Superiore, Pisa, Italy.

11. References

Ahissar, M. and Hochstein, S. (1993). Attentional control of early perceptual learning. *Proc Natl Acad Sci U S A,* Vol. 90, No. 12, pp. 5718-5722.

Amar, M., Lucas-Meunier, E., Baux, G. and Fossier, P. (2010). Blockade of different muscarinic receptor subtypes changes the equilibrium between excitation and inhibition in rat visual cortex. *Neuroscience,* Vol. 169, No. 4, pp. 1610-1620.

Antonini, A. and Stryker, M.P. (1993). Rapid remodeling of axonal arbors in the visual cortex. *Science,* Vol. 260, No. 5115, pp. 1819-1821.

Baroncelli, L., Sale, A., Viegi, A., Maya-Vetencourt, J.F., De Pasquale, R., Baldini, S. and Maffei, L. (2010). Experience-dependent reactivation of ocular dominance plasticity in the adult visual cortex. *Exp Neurol,* Vol. 226, No. 1, pp. 100-109.

Bartoletti, A., Medini, P., Berardi, N. and Maffei, L. (2004). Environmental enrichment prevents effects of dark-rearing in the rat visual cortex. *Nat Neurosci,* Vol. 7, No. 3, pp. 215-216.

Bavelier, D., Levi, D.M., Li, R.W., Dan, Y. and Hensch, T.K. (2010). Removing brakes on adult brain plasticity: from molecular to behavioral interventions. *J Neurosci,* Vol. 30, No. 45, pp. 14964-14971.

Bavelier, D. and Neville, H.J. (2002). Cross-modal plasticity: where and how? *Nat Rev Neurosci,* Vol. 3, No. 6, pp. 443-452.

Bear, M.F. (1996). NMDA-receptor-dependent synaptic plasticity in the visual cortex. *Prog Brain Res,* Vol. 108, No. pp. 205-218.

Bear, M.F. and Singer, W. (1986). Modulation of visual cortical plasticity by acetylcholine and noradrenaline. *Nature,* Vol. 320, No. 6058, pp. 172-176.

Beaver, C.J., Ji, Q., Fischer, Q.S. and Daw, N.W. (2001). Cyclic AMP-dependent protein kinase mediates ocular dominance shifts in cat visual cortex. *Nat Neurosci,* Vol. 4, No. 2, pp. 159-163.

Bedny, M., Pascual-Leone, A., Dodell-Feder, D., Fedorenko, E. and Saxe, R. (2011). Language processing in the occipital cortex of congenitally blind adults. *Proc Natl Acad Sci U S A,* Vol. 108, No. 11, pp. 4429-4434.

Berardi, N., Pizzorusso, T. and Maffei, L. (2000). Critical periods during sensory development. *Curr Opin Neurobiol,* Vol. 10, No. 1, pp. 138-145.

Blakemore, C. and Price, D.J. (1987). Effects of dark-rearing on the development of area 18 of the cat's visual cortex. *J Physiol,* Vol. 384, No. pp. 293-309.

Brocher, S., Artola, A. and Singer, W. (1992). Agonists of cholinergic and noradrenergic receptors facilitate synergistically the induction of long-term potentiation in slices of rat visual cortex. *Brain Res,* Vol. 573, No. 1, pp. 27-36.

Caleo, M., Restani, L., Gianfranceschi, L., Costantin, L., Rossi, C., Rossetto, O., Montecucco, C. and Maffei, L. (2007). Transient synaptic silencing of developing striate cortex has persistent effects on visual function and plasticity. *J Neurosci,* Vol. 27, No. 17, pp. 4530-4540.

Cancedda, L., Putignano, E., Sale, A., Viegi, A., Berardi, N. and Maffei, L. (2004). Acceleration of visual system development by environmental enrichment. *J Neurosci,* Vol. 24, No. 20, pp. 4840-4848.

Castren, E., Zafra, F., Thoenen, H. and Lindholm, D. (1992). Light regulates expression of brain-derived neurotrophic factor mRNA in rat visual cortex. *Proc Natl Acad Sci U S A,* Vol. 89, No. 20, pp. 9444-9448.

Cerri, C., Fabbri, A., Vannini, E., Spolidoro, M., Costa, M., Maffei, L., Fiorentini, C. and Caleo, M. (2011). Activation of Rho GTPases triggers structural remodeling and functional plasticity in the adult rat visual cortex. *J Neurosci,* Vol. 31, No. 42, pp. 15163-15172.

Cerri, C., Restani, L. and Caleo, M. (2010). Callosal contribution to ocular dominance in rat primary visual cortex. *Eur J Neurosci,* Vol. 32, No. 7, pp. 1163-1169.

Chen, J.L., Lin, W.C., Cha, J.W., So, P.T., Kubota, Y. and Nedivi, E. (2011). Structural basis for the role of inhibition in facilitating adult brain plasticity. *Nat Neurosci,* Vol. 14, No. 5, pp. 587-594.

Chollet, F., Tardy, J., Albucher, J.F., Thalamas, C., Berard, E., Lamy, C., Bejot, Y., Deltour, S., Jaillard, A., Niclot, P., Guillon, B., Moulin, T., Marque, P., Pariente, J., Arnaud, C. and Loubinoux, I. (2011). Fluoxetine for motor recovery after acute ischaemic stroke (FLAME): a randomised placebo-controlled trial. *Lancet Neurol,* Vol. 10, No. 2, pp. 123-130.

Cohen, L.G., Celnik, P., Pascual-Leone, A., Corwell, B., Falz, L., Dambrosia, J., Honda, M., Sadato, N., Gerloff, C., Catala, M.D. and Hallett, M. (1997). Functional relevance of cross-modal plasticity in blind humans. *Nature,* Vol. 389, No. 6647, pp. 180-183.

Cohen, L.G., Weeks, R.A., Sadato, N., Celnik, P., Ishii, K. and Hallett, M. (1999). Period of susceptibility for cross-modal plasticity in the blind. *Ann Neurol,* Vol. 45, No. 4, pp. 451-460.

Crist, R.E., Kapadia, M.K., Westheimer, G. and Gilbert, C.D. (1997). Perceptual learning of spatial localization: specificity for orientation, position, and context. *J Neurophysiol,* Vol. 78, No. 6, pp. 2889-2894.

Di Cristo, G., Berardi, N., Cancedda, L., Pizzorusso, T., Putignano, E., Ratto, G.M. and Maffei, L. (2001). Requirement of ERK activation for visual cortical plasticity. *Science,* Vol. 292, No. 5525, pp. 2337-2340.

Diao, Y.C., Wang, Y.K. and Pu, M.L. (1983). Binocular responses of cortical cells and the callosal projection in the albino rat. *Exp Brain Res,* Vol. 49, No. 3, pp. 410-418.

Doucet, M.E., Bergeron, F., Lassonde, M., Ferron, P. and Lepore, F. (2006). Cross-modal reorganization and speech perception in cochlear implant users. *Brain,* Vol. 129, No. Pt 12, pp. 3376-3383.

Elberger, A.J. (1984). The existence of a separate, brief critical period for the corpus callosum to affect visual development. *Behav Brain Res,* Vol. 11, No. 3, pp. 223-231.

Fagiolini, M. and Hensch, T.K. (2000). Inhibitory threshold for critical-period activation in primary visual cortex. *Nature,* Vol. 404, No. 6774, pp. 183-186.

Fagiolini, M., Pizzorusso, T., Berardi, N., Domenici, L. and Maffei, L. (1994). Functional postnatal development of the rat primary visual cortex and the role of visual experience: dark rearing and monocular deprivation. *Vision Res,* Vol. 34, No. 6, pp. 709-720.

Francis, D., Diorio, J., Liu, D. and Meaney, M.J. (1999). Nongenomic transmission across generations of maternal behavior and stress responses in the rat. *Science,* Vol. 286, No. 5442, pp. 1155-1158.

Frenkel, M.Y. and Bear, M.F. (2004). How monocular deprivation shifts ocular dominance in visual cortex of young mice. *Neuron,* Vol. 44, No. 6, pp. 917-923.

Friedman, D.S., Repka, M.X., Katz, J., Giordano, L., Ibironke, J., Hawse, P. and Tielsch, J.M. (2009). Prevalence of amblyopia and strabismus in white and African American children aged 6 through 71 months the Baltimore Pediatric Eye Disease Study. *Ophthalmology,* Vol. 116, No. 11, pp. 2128-2134 e2121-2122.

Fu, M. and Zuo, Y. (2011). Experience-dependent structural plasticity in the cortex. *Trends Neurosci,* Vol. 34, No. 4, pp. 177-187.

Gianfranceschi, L., Siciliano, R., Walls, J., Morales, B., Kirkwood, A., Huang, Z.J., Tonegawa, S. and Maffei, L. (2003). Visual cortex is rescued from the effects of dark rearing by overexpression of BDNF. *Proc Natl Acad Sci U S A,* Vol. 100, No. 21, pp. 12486-12491.

Gu, Q. and Singer, W. (1993). Effects of intracortical infusion of anticholinergic drugs on neuronal plasticity in kitten striate cortex. *Eur J Neurosci,* Vol. 5, No. 5, pp. 475-485.

Gu, Q. and Singer, W. (1995). Involvement of serotonin in developmental plasticity of kitten visual cortex. *Eur J Neurosci,* Vol. 7, No. 6, pp. 1146-1153.

Guzzetta, A., Baldini, S., Bancale, A., Baroncelli, L., Ciucci, F., Ghirri, P., Putignano, E., Sale, A., Viegi, A., Berardi, N., Boldrini, A., Cioni, G. and Maffei, L. (2009). Massage accelerates brain development and the maturation of visual function. *J Neurosci,* Vol. 29, No. 18, pp. 6042-6051.

Harauzov, A., Spolidoro, M., DiCristo, G., De Pasquale, R., Cancedda, L., Pizzorusso, T., Viegi, A., Berardi, N. and Maffei, L. (2010). Reducing intracortical inhibition in the adult visual cortex promotes ocular dominance plasticity. *J Neurosci,* Vol. 30, No. 1, pp. 361-371.

He, H.Y., Hodos, W. and Quinlan, E.M. (2006). Visual deprivation reactivates rapid ocular dominance plasticity in adult visual cortex. *J Neurosci,* Vol. 26, No. 11, pp. 2951-2955.

Hensch, T.K. (2005). Critical period plasticity in local cortical circuits. *Nat Rev Neurosci,* Vol. 6, No. 11, pp. 877-888.

Hensch, T.K., Fagiolini, M., Mataga, N., Stryker, M.P., Baekkeskov, S. and Kash, S.F. (1998). Local GABA circuit control of experience-dependent plasticity in developing visual cortex. *Science,* Vol. 282, No. 5393, pp. 1504-1508.

Hofer, S.B., Mrsic-Flogel, T.D., Bonhoeffer, T. and Hubener, M. (2009). Experience leaves a lasting structural trace in cortical circuits. *Nature,* Vol. 457, No. 7227, pp. 313-317.

Holmes, J.M. and Clarke, M.P. (2006). Amblyopia. *Lancet,* Vol. 367, No. 9519, pp. 1343-1351.

Huang, C.B., Zhou, Y. and Lu, Z.L. (2008). Broad bandwidth of perceptual learning in the visual system of adults with anisometropic amblyopia. *Proc Natl Acad Sci U S A,* Vol. 105, No. 10, pp. 4068-4073.

Huang, Z.J., Kirkwood, A., Pizzorusso, T., Porciatti, V., Morales, B., Bear, M.F., Maffei, L. and Tonegawa, S. (1999). BDNF regulates the maturation of inhibition and the critical period of plasticity in mouse visual cortex. *Cell,* Vol. 98, No. 6, pp. 739-755.

Hubel, D.H. and Wiesel, T.N. (1970). The period of susceptibility to the physiological effects of unilateral eye closure in kittens. *J Physiol,* Vol. 206, No. 2, pp. 419-436.

Imamura, K. and Kasamatsu, T. (1991). Ocular dominance plasticity restored by NA infusion to aplastic visual cortex of anesthetized and paralyzed kittens. *Exp Brain Res,* Vol. 87, No. 2, pp. 309-318.

Jiang, B., Huang, Z.J., Morales, B. and Kirkwood, A. (2005). Maturation of GABAergic transmission and the timing of plasticity in visual cortex. *Brain Res Brain Res Rev,* Vol. 50, No. 1, pp. 126-133.

Kasamatsu, T. and Pettigrew, J.D. (1979). Preservation of binocularity after monocular deprivation in the striate cortex of kittens treated with 6-hydroxydopamine. *J Comp Neurol,* Vol. 185, No. 1, pp. 139-161.

Kasamatsu, T., Pettigrew, J.D. and Ary, M. (1979). Restoration of visual cortical plasticity by local microperfusion of norepinephrine. *J Comp Neurol,* Vol. 185, No. 1, pp. 163-181.

Kasamatsu, T., Watabe, K., Heggelund, P. and Scholler, E. (1985). Plasticity in cat visual cortex restored by electrical stimulation of the locus coeruleus. *Neurosci Res,* Vol. 2, No. 5, pp. 365-386.

Katz, L.C. and Shatz, C.J. (1996). Synaptic activity and the construction of cortical circuits. *Science,* Vol. 274, No. 5290, pp. 1133-1138.

Kirkwood, A. (2000). Serotonergic control of developmental plasticity. *Proc Natl Acad Sci U S A,* Vol. 97, No. 5, pp. 1951-1952.

Kirkwood, A., Rozas, C., Kirkwood, J., Perez, F. and Bear, M.F. (1999). Modulation of long-term synaptic depression in visual cortex by acetylcholine and norepinephrine. *J Neurosci,* Vol. 19, No. 5, pp. 1599-1609.

Kojic, L., Gu, Q., Douglas, R.M. and Cynader, M.S. (1997). Serotonin facilitates synaptic plasticity in kitten visual cortex: an in vitro study. *Brain Res Dev Brain Res,* Vol. 101, No. 1-2, pp. 299-304.

Lambertz, N., Gizewski, E.R., de Greiff, A. and Forsting, M. (2005). Cross-modal plasticity in deaf subjects dependent on the extent of hearing loss. *Brain Res Cogn Brain Res,* Vol. 25, No. 3, pp. 884-890.

LeVay, S., Wiesel, T.N. and Hubel, D.H. (1980). The development of ocular dominance columns in normal and visually deprived monkeys. *J Comp Neurol,* Vol. 191, No. 1, pp. 1-51.

Levelt, C.N. and Hubener, M. (2012). Critical-Period Plasticity in the Visual Cortex. *Annu Rev Neurosci,* Vol. No.

Levi, D.M. and Li, R.W. (2009). Perceptual learning as a potential treatment for amblyopia: a mini-review. *Vision Res,* Vol. 49, No. 21, pp. 2535-2549.

Li, R.W., Ngo, C., Nguyen, J., Levi, D.M. (2011). Video-game play indices plasticity in the visual system of adults with amblyopia. *PLoS Biol,* Vol. 9, No. 8, pp. e1001135.

Lloyd, I.C., Ashworth, J., Biswas, S. and Abadi, R.V. (2007). Advances in the management of congenital and infantile cataract. *Eye (Lond),* Vol. 21, No. 10, pp. 1301-1309.

Majewska, A. and Sur, M. (2003). Motility of dendritic spines in visual cortex in vivo: changes during the critical period and effects of visual deprivation. *Proc Natl Acad Sci U S A,* Vol. 100, No. 26, pp. 16024-16029.

Mataga, N., Imamura, K. and Watanabe, Y. (1992). L-threo-3,4-dihydroxyphenylserine enhanced ocular dominance plasticity in adult cats. *Neurosci Lett,* Vol. 142, No. 2, pp. 115-118.

Mataga, N., Mizuguchi, Y. and Hensch, T.K. (2004). Experience-dependent pruning of dendritic spines in visual cortex by tissue plasminogen activator. *Neuron,* Vol. 44, No. 6, pp. 1031-1041.
Maurer, D. and Hensch, T.K. (2012). Amblyopia: Background to the special issue on stroke recovery. *Dev Psychobiol,* Vol. 54, No. 3, pp. 224-238.
Maya-Vetencourt, J.F., Baroncelli, L., Viegi, A., Tiraboschi, E., Castren, E., Cattaneo, A. and Maffei, L. (2012). IGF-1 restores visual cortex plasticity in adult life by reducing local GABA levels. *Neural Plasticity,* Vol. No.
Maya-Vetencourt, J.F., Sale, A., Viegi, A., Baroncelli, L., De Pasquale, R., O'Leary, O.F., Castren, E. and Maffei, L. (2008). The antidepressant fluoxetine restores plasticity in the adult visual cortex. *Science,* Vol. 320, No. 5874, pp. 385-388.
Maya-Vetencourt, J.F., Tiraboschi, E., Spolidoro, M., Castren, E. and Maffei, L. (2011). Serotonin triggers a transient epigenetic mechanism that reinstates adult visual cortex plasticity in rats. *Eur J Neurosci,* Vol. 33, No. 1, pp. 49-57.
Milazzo, S., Turut, P. and Bremond-Gignac, D. (2011). [Infantile cataract and surgical management]. *J Fr Ophtalmol,* Vol. 34, No. 3, pp. 192-197.
Mizuno, H., Hirano, T. and Tagawa, Y. (2007). Evidence for activity-dependent cortical wiring: formation of interhemispheric connections in neonatal mouse visual cortex requires projection neuron activity. *J Neurosci,* Vol. 27, No. 25, pp. 6760-6770.
Morales, B., Choi, S.Y. and Kirkwood, A. (2002). Dark rearing alters the development of GABAergic transmission in visual cortex. *J Neurosci,* Vol. 22, No. 18, pp. 8084-8090.
Moreau, A.W., Amar, M., Le Roux, N., Morel, N. and Fossier, P. (2010). Serotoninergic fine-tuning of the excitation-inhibition balance in rat visual cortical networks. *Cereb Cortex,* Vol. 20, No. 2, pp. 456-467.
Morishita, H., Miwa, J.M., Heintz, N. and Hensch, T.K. (2010). Lynx1, a cholinergic brake, limits plasticity in adult visual cortex. *Science,* Vol. 330, No. 6008, pp. 1238-1240.
O'Donnell, C., Nolan, M.F. and van Rossum, M.C. (2011). Dendritic spine dynamics regulate the long-term stability of synaptic plasticity. *J Neurosci,* Vol. 31, No. 45, pp. 16142-16156.
Paramei, G.V. and Sabel, B.A. (2008). Contour-integration deficits on the intact side of the visual field in hemianopia patients. *Behav Brain Res,* Vol. 188, No. 1, pp. 109-124.
Pettigrew, J.D. and Kasamatsu, T. (1978). Local perfusion of noradrenaline maintains visual cortical plasticity. *Nature,* Vol. 271, No. 5647, pp. 761-763.
Pham, T.A., Impey, S., Storm, D.R. and Stryker, M.P. (1999). CRE-mediated gene transcription in neocortical neuronal plasticity during the developmental critical period. *Neuron,* Vol. 22, No. 1, pp. 63-72.
Pinto, L., Drechsel, D., Schmid, M.T., Ninkovic, J., Irmler, M., Brill, M.S., Restani, L., Gianfranceschi, L., Cerri, C., Weber, S.N., Tarabykin, V., Baer, K., Guillemot, F., Beckers, J., Zecevic, N., Dehay, C., Caleo, M., Schorle, H. and Gotz, M. (2009). AP2gamma regulates basal progenitor fate in a region- and layer-specific manner in the developing cortex. *Nat Neurosci,* Vol. 12, No. 10, pp. 1229-1237.
Polat, U., Ma-Naim, T., Belkin, M. and Sagi, D. (2004). Improving vision in adult amblyopia by perceptual learning. *Proc Natl Acad Sci U S A,* Vol. 101, No. 17, pp. 6692-6697.
Putignano, E., Lonetti, G., Cancedda, L., Ratto, G., Costa, M., Maffei, L. and Pizzorusso, T. (2007). Developmental downregulation of histone posttranslational modifications regulates visual cortical plasticity. *Neuron,* Vol. 53, No. 5, pp. 747-759.

Restani, L., Cerri, C., Pietrasanta, M., Gianfranceschi, L., Maffei, L. and Caleo, M. (2009). Functional masking of deprived eye responses by callosal input during ocular dominance plasticity. *Neuron,* Vol. 64, No. 5, pp. 707-718.

Roder, B., Teder-Salejarvi, W., Sterr, A., Rosler, F., Hillyard, S.A. and Neville, H.J. (1999). Improved auditory spatial tuning in blind humans. *Nature,* Vol. 400, No. 6740, pp. 162-166.

Sadato, N., Pascual-Leone, A., Grafman, J., Ibanez, V., Deiber, M.P., Dold, G. and Hallett, M. (1996). Activation of the primary visual cortex by Braille reading in blind subjects. *Nature,* Vol. 380, No. 6574, pp. 526-528.

Sale, A., Berardi, N., Spolidoro, M., Baroncelli, L. and Maffei, L. (2010). GABAergic inhibition in visual cortical plasticity. *Front Cell Neurosci,* Vol. 4, No. pp. 10.

Silingardi, D., Scali, M., Belluomini, G. and Pizzorusso, T. (2010). Epigenetic treatments of adult rats promote recovery from visual acuity deficits induced by long-term monocular deprivation. *Eur J Neurosci,* Vol. 31, No. 12, pp. 2185-2192.

Singer, W. (1990). The formation of cooperative cell assemblies in the visual cortex. *J Exp Biol,* Vol. 153, No. pp. 177-197.

Singer, W. (1995). Development and plasticity of cortical processing architectures. *Science,* Vol. 270, No. 5237, pp. 758-764.

Spolidoro, M., Baroncelli, L., Putignano, E., Maya-Vetencourt, J.F., Viegi, A. and Maffei, L. (2011). Food restriction enhances visual cortex plasticity in adulthood. *Nat Commun,* Vol. 2, No. pp. 320.

Sugiyama, S., Di Nardo, A.A., Aizawa, S., Matsuo, I., Volovitch, M., Prochiantz, A. and Hensch, T.K. (2008). Experience-dependent transfer of Otx2 homeoprotein into the visual cortex activates postnatal plasticity. *Cell,* Vol. 134, No. 3, pp. 508-520.

Taha, S., Hanover, J.L., Silva, A.J. and Stryker, M.P. (2002). Autophosphorylation of alphaCaMKII is required for ocular dominance plasticity. *Neuron,* Vol. 36, No. 3, pp. 483-491.

Tropea, D., Majewska, A.K., Garcia, R. and Sur, M. (2010). Structural dynamics of synapses in vivo correlate with functional changes during experience-dependent plasticity in visual cortex. *J Neurosci,* Vol. 30, No. 33, pp. 11086-11095.

Wallace, W. and Bear, M.F. (2004). A morphological correlate of synaptic scaling in visual cortex. *J Neurosci,* Vol. 24, No. 31, pp. 6928-6938.

Wang, Y., Gu, Q. and Cynader, M.S. (1997). Blockade of serotonin-2C receptors by mesulergine reduces ocular dominance plasticity in kitten visual cortex. *Exp Brain Res,* Vol. 114, No. 2, pp. 321-328.

Wiesel, T.N. and Hubel, D.H. (1963). Single-Cell Responses in Striate Cortex of Kittens Deprived of Vision in One Eye. *J Neurophysiol,* Vol. 26, No. pp. 1003-1017.

Xu, T., Yu, X., Perlik, A.J., Tobin, W.F., Zweig, J.A., Tennant, K., Jones, T. and Zuo, Y. (2009). Rapid formation and selective stabilization of synapses for enduring motor memories. *Nature,* Vol. 462, No. 7275, pp. 915-919.

Yu, H., Majewska, A.K. and Sur, M. (2011). Rapid experience-dependent plasticity of synapse function and structure in ferret visual cortex in vivo. *Proc Natl Acad Sci U S A,* Vol. 108, No. 52, pp. 21235-21240.

Zito, K., Scheuss, V., Knott, G., Hill, T. and Svoboda, K. (2009). Rapid functional maturation of nascent dendritic spines. *Neuron,* Vol. 61, No. 2, pp. 247-258.

Chapter 14

Environmental Influences on Visual Cortex Development and Plasticity

Alessandro Sale, Nicoletta Berardi and Lamberto Maffei

Additional information is available at the end of the chapter

http://dx.doi.org/10.5772/48522

1. Introduction

The term "plasticity" refers to the ability of the nervous system to reorganize its connections functionally and structurally in response to changes in environmental experience, underlying the adaptive development and remodeling of neuronal circuitry. The primary visual cortex (V1) has been for decades the election model for studying experience-dependent plasticity in the brain. The pioneering experiments performed by Hubel and Wiesel showed how dramatically can early sensory deprivation affect the anatomy and physiology of the visual cortex. They reported that, early in development, reducing the visual input to one eye by means of lid suture, a treatment classically referred to as monocular deprivation (MD), disrupts the ocular dominance (OD) of V1 cells, with a loss of neurons driven by the deprived eye and a strong increment in the number of cells driven by the open eye, and reduces the number of binocular neurons [1]. Anatomically, the imbalance of activity between the two eyes results in the shrinkage of deprived eye ocular dominance columns, regions in V1 layer IV which receive thalamic inputs driven by the closed eye, and in the expansion of open eye ocular dominance columns [2-5], accompanied by a rapid remodeling of cortical horizontal connections [6]. Behaviorally, long-term MD is associated with a poor development of visual acuity (VA) and contrast sensitivity for the deprived eye and a loss of binocular vision. Strikingly, the same manipulation of visual experience appeared to be totally ineffective in the adult [4], leading to the characterization of a classic example or critical period, a time-window early in life in which the brain displays enhanced neural plasticity in response to experience [7-12].

In parallel to this seminal work based on a sensory deprivation approach, fundamental contributions to our knowledge of the effects of experience on the brain have been provided by the environmental enrichment (EE) paradigm, first introduced by the group of Rosenzweig and colleagues, in California. Originally defined as "a combination of complex inanimate and social stimulation" [13], EE consists in wide and attractive cages where the animals are reared in large social groups and in presence of a variety of objects (e.g. toys, tunnels, nesting material, stairs) that are frequently changed by the experimenter to stimulate explorative behavior, curiosity and attentional processes. A further, essential component of EE is the opportunity for the animals to attain sustained levels of voluntary physical exercise on one or more running wheels. EE definition is based on the comparison with alternative rearing conditions, such as the standard condition (SC), in which the animals are reared in small social groups and in very simple cages where no particular objects other than nesting material, food and water are present, or the so-called impoverished condition (IC), in which even social interactions are impossible because the animals are reared alone in individual cages, otherwise identical to those used for SC. With respect to their standard-reared or impoverished companions, enriched animals have the opportunity for enhanced social interaction, multi-sensorial stimulation and increased levels of physical activity, with the additional advantage that they are totally free to choose when and how much to experience the environmental richness, without the contingencies and risks typically associated with living in the wild [14].

In over fifty years of research in the field, a great number of studies have documented the positive impact of EE on the morphology, chemistry and physiology of the brain [14-17]. Initial experiments by Rosenzweig et al. [18] showed that after 30 days of exposition to an enriched living condition the cortex of enriched rats increased robustly in thickness and weight compared with that of standard reared animals. These changes occurred in the entire dorsal cortex, including frontal, parietal and occipital cortex. Since then, many studies have reported various anatomical changes associated with enriched living conditions, including nearly all structural components analyzed, such as increased dendritic arborization and length of dendritic spines [19-21], augmented synaptic size and number [22, 23] and increased postsynaptic thickening [24] and gliogenesis [25].

More recently, EE studies have regained special interest with the fall of the dogma regarding the postulated incapability of adult brain to generate new neurons. Although, in mammals, the majority of neurons are generated by the time of birth, some brain structures, with the paradigmatic examples of the granule cells of olfactory bulb and hippocampal dentate gyrus, maintain this potentiality for neurogenesis even after sexual maturity [26, 27], a property that has been demonstrated not only in rodents but also in monkeys [28] and, remarkably, in humans [29]. Numerous studies have shown that exposure to an enriched environment produces a significant increase in hippocampal neurogenesis [30]. A similar effect is induced by enhanced levels of physical exercise through running [31, 32], but the two conditions appear to act with distinct mechanisms: while voluntary exercise alone in a standard cage increases neurogenesis with an increment in both proliferation and survival of new-generated neurons, exposure to an enriched environment is only able to increase the number of surviving newborn cells, leaving the proportion of newly born cells unaffected. It has been suggested that to induce a shortening of the cell cycle or to elicit additional quiescent cells to enter the cell cycle (both effects resulting in increased amount of cell proliferation and neurogenesis) one specific type of very focused activity is needed, such as running. Running levels are probably not increased in the enriched condition to the same levels occurring with standard cage running. Interestingly, running increases brain uptake of the insuline-like growth factor I (IGF-I) [33], and IGF-I has been shown to accelerate cell cycle in the embryonic cerebral cortex [34]. If present at the level of adult brain neurogenesis, this effect could explain the strong influence elicited by sustained levels of voluntary running on hippocampal cell proliferation. The ability of EE to interact with the programs of nerve cell renewal extends beyond the influence on neurogenesis, including the capability to reduce apoptotic cell death in the hippocampus under both natural conditions and following excitotoxic insults [35]. These results challenge the traditional view that the anatomical structure of the brain is immutable under non-pathological conditions, revealing an unexpected plasticity induced by environmental stimulation at the structural level.

One striking peculiarity of EE is its ability to improve learning and memory functions, and with a specific reduction of the cognitive decline associated with aging [36, 37]. This last effect is related to a robust facilitation of hippocampal LTP, a widely accepted synaptic plasticity model of learning and memory [38] and linked with general signs of "cellular health" in the hippocampus, such as increased levels of synaptophysin [39, 40], a glycoprotein found in membranes of neurotransmitter-containing presynaptic vesicles, a reduced load of lipofuscin deposits [41], which are good indicators of chronic oxidative stress [42], and the pronounced induction of hippocampal neurogenesis [41]. EE positively affects also emotional and stress reactivity, both in normal animals and in strains of mice considered pathologically anxious [43]. Interestingly, the effects of EE are not restricted to the cerebral cortex, as demonstrated by a recent work in which this paradigm has been used to investigate the effects of lifestyle change on metabolic parameters [44]. Enriched mice showed decreased leptin, reduced adipose mass, and increased food intake compared to standard-reared animals, demonstrating that the leptin-hypothalamic axis can be enhanced by environmental stimulation.

At the molecular level, studies based on gene chip analysis have revealed that a large number of genes related to neuronal structure, synaptic transmission and plasticity, neuronal excitability and neuroprotection change their expression levels in response to EE [45]. One group of molecules particularly sensitive to experience are neurotrophins, a family of secreted factors critically involved in structural and functional plasticity during development and in adulthood [46].

An important line of research deals with the potential therapeutic effects of EE: indeed, it has been shown that enriching the housing environment delays the progression of, and facilitates recovery from, various nervous system dysfunctions, including neurodevelopmental disorders, neurodegenerative diseases, different types of brain injury and psychiatric disorders [47-54]. These studies have profound consequences for humans. The development of intervention protocols aimed at maintaining a healthy and active lifestyle has been effectively encouraged by the results of basic research on EE. For example, strong correlative and epidemiological evidence shows that living habits, including occupation, leisure activities and physical exercise, have a direct effect on the risk of cognitive decline, with an increasing number of results indicating that a higher level and variety of mental and physical activity is associated with lower cognitive decline and reduced risk for dementia (for a review, [55]).

2. Environmental enrichment and visual system development

2.1. Acceleration of visual system development by EE

Most studies addressing the effects elicited by EE focused on the adult brain, leaving almost unexplored the question whether an enhanced environmental stimulation can also affect processes governing the development of the brain architecture. In Neuroscience and developmental Psychobiology, this is a fundamental issue dealing with the classic debate about the role of Nature and Nurture, or, in more biological terms, Genes and Environment, in the construction of brain structure and its functional output, the behavior.

The scarce interest attracted by early EE studies can be possibly attributed to the fact that pre-weaning enrichment is characterized by very little amounts of voluntary physical exercise, as the pups are too inert to engage in sustained motor activities. Since increased levels of physical activity are thought to be an essential component of the enrichment protocol [16], this can explain why the possibility to evoke neural and behavioral changes through pre-weaning enrichment have been considered quite limited. For instance, differently from adult animals, hippocampal neurogenesis was not found to be promoted by an intensive preweaning EE protocol consisting of increasing complex combinations of tactile, olfactory, visual, acoustic and vestibular stimuli to which pups were exposed from post-natal day 7 (P7) until P21 [56]. However, since early EE provides increased levels of polysensory stimulation occurring during a period of high anatomical and functional rearrangement of the cerebral cortex, it might be expected to elicit brain changes through experience-dependent plasticity processes.

Some years ago, we started in Pisa a series of studies in which we focused on visual system maturation in environmentally enriched rodents as a paradigmatic model to probe the impact of experience-dependent stimulation on central nervous system development. This approach has proved quite fruitful, allowing us to open a window on the dynamic building of the brain according to different levels of environmental stimulation.

One sensitive parameter which allows researchers to faithfully follow visual system maturation is the progressive increase of visual acuity that occurs during the first postnatal weeks (in rodents), months (in monkeys) or years (in humans). The time course of this process, which results in the ability to perceive fine spatial details in the visual world, turned out to be highly susceptible to the influence exerted by EE, with a one- (in the mouse) or two- (in the rat) week acceleration displayed by both mice and rats exposed to EE since birth [57, 58]. In the timescale of human visual development this is a strong effect, if one considers that is corresponds to an acceleration of about two years in the five-year period normally required for a child to reach adult-like visual acuity values. At the synaptic plasticity level, EE induces a faster closure of the time-window during which it is possible, early in development, to induce LTP in visual cortical slices through theta-frequency stimulation from the white-matter [57]. Moreover, the functional effects of EE are preceded by a very early increase in the visual cortex of the expression of brain-derived neurotrophic factor (BDNF), a neurotrophin strongly involved in the maturation of brain circuitries. BDNF increase at P7 is accompanied by an enhanced expression of the GABA biosynthetic enzymes, GAD65 and 67, detectable both at P7 and P15. These findings led us to compare our results (see [14]) with those previously found in BDNF overexpressing mice. In these animals, BDNF expression in the visual cortex is higher than in wt mice starting from very early postnatal ages and this correlates with a precocious development of intracortical GABAergic inhibition, as shown by the faster developmental increase in inhibitory postsynaptic currents and GABA biosynthetic enzyme GAD65 in the perisomatic region of pyramidal cells [59]. This early development of GABAergic inhibition is accompanied by an accelerated maturation of visual acuity, likely due to the refinement of visual receptive fields under the direct control of inhibitory interneurons. Thus, EE effects on BDNF and GABA biosynthetic enzymes provide an explanation for EE action on visual cortical development and confirm the role of neurotrophins and of the intracortical GABAergic inhibition as determinants of visual functional development.

Application of EE paradigms allowed us also to demonstrate a key role in visual development of another molecule, insuline-like growth factor-I (IGF-I). IGF-I expression is increased at P18 in the visual cortex of rats raised in EE compared to standard-reared animals, and exogenous IGF-I supply mimics, whereas blocking IGF-I action prevents, the EE effects on visual acuity maturation [60]. It is possible that BDNF and IGF-I signaling may eventually converge on the same pathways, as suggested by results showing that the CREB/CRE-mediated gene expression, which is regulated by both molecules [61, 62], is developmentally accelerated in the visual cortex of enriched animals, while chronic injections of control animals with rolipram, a pharmacological treatment increasing the phosphorylation of CREB, partially mimic the EE outcome on visual acuity maturation [57]. Another biochemical pathway shared by BDNF and IGF-I might be regulation of the inhibitory GABAergic system, since cortical interneurons respond to IGF-I infusion increasing GAD65 expression in their synaptic terminals [60].

The precociousness of EE effects on BDNF and GAD65/67 challenges the intuitive view by which the development of a particular sensory system should be strictly dependent on experience of the same sensory modality. Indeed, the increase in BDNF and GAD enzymes does not require vision at all, if one considers that it is clearly evident before eye opening and even before photoreceptor formation. This is confirmed by results obtained in enriched rats raised in darkness during development [63]. It is well known that rearing mammals in total darkness affects the maturation of visual cortical circuits, prolonging the duration of the critical period and impairing the process of visual acuity maturation until normal visual experience is re-established [64, 65]. We found that both effects of dark rearing were completely counteracted by EE [63]. Once again, the effect is very similar to that found in BDNF over-expressing mice, where a full rescue of the typical dark-rearing phenotype has been reported [66].

The impact of EE on visual system development turned out not to be restricted to the cerebral cortex, but was clearly present also at the level of the retina, a peripheral part of the central nervous system traditionally considered little or not plastic at all in response to changes of sensory inputs. This classic concept has been mostly based on results showing that retinal acuity, i.e. the spatial discrimination limit of the retinal output, determined with electroretinogram, is unresponsive to visual deprivation in cats, rats and humans [64, 67, 68]. However, when probed with EE, retinal development resulted to be robustly accelerated, both when taking into account retinal acuity development [58] and when analyzing the process of retinal ganglion cell dendrite segregation into ON and OFF sublaminae [69]. The molecular alphabet underlying these changes appears to be the same followed by the visual cortex: levels of retinal IGF-I and BDNF are precociously increased in the retinal ganglion cell layer of developing rats raised under enriched conditions, and separately blocking IGF-I or BDNF action prevents EE effects [58, 69]. Interestingly, the possibility to evoke retinal plasticity is not a prerogative of an enhanced environmental stimulation, as both the anatomical and physiological maturation of retinal circuits is also altered by a complete lack of visual experience in mice [70, 71].

2.2. Maternal enrichment effects

The precociousness of the effects elicited by EE on brain development led us to hypothesize that they might be mediated by maternal behavior differences between enriched and non-enriched dams. What else, indeed, might cause a P7 increase of BDNF in pups spending the whole time in the nest, with no exploration of the enriched surroundings and no visual experience of it? Experience acquired between birth and weaning is essential in promoting and regulating neural development and behavioral traits of the newborn in both rodents and primates [72]. During this critical period of high developmental plasticity, maternal influence can be considered one of the most important sources of sensory experience for the developing subject [73-75], regulating physical growth and promoting the neural maturation of brain structures [72, 76, 77]. Our hypothesis of a critical involvement of maternal behavior in early EE effects has found experimental support in a detailed quantitative study of maternal care in different environmental conditions, which showed that enriched pups receive higher levels of maternal stimulation compared to standard-reared animals [78]. More specifically, enriched rats experience a continuous physical contact due to the presence of adult females in the nest and are also provided with increased levels of licking and grooming, a fundamental source of tactile stimulation. Thus, living in an EE setting provides the animals with an additional source of stimulation other than the social, cognitive and motor components: maternal touch. More recently [79], we were able to reproduce the EE-dependent acceleration of visual development by providing standard-reared rat pups, during their first ten postnatal days of life, with a tactile stimulation (massage) mimicking maternal behavior, a procedure previously shown to compensate for the deleterious effects of long-lasting maternal deprivation (Figure 1) [80-82]. In addition to an accelerated maturation of visual acuity, stimulated pups exhibited increased IGF-I levels at P18, and blocking the IGF-I action prevented its effects on visual system development [79].

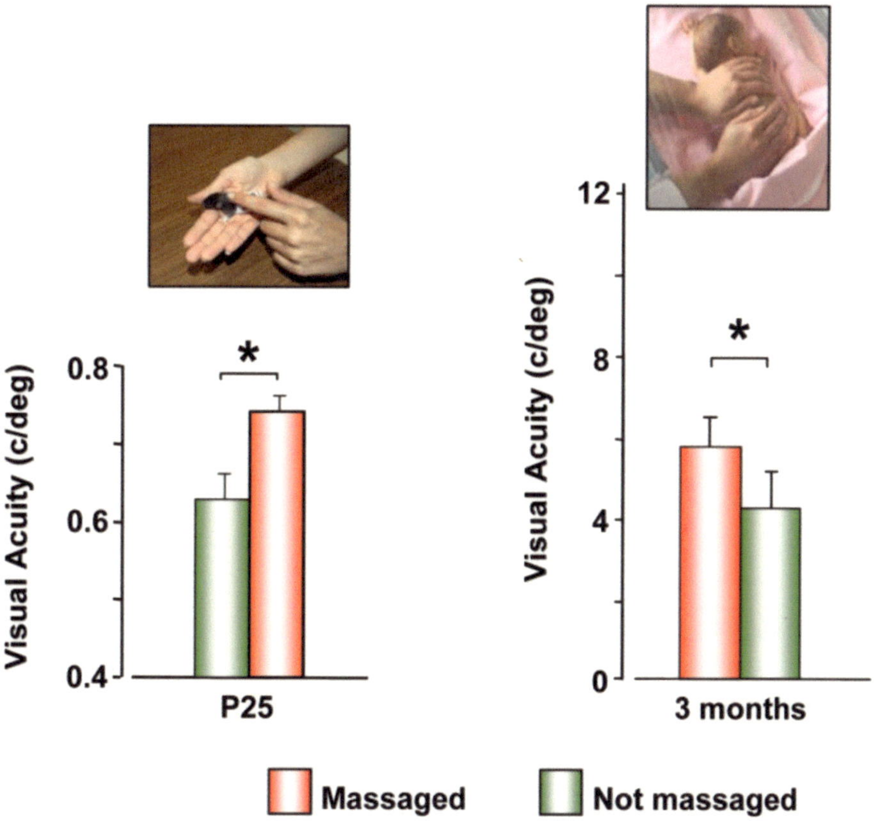

Figure 1. Massage therapy promotes visual acuity maturation in pre-term infants and rat pups. In rat pups, massage was performed during the first twelve postnatal days, three times per day. Stimulated rats exhibited higher visual acuity values compared to non-stimulated controls at postnatal day (P) 25. In pre-term babies, massage therapy started on day 10 after birth and continued for a total of ten days. During tactile stimulation, the infants were placed prone and given moderate pressure stroking with the flats of the fingers of both hands. In addition, passive flexion/extension movements of the limbs were applied in sequence. Visual acuity in massaged infants was significantly higher than in controls at 3 months. Asterisks indicate statistical significance. Data replotted from Guzzetta et al. [79].

Since the essence of EE embodies the concept of "optimization" of sensory-motor stimulation rather than its "alteration or reduction", this paradigm is an ideal candidate for application to humans. In parallel to the effects obtained in massaged rats, Guzzetta et al. [79] reported that enriching the environment in terms of body massage ('massage therapy') accelerates brain development in healthy pre-term infants (gestational age between 30 and 33 weeks). Massaged infants exhibited a faster developmental reduction in the latency of flash visual evoked potentials (VEPs) and an increase in behavioral visual acuity, which persisted above two months after the end of the treatment. Moreover, a faster EEG maturation was evident in massaged babies, as shown by the more rapid shortening of the interbust intervals, a reliable index of the developmental stage of the brain electrical activity. Interestingly, massaged babies did not exhibit the change in EEG spectral power found in the comparison group [83], confirming that massage intervention affects the maturation of brain electrical activity and suggesting that if may favor a process more similar to that observed in utero in term infants. In good agreement with results obtained in the animal model, massaged infants displayed increased levels of plasma IGF-1 [79]. The results of these studies, which are one of the first attempts to rigorously investigate the effects of early EE on human brain, emphasize the role of mother Nurture as a driving force for brain development in humans.

Maternal influence on the offspring development not only takes the form of maternal care given to pups during the first postnatal weeks, but it also includes the complex supply of nutrients, hormones and respiratory gases provided by the mother to the fetus during pregnancy, through placental exchanges [84]. The extent to which different environmental conditions experienced by the mother during pregnancy affect fetal development is still debated. For many years, the best documented effects were only those elicited by prenatal stress protocols, which have a well established role in growth retardation and structural malformations of the offspring [85, 86]. We found that the ability of EE to modulate growth factors critical for central nervous system development is present also during prenatal life (Figure 2).

Indeed, enriching female rats for the entire length of gestation results in faster dynamics of neural progenitor migration and spontaneous apoptosis in the retinal ganglion cell layer, an effect mediated also in this case by IGF-I [87]. We proposed a model in which sustained physical exercise during pregnancy increases IGF-I in the mother, promoting placental transfer of nutrients to the fetus; this would in turn lead to increased amounts of IGF-I autonomously produced by the fetus, resulting in the accelerated development detectable at retinal level (Figure 2). The influence exerted by maternal enrichment during pregnancy on the fetus is not restricted to the visual system. The hippocampus of pups born from enriched mothers, indeed, displays increased expression of BDNF [88] and increased proliferation of progenitor cells in the granule layer [89], resulting in improved cognitive functions when the animals reach adult ages [90].

3. Impact of EE on adult visual system plasticity

3.1. Amblyopia recovery in enriched animals

When visual functions mature up to their adult-like levels, the critical period for plasticity in the visual cortex closes and the possibility to induce further functional and structural changes by manipulating sensory experience abruptly wanes. This poses enduring brakes to the potential for recovery from defective development and for functional rehabilitation. Overcoming the obstacles which limit plasticity in the adult brain is a fundamental goal of both basic and clinical research in Neuroscience [91].

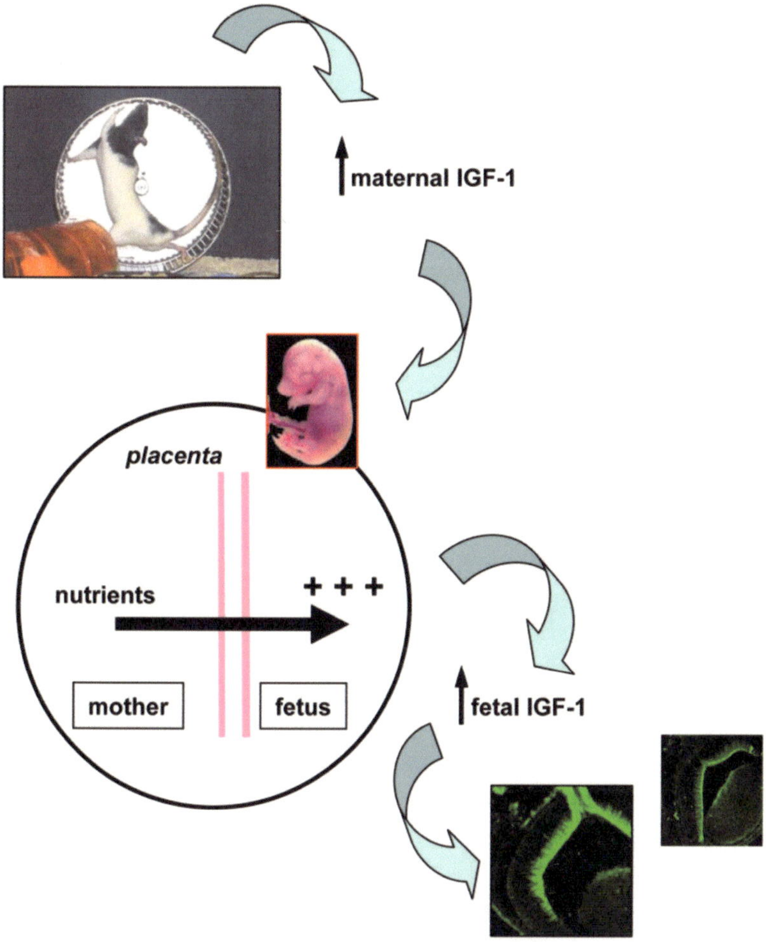

Figure 2. **Prenatal enrichment modulates retinal development in the fetus.** The figure depicts a possible explicative model for the effects elicited by maternal enrichment during pregnancy on retinal development. Increased levels of physical exercise in gestating dams lead to higher amounts of circulating IGF-I in the maternal blood stream, stimulating the supply of nutrients transferred to the fetus through the placental barrier. The enhancement in glucose and placental lactogens received by the fetus stimulates the autonomous production of IGF-1 in fetal tissues, with an increased expression detectable in the ganglion cell layer of the retina. IGF, in turn, stimulates the maturation of retinal circuitries. The photographs depict two examples of one enriched (left) and one non-enriched (right) retinal sections immunostained for double-cortin, which labels migrating cells and is a good marker of the temporal and spatial distribution of neural progenitors during the early developmental stages of the rat retina. Modified from Sale et al. [87].

The decay of plasticity levels in the adult visual system is not absolute, of course, but is dependent on the kind of stimuli and neural processes under investigation. A striking example of use-dependent plasticity in the adult visual cortex has been described in the work of Bear and colleagues which showed that repeated exposure to grating stimuli of a single orientation results in a long-lasting increase of VEP amplitudes in response to the test stimulus [92]. Another well defined phenomenon is the shift in orientation or spatial frequency selectivity displayed by neurons in the cat primary visual cortex after a period of adaptation consisting in the presentation of a stimulus at non-preferred orientations or spatial frequencies [93, 94]. Despite these and other [95] remarkable examples of adult V1 plasticity, however, the possibility of recovery from the consequences of an altered visual experience extending beyond the end of critical periods is extremely limited. One paradigmatic example of an enduring loss of visual abilities which is still orphan of treatment is amblyopia (lazy eye), a severe condition with an estimated prevalence of 1-5% in the total world population [96]. Amblyopia is caused by a marked functional imbalance between the two eyes occurring early in development and due to an unequal refractive power in the two eyes (anisometropia), an abnormal alignment of ocular axes (strabismus) or visual clouding caused, for instance, by congenital cataract [97]. If the cause of visual impairment is not rapidly removed, amblyopic subjects develop a dramatic degradation of visual acuity and contrast sensitivity in the anisometropic, strabismic or cataract affected eye and experience a broad range of other perceptual deficits, including stereopsis defects [96, 98, 99]. These deficits are attributed to the alteration in ocular dominance and binocularity of neurons in the developing visual cortex caused by the imbalance between the inputs form the two eyes.

While it is generally accepted that recovery of visual functions is possible only if normal visual experience is re-established early in development, recent studies in rodents have shown new therapeutic possibilities for the treatment of adult subjects [100]. In animal models like rats and mice, amblyopia can be easily induced by imposing a long-term occlusion of vision through one eye by an enduring MD procedure starting at the peak of plasticity early in development and protracted until adulthood. In the effort to challenge the critical period dogma, we showed that adult amblyopic rats transferred to an EE setting for three weeks undergo a full recovery of visual functions [101]. Immediately before starting the EE procedure, all rats were subjected to reverse suture, which consists in the re-opening of the long-term deprived (amblyopic) eye and the concomitant closure of the eyelids in the fellow eye, a procedure that, analogously to the so-called patching therapy in humans [102], is aimed at penalizing the preferred eye and forcing the brain to use visual inputs carried by the amblyopic eye. Reverse suture is very effective in promoting recovery form amblyopia if performed during the critical period but it is ineffective in adult subjects. On the contrary, reverse suture in animals exposed to EE was found to promote a complete rescue of ocular dominance and visual acuity, with beneficial effects detectable at both the electrophysiological and behavioral level and outlasting the end of the treatment for at least ten days. Recovery of plasticity in enriched animals was accompanied by a three-fold reduction in GABA-release detected in the visual cortex contralateral to the previously deprived eye by means of in vivo brain microdialysis, without any significant change in the release of glutamate. Moreover, the beneficial effects elicited by EE were totally counteracted by intracortical infusion of the benzodiazepine Diazepam, revealing a key role for decreased GABAergic transmission in driving amblyopia rescue in enriched animals. This was one of the first demonstrations that reducing the inhibition-excitation balance reinstates plasticity in the adult brain [103], as subsequently confirmed by another study in which a pharmacological reduction of inhibition through intracortical infusion of either MPA (an inhibitor of GABA synthesis) or picrotoxin (a GABAA antagonist) was reported to reactivate plasticity in response to MD in adult rats [104] (Figure 3).

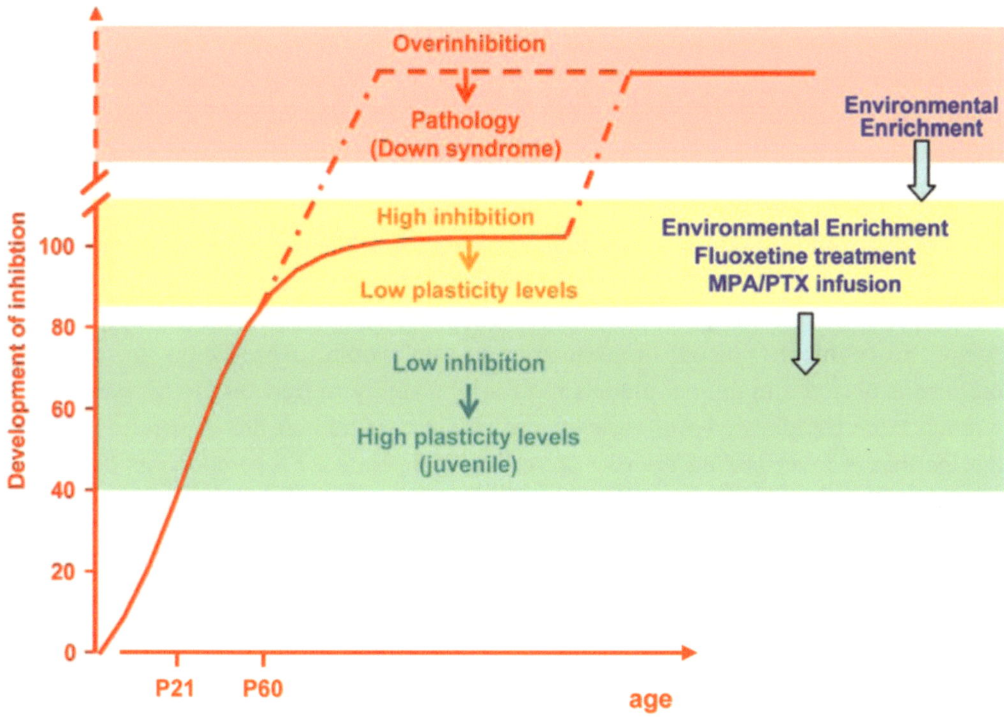

Figure 3. Developmental increase of brain GABAergic inhibition levels is paralleled by a progressive reduction of experience-dependent plasticity. Plasticity is high during early development (green block) and very low in the adult brain (yellow block). Anomalous increases in the strength of inhibitory neural circuits may lead to overinhibition linked to permanent deficits in synaptic plasticity and neural development, like in the Down syndrome. Reducing GABAergic inhibition with environmental enrichment, fluoxetine or pharmacological treatments (blockers of GABA synthesis or GABA receptor antagonists) can increase plasticity in the adult brain, enabling plasticity in V1 and favoring recovery from amblyopia. The capability of EE to reduce GABAergic inhibition makes this paradigm eligible for therapeutic applications also in the treatment of developmental intellectual disabilities. Plasticity levels have been normalized to the normal adult values (red curve). Modified from Sale et al. [113].

In amblyopia, one case of particularly relevant clinical interest is that of those patients who loose their better eye due to an accident or ocular illnesses, thus becoming severely visually impaired. It has been reported that the visual acuity of the amblyopic eye can display partial spontaneous recovery following loss of vision in the fellow eye [105-109], but the occurrence of this fortunate response is unpredictable and which factors promote improvement under similar circumstances remains totally unknown. We recently addressed the possibility to rescue visual acuity in long-term deprived adult rats exposed to EE immediately after silencing of retino-thalamic projections of the fellow (non amblyopic) eye due to optic nerve dissection [110]. While no spontaneous rescue of visual abilities was detected in animals reared under standard environmental conditions, a full recovery of visual acuity was achieved in monocular rats exposed to EE, an effect accompanied by lower numbers of GAD67+ cells and increased BDNF in the visual cortex. Thus, an enhanced environmental stimulation can promote visual cortex plasticity and functional recovery even in a condition in which competition between the two eyes is completely suppressed. However, this effect fits also well with a competition-based model, because stronger inputs from the fellow eye could mask activity in the weaker connections from the amblyopic eye until they are selectively silenced by optic nerve dissection.

Since it is currently thought that the inhibition-excitation balance is also impaired during development in amblyopic human subjects and that excessive inhibition levels are involved in the degradation of their spatial vision abilities [111, 112], EE appears as a very promising strategy to counteract visual impairments in amblyopia. Application to clinics of these results obtained in animal models requires the ability to transfer the EE paradigm in the much more complicated and variegated dimension of human life. A fruitful approach might be that of investigating the role of various independent EE components (e.g. social, sensory, motor) in reproducing the beneficial effects elicited by the entire enriched experience, and then designing therapeutic approaches based on the most promising and effective variables.

Recently, we followed this route by separately assessing the efficacy of physical exercise, increased levels of social interaction and enhanced visual stimulation for their potential in promoting recovery from amblyopia in adult rats [114]. Our results show a full recovery of ocular dominance and visual acuity either in both animals experiencing high levels of voluntary motor activity in a running wheel and in rats exposed to a protocol of visual enrichment inside a rotating fluorescent drum specifically designed to maximize stimulation of V1 cortical neurons (Figure 4). The strong involvement of visual experience in the recovery process was further indicated by the demonstration that amblyopic animals placed under classic EE conditions, but completely deprived from visual stimulation, failed to recover normal visual functions, and that using EE in no-reverse sutured animals in which the long-term deprived eye was maintained closed, prevented the animals to differentiate their visual function abilities from untreated controls. In contrast to motor and visual enrichment, enhancing social stimulation alone was not able to induce restoration of normal visual acuity and ocular dominance (Figure 4). Recovery from amblyopia was faithfully associated with a reduction of GABAergic intracortical inhibition, as revealed by decreased GABA release in synaptosome analysis. Thus, potentiation of single components typically present in EE is able to reproduce the effect of visual function recovery from amblyopia previously reported in classically-enriched animals [101, 114]. These findings should encourage the implementation of new environmental strategies devoted to promote stimulation of the amblyopic eye in adult patients as a way to increase their chance of visual functional improvements.

3.2. Visual perceptual learning and amblyopia

The possibility to reinstate plasticity in the adult visual cortex by using a non-invasive procedure such as EE is appealing. A growing body of evidence in humans shows that experimental paradigms akin to EE, such as playing videogames or practicing visual perceptual learning (PL), are effective in promoting recovery from amblyopia in adulthood [115-118].

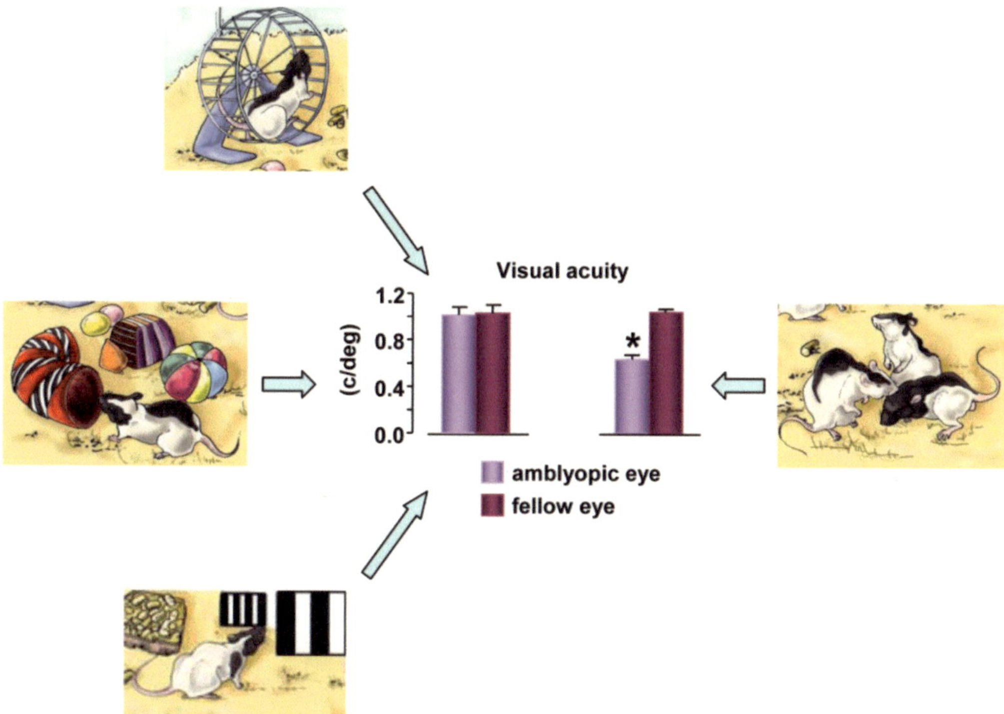

Figure 4. Impact of motor, social and sensory components on recovery from amblyopia in adult rats. Adult amblyopic rats were subjected for three weeks to either motor enrichment (consisting of a standard cage equipped with a running wheel connected to an automatic device recording the number of wheel turns), visual enrichment (consisting of a standard cage positioned at the centre of a rotating fluorescent drum where specific visual patterns were drawn), social stimulation (consisting of a slightly bigger standard cage where numerous rats where housed together), or visual perceptual learning (see Figure 5 for more details). A complete rescue of visual acuity in the amblyopic eye was achieved by rats performing physical exercise on a running wheel, in animals exposed to visual enrichment and in animals engaged in visual perceptual learning. This effect was also accompanied by a reduced inhibition/excitation balance in the visual cortex. In contrast, no recovery occurred in socially enriched rats or in animals practicing a purely associative visual task. Asterisk indicates statistical significance. Data replotted from Baroncelli et al. [114].

The cellular and molecular mechanisms underlying PL effects are still scarcely known. We reported that visual PL induces long-term potentiation (LTP) of intracortical synaptic responses in rat V1 [119], in agreement with Cooke and Bear [120]. To elicit visual PL, we first trained a group of adult animals to practice in a forced-choice visual discrimination task that requires them to distinguish between two vertical gratings differing only for their spatial frequency; then, we made the two stimuli progressively more similar to each other, until the animal performance reached a steady plateau (Figure 5A). This task requires activation of V1 circuitries, as indicated by the strong selectivity of PL for the orientation of gratings employed during training (Figure 5B). Control animals only learned the association task, i.e. they were only required to discriminate between a grating and a homogeneous grey panel, matching the overall swim time and number of training days in the water maze with those of PL rats (Figure 5A). Within 1 h from the last discrimination trial, LTP from layer II-III of V1 slices appeared occluded in PL animals compared to controls, both when testing its inducibility in vertical connections (stimulating electrode placed in layer IV) and when stimulating at the level of horizontal connections (stimulating electrode placed in layer II/III) (Figure 5A). Moreover, a significant shift toward increased amplitude of fEPSPs was found in the input/output curves of trained animals compared to controls. Thus, the data fulfill two of the most commonly accepted criteria used to relate LTP with learning, i.e.occlusion and mimicry, demonstrating that the improvements displayed by PL rats in discriminating visual gratings of progressively closer spatial frequencies can be explained in terms of long-term increments of synaptic efficacy in V1, the same cortical area at work during perception. This is consistent with the critical role for LTP in mediating learning processes previously reported in other brain areas such as the amygdala, the hippocampus and the motor cortex [122-124]. An impact on V1 LTP appears to be a common prerogative of visual PL and EE. Indeed, enriched rats also show an enhancement of thalamocortical LTP triggered by theta-burst stimulation (TBS) of the dorsal lateral geniculate nucleus of the thalamus [125], leading to an enhancement in VEP responses to visual stimulation across a wide range of contrasts.

Since potentiation of synaptic transmission might help the recovery process of visual responses for the long-term deprived eye, practice with visual PL through the amblyopic eye is expected to favor a functional rescue in amblyopic animals. In agreement with evidence on human subjects, a marked recovery of visual functions was evident in amblyopic rats subjected to visual PL, while no recovery occurred in two control groups in which the treatment did not induce LTP in V1, i.e. in rats that only learned the associative visual task and in animals that were trained only until the first step of the discrimination procedure between the test and the reference grating, without proceeding further with a progression of finer discrimination trials [114] (Figure 5A). Recovery of visual abilities in PL animals was accompanied by a robust decrease of the inhibition-excitation balance, which could pave the way for future therapeutic attempts in humans based on a manipulation of the GABAergic tone. In line with this, repetitive transcranial magnetic stimulation, a treatment increasing cortical excitability, transiently improves contrast sensitivity in adult amblyopes [126].

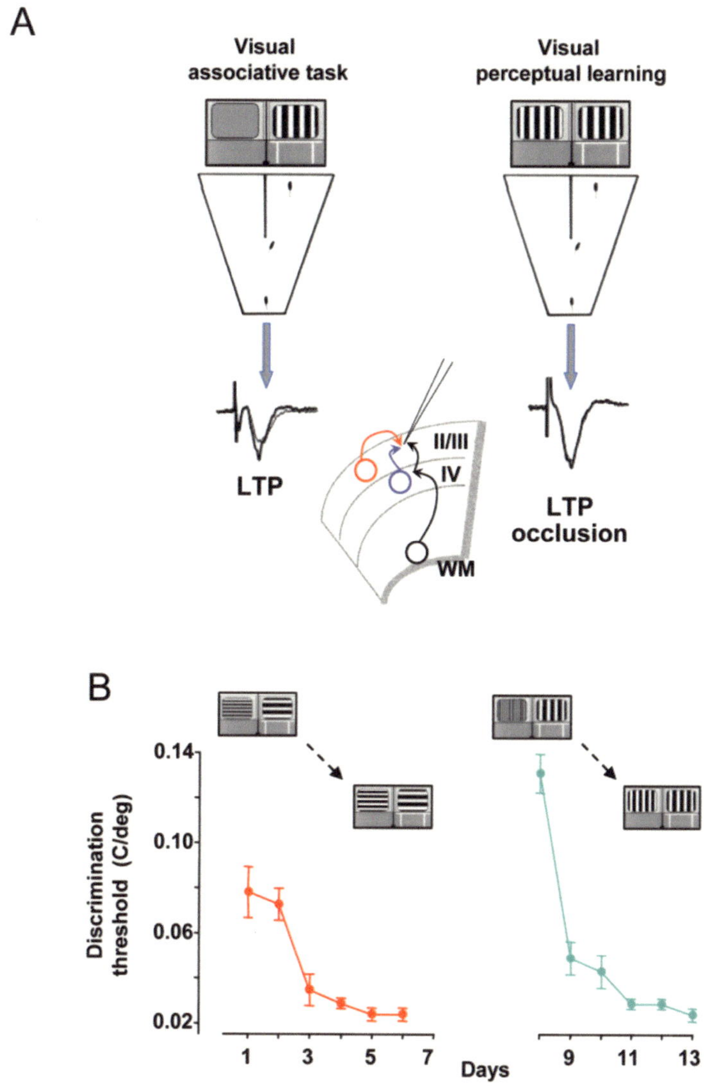

Figure 5. Visual perceptual learning induces long-term potentiation in the primary visual cortex. A) A modified version of the visual water box task [57, 121] was used to induce visual perceptual learning in a group of adult rats that were first trained to distinguish a low 0.117 cycles per degree (c/deg) spatial frequency (SF) grating (reference grating) from a 0.712 c/deg SF grating (test grating) (right panel) and then learned to distinguish the two gratings when they became more and more similar to each other. A group of control animals was trained to distinguish the reference grating from a homogeneous grey (left panel). After training, LTP from layer II-III of V1 slices was occluded in PL animals compared to controls, at the level of both vertical (blue arrow) and horizontal (red arrow) connections. Sample traces from PL and control slices 5 min before (thin line) and 25 min after (thick line) induction of LTP are shown. **B)** Visual perceptual learning is specific for stimulus orientation. The graphs show daily discrimination threshold values obtained in PL animals trained in discriminating first horizontal gratings and then tested with vertical. After the orientation change, the animals displayed a marked impairment in their discrimination abilities. Data replotted from Sale et al. [119].

3.3. Serotonin: A master regulator of adult neural plasticity

The capability of EE to reinstate juvenile-like plasticity in the adult brain is not limited to its effects on amblyopia. Indeed, the visual cortex of enriched rats displays a remarkable reactivation of ocular dominance plasticity in response to MD [127, 128]. The ocular dominance shift of cortical neurons is detectable using both VEPs and single-unit recordings. While, also in this case, recovery of plasticity is paralleled by a marked reduction of the inhibitory tone and an increase in the number of BDNF-expressing neurons in the visual cortex, a crucial role for the neurotransmitter serotonin in triggering the plastic changes elicited by exposure to EE has been identified. Indeed, EE elicits a twofold enhancement of serotoninergic transmission in the visual cortex and infusion of a serotonin synthesis inhibitor not only blocks plasticity in response to MD but also completely counteracts the effects produced by EE on GABAergic inhibition and BDNF [127]. This led us to put forward a model in which serotonin, probably enhanced by a more sustained attention and arousal level promoted by living in the enriched condition, is the first trigger in the chain of plastic changes set in motion by EE, eliciting the decrease of GABA-mediated intracortical inhibition and, in parallel or in series, the enhancement of BDNF levels (Figure 6).

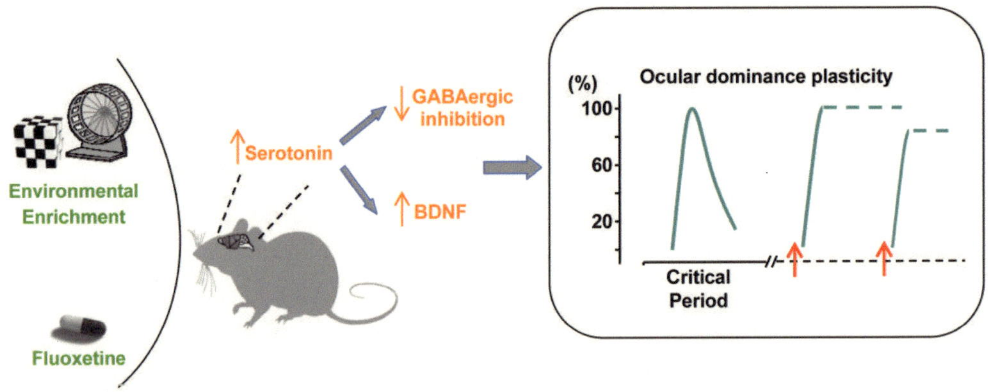

Figure 6. A critical role for serotonin in restoring ocular dominance plasticity in the adult visual cortex. Enhancing serotonergic transmission through exposure to environmental enrichment or administration of a chronic treatment with fluoxetine reinstates ocular dominance plasticity in adult rats. We propose a model in which serotonin drives a reduction of GABAergic inhibition and an increase in BDNF levels in the visual cortex. The graph on the right depicts the time course of the critical period for plasticity in response to monocular deprivation in rodents, and the reopening of plasticity achievable, though to a slightly reduced extent, at multiple distinct ages in adulthood (red arrows). Ocular dominance plasticity is normalized to the critical period peak's level.

The central role of serotonin in promoting adult visual cortex plasticity has been further demonstrated in animals chronically treated with fluoxetine, a selective serotonin reuptake inhibitor (SSRI) widely prescribed in the treatment of depression and various psychiatric disorders. The authors showed that fluoxetine delivered in the drinking water induces a full reinstatement of ocular dominance plasticity in response to MD (Figures 3 and 6) and a complete recovery of visual functions from amblyopia. As found for enriched rats, these functional effects are associated with a marked reduction of GABAergic inhibition and are completely prevented by cortical Diazepam administration [129]. The reduction of inhibition triggered by fluoxetine provides a permissive environment for structural changes, such as the addition of new synapse-bearing branch spine tips [130]. In light of these promising results, fluoxetine appears to behave as a powerful enviromimetic [131], a drug that can be successfully exploited, alone or in combination with EE, to reproduce or to strengthen the positive effects elicited by the environment on brain health and plasticity.

4. Life-long beneficial outcome of EE: from developmental disorders to the aging brain

As underscored by the effects on amblyopia, the non invasive nature of EE makes this paradigm eligible for application in the domain of brain dysfunctions. The beneficial impact of EE does not only apply to the case of diseases deriving form alterations of sensory experience, but it also extends to genetically programmed states of brain disability.

One paradigmatic example is that of Down syndrome, the most common genetic cause of mental retardation [76] caused by triplication of chromosome 21. People with Down syndrome have a marked cognitive impairment [132, 133], and a number of attention and visual deficits [134-136] together with various disturbances in learning and memory abilities [132, 133]. The most widely animal study of Down syndrome is the Ts65Dn mouse, which carries triplication of a segment of Chr16, syntenic with human Chr21 [137, 138]. This model recapitulates the main hallmarks of the syndrome phenotype, including craniofacial abnormalities, impaired learning abilities and attention and visual function deficits (e.g., [139-141]. Moreover, in vivo cellular analyses, which are of course prevented in humans but easily conducted in the animal model, have allowed a substantial advancement in our knowledge concerning the mechanisms underlying neural impairments in Ts65Dn mice. In particular, a critical role for excessive levels of brain inhibition emerges, with an ensuing failure of long-term synaptic plasticity in the hippocampus [142-145]. This is in agreement with results obtained in post-mortem tissue from people with Down syndrome, which displays an impaired balance between excitatory and inhibitory systems (see [146]. The central role of overinhibition in Down syndrome pathogenesis is confirmed by the demonstration that administration of non-competitive antagonists of GABA-A receptors reverses spatial learning disabilities and LTP deficits in Ts65Dn mice [146]. Since EE is effective in reducing GABAergic inhibition, we have tested its potential for therapeutic application in the Ts65Dn model of the syndrome. Our findings show that EE promotes recovery from cognitive impairment and synaptic plasticity failure and induces a full rescue of visual acuity, ocular dominance and visual neuronal response latencies in Ts65Dn mice compared to their littermates reared in standard conditions, an effect accompanied by normalization of GABA release in hippocampal and visual cortex synaptosomes [147].

On the opposite end of lifetime, severe functional deterioration can also occur during the aging process, across multiple systems including cognitive and sensory-motor domains. These deficits can, at least in part, be attributed to a progressive decay of neural plasticity in the elderly [148]. Interestingly, an enhanced environmental stimulation is able to restore ocular dominance plasticity not only in young adults [127], but also in the aging visual cortex, though to a slightly lower extent [149]. Plasticity in response to one week of MD is detectable at both the level of subthreshold modifications of postsynaptic potentials (by means of VEPs) and that of spike properties of cortical neurons (by means of single-unit recordings). In agreement to our previous results in younger animals, the number of GAD67+ cells was decreased while density of extracellular matrix PNNs increased in the visual cortex of aged enriched rats compared to age-matched standard-reared animals, demonstrating that the brain retains its capacity to undergo plastic changes elicited by a rich environmental experience without substantial changes in the underlying molecular machinery. This effect on neural plasticity offers an attractive explanation for the well known positive effects elicited by EE in the aging brain (e.g. [40, 148, 150]. Accordingly, intervention protocols aimed at promoting an active lifestyle in aging people should be encouraged.

5. Concluding remarks and future research lines

The data reviewed in this chapter have shown that EE is a powerful tool to modulate the development of the central nervous system and to boost plasticity in the adult cerebral cortex. The great success of this approach should not be hailed as a miracle, as it stands on the reliable EE ability to impact at multiple molecular substrate levels in the brain, including stimulation of maturational processes by enhanced activation of growth factors, reopening of plasticity windows through reduced intracortical inhibition and upregulation of plastic structural and functional changes by neurotrophin increments, which could in turn promote the expression of genes specifically involved in brain plasticity. We believe that the combination of a proper pharmacotherapy with non invasive strategies of environmental stimulation aimed at enhancing the spontaneous reparative potential held by the brain might emerge as the election curative approach for several neurological diseases.

Author details

Alessandro Sale*, Nicoletta Berardi and Lamberto Maffei
Institute of Neuroscience, National Research Council (CNR), Pisa, Italy
Department of Psychology, Florence University, Florence, Italy

Lamberto Maffei
Laboratory of Neurobiology, Scuola Normale Superiore, Pisa, Italy

---

* Corresponding Author

6. References

[1] Wiesel TN, Hubel DH (1963) Single-Cell Responses in Striate Cortex of Kittens Deprived of Vision in One Eye. J Neurophysiol 26: 1003-1017.
[2] Hubel DH, Wiesel TN, LeVay S (1977) Plasticity of ocular dominance columns in monkey striate cortex. Philos Trans R Soc Lond B Biol Sci 278: 377-409.
[3] Shatz CJ, Stryker MP (1978) Ocular dominance in layer IV of the cat's visual cortex and the effects of monocular deprivation. J Physiol 281: 267-283.
[4] LeVay S, Wiesel TN, Hubel DH (1980) The development of ocular dominance columns in normal and visually deprived monkeys. J Comp Neurol 191: 1-51.
[5] Antonini A, Stryker MP (1993) Rapid remodeling of axonal arbors in the visual cortex. Science 260: 1819-1821.
[6] Trachtenberg JT, Stryker MP (2001) Rapid anatomical plasticity of horizontal connections in the developing visual cortex. J Neurosci 21: 3476-3482.
[7] Berardi N, Pizzorusso T, Maffei L (2000) Critical periods during sensory development. Curr Opin Neurobiol 10: 138-145.
[8] Knudsen EI (2004) Sensitive periods in the development of the brain and behavior. J Cogn Neurosci 16: 1412-1425.
[9] Levelt CN, Hubener M Critical-Period Plasticity in the Visual Cortex. Annu Rev Neurosci.
[10] Hensch TK (2005) Critical period plasticity in local cortical circuits. Nat Rev Neurosci 6: 877-888.
[11] Hensch TK (2005) Critical period mechanisms in developing visual cortex. Curr Top Dev Biol 69: 215-237.
[12] Berardi N, Pizzorusso T, Ratto GM, Maffei L (2003) Molecular basis of plasticity in the visual cortex. Trends Neurosci 26: 369-378.
[13] Rosenzweig MR, Bennett EL, Hebert M, Morimoto H (1978) Social grouping cannot account for cerebral effects of enriched environments. Brain Res 153: 563-576.
[14] Sale A, Berardi N, Maffei L (2009) Enrich the environment to empower the brain. Trends Neurosci 32: 233-239.
[15] Rosenzweig MR, Bennett EL (1996) Psychobiology of plasticity: effects of training and experience on brain and behavior. Behav Brain Res 78: 57-65.
[16] van Praag H, Kempermann G, Gage FH (2000) Neural consequences of environmental enrichment. Nat Rev Neurosci 1: 191-198.
[17] Diamond MC (2001) Response of the brain to enrichment. An Acad Bras Cienc 73: 211-220.
[18] Rosenzweig MR, Bennett EL, Krech D (1964) Cerebral Effects of Environmental Complexity and Training among Adult Rats. J Comp Physiol Psychol 57: 438-439.
[19] Holloway RL, Jr. (1966) Dendritic branching: some preliminary results of training and complexity in rat visual cortex. Brain Res 2: 393-396.

[20] Globus A, Rosenzweig MR, Bennett EL, Diamond MC (1973) Effects of differential experience on dendritic spine counts in rat cerebral cortex. J Comp Physiol Psychol 82: 175-181.

[21] Greenough WT, Volkmar FR, Juraska JM (1973) Effects of rearing complexity on dendritic branching in frontolateral and temporal cortex of the rat. Exp Neurol 41: 371-378.

[22] Mollgaard K, Diamond MC, Bennett EL, Rosenzweig MR, Lindner B (1971) Quantitative synaptic changes with differential experience in rat brain. Int J Neurosci 2: 113-127.

[23] Black JE, Isaacs KR, Anderson BJ, Alcantara AA, Greenough WT (1990) Learning causes synaptogenesis, whereas motor activity causes angiogenesis, in cerebellar cortex of adult rats. Proc Natl Acad Sci U S A 87: 5568-5572.

[24] Diamond MC, Krech D, Rosenzweig MR (1964) The Effects of an Enriched Environment on the Histology of the Rat Cerebral Cortex. J Comp Neurol 123: 111-120.

[25] Diamond MC, Law F, Rhodes H, Lindner B, Rosenzweig MR, Krech D, Bennett EL (1966) Increases in cortical depth and glia numbers in rats subjected to enriched environment. J Comp Neurol 128: 117-126.

[26] Gueneau G, Privat A, Drouet J, Court L (1982) Subgranular zone of the dentate gyrus of young rabbits as a secondary matrix. A high-resolution autoradiographic study. Dev Neurosci 5: 345-358.

[27] Kuhn HG, Dickinson-Anson H, Gage FH (1996) Neurogenesis in the dentate gyrus of the adult rat: age-related decrease of neuronal progenitor proliferation. J Neurosci 16: 2027-2033.

[28] Gould E, Reeves AJ, Fallah M, Tanapat P, Gross CG, Fuchs E (1999) Hippocampal neurogenesis in adult Old World primates. Proc Natl Acad Sci U S A 96: 5263-5267.

[29] Eriksson PS, Perfilieva E, Bjork-Eriksson T, Alborn AM, Nordborg C, Peterson DA, Gage FH (1998) Neurogenesis in the adult human hippocampus. Nat Med 4: 1313-1317.

[30] Kempermann G, Kuhn HG, Gage FH (1997) More hippocampal neurons in adult mice living in an enriched environment. Nature 386: 493-495.

[31] van Praag H, Kempermann G, Gage FH (1999) Running increases cell proliferation and neurogenesis in the adult mouse dentate gyrus. Nat Neurosci 2: 266-270.

[32] van Praag H, Christie BR, Sejnowski TJ, Gage FH (1999) Running enhances neurogenesis, learning, and long-term potentiation in mice. Proc Natl Acad Sci U S A 96: 13427-13431.

[33] Carro E, Nunez A, Busiguina S, Torres-Aleman I (2000) Circulating insulin-like growth factor I mediates effects of exercise on the brain. J Neurosci 20: 2926-2933.

[34] Hodge RD, D'Ercole AJ, O'Kusky JR (2004) Insulin-like growth factor-I accelerates the cell cycle by decreasing G1 phase length and increases cell cycle reentry in the embryonic cerebral cortex. J Neurosci 24: 10201-10210.

[35] Young D, Lawlor PA, Leone P, Dragunow M, During MJ (1999) Environmental enrichment inhibits spontaneous apoptosis, prevents seizures and is neuroprotective. Nat Med 5: 448-453.
[36] Mohammed AH, Henriksson BG, Soderstrom S, Ebendal T, Olsson T, Seckl JR (1993) Environmental influences on the central nervous system and their implications for the aging rat. Behav Brain Res 57: 183-191.
[37] Mohammed AH, Zhu SW, Darmopil S, Hjerling-Leffler J, Ernfors P, Winblad B, Diamond MC, Eriksson PS, Bogdanovic N (2002) Environmental enrichment and the brain. Prog Brain Res 138: 109-133.
[38] Lynch MA (2004) Long-term potentiation and memory. Physiol Rev 84: 87-136.
[39] Saito S, Kobayashi S, Ohashi Y, Igarashi M, Komiya Y, Ando S (1994) Decreased synaptic density in aged brains and its prevention by rearing under enriched environment as revealed by synaptophysin contents. J Neurosci Res 39: 57-62.
[40] Frick KM, Fernandez SM (2003) Enrichment enhances spatial memory and increases synaptophysin levels in aged female mice. Neurobiol Aging 24: 615-626.
[41] Kempermann G, Gast D, Gage FH (2002) Neuroplasticity in old age: sustained fivefold induction of hippocampal neurogenesis by long-term environmental enrichment. Ann Neurol 52: 135-143.
[42] Terman A, Brunk UT (1998) Lipofuscin: mechanisms of formation and increase with age. Apmis 106: 265-276.
[43] Chapillon P, Patin V, Roy V, Vincent A, Caston J (2002) Effects of pre- and postnatal stimulation on developmental, emotional, and cognitive aspects in rodents: a review. Dev Psychobiol 41: 373-387.
[44] Mainardi M, Scabia G, Vottari T, Santini F, Pinchera A, Maffei L, Pizzorusso T, Maffei M A sensitive period for environmental regulation of eating behavior and leptin sensitivity. Proc Natl Acad Sci U S A 107: 16673-16678.
[45] Rampon C, Jiang CH, Dong H, Tang YP, Lockhart DJ, Schultz PG, Tsien JZ, Hu Y (2000) Effects of environmental enrichment on gene expression in the brain. Proc Natl Acad Sci U S A 97: 12880-12884.
[46] Pham TM, Winblad B, Granholm AC, Mohammed AH (2002) Environmental influences on brain neurotrophins in rats. Pharmacol Biochem Behav 73: 167-175.
[47] Nithianantharajah J, Hannan AJ (2006) Enriched environments, experience-dependent plasticity and disorders of the nervous system. Nat Rev Neurosci 7: 697-709.
[48] Berardi N, Braschi C, Capsoni S, Cattaneo A, Maffei L (2007) Environmental enrichment delays the onset of memory deficits and reduces neuropathological hallmarks in a mouse model of Alzheimer-like neurodegeneration. J Alzheimers Dis 11: 359-370.
[49] Fischer A, Sananbenesi F, Wang X, Dobbin M, Tsai LH (2007) Recovery of learning and memory is associated with chromatin remodelling. Nature 447: 178-182.
[50] Johansson BB (1996) Functional outcome in rats transferred to an enriched environment 15 days after focal brain ischemia. Stroke 27: 324-326.

[51] Koopmans GC, Brans M, Gomez-Pinilla F, Duis S, Gispen WH, Torres-Aleman I, Joosten EA, Hamers FP (2006) Circulating insulin-like growth factor I and functional recovery from spinal cord injury under enriched housing conditions. Eur J Neurosci 23: 1035-1046.

[52] Comeau W, Gibb R, Hastings E, Cioe J, Kolb B (2008) Therapeutic effects of complex rearing or bFGF after perinatal frontal lesions. Dev Psychobiol 50: 134-146.

[53] Soeda F, Tanaka A, Shirasaki T, Takahama K An enriched environment mitigates the brain-disruptive effects of prenatal diethylstilbestrol exposure in mice. Neuroscience 169: 223-228.

[54] Kovesdi E, Gyorgy AB, Kwon SK, Wingo DL, Kamnaksh A, Long JB, Kasper CE, Agoston DV The effect of enriched environment on the outcome of traumatic brain injury; a behavioral, proteomics, and histological study. Front Neurosci 5: 42.

[55] Nithianantharajah J, Hannan AJ (2009) The neurobiology of brain and cognitive reserve: mental and physical activity as modulators of brain disorders. Prog Neurobiol 89: 369-382.

[56] Kohl Z, Kuhn HG, Cooper-Kuhn CM, Winkler J, Aigner L, Kempermann G (2002) Preweaning enrichment has no lasting effects on adult hippocampal neurogenesis in four-month-old mice. Genes Brain Behav 1: 46-54.

[57] Cancedda L, Putignano E, Sale A, Viegi A, Berardi N, Maffei L (2004) Acceleration of visual system development by environmental enrichment. J Neurosci 24: 4840-4848.

[58] Landi S, Sale A, Berardi N, Viegi A, Maffei L, Cenni MC (2007) Retinal functional development is sensitive to environmental enrichment: a role for BDNF. Faseb J 21: 130-139.

[59] Huang ZJ, Kirkwood A, Pizzorusso T, Porciatti V, Morales B, Bear MF, Maffei L, Tonegawa S (1999) BDNF regulates the maturation of inhibition and the critical period of plasticity in mouse visual cortex. Cell 98: 739-755.

[60] Ciucci F, Putignano E, Baroncelli L, Landi S, Berardi N, Maffei L (2007) Insulin-like growth factor 1 (IGF-1) mediates the effects of enriched environment (EE) on visual cortical development. PLoS ONE 2: e475.

[61] Santos AR, Comprido D, Duarte CB Regulation of local translation at the synapse by BDNF. Prog Neurobiol 92: 505-516.

[62] Zheng WH, Quirion R (2006) Insulin-like growth factor-1 (IGF-1) induces the activation/phosphorylation of Akt kinase and cAMP response element-binding protein (CREB) by activating different signaling pathways in PC12 cells. BMC Neurosci 7: 51.

[63] Bartoletti A, Medini P, Berardi N, Maffei L (2004) Environmental enrichment prevents effects of dark-rearing in the rat visual cortex. Nat Neurosci 7: 215-216.

[64] Fagiolini M, Pizzorusso T, Berardi N, Domenici L, Maffei L (1994) Functional postnatal development of the rat primary visual cortex and the role of visual experience: dark rearing and monocular deprivation. Vision Res 34: 709-720.

[65] Timney B, Mitchell DE, Giffin F (1978) The development of vision in cats after extended periods of dark-rearing. Exp Brain Res 31: 547-560.

[66] Gianfranceschi L, Siciliano R, Walls J, Morales B, Kirkwood A, Huang ZJ, Tonegawa S, Maffei L (2003) Visual cortex is rescued from the effects of dark rearing by overexpression of BDNF. Proc Natl Acad Sci U S A 100: 12486-12491.

[67] Baro JA, Lehmkuhle S, Kratz KE (1990) Electroretinograms and visual evoked potentials in long-term monocularly deprived cats. Invest Ophthalmol Vis Sci 31: 1405-1409.

[68] Fine I, Wade AR, Brewer AA, May MG, Goodman DF, Boynton GM, Wandell BA, MacLeod DI (2003) Long-term deprivation affects visual perception and cortex. Nat Neurosci 6: 915-916.

[69] Landi S, Cenni MC, Maffei L, Berardi N (2007) Environmental enrichment effects on development of retinal ganglion cell dendritic stratification require retinal BDNF. PLoS One 2: e346.

[70] Tian N, Copenhagen DR (2001) Visual deprivation alters development of synaptic function in inner retina after eye opening. Neuron 32: 439-449.

[71] Tian N, Copenhagen DR (2003) Visual stimulation is required for refinement of ON and OFF pathways in postnatal retina. Neuron 39: 85-96.

[72] Fleming AS, O'Day DH, Kraemer GW (1999) Neurobiology of mother-infant interactions: experience and central nervous system plasticity across development and generations. Neurosci Biobehav Rev 23: 673-685.

[73] Hofer MA (1984) Relationships as regulators: a psychobiologic perspective on bereavement. Psychosom Med 46: 183-197.

[74] Ronca AE, Lamkin CA, Alberts JR (1993) Maternal contributions to sensory experience in the fetal and newborn rat (Rattus norvegicus). J Comp Psychol 107: 61-74.

[75] Liu D, Diorio J, Day JC, Francis DD, Meaney MJ (2000) Maternal care, hippocampal synaptogenesis and cognitive development in rats. Nat Neurosci 3: 799-806.

[76] Champagne DL, Bagot RC, van Hasselt F, Ramakers G, Meaney MJ, de Kloet ER, Joels M, Krugers H (2008) Maternal care and hippocampal plasticity: evidence for experience-dependent structural plasticity, altered synaptic functioning, and differential responsiveness to glucocorticoids and stress. J Neurosci 28: 6037-6045.

[77] Meaney MJ, Szyf M (2005) Maternal care as a model for experience-dependent chromatin plasticity? Trends Neurosci 28: 456-463.

[78] Sale A, Putignano E, Cancedda L, Landi S, Cirulli F, Berardi N, Maffei L (2004) Enriched environment and acceleration of visual system development. Neuropharmacology 47: 649-660.

[79] Guzzetta A, Baldini S, Bancale A, Baroncelli L, Ciucci F, Ghirri P, Putignano E, Sale A, Viegi A, Berardi N, Boldrini A, Cioni G, Maffei L (2009) Massage accelerates brain development and the maturation of visual function. J Neurosci 29: 6042-6051.

[80] Burton CL, Chatterjee D, Chatterjee-Chakraborty M, Lovic V, Grella SL, Steiner M, Fleming AS (2007) Prenatal restraint stress and motherless rearing disrupts expression

of plasticity markers and stress-induced corticosterone release in adult female Sprague-Dawley rats. Brain Res 1158: 28-38.

[81] Chatterjee D, Chatterjee-Chakraborty M, Rees S, Cauchi J, de Medeiros CB, Fleming AS (2007) Maternal isolation alters the expression of neural proteins during development: 'Stroking' stimulation reverses these effects. Brain Res 1158: 11-27.

[82] Schanberg SM, Field TM (1987) Sensory deprivation stress and supplemental stimulation in the rat pup and preterm human neonate. Child Dev 58: 1431-1447.

[83] Guzzetta A, D'Acunto MG, Carotenuto M, Berardi N, Bancale A, Biagioni E, Boldrini A, Ghirri P, Maffei L, Cioni G The effects of preterm infant massage on brain electrical activity. Dev Med Child Neurol 53 Suppl 4: 46-51.

[84] Anthony RV, Pratt SL, Liang R, Holland MD (1995) Placental-fetal hormonal interactions: impact on fetal growth. J Anim Sci 73: 1861-1871.

[85] Seckl JR (2004) Prenatal glucocorticoids and long-term programming. Eur J Endocrinol 151 Suppl 3: U49-62.

[86] Mulder EJ, Robles de Medina PG, Huizink AC, Van den Bergh BR, Buitelaar JK, Visser GH (2002) Prenatal maternal stress: effects on pregnancy and the (unborn) child. Early Hum Dev 70: 3-14.

[87] Sale A, Cenni MC, Ciucci F, Putignano E, Chierzi S, Maffei L (2007) Maternal enrichment during pregnancy accelerates retinal development of the fetus. PLoS One 2: e1160.

[88] Parnpiansil P, Jutapakdeegul N, Chentanez T, Kotchabhakdi N (2003) Exercise during pregnancy increases hippocampal brain-derived neurotrophic factor mRNA expression and spatial learning in neonatal rat pup. Neurosci Lett 352: 45-48.

[89] Bick-Sander A, Steiner B, Wolf SA, Babu H, Kempermann G (2006) Running in pregnancy transiently increases postnatal hippocampal neurogenesis in the offspring. Proc Natl Acad Sci U S A 103: 3852-3857.

[90] Koo JW, Park CH, Choi SH, Kim NJ, Kim HS, Choe JC, Suh YH (2003) The postnatal environment can counteract prenatal effects on cognitive ability, cell proliferation, and synaptic protein expression. Faseb J 17: 1556-1558.

[91] Bavelier D, Levi DM, Li RW, Dan Y, Hensch TK Removing brakes on adult brain plasticity: from molecular to behavioral interventions. J Neurosci 30: 14964-14971.

[92] Frenkel MY, Sawtell NB, Diogo AC, Yoon B, Neve RL, Bear MF (2006) Instructive effect of visual experience in mouse visual cortex. Neuron 51: 339-349.

[93] Ghisovan N, Nemri A, Shumikhina S, Molotchnikoff S (2008) Visual cells remember earlier applied target: plasticity of orientation selectivity. PLoS One 3: e3689.

[94] Marshansky S, Shumikhina S, Molotchnikoff S Repetitive adaptation induces plasticity of spatial frequency tuning in cat primary visual cortex. Neuroscience 172: 355-365.

[95] Sawtell NB, Frenkel MY, Philpot BD, Nakazawa K, Tonegawa S, Bear MF (2003) NMDA receptor-dependent ocular dominance plasticity in adult visual cortex. Neuron 38: 977-985.

[96] Holmes JM, Clarke MP (2006) Amblyopia. Lancet 367: 1343-1351.
[97] Mittelman D (2003) Amblyopia. Pediatr Clin North Am 50: 189-196.
[98] Kiorpes L (2006) Visual processing in amblyopia: animal studies. Strabismus 14: 3-10.
[99] Levi DM (2006) Visual processing in amblyopia: human studies. Strabismus 14: 11-19.
[100] Baroncelli L, Maffei L, Sale A New perspectives in amblyopia therapy on adults: a critical role for the excitatory/inhibitory balance. Front Cell Neurosci 5: 25.
[101] Sale A, Maya Vetencourt JF, Medini P, Cenni MC, Baroncelli L, De Pasquale R, Maffei L (2007) Environmental enrichment in adulthood promotes amblyopia recovery through a reduction of intracortical inhibition. Nat Neurosci 10: 679-681.
[102] Wu C, Hunter DG (2006) Amblyopia: diagnostic and therapeutic options. Am J Ophthalmol 141: 175-184.
[103] Baroncelli L, Braschi C, Spolidoro M, Begenisic T, Maffei L, Sale A Brain plasticity and disease: a matter of inhibition. Neural Plast 2011: 286073.
[104] Harauzov A, Spolidoro M, DiCristo G, De Pasquale R, Cancedda L, Pizzorusso T, Viegi A, Berardi N, Maffei L Reducing intracortical inhibition in the adult visual cortex promotes ocular dominance plasticity. J Neurosci 30: 361-371.
[105] Fronius M, Cirina L, Cordey A, Ohrloff C (2005) Visual improvement during psychophysical training in an adult amblyopic eye following visual loss in the contralateral eye. Graefes Arch Clin Exp Ophthalmol 243: 278-280.
[106] El Mallah MK, Chakravarthy U, Hart PM (2000) Amblyopia: is visual loss permanent? Br J Ophthalmol 84: 952-956.
[107] Hamed LM (1991) Strabismus presenting after cataract surgery. Ophthalmology 98: 247-252.
[108] Vereecken EP, Brabant P (1984) Prognosis for vision in amblyopia after the loss of the good eye. Arch Ophthalmol 102: 220-224.
[109] Wilson ME (1992) Adult amblyopia reversed by contralateral cataract formation. J Pediatr Ophthalmol Strabismus 29: 100-102.
[110] Tognini P MI, Bonaccorsi J, Cenni MC, Sale A, Maffei L (2012) Environmental Enrichment Promotes Plasticity and Visual Acuity Recovery in Adult Monocular Amblyopic Rats. PLoS ONE 7(4): e34815. .
[111] Levi DM, Hariharan S, Klein SA (2002) Suppressive and facilitatory spatial interactions in amblyopic vision. Vision Res 42: 1379-1394.
[112] Polat U, Bonneh Y, Ma-Naim T, Belkin M, Sagi D (2005) Spatial interactions in amblyopia: effects of stimulus parameters and amblyopia type. Vision Res 45: 1471-1479.
[113] Sale A, Berardi N, Spolidoro M, Baroncelli L, Maffei L GABAergic inhibition in visual cortical plasticity. Front Cell Neurosci 4: 10.
[114] Baroncelli L BJ, Milanese M, Bonifacino T, Giribaldi F, Manno I, Cenni MC, Berardi N, Bonanno G, Maffei L, Sale A (2012) Enriched experience and recovery from amblyopia in adult rats: Impact of motor, social and sensory components Neuropharmacology 62: 2388-2397.

[115] Levi DM, Li RW (2009) Perceptual learning as a potential treatment for amblyopia: a mini-review. Vision Res 49: 2535-2549.

[116] Astle AT, Webb BS, McGraw PV Can perceptual learning be used to treat amblyopia beyond the critical period of visual development? Ophthalmic Physiol Opt 31: 564-573.

[117] Li RW, Ngo C, Nguyen J, Levi DM Video-game play induces plasticity in the visual system of adults with amblyopia. PLoS Biol 9: e1001135.

[118] Green CS, Bavelier D Learning, attentional control, and action video games. Curr Biol 22: R197-206.

[119] Sale A, De Pasquale R, Bonaccorsi J, Pietra G, Olivieri D, Berardi N, Maffei L Visual perceptual learning induces long-term potentiation in the visual cortex. Neuroscience 172: 219-225.

[120] Cooke SF, Bear MF Visual experience induces long-term potentiation in the primary visual cortex. J Neurosci 30: 16304-16313.

[121] Prusky GT, West PW, Douglas RM (2000) Behavioral assessment of visual acuity in mice and rats. Vision Res 40: 2201-2209.

[122] Rogan MT, Staubli UV, LeDoux JE (1997) Fear conditioning induces associative long-term potentiation in the amygdala. Nature 390: 604-607.

[123] Rioult-Pedotti MS, Friedman D, Donoghue JP (2000) Learning-induced LTP in neocortex. Science 290: 533-536.

[124] Whitlock JR, Heynen AJ, Shuler MG, Bear MF (2006) Learning induces long-term potentiation in the hippocampus. Science 313: 1093-1097.

[125] Mainardi M, Landi S, Gianfranceschi L, Baldini S, De Pasquale R, Berardi N, Maffei L, Caleo M Environmental enrichment potentiates thalamocortical transmission and plasticity in the adult rat visual cortex. J Neurosci Res 88: 3048-3059.

[126] Thompson B, Mansouri B, Koski L, Hess RF (2008) Brain plasticity in the adult: modulation of function in amblyopia with rTMS. Curr Biol 18: 1067-1071.

[127] Baroncelli L, Sale A, Viegi A, Maya Vetencourt JF, De Pasquale R, Baldini S, Maffei L Experience-dependent reactivation of ocular dominance plasticity in the adult visual cortex. Exp Neurol 226: 100-109.

[128] Baroncelli L, Braschi C, Spolidoro M, Begenisic T, Sale A, Maffei L Nurturing brain plasticity: impact of environmental enrichment. Cell Death Differ 17: 1092-1103.

[129] Maya Vetencourt JF, Sale A, Viegi A, Baroncelli L, De Pasquale R, O'Leary OF, Castren E, Maffei L (2008) The antidepressant fluoxetine restores plasticity in the adult visual cortex. Science 320: 385-388.

[130] Chen JL, Lin WC, Cha JW, So PT, Kubota Y, Nedivi E Structural basis for the role of inhibition in facilitating adult brain plasticity. Nat Neurosci 14: 587-594.

[131] McOmish CE, Hannan AJ (2007) Enviromimetics: exploring gene environment interactions to identify therapeutic targets for brain disorders. Expert Opin Ther Targets 11: 899-913.

[132] Nadel L (2003) Down's syndrome: a genetic disorder in biobehavioral perspective. Genes Brain Behav 2: 156-166.

[133] Pennington BF, Moon J, Edgin J, Stedron J, Nadel L (2003) The neuropsychology of Down syndrome: evidence for hippocampal dysfunction. Child Dev 74: 75-93.

[134] Brown JH, Johnson MH, Paterson SJ, Gilmore R, Longhi E, Karmiloff-Smith A (2003) Spatial representation and attention in toddlers with Williams syndrome and Down syndrome. Neuropsychologia 41: 1037-1046.

[135] Clark D, Wilson GN (2003) Behavioral assessment of children with Down syndrome using the Reiss psychopathology scale. Am J Med Genet A 118A: 210-216.

[136] John FM, Bromham NR, Woodhouse JM, Candy TR (2004) Spatial vision deficits in infants and children with Down syndrome. Invest Ophthalmol Vis Sci 45: 1566-1572.

[137] Gardiner K, Fortna A, Bechtel L, Davisson MT (2003) Mouse models of Down syndrome: how useful can they be? Comparison of the gene content of human chromosome 21 with orthologous mouse genomic regions. Gene 318: 137-147.

[138] Seregaza Z, Roubertoux PL, Jamon M, Soumireu-Mourat B (2006) Mouse models of cognitive disorders in trisomy 21: a review. Behav Genet 36: 387-404.

[139] Holtzman DM, Santucci D, Kilbridge J, Chua-Couzens J, Fontana DJ, Daniels SE, Johnson RM, Chen K, Sun Y, Carlson E, Alleva E, Epstein CJ, Mobley WC (1996) Developmental abnormalities and age-related neurodegeneration in a mouse model of Down syndrome. Proc Natl Acad Sci U S A 93: 13333-13338.

[140] Escorihuela RM, Vallina IF, Martinez-Cue C, Baamonde C, Dierssen M, Tobena A, Florez J, Fernandez-Teruel A (1998) Impaired short- and long-term memory in Ts65Dn mice, a model for Down syndrome. Neurosci Lett 247: 171-174.

[141] Scott-McKean JJ, Chang B, Hurd RE, Nusinowitz S, Schmidt C, Davisson MT, Costa AC The mouse model of Down syndrome Ts65Dn presents visual deficits as assessed by pattern visual evoked potentials. Invest Ophthalmol Vis Sci 51: 3300-3308.

[142] Siarey RJ, Carlson EJ, Epstein CJ, Balbo A, Rapoport SI, Galdzicki Z (1999) Increased synaptic depression in the Ts65Dn mouse, a model for mental retardation in Down syndrome. Neuropharmacology 38: 1917-1920.

[143] Kleschevnikov AM, Belichenko PV, Villar AJ, Epstein CJ, Malenka RC, Mobley WC (2004) Hippocampal long-term potentiation suppressed by increased inhibition in the Ts65Dn mouse, a genetic model of Down syndrome. J Neurosci 24: 8153-8160.

[144] Fernandez F, Morishita W, Zuniga E, Nguyen J, Blank M, Malenka RC, Garner CC (2007) Pharmacotherapy for cognitive impairment in a mouse model of Down syndrome. Nat Neurosci 10: 411-413.

[145] Best TK, Cramer NP, Chakrabarti L, Haydar TF, Galdzicki Z Dysfunctional hippocampal inhibition in the Ts65Dn mouse model of Down syndrome. Exp Neurol 233: 749-757.

[146] Rissman RA, Mobley WC Implications for treatment: GABAA receptors in aging, Down syndrome and Alzheimer's disease. J Neurochem 117: 613-622.

[147] Begenisic T, Spolidoro M, Braschi C, Baroncelli L, Milanese M, Pietra G, Fabbri ME, Bonanno G, Cioni G, Maffei L, Sale A Environmental enrichment decreases GABAergic inhibition and improves cognitive abilities, synaptic plasticity, and visual functions in a mouse model of Down syndrome. Front Cell Neurosci 5: 29.

[148] Burke SN, Barnes CA (2006) Neural plasticity in the ageing brain. Nat Rev Neurosci 7: 30-40.
[149] Scali M, Baroncelli L, Cenni MC, Sale A, Maffei L A rich environmental experience reactivates visual cortex plasticity in aged rats. Exp Gerontol 47: 337-341.
[150] Kempermann G, Kuhn HG, Gage FH (1998) Experience-induced neurogenesis in the senescent dentate gyrus. J Neurosci 18: 3206-3212.

Chapter 15

Adaptation and Neuronal Network in Visual Cortex

Lyes Bachatene, Vishal Bharmauria and Stéphane Molotchnikoff

Additional information is available at the end of the chapter

http://dx.doi.org/10.5772/46011

1. Introduction

Complex mechanisms from retina to different visual areas allow us to read these lines. The visual system is inevitable for the way we interact with our surroundings as majority of our impressions, memories, feelings are bound to the visual perception. Millions of cortical neurons are implicated and programmed specifically to frame this incredible interface (perception) for us to interact with the world. Neurons in the visual cortex respond essentially to the variations in luminance occurring within their receptive fields, where each neuron fires maximally by acting as a filter for stimulus features such as orientation, motion, direction and velocity, with an appropriate combination of these properties [1-5].

The seminal work of Hubel and Wiesel on the visual cortex of cat [1, 2, 6-8], has been instrumental in establishing the anatomical and physiological aspects of the visual cortex. Many studies by various investigators on the visual cortex of different animals, thereafter, have been phenomenal in understanding the brain in general and the vision in particular; yet, neuronal mechanisms involved in processing of stimuli still elude our complete understanding of cortical functioning. These findings have been crucial in unravelling the organization of the visual cortex. The visual cortex reorganises itself in the postnatal development, within a specific period called 'the critical period' [9], which is a period characterised with pronounced brain plasticity. In recent years, the focus of the research has been to comprehend the 'reorganization' of neuronal framework, especially after the so called 'critical period' [10-12] in response to various conditions and its ability to adapt accordingly. This amazing tendency of brain to change its neuronal connections and properties is termed 'plasticity' [13]. Two common approaches to study the reorganization of visual cortex are frequently applied: deprivation and induced adaptation. Deprivation refers to the removal of sensory inputs, whereas induced adaptation refers to the forceful application of a sensory input. Consequently, neurons communicate dynamically with each other in a specific way self-assembling, auto-calibrating, memorizing and adapting to different stimuli properties, thus responding accordingly to several experiences [14-16].

The aim of this chapter is to primarily focus on how the linkage between cells changes following plastic modifications of cortical neuronal properties, that is, how the reorganization of the cortical network is modulated following adaptation-induced plasticity, as it is inferred by cross-correlating the action potentials of the neurons in the primary visual cortex. We begin with the general architecture of visual cortex (particularly cat visual cortex), followed by a brief introduction to plasticity and adaptation. Then, we cite an example of modification of the neuronal connections before and after adaptation as revealed by cross-correlation method. Based on this example, we propose a model for changing functional connections prior and post adaptation and conclude with how neurons change their functional relationships when forcefully adapted to a non-optimal stimulus.

2. Visual system: Organization

2.1. Introduction

Visual area constitutes about 25 % of the cortex in humans with approximately 5 billion neurons. The study of the visual cortex has revealed many of these visual regions such as V1, V2, V3, V4 and MT on the basis of their anatomical architecture, topography and physiological properties [17, 18]. These regions are involved in processing of multitude of informations (shape, orientation, color, movement, size etc) resulting from the visual pathways, thus making up an image applied to retina.

The cortical area of higher mammals such as cats, monkeys and humans is generally divided into modules of selectivity (e.g. the visual cortex is divided into areas of selectivity called orientation columns). Several characteristics of the visual system of mammals appear to be common to many species [19, 20], though the neurons are distributed in a salt and pepper fashion in the visual cortex of lower animals such as rats and mice, lacking the orientation domains [21, 22]. Research on animal models is used on a large scale to study and investigate the structure and function of the visual system. Monkeys, cats, and mice are commonly used in neurophysiological experiments for understanding cortical mechanisms in general and visual pathways in particular [23].

2.2. From retina to visual areas

Visual perception begins in the retina where the received light is transformed into electrical signal by a biochemical cascade produced in the rods and cones. The retinal ganglion cells relay the message to the lateral geniculate body (LGN) which consists of six layers [24]. Each layer receives information from the retinal hemi-field of one eye. The axon terminals of ganglion cells which project on each layer form a precise retinotopic map. This retinotopy denotes the spatial organization of neuronal responses to visual stimuli. Indeed, in many parts of the brain, neurons that respond to stimulation from a given portion of the visual field are located right next to the neurons whose receptive fields cover adjacent portions.

Therefore, all the neurons in these brain regions form a topographical map of the visual field from its projection onto the retina.

From the LGN, axons are organized into thalamocortical fibres forming the optic radiations. These optic radiations project onto the cortex in specialized visual areas. The distribution of fibres in the cortex can reproduce the visual field on the cortical layer, and the stimulation of a small cortical area leads to the appearance of bright spots called 'phosphenes' [25] in a specific location of the visual field. Visual areas begin in the occipital lobe, and the primary visual cortex or area 17 is the main entrance to cortex for thalamic relay cells [24]. The primary visual cortex is organized into functional modules. Neurons with similar receptive fields are organized into columns [26, 27]. Visual neurons have other fundamental properties, such as the direction selectivity of cells in the layer IVβ, and the selectivity for speed [3, 6]. There is another system of alternating columns, which corresponds to the separation of afferents from both eyes. These are the ocular dominance columns. The ocular dominance columns represent bands of cortical tissue alternately occupied by afferents from the left eye or right eye [28-30]. These bands are particularly pronounced at the cortical layer IV, which receives the afferent endings of the lateral geniculate nucleus. Thus the visual cortex is organized into functional maps of orientation, spatial frequency, ocular dominance, temporal frequency which are interrelated to each other [31-33].

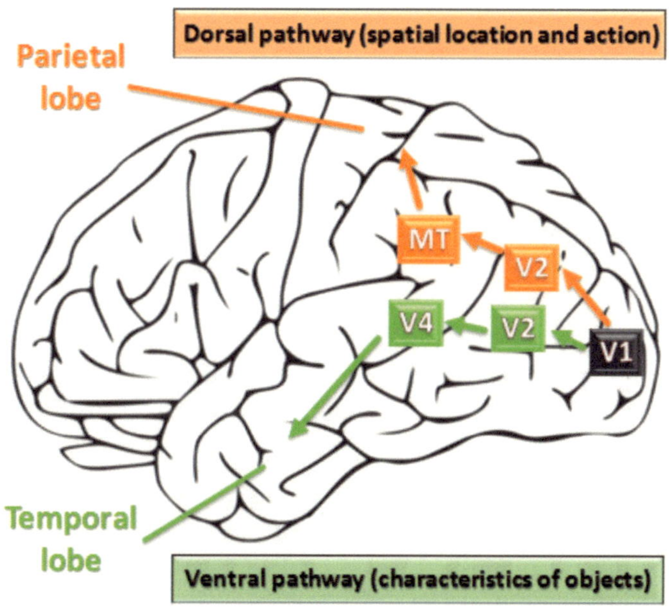

Figure 1. Parallel organization of the visual system

Many findings have led to the discovery of thirty different cortical areas that contribute to visual perception. The primary areas (V1) and secondary areas (V2) are surrounded by many other tertiary or associative visual areas such as V3, V4, V5 (or MT) involved in processing various attributes of trigger features [18, 34]. Areas V3 and V3A are selective to the form of stimuli [35], and neurons of area V4 are selective to colors [36]. Area V5 or MT (middle temporal) is an area where majority of cells are sensitive to motion and direction, and none of which are selective to color [37].

Moreover, the parallel organization of visual system is involved in the establishment of two major visual pathways: Ventral and dorsal pathways which are indispensable for the object recognition [38, 39]. Figure 1 illustrates the parallel organization of visual system, two major pathways: Green part corresponds to the ventral pathway in the cortex ending in the temporal lobe [38, 40]. It is involved in the processing of information on the characteristics of the objects (shapes, colours, materials), that is, object recognition including faces. Orange part corresponds to the dorsal pathway in the cortex ending in the parietal lobe [38, 40]. This path is associated with spatial vision (action / location) of objects, and is involved in processing of action in space.

3. Neuron types in primary visual cortex

3.1. Pyramidal cells and interneurons

The grey matter in the primary visual cortex is divided into six layers namely I, II, III, IV, V, VI (Figure 2) which comprise of different types of neurons [41, 42]. Two types of neurons are mainly observed: pyramidal cells and interneurons which can be physiologically separated and are the focus of interest in this chapter, that is, how they modify their properties and change linkage with each other post-adaptation. Pyramidal cells are excitatory neurons projecting onto other brain regions [43, 44] whereas stellate cells which are the recipient cells from the relay cells of the LGN correspond to the local excitatory interneurons [45]. In addition, there are interneurons that are inhibitory in nature [45]. Figure 2 illustrates the layers and cell types in primary visual cortex. Each layer has specific cell types and connectivity in primary visual cortex. Layer IV contains many stellate cells, small neurons with dendrites arranged radially around the cell body. Pyramidal cells are found in layers II-III, V and VI and are the only type of neurons that send axons outside the cortex. These neurons exhibit two levels of their dendritic extension: basal level close to the cell body and relatively long apical dendritic branches extending sometimes over the entire thickness of the cortex.

Classically, spike waveforms allow cells' distinction into two functional cell-groups, that is, excitatory pyramidal cells and inhibitory interneurons [11, 46, 47]. Figure 3 illustrates a typical example of cells distinguished based on their waveforms: fast spike and regular spike. Figure 3a corresponds to a fast spike with steeper ascending slope of the action potential and represents the putative interneuron [11], whereas Figure 3b corresponds to a regular spike which exhibits a slower ascending slope and represents the putative pyramidal cell [11].

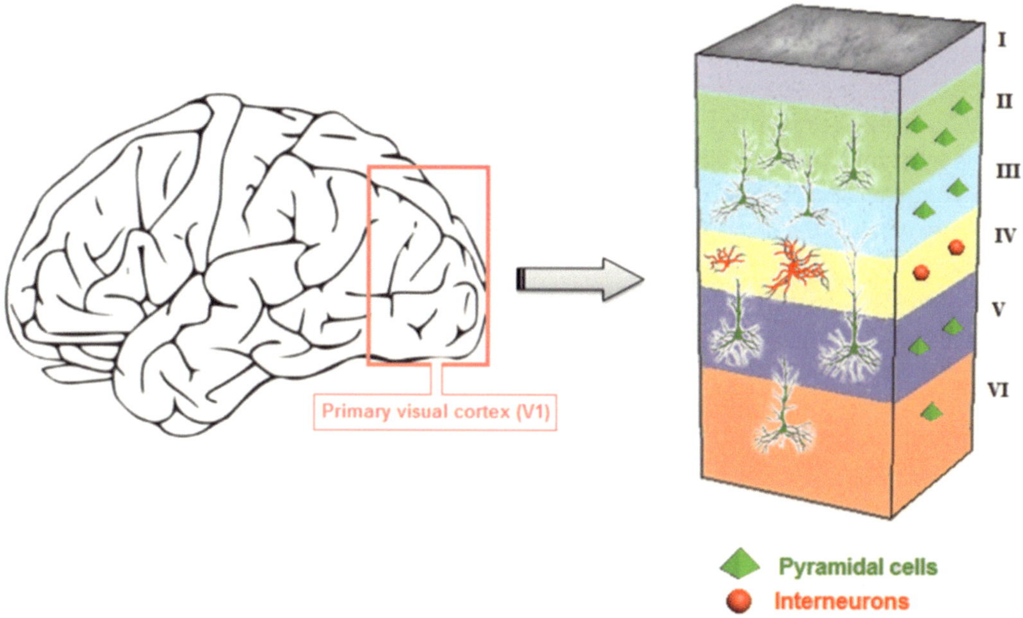

Figure 2. Organization of the primary visual cortex

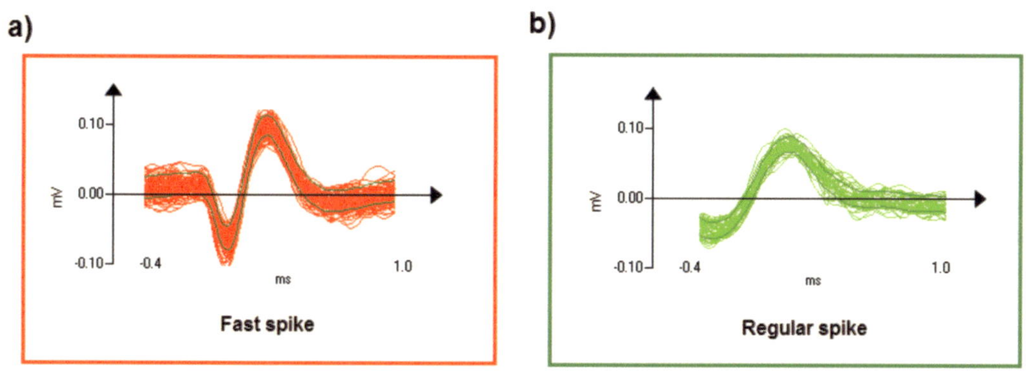

Figure 3. Spike waveforms for putative interneurons (a) and putative pyramidal cells (b)

3.2. Receptive fields

Visual information from the LGN cells firstly projects onto the stellate interneurons in layer IV, which have concentric receptive fields similar to those of LGN neurons [24, 48]. Neurons of layer IV project vertically onto other cortical layers. In layers II / III, cortical cells exhibit a radical transformation of the receptive field organization, where cells respond preferentially to stimuli with properties such as a bar or an edge that has specific characteristics namely orientation, direction, length, width, and motion [3, 6, 49].

Cells in these layers are classified into simple, complex and hypercomplex cells based on their dark or light-edge properties [6]. Simple cell is a cell which has an ON-OFF sub field, that is, it responds to ON or OFF stimuli in the receptive field and has adjacent excitatory and inhibitory areas [6]. Complex neurons have receptive fields larger than those of simple neurons. They are also selective for orientation, but the precise position of the stimulus within the receptive field is less critical because they have no defined ON or OFF sub-areas. That is why a movement of the stimulus through the receptive field is a potent stimulus for some complex neurons [6, 50, 51]. A complex cell does not have adjacent excitatory and inhibitory areas in the receptive field and responds to whole of the receptive field regardless of the exactitude of the stimulus area, though complex cells can be direction-specific [6]. A hypercomplex cell appears to result, when the axons of complex neurons with different orientations converge on it. A hypercomplex cell is selective to lines of a defined length, and if the stimulus exceeds this length the response is diminished due to inhibitory extremities in addition to antagonistic flanks [6].

Neurons in primary visual cortex are connected laterally and vertically to each other. Lateral or horizontal connections are specified as long range connections between neurons preferring similar stimulus features [52, 53] which are functionally connected to each other at large distance [54, 55]. Vertical connections are specified as inputs to layers II and III from layer IV of the visual cortex [56, 57] which receives its inputs from LGN [58]. From layers II and III, the connections descend to layers V and VI [57].

Cats have a high performance visual system close to that of primates, making it a very coveted subject for researches to reveal the functional aspects of this complex system [59, 60]. Approaches to study the visual system are based on functional electrophysiology, where animals are anaesthetized and paralyzed for electrophysiological recordings by lowering microelectrodes into regions of interest within the visual area and visually stimulating the neurons [6, 11, 49, 61].

4. Plasticity and adaptation in the visual cortex

Neurons in the mammalian visual cortex are tuned to respond to visual stimuli such as contour orientation, motion, direction, and speed [3, 6, 59]. Preference for orientation in orientation columns is considered relatively stable in the primary visual cortex (V1) as an emergent property that is established early in the life, following the so-called critical period [9].

Studies from various laboratories have shown that in a fully mature brain, neuronal network restructures itself beyond the postnatal critical period that follows birth [11, 49, 61-65]. Recent investigations revealed the ability of visual neurons to respond to different stimuli conditions (deprivation or imposition) by changing their optimal properties acquired after birth. This adaptation of neurons for visual perception suggests the existence of neuronal plasticity in adults, hence a mature brain.

Adaptation-induced-plasticity of orientation in primary visual cortex is characterized by authors as the ability of cortical neurons to change their preferred orientation following a long [11, 61, 63] or short [62, 65] exposure to a non-preferred orientation for the primary visual cortex neurons in cats, e.g. Long adaptation leads to the shift of orientation tuning towards attractive direction [61]. In a similar fashion, repetitive adaptation to a non-preferred spatial frequency reveals the spatial frequency tuning shifts in cat visual cortex [49]. In general, imposing a particular stimulus induces instructive process to modify neuronal properties, for example, when in the visual cortex of awake mice a single orientation grating stimulus is repeatedly presented; it leads to augmentation of responses evoked exclusively by testing stimulus, that is, the experience led to enhancement of response [66]. In experiments where animals are anaesthetized (e.g. a cat in the experiment described later on) the shifts of peaks of tuning curves following adaptation (described in figure 4) are not attributed to attention modulations. Consequently, these shifts result from basic neuronal processes outside the frame of attentional processes that might impact response magnitudes.

Adaptation studies in recent years have presented a more complex picture where prolonged exposure to a non-preferred orientation has shown modifications in neurons' preferred orientations. After adaptation to a non preferred orientation, obtained tuning curve for the new preferred orientation (after adaptation) can shift in two directions relative to the original preferred orientation: attractive or repulsive [11, 61, 63, 64]. An attractive shift is a shift of the tuning curve towards the adapting orientation. On the other hand; a repulsive shift is a shift of the tuning curve in the opposite side of the adapting orientation. Figure 4 illustrates types of shifts post-adaptation. Figure 4a corresponds to an attractive shift, in which blue tuning curve represents control optimal orientation (before adaptation), and red tuning curve represents new optimal orientation (after adaptation).The tuning curve shifted towards the adapting orientation. Figure 4b corresponds to the repulsive shift, in which blue tuning curve represents control optimal orientation (before adaptation), and red tuning curve represents new optimal orientation (after adaptation). The tuning curve shifted away from the adapting orientation. Red arrows depict adapting orientation (non-preferred orientation in control).

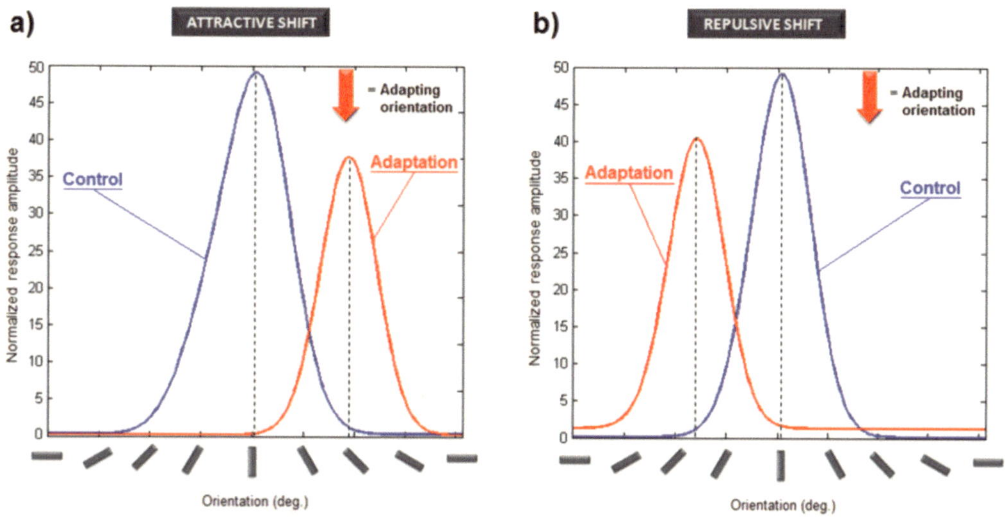

Figure 4. Types of shifts post-adaptation

Attractive shifts are more frequent than repulsive shifts in longer adaptation durations (≥ 6 min) [11, 61]. Repeated or prolonged exposure to an adapter diminished neuronal responses evoked by the original optimal properties, furthermore in parallel, if it is the neuron's preferred stimulus [61]. Optical imaging investigations in recent years have also revealed the impact of adaptation-induced-plasticity, showing that orientation maps in V1 can be modified by imposing one particular orientation [62, 65, 67].

5. Crosscorrelograms and neuronal relationships in visual cortex

As reviewed above [11, 49, 61-65], adaptation- induced studies on visual cortex can reveal a great deal about the functioning of the visual cortex. Crosscorrelogram analysis is an efficient tool to establish the functional connectivity between neurons. Ever since the crosscorrelogram approach was introduced [68], it has proved to be an invaluable tool to determine how specific neurons interact with each other. A crosscorrelogram is a histogram used to infer the connectivity between two neurons, where one neuron is reference and other target. The histogram shows us when the spikes of target neuron are related in time to the spikes of reference neuron. The technique has been instrumental in revealing widespread incidences of neuronal synchrony and neuronal time-relationships among various cortical areas [64, 70-78]. For instance, as revealed by crosscorrelogram analysis, synchrony has been reported to be strong between cells with similar preferred parameters due in part to specific connections between cortical domains having similar tuning properties. Thus, based on the crosscorrelogram analysis, the functional network connections can be established between the neurons [58, 71, 79-81].

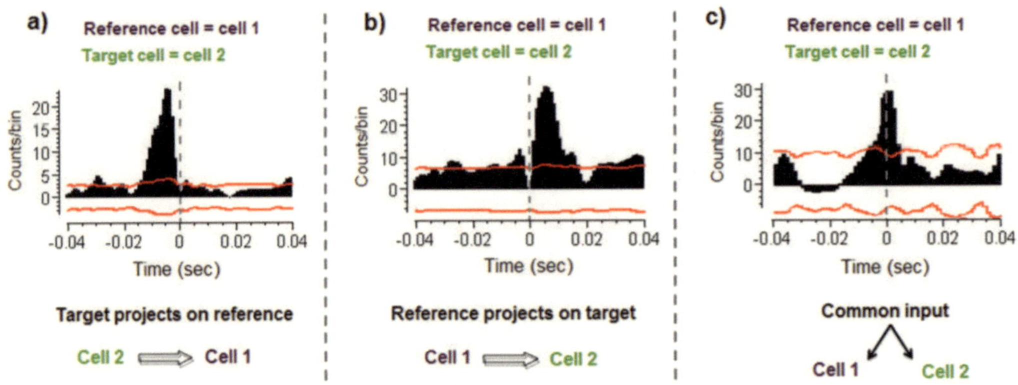

Figure 5. Crosscorrelograms between two neurons (reference and target)

A typical crosscorrelogram between two neurons to interpret the relation between them is obtained by keeping one of the neurons as reference and calculating the spikes of the other neuron with reference to it. An investigator generally is interested in one of the following patterns as illustrated in figure 5, while he is interpreting crosscorrelograms. Figure 5 illustrates the time relations between two neurons as revealed by shifted and corrected crosscorrelograms when one neuron is reference and other target. A shifted crosscorrelogram is a histogram obtained, when the spikes of the reference cell are shifted by one or two cycles of stimulation. This eliminates the possibility of stimulus-induced-relationship between two neurons. After this the shifted crosscorrelogram is subtracted (corrected) to remove the stimulus-locked -component. Figure 5a corresponds to target cell projecting onto the reference cell. Target neuron fires few milliseconds before the reference cell since the peak of the crosscorrelogram appears few milliseconds before zero, that is, offset from zero, within 5ms. This means there is an excitation from target to the reference cell [79, 81]. Figure 5b corresponds to the reference cell projecting onto the target cell. Target neuron fires few milliseconds after the reference cell since the peak of the crosscorrelogram appears few milliseconds after zero, within 5ms. This means the excitation is from reference cell to the target cell [79, 81]. Figure 5c corresponds to the synchrony between two neurons, as the peak straddles zero [73, 82]. This means there is a common excitatory input to both neurons most likely from other neuron or neurons. Though, various time windows have been taken into consideration ranging from 3ms to 10 ms [72, 79] to reveal the functional connections between the involved neurons, but a time window within 5ms is most frequently used.

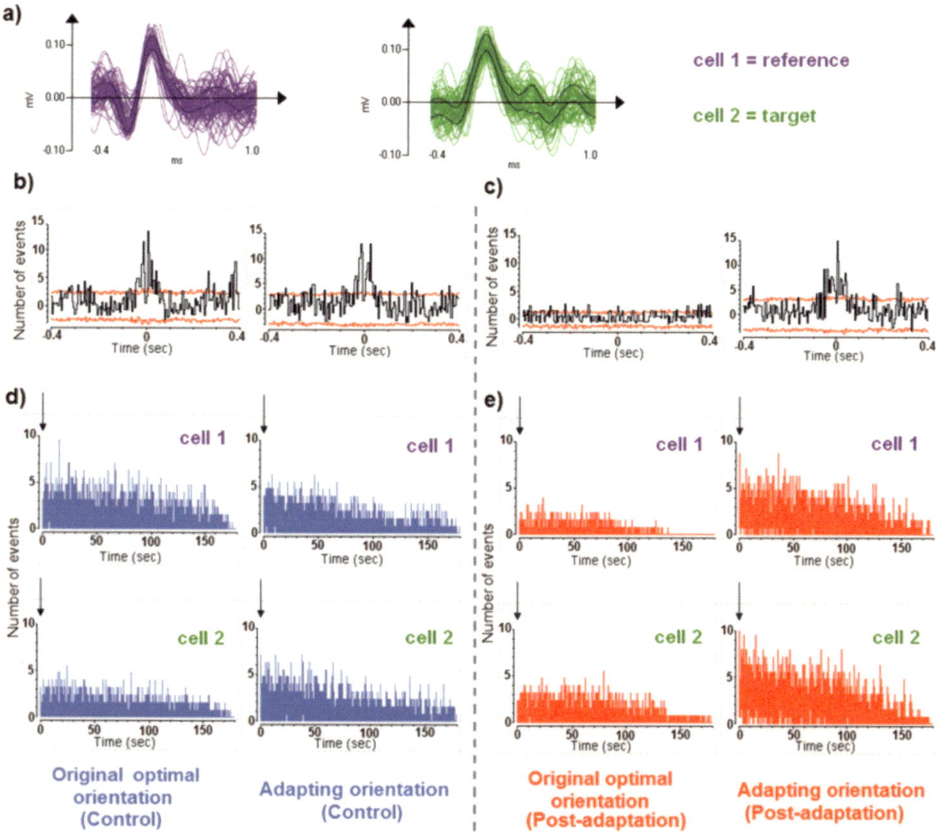

Figure 6. Differential effects of adaptation on synchrony for responses evoked by original orientation and adapting orientation

Figure 6 corresponds to differential effects of adaptation on synchrony for responses evoked by original orientation and adapting orientation. Figure 6a represents respective spike-waveforms for cell 1 and cell 2. Figure 6b shows crosscorrelograms between cell 1 and cell 2 before adaptation (control). The centered peak corresponds to synchrony. Fig 6c represents crosscorrelograms between cell 1 and cell 2 after adaptation. Synchrony disappeared for original optimal orientation while it persists for responses evoked by adapter. Figure 6d shows respective Peri-Stimulus Time Histograms (PSTH's) for cells in control (before adaptation). Figure 6e corresponds to respective Peri-Stimulus Time Histograms (PSTH's) for cells after adaptation. The downward black arrows indicate onset of the drifting sine-wave patch positioned in the receptive field.

Since adaptation modifies the optimal properties of neurons, whether orientation, direction or spatial frequency, it seems reasonable to postulate that these modifications following adaptation induce a rapid reorganization of the inter-neuronal relationships, as revealed by crosscorrelogram analyses. For instance, a recipient neuron programmed since birth to be connected to a specific neuron that responds optimally to one specific property, all of a sudden starts responding optimally to another stimulus, and begins participating in a different network with other neuron- as if breaking its allegiance to the neuron it is programmed to be connected since birth.

6. Network formation

Neurons do not respond in isolation to the trigger features, but in coordination with surrounding neurons. Thus, they encode stimuli features by forming cell assemblies, where in the involved neurons are time related with each other. Recent investigations have revealed the ability of visual neurons to respond to different stimuli conditions by changing their optimal properties acquired after birth. Most of these studies have been done by visual deprivation [9, 83-86], whereas only a few have centered on induced adaptation [11, 62, 64, 87]. This adaptation of neurons to non-optimal stimuli suggests the adaptability of neuronal code to visual stimuli.

Neuronal connections in the cortex generally occur locally [79, 88]. Visual cortex is a highly specialized functional area where the neurons coordinate locally to encode the visual scenes [89, 90, 91]. To reveal how this local circuitry of different neurons in visual cortex is set up and modulated in response to different visual stimuli is of prime importance to understand the mechanisms of information processing. Crosscorrelogram strategy discussed above can be effectively applied to form a neuronal network in response to visual stimuli. Thus, it can be an efficient tool in deciphering the changes in the neuronal code post-adaptation, hence, the mechanisms of plastic modifications can be revealed.

For example, in the Figure 7 we show the network of connections prior and post adaptation between three neurons recorded simultaneously from the same electrode lowered into the primary visual cortex of an anaesthetized cat. In this experiment, a stimulating sine-wave drifting grating was set to excite cells optimally. Shifted and corrected crosscorrlegrams

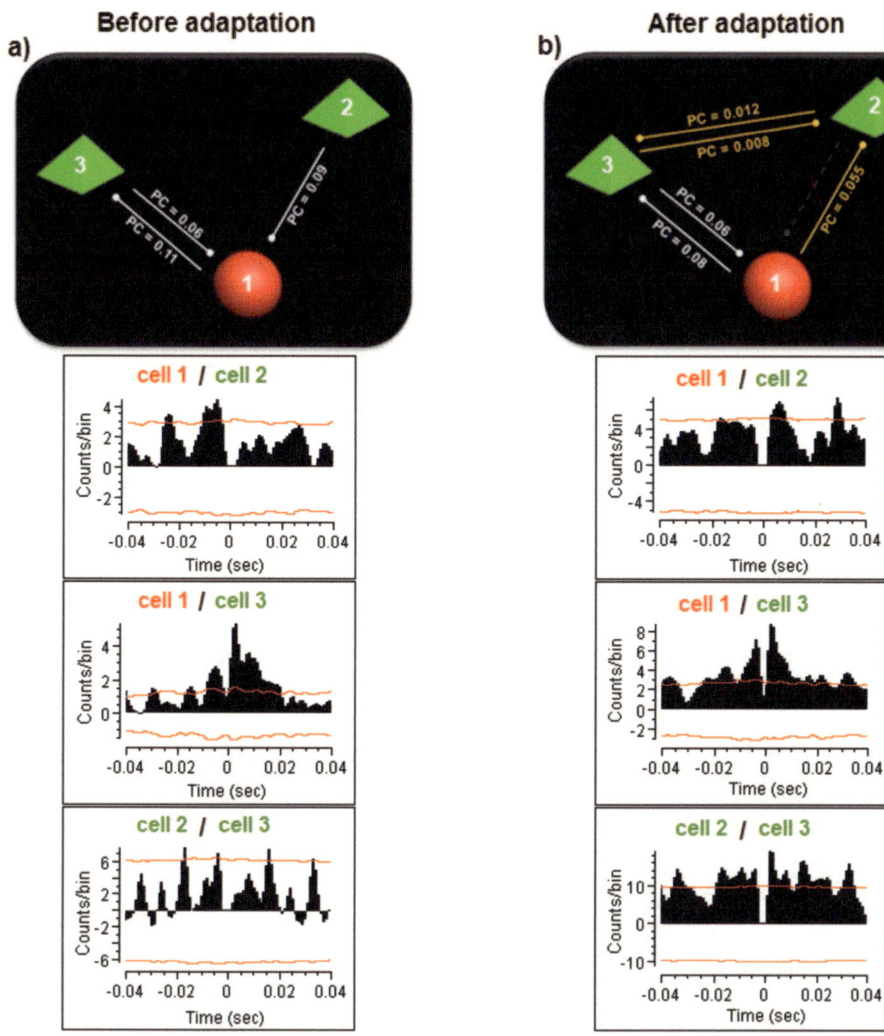

Figure 7. Functional relationships between simultaneously recorded cells before and after adaptation

between all the involved neurons were obtained. A time window of 5 ms before or after the zero in the shifted and corrected crosscorrelogram is taken into account for the projection to be valid. The physiological connectivity (synaptic connections, common input) between cells occurs on very small time scales, less than 3 ms [79, 81]. Since we consider a time window of 10 ms in crosscorrelograms for establishing connections, therefore, this connectivity only reflects that the cells function (irrespective of physical connectivity) in coordination with each other in a time-window of 10 ms following a presented stimulus. Figure 7a illustrates the functional connections between three neurons as revealed by their respective crosscorrelograms (shifted and corrected). White projections correspond to established connections before adaptation. Figure 7b illustrates the new functional connections between same neurons as revealed by their respective crosscorrelograms (shifted and corrected). Yellow projection corresponds to the new connection established after adaptation. Dotted gray projection represents the disappeared projection. PC corresponds to the probability coefficient of the connections. Solid green pyramid represents a pyramidal cell and the solid red sphere represents an interneuron. Red curve line indicates 95% significance level.

This changing of connections indicates that the functional relationships between neurons are modified depending on the stimulus features. For instance, following the forceful presentation of a particular stimulus (in this example a different orientation) results in disappearance of some relationships, and appearance of new relationships.

Based on the above example, we hypothesize and propose a model how the network of neurons is modulated prior and post adaptation as revealed by the functional time-relationship of neurons between them. Figure 8 depicts the functional connections between the same neurons before and after adaptation. White projections in figure 8a show the projections that cells have onto each other before adaptation, whereas figure 8b depicts how the network changes in the same group of neurons after adaptation. Some of the connections between the cells remain distinct (white projections) whereas some connections disappear (dotted gray arrows) with appearing new connections (yellow projections).

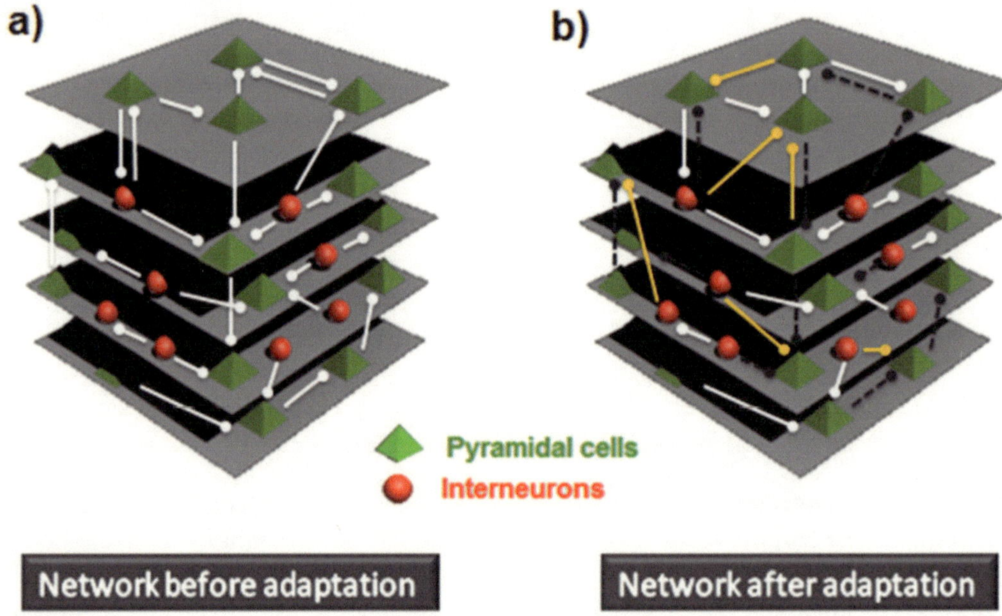

Figure 8. Network model before and after adaptation

7. Conclusion

This chapter reviewed the changes in the cellular properties post-adaptation. Indeed, the optimal trigger features may change following the prolonged application of a stimulus to which the cell responded feebly before adaptation. This phenomenon has been virtually observed in all mammals which have been tested so far. Also in parallel, following adaptation the inter-neuronal relationships are modified. This suggests that the entire cortical network reorganises itself post adaptation, that is, a new cortex is formed, as if designed for changed properties.

To sum it up, it is of prime importance to understand the plastic modifications of brain for various fundamental and medical reasons. This chapter underlined the importance of imposed adaptation studies within brain, particularly in primary visual cortex based on the crosscorrelogram analysis, framing a premise to better understand the functional connectivity [79, 92] and mechanisms in local neuronal circuits between various identified neurons, at least between the pyramidal cells and interneurons before and after adaptation. and post adaptation, thus, could help us to decipher the mechanisms of information processing, hence the neuronal codes governing them.

Author details

Lyes Bachatene* and Vishal Bharmauria*
Department of Biological Sciences, University of Montreal, Montreal, Canada

Stéphane Molotchnikoff**
Department of Biological Sciences, University of Montreal, Montreal, Canada

8. References

[1] Hubel DH, Wiesel TN (1959) Receptive Fields of Single Neurones in the Cat's Striate Cortex. J Physiol. 148: 574-591.
[2] Hubel DH, Wiesel TN (1968) Receptive Fields and Functional Architecture of Monkey Striate Cortex. J Physiol. 195: 215-243.
[3] Movshon JA (1975) The Velocity Tuning of Single Units in Cat Striate Cortex. J Physiol. 249: 445-468.
[4] Martinez LM, Wang Q, Reid RC, Pillai C, Alonso JM, Sommer FT, Hirsch JA (2005) Receptive Field Structure Varies with Layer in the Primary Visual Cortex. Nat Neurosci. 8: 372-379.
[5] Bishop PO, Henry GH (1972) Striate Neurons: Receptive Field Concepts. Invest Ophthalmol. 11: 346-354.
[6] Hubel DH, Wiesel TN (1962) Receptive Fields, Binocular Interaction and Functional Architecture in the Cat's Visual Cortex. J Physiol.160: 106-154.
[7] Hubel DH, Wiesel TN (1963a) Shape and Arrangement of Columns in Cat's Striate Cortex. J Physiol. 165: 559-568.
[8] Hubel DH, Wiesel TN (1963b) Receptive Fields of Cells in Striate Cortex of Very Young, Visually Inexperienced Kittens. J Neurophysiol. 26: 994-1002.

* Both Authors Contributed Equally
** Corresponding Author

[9] Tanaka S, Tani T, Ribot J, O'Hashi K, Imamura K (2009) A Postnatal Critical Period for Orientation Plasticity in the Cat Visual Cortex. PLoS One. 4: e5380.

[10] Chiu C, Weliki M. 2003 The role of neural activity in the development of orientation selectivity. The visual neurosciences. 117–125Cambridge, MA: MIT Press. pp.

[11] Bachatene L, Bharmauria V, Rouat J, Molotchnikoff S (2012) Adaptation-induced Plasticity and Spike Waveforms in Cat Visual Cortex. Neuroreport. 23: 88-92.

[12] Southwell DG, Froemke RC, Alvarez-Buylla A, Stryker MP, Gandhi SP (2010) Cortical Plasticity Induced by Inhibitory Neuron Transplantation. Science. 327: 1145-1148.

[13] Buonomano DV, Merzenich MM (1998) Cortical Plasticity: From Synapses to Maps. Annu Rev Neurosci. 21: 149-186.

[14] Laughlin SB, Sejnowski TJ (2003) Communication in Neuronal Networks. Science. 301: 1870-1874.

[15] Singer W (2011) Dynamic Formation of Functional Networks by Synchronization. Neuron. 69: 191-193.

[16] Buzsáki G (2010) Neural Syntax: Cell Assemblies, Synapsembles, and Readers. Neuron. 68: 362-385.

[17] Kujovic M, Zilles K, Malikovic A, Schleicher A, Mohlberg H, Rottschy C, Eickhoff SB, Amunts K (2012) Cytoarchitectonic Mapping of the Human Dorsal Extrastriate Cortex. Brain Struct Funct. [Epub ahead of print]

[18] Felleman DJ, Van Essen DC (1991) Distributed Hierarchical Processing in the Primate Cerebral Cortex. Cereb Cortex. 1: 1-47.

[19] Kaschube M, Schnabel M, Löwel S, Coppola DM, White LE, Wolf F (2010) Universality in the Evolution of Orientation Columns in the Visual Cortex. Science. 330: 1113-1116.

[20] Tyler CJ, Dunlop SA, Lund RD, Harman AM, Dann JF, Beazley LD, Lund JS (1998) Anatomical Comparison of the Macaque and Marsupial Visual Cortex: Common Features That May Reflect Retention of Essential Cortical Elements. J Comp Neurol. 400: 449-468.

[21] Ohki K, Chung S, Ch'ng YH, Kara P, Reid RC (2005) Functional Imaging with Cellular Resolution Reveals Precise Micro-architecture in Visual Cortex. Nature. 433: 597-603.

[22] Van Hooser SD (2007) Similarity and Diversity in Visual Cortex: Is There a Unifying Theory of Cortical Computation? Neuroscientist. 13: 639-656.

[23] Casagrande VA, Xu X (2004) Parallel visual pathways: a comparative perspective. The Visual Neurosciences. pp. 494-506 Cambridge, MA: MIT Press.

[24] Gilbert CD, Wiesel TN (1979) Morphology and Intracortical Projections of Functionally Characterised Neurones in the Cat Visual Cortex. Nature. 280: 120-125.

[25] Davis FA, Bergen D, Schauf C, McDonald I, Deutsch W (1976) Movement Phosphenes in Optic Neuritis: A New Clinical Sign. Neurology. 26: 1100-1104.

[26] Hubel DH, Wiesel TN, Stryker MP (1977) Orientation Columns in Macaque Monkey Visual Cortex Demonstrated by the 2-Deoxyglucose Autoradiographic Technique. Nature. 269: 328-330.

[27] Blasdel GG, Salama G (1986) Voltage-sensitive Dyes Reveal a Modular Organization in Monkey Striate Cortex. Nature. 321: 579-585.

[28] Adams DL, Sincich LC, Horton JC (2007) Complete Pattern of Ocular Dominance Columns in Human Primary Visual Cortex. J Neurosci. 27: 10391-10403.
[29] Horton JC, Hocking DR (1996) Intrinsic Variability of Ocular Dominance Column Periodicity in Normal Macaque Monkeys. J Neurosci. 16: 7228-7239.
[30] Shatz CJ, Stryker MP (1978) Ocular Dominance in Layer IV of the Cat's Visual Cortex and the Effects of Monocular Deprivation. J Physiol. 281: 267-283.
[31] Carandini M, Sengpiel F (2004) Contrast Invariance of Functional Maps in Cat Primary Visual Cortex. J Vis. 4: 130-143.
[32] Issa NP, Trepel C, Stryker MP (2000) Spatial Frequency Maps in Cat Visual Cortex. J Neurosci. 20: 8504-8514.
[33] Issa NP, Rosenberg A, Husson TR (2008) Models and Measurements of Functional Maps in V1. J Neurophysiol. 99: 2745-2754.
[34] Van Essen DC, Felleman DJ, DeYoe EA, Olavarria J, Knierim J (1990) Modular and Hierarchical Organization of Extrastriate Visual Cortex in the Macaque Monkey. Cold Spring Harb Symp Quant Biol. 55: 679-696.
[35] Essen DC, Zeki SM (1978) The Topographic Organization of Rhesus Monkey Prestriate Cortex. J Physiol. 277: 193-226.
[36] Heywood CA, Gadotti A, Cowey A (1992) Cortical Area V4 and its Role in the Perception of Color. J Neurosci. 12: 4056-4065.
[37] Born RT, Bradley DC (2005) Structure and Function of Visual Area MT. Annu Rev Neurosci. 28: 157-189.
[38] Mishkin, M., Ungerleider, L., & Macko, K (1983) Object Vision and Spatial Vision: Two Cortical Pathways.Trends in Neuroscience. 6: 414-417.
[39] DiCarlo JJ, Zoccolan D, Rust NC (2012) How Does the Brain Solve Visual Object Recognition? Neuron. 73: 415-434.
[40] Milner, D. A., & Goodale, M. (1995).The visual brain in action. Oxford University Press
[41] Lin CS, Friedlander MJ, Sherman SM (1979) Morphology of Physiologically Identified Neurons in the Visual Cortex of the Cat. Brain Res. 172: 344-348.
[42] Peters A (1984) Identified neurons in visual cortex.Trends in Neurosci. 7 :375–378
[43] González-Burgos G, Krimer LS, Povysheva NV, Barrionuevo G, Lewis DA (2005) Functional Properties of Fast Spiking Interneurons and their Synaptic Connections with Pyramidal Cells in Primate Dorsolateral Prefrontal Cortex. J Neurophysiol. 93: 942-953.
[44] Povysheva NV, Gonzalez-Burgos G, Zaitsev AV, Kröner S, Barrionuevo G, Lewis DA, Krimer LS (2006) Properties of Excitatory Synaptic Responses in Fast-spiking Interneurons and Pyramidal Cells From Monkey and Rat Prefrontal Cortex. Cereb Cortex. 16: 541-552.
[45] Markram H, Toledo-Rodriguez M, Wang Y, Gupta A, Silberberg G, Wu C (2004) Interneurons of the Neocortical Inhibitory System. Nat Rev Neurosci. 5: 793-807.
[46] Ison MJ, Mormann F, Cerf M, Koch C, Fried I, Quiroga RQ (2011) Selectivity of Pyramidal Cells and Interneurons in the Human Medial Temporal Lobe. J Neurophysiol. 106: 1713-1721.

[47] Wilson FA, O'Scalaidhe SP, Goldman-Rakic PS (1994) Functional Synergism Between Putative Gamma-Aminobutyrate-Containing Neurons and Pyramidal Neurons in Prefrontal Cortex. Proc Natl Acad Sci U S A. 91: 4009-4013.

[48] Gilbert CD (1977) Laminar Differences in Receptive Field Properties of Cells in Cat Primary Visual Cortex. J Physiol. 268: 391-421.

[49] Marshansky S, Shumikhina S, Molotchnikoff S (2011) Repetitive Adaptation Induces Plasticity of Spatial Frequency Tuning in Cat Primary Visual Cortex. Neuroscience. 172: 355-365.

[50] Wilson JR, Sherman SM (1976) Receptive-field Characteristics of Neurons in Cat Striate Cortex: Changes with Visual Field Eccentricity. J Neurophysiol. 39: 512-533.

[51] Pettigrew JD, Nikara T, Bishop PO (1968) Responses to Moving Slits by Single Units in Cat Striate Cortex. Exp Brain Res. 6: 373-390.

[52] Das A, Gilbert CD (1995) Long-range Horizontal Connections and Their Role in Cortical Reorganization Revealed by Optical Recording of Cat Primary Visual Cortex. Nature. 375: 780-784.

[53] Sompolinsky H, Golomb D, Kleinfeld D (1990) Global Processing of Visual Stimuli in a Neural Network of Coupled Oscillators. Proc Natl Acad Sci U S A. 87: 7200-7204.

[54] Ts'o DY, Gilbert CD, Wiesel TN (1986) Relationships Between Horizontal Interactions and Functional Architecture in Cat Striate Cortex as Revealed by Cross-correlation Analysis. J Neurosci. 6: 1160-1170.

[55] Hata Y, Tsumoto T, Sato H, Tamura H (1991) Horizontal Interactions between Visual Cortical Neurones Studied by Cross-correlation Analysis in the Cat. J Physiol. 441: 593-614.

[56] Yoshimura Y, Sato H, Imamura K, Watanabe Y (2000) Properties of Horizontal and Vertical Inputs to Pyramidal Cells in the Superficial Layers of the Cat Visual Cortex. J Neurosci. 20: 1931-1940.

[57] Stratford KJ, Tarczy-Hornoch K, Martin KA, Bannister NJ, Jack JJ (1996) Excitatory Synaptic Inputs to Spiny Stellate Cells in Cat Visual Cortex. Nature. 382: 258-261.

[58] Alonso JM, Usrey WM, Reid RC (1996) Precisely Correlated Firing in Cells of the Lateral Geniculate Nucleus. Nature. 383: 815-819.

[59] De Weerd P, Vandenbussche E, De Bruyn B, Orban GA (1990) Illusory Contour Orientation Discrimination in the Cat. Behav Brain Res. 39: 1-17.

[60] Bravo M, Blake R, Morrison S (1988) Cats See Subjective Contours. Vision Res. 28: 861-865.

[61] Ghisovan N, Nemri A, Shumikhina S, Molotchnikoff S (2009) Long Adaptation Reveals Mostly Attractive Shifts of Orientation Tuning in Cat Primary Visual Cortex. Neuroscience.164: 1274-1283.

[62] Dragoi V, Sharma J, Sur M (2000) Adaptation-induced Plasticity of Orientation Tuning in Adult Visual Cortex. Neuron. 28: 287-298.

[63] Nemri A, Ghisovan N, Shumikhina S, Molotchnikoff S (2009) Adaptive Behavior of Neighboring Neurons During Adaptation-induced Plasticity of Orientation Tuning in VI. BMC Neurosci. 10: 147.

[64] Ghisovan N, Nemri A, Shumikhina S, Molotchnikoff S (2008) Visual Cells Remember Earlier Applied Target: Plasticity of Orientation Selectivity. PLoS One. 3: e3689.

[65] Dragoi V, Rivadulla C, Sur M (2001) Foci of Orientation Plasticity in Visual Cortex. Nature. 411: 80-86.

[66] Frenkel MY, Sawtell NB, Diogo AC, Yoon B, Neve RL, Bear MF (2006) Instructive Effect of Visual Experience in Mouse Visual Cortex. Neuron. 51: 339-349.

[67] Voussoughi A, Shumikhina S, Milleret C, Molotchnikoff S (2010) Adaptation Modifies the Organization of Orientation Maps in Adult Cat Visual Cortex. II. Pinwhell Reorganization. Soc. Neurosci:371.22

[68] Perkel DH, Gerstein GL, Moore GP (1967) Neuronal Spike Trains and Stochastic Point Processes. I. The Single Spike Train. Biophys J. 7: 391-418.

[69] König P, Engel AK (1995) Correlated Firing in Sensory-Motor Systems. Curr Opin Neurobiol. 5: 511-519.

[70] Singer W, Engel AK, Kreiter AK, Munk MH, Neuenschwander S, Roelfsema PR (1997) Neuronal Assemblies: Necessity, Signature and Detectability. Trends Cogn Sci. 1: 252-261.

[71] Alloway KD, Roy SA (2002) Conditional Cross-correlation Analysis of Thalamocortical Neurotransmission. Behav Brain Res.135: 191-196.

[72] Singer W, Gray CM (1995) Visual Feature Integration and the Temporal Correlation Hypothesis. Annu Rev Neurosci. 18: 555-586.

[73] Shumikhina S, Guay J, Duret F, Molotchnikoff S (2004) Contextual Modulation of Synchronization to Random Dots in the Cat Visual Cortex. Exp Brain Res. 158: 223-232.

[74] König P, Engel AK, Singer W (1996) Integrator or Coincidence Detector? The Role of the Cortical Neuron Revisited. Trends Neurosci. 19: 130-137.

[75] Softky WR, Koch C (1993) The Highly Irregular Firing of Cortical Cells is Inconsistent with Temporal Integration of Random EPSPs. J Neurosci. 13: 334-350.

[76] Abeles M. (1982) Local cortical circuits: an electrophysiological study. 67-69 Berlin:Springer-Verlag.

[77] Takahashi N, Kitamura K, Matsuo N, Mayford M, Kano M, Matsuki N, Ikegaya Y (2012) Locally Synchronized Synaptic Inputs. Science. 335: 353-356.

[78] Duret F, Shumikhina S, Molotchnikoff S (2006) Neuron Participation in a Synchrony-encoding Assembly. BMC Neurosci. 7: 72.

[79] Barthó P, Hirase H, Monconduit L, Zugaro M, Harris KD, Buzsáki G (2004) Characterization of Neocortical Principal Cells and Interneurons by Network Interactions and Extracellular Features. J Neurophysiol. 92: 600-608.

[80] Yoshimura Y, Callaway EM (2005) Fine-scale Specificity of Cortical Networks Depends on Inhibitory Cell Type and Connectivity. Nat Neurosci. 8: 1552-1559.

[81] Csicsvari J, Hirase H, Czurko A, Buzsáki G (1998) Reliability and State Dependence of Pyramidal Cell-interneuron Synapses in the Hippocampus: An Ensemble Approach in the Behaving Rat. Neuron. 21: 179-189.

[82] Ghisovan N, Nemri A, Shumikhina S, Molotchnikoff S (2008) Synchrony between Orientation-selective Neurons is Modulated During Adaptation-induced Plasticity in Cat Visual Cortex. BMC Neurosci. 9: 60.

[83] He HY, Hodos W, Quinlan EM (2006) Visual Deprivation Reactivates Rapid Ocular Dominance Plasticity in Adult Visual Cortex. J Neurosci. 26: 2951-2955.

[84] Daw NW, Fox K, Sato H, Czepita D (1992) Critical Period for Monocular Deprivation in the Cat Visual Cortex. J Neurophysiol. 67: 197-202

[85] Yaka R, Yinon U, Wollberg Z (1999) Auditory Activation of Cortical Visual Areas in Cats After Early Visual Deprivation. Eur J Neurosci. 11: 1301-1312.

[86] Mower GD, Christen WG (1985) Role of Visual Experience in Activating Critical Period in Cat Visual Cortex. J Neurophysiol. 53: 572-589.

[87] Gutnisky DA, Dragoi V (2008) Adaptive Coding of Visual Information in Neural Populations.Nature. 452: 220-4.

[88] Angulo MC, Staiger JF, Rossier J, Audinat E (2003) Distinct Local Circuits Between Neocortical Pyramidal Cells and Fast-spiking Interneurons in Young Adult Rats. J Neurophysiol. 89: 943-953.

[89] Lee WC, Reid RC (2011) Specificity and Randomness: Structure-function Relationships in Neural Circuits. Curr Opin Neurobiol. 21: 801-807.

[90] Kampa BM, Roth MM, Göbel W, Helmchen F (2011) Representation of Visual Scenes by Local Neuronal Populations in Layer 2/3 of Mouse Visual Cortex. Front Neural Circuits. 5: 18.

[91] Wallace DJ, Kerr JN (2010) Chasing the Cell Assembly. Curr Opin Neurobiol. 20: 296-305.

[92] Holmgren C, Harkany T, Svennenfors B, Zilberter Y (2003) Pyramidal Cell Communication Within Local Networks in Layer 2/3 of Rat Neocortex. J Physiol. 551: 139-153.

Chapter 16

New Pictures of the Structure and Plasticity of Orientation Columns in the Visual Cortex

Shigeru Tanaka

Additional information is available at the end of the chapter

http://dx.doi.org/10.5772/48396

1. Introduction

Orientation selectivity of neurons in the primary visual cortex is thought to be an important requisite for the preprocessing of visual information, which is followed by more complex information processing and representation in the extrastriate cortex for visual perception. It is widely accepted that neurons in the primary visual cortex optimally responding to similar stimulus orientations are clustered in a manner of straight columns extending from the superficial to deep layers (Hubel & Wiesel, 1962, 1963a). The cerebral cortex is, however, folded inside a skull, which makes gyri and fundi. Particularly, in cats, area 17 (primary visual cortex) is located on the curved cortex called the lateral gyrus (Tusa et al., 1978). These facts raise questions of how the tangential arrangement of orientation columns is reconciled with the curvature of the gyrus, and whether the columns penetrate the cortex from the superficial to deep layers. In the first part of this chapter, we show a possible configuration of feature representation in the visual cortex using a three-dimensional (3D) self-organization model, and then confirm the predicted 3D orientation representation using multi-slice, high-resolution functional magnetic resonance imaging (fMRI) performed in the cat visual cortex (Tanaka et al., 2011). We obtained a close agreement in orientation representation between theoretical predictions and experimental observations. These studies demonstrated that in the curved cortex, preferred orientations are represented by wedge-like orientation columns which do not necessarily penetrate from superficial to deep layers, whereas in the flat cortex, preferred orientations are tended to be represented by classical straight columns.

On the other hand, numerous studies have been devoted to solving a question of how orientation selectivity is established and elaborated in early life. It is believed that orientation selectivity innately emerges prior to visual experience (Albus & Wolf, 1984;

Blakemore & Van Sluyters, 1975; Crair et al., 1998; Hubel & Wiesel, 1963b), but there has been a debate on the issue whether visual experience can modify orientation selectivity. Historically, Blakemore & Cooper (1970) reported that orientation-restricted visual experience modified response properties of visual cortical neurons so as to respond selectively to experienced orientations, which suggests a validity of the instruction hypothesis: Preferred orientations of neurons shift to experienced orientations (Rauschecker & Singer, 1981). Later, Stryker et al. (1978) and Carlson et al. (1986) claimed an objection against this hypothesis and proposed the suppression hypothesis: Neurons innately selective for inexperienced orientations only diminish their responsiveness while preferred orientations do not change. The current consensus of orientation plasticity in early life favors the suppression hypothesis. However, considering that visual experience for a few days under monocular deprivation shifts ocular dominance of visual cortical neurons towards an open eye (Wiesel & Hubel, 1963), one may not feel that the selection hypothesis is convincing. In the second part of this chapter, we show data obtained from *in vivo* intrinsic signal optical imaging in the visual cortex of kittens reared with head-mounted cylindrical-lens-fitted goggles for stable exposure to a single orientation (Tanaka et al., 2004, 2006, 2007). It was revealed that single-orientation exposure expands the cortical territory that represents the exposed orientation, as a previous study by Sengpiel et al. (1999). However, the degree of overrepresentation of the exposed orientation was more prominent in our data due to several differences of visual experience manipulation. Also, we show an age-dependent sensitive period profile for orientation selectivity in the visual cortex of goggle-reared kittens (Tanaka et al. 2009).

2. Theory and experiment on 3D orientation representation

We employed a self-organization model with minimal assumptions to describe the formation of joint maps of the preferred orientation, preferred direction, ocular dominance and retinotopy. We performed computer simulation using a structural annealing: Simulation was started only in the middle layer at the beginning and then the simulation range was expanded gradually to other layers. This annealing method well reproduced orientation columns vertically spanning all the layers in the flat cortex, consistent with widely accepted columnar organization. On the other hand, in the curved parts, orientation straight columns were disrupted and preferred orientations were clustered in wedge-like forms. It was likely that preferred directions are reversed in the deeper layers. Singularities associated with orientation representation appeared as warped lines in the 3D model cortex. Direction reversal appeared on the sheets that were delimited by orientation-singularity lines. These structures emerged from the balance between periodic arrangements of preferred orientations and vertical alignment of the same orientations. Then, to examine the biological plausibility of the simulation results, we attempted to visualize orientation representation in the cat visual cortex using multi-slice, high-resolution fMRI. We obtained a close agreement in orientation representation between theoretical predictions and experimental observations (Tanaka et al., 2011).

2.1. Mathematical modeling

We extended the previously reported model (Nakagama & Tanaka, 2004) to describe the formation of orientation, direction, ocular dominance and retinotopic representation in the 3D primary visual cortex. For simplicity, among 6 layers of the visual cortex, we omitted layer 1, in which massive fibers are running tangentially and neurons exist sparsely. In the other 5 layers, we assumed that each neuron represents *a priori* a set of visual features such as ocular dominance, orientation preference, direction-of-motion preference and the center of the receptive field for simplicity. The cortical arrangement of the visual features was modified by local intracortical interaction among neurons, which change an initial random arrangement of visual features to form an orderly arrangement over the 3D primary visual cortex.

2.1.1. Three-dimensional model visual cortex and visual feature space

One of the purposes of this study is to investigate the effect of the global curvature of the visual cortex on visual feature representation. For this purpose, we assumed a "stadium-shape" of the model cortex with a finite thickness, which is embedded inside a box composed of 128 × 128 × 72 voxels. Each voxel represents a cortical neuron. The outer and inner surfaces, respectively, correspond to the cortical surface and the boundary between the gray and white matter. The model cortical depth was set at 30 voxels with a 6-voxel thickness of each layer from layer 2 to layer 6. We assumed the thickness of the model cortex to be 2 mm, meaning one voxel is 66 μm. The periodic boundary condition was adopted to minimize a small-size effect. The feature space (FS) is given by the direct product of the space of the visual field (VF), the circular symmetric space of the preferred direction (PD) and the space of ocular dominance (OD): FS = VF×PD×OD. Space VF is the 2D visual field (26×54 grids), in which the position of a receptive field center of a cortical neuron is defined. The periodic boundary condition was imposed on space VF so as to be consistent with the periodic boundary condition imposed on the model visual cortex. The preferred orientation is defined as the axis orthogonal to the preferred direction of motion. The space OD is subdivided into five groups, in which groups 1 and 5 are driven exclusively by either of the two eyes, group 3 is driven by the two eyes equally, and groups 2 and 4 receive imbalanced inputs from the two eyes.

2.1.2. Energy function

We assume that a neuron located at j in the model visual cortex represents a set of visual features (k, θ, μ), where k, θ and μ indicate the position of the receptive field, preferred direction and ocular dominance, respectively. The ocular dominance μ takes a value out of $-1, -1/2, 0, 1/2$, and 1 : $\mu = 1$ represents exclusively the left-eye dominance and $\mu = -1$ exclusively the right-eye dominance. The preferred direction θ takes one of 16 values out of $0, \pi/8, 2\pi/8, \ldots,$ and $15\pi/8$. The preferred orientation was assumed to be orthogonal to the preferred direction and invariant under rotational transformation by π. When a cortical neuron j represents (k, θ, μ), $\sigma_{j,k,\theta,\mu}$ takes 1, and otherwise, 0. Here we assume that any cortical neuron is supposed to represent only one set of visual features. The state of the visual feature arrangements is characterized by the energy function:

$$H = -\sum_{j,j'}\sum_{k,\theta,\mu}\sum_{k',\theta',\mu'} V_{j,j'}\Gamma_{k,\theta,\mu;k',\theta',\mu'}\sigma_{j,k,\theta,\mu}\sigma_{j',k',\theta',\mu'} + c\sum_{l=2}^{6}\sum_{k,\theta,\mu}\left(\sum_{j\in l\text{-th layer}}\sigma_{j,k,\theta,\mu}\right)^2, \quad (1)$$

where $V_{j,j'}$ represents the 3D cortical interaction between a pair of visual features represented by neurons j and j'. This interaction is determined by the convolution of the dendritic arbor function with the axonal arbor function. It is know that in the adult cortex, there are long-range tangential and inter-layer connections. However, we assume that the axonal arbor of nearby cortical neurons mainly works for column formation in the early developmental stage, and we omit the long-range connections. This assumption indicates that the interaction does not depend on the global morphology of the cortex and is identical for any positions either in the superficial layers or deep layers. Therefore, we identify the cortical interaction as the dendritic integration, which is simply given by the Gaussian function:

$$V_{j,j'} = \frac{1}{2\pi\lambda_v^2}\exp\left(-\frac{d_{j,j'}^2}{2\lambda_v^2}\right), \quad (2)$$

where λ_v is the excitatory interaction length in the cortex (λ_v =2.0 corresponding to 132 μm), and $d_{j,j'}$ indicates the distance between cortical neurons j and j'. $\Gamma_{k,\theta,\mu;k',\theta',\mu'}$ represents the correlation function of input signals. The second term of Eq. (1) represents a constraint on the representation of the visual features to avoid imbalanced representation and results in each layer covering all the feature space as uniformly as possible. The constraint is imposed layer by layer. The sum of j is taken over all neurons located within the l-th layer of the model cortex. The strength of constraint c was set at 0.008.

The correlation function of input signals $\Gamma_{k,\theta,\mu;k',\theta',\mu'}$ is modeled by assuming that local components of visual images obey white noise regarding the position and direction of motion with a strength of correlation between the two eyes r, and that the input signal receptive field is given by the product of the positional Gaussian function and the directional cosine series. After short calculations, the correlation functiont is rewritten as

$$\Gamma_{k,\theta,\mu;k',\theta',\mu'} = S_{k,k'}\Psi_{\theta,\theta'}O_{\mu,\mu'}, \quad (3)$$

where $S_{k,k'}$, $\Psi_{\theta,\theta'}$ and $O_{\mu,\mu'}$ represent component correlation functions regarding the position of receptive field centers in the visual field, direction of motion and ocular dominance, respectively. These component correlation functions are given by

$$S_{k,k'} = \exp\left(-\frac{d_{k,k'}^2}{2\lambda_{corr}^2}\right), \quad (4)$$

$$\Psi_{\theta,\theta'} = 2a_0^2 + \sum_{m=1}^{\infty} a_m^2 \cos m\left(\theta - \theta'\right), \tag{5}$$

$$\mathrm{O}_{\mu,\mu'} = \frac{(1+r)+\left(1-r\right)\mu\mu'}{2}. \tag{6}$$

Here, λ_{corr} is the positional correlation length equal to $\sqrt{2}\lambda_{ref}$, which is set at 1.0. The directional component of the correlation function is given as a Fourier cosine series. The order of m=1 represents the correlation between a pair of preferred directions, whereas the order of m=2 represents the correlation between a pair of preferred axes of motion, which are orthogonal to the preferred orientations.

2.1.3. Computer simulation

At the beginning of the simulation, we randomize visual features in the model cortex. In the middle layer of the cortex, neurons receive random inputs from either eye ($\mu = +1$ or -1), because the layer is geniculocortical input layer. In the other layers, neurons receive random inputs with ocular dominance of either of −1, −1/2, 0, 1/2, or 1, and preferred direction of either of 0, π / 8, 2π / 8, ···, or 15π / 8. The RF center position is also randomized retaining rough retinotopy according to the probability:

$$A_{k;j} = \exp\left(-\frac{d_{J_k;j}^2}{2\lambda_{\mathrm{Ret}}^2}\right), \tag{7}$$

where $d_{J_k;j}$ represents the distance between cortical position j and position J_k that retinotopically corresponds to the position k in the visual field, where λ_{Ret} represents the roughness of retinotopy (λ_{Ret} = 3.5). For each trial of updating visual features in the simulation, a new candidate for a set of visual features is selected according to the same probability distribution as in the initial randomization, and then the old set of features is replaced with the new one according to the probability determined by the energy difference between the states before and after the trial of replacement:

$$\Pr(\mathit{before} \to \mathit{after}) = \frac{1}{1+\exp[\beta(H^{\mathit{after}} - H^{\mathit{before}})]}. \tag{8}$$

Here, H^{before} and H^{after} represent the energy before and after the trial of replacement, respectively. The parameter β, which determines the steepness of the logistic function of the right-hand side of Eq. (8) in the transition region, was set at $\beta = \infty$. Thereby, the probability takes 1 when H^{after} is smaller than H^{before}, otherwise 0. The repetition of the update procedure likely decreases the energy of the system and realizes an equilibrium cortical arrangement of visual features when the change in energy becomes negligibly small.

In the present model, in which the cortical interaction function is isotropic, clustering of similar visual features occurs but columnar organization cannot be formed even in flat parts of the model visual cortex when the simulation is carried out to update features sampled randomly from the entire model cortex. So, we carried out the simulation according to the following schedule of spatial simulated annealing that we call hereafter, which assists the formation of iso-orientation domains continuously extending from layer 2 to layer 6. For simulation step t in the interval of $1 \le t < T_1$, simulation was performed only in the middle layer whose upper and lower boundaries were located at 13 and 18 voxels from the bottom of the model cortex. For $T_1 \le t \le T_2$, the inner boundary z^{inner} and the outer boundary z^{outer} of the simulation range in the depth direction was gradually changed as $z^{inner} = 13 - \left\lceil 12 \times \frac{t - T_1}{T_2 - T_1} \right\rceil$, and $z^{outer} = 18 + \left\lceil 12 \times \frac{t - T_1}{T_2 - T_1} \right\rceil$. For $T_2 < t$, simulation was carried out in all model visual cortex. Here, one simulation step is defined as the trial numbers of updating features by the total number of voxels within which simulation is conducted. That is, for 1 simulation step, each voxel is tried to be updated, on average, once. Parameters T_1 and T_2 were set at 100 and 350 simulation steps. Thus, columnar structures of visual features are likely formed owing to the spatial simulated annealing, even if we do not assume anisotropic cortical interaction.

2.1.4. *Analyses of cortical feature representations*

An output response of neuron j to the presentation of visual images through either eye is given by the integration of evoked activities at nearby neurons through the dendrite. Therefore, the output neuronal response is expressed by

$$\eta^{out}_{j;k,\theta,\mu} = \sum_{j',l,\varphi} V_{j;j'} \, \sigma_{j';l,\varphi,\mu} \, R_{l,\varphi;k,\theta}. \tag{9}$$

Here we suppose that a global stimulus like an oriented grating stimulus moving in the direction θ is presented to both eyes. The direction tuning curve of model cortical neuron j is defined by

$$\varsigma^{dir}_j(\theta) = \sum_{k,\mu} \eta^{out}_{j;k,\theta,\mu}. \tag{10}$$

The preferred direction of the neuron j is determined when $\varsigma^{dir}_j(\theta)$ takes the maximum at $\theta = \theta^{pref}_j$. The orientation tuning curve of model cortical neuron j is defined by the sum of responses to opposite directions orthogonal to the stimulus orientation ϕ as follows:

$$\varsigma^{ori}_j(\phi) = \frac{1}{2} \sum_{k,\mu} \left(\eta^{out}_{j;k,\phi-\pi/2,\mu} + \eta^{out}_{j;k,\phi+\pi/2,\mu} \right). \tag{11}$$

The preferred orientation of this neuron is determined when the orientation tuning curve $\varsigma^{ori}_j(\phi)$ takes the maximum at $\phi = \phi^{pref}_j$. The ocular dominance of neuronal responses is defined by the contrast form of responses to the left- and right-eye stimuli as follows:

$$O_j = \frac{\sum_{k,\theta,\mu} \mu \eta^{out}_{j;k,\theta,\mu}}{\sum_{k,\theta,\mu} \eta^{out}_{j;k,\theta,\mu}}. \tag{12}$$

To analyze orientation and direction singularities, we calculate an absolute value of the gradient vector for the preferred orientation, $\left|\vec{\nabla}\phi_j^{pref}\right| = \sqrt{\left(\partial_x\phi_j^{pref}\right)^2 + \left(\partial_y\phi_j^{pref}\right)^2 + \left(\partial_z\phi_j^{pref}\right)^2}$, and that for the preferred direction, $\left|\vec{\nabla}\theta_j^{pref}\right| = \sqrt{\left(\partial_x\theta_j^{pref}\right)^2 + \left(\partial_y\theta_j^{pref}\right)^2 + \left(\partial_z\theta_j^{pref}\right)^2}$, at position $\left(x_j, y_j, z_j\right)$ in the model cortex. Gradient vector components of any given function ψ_j are given by

$$\begin{aligned}
\partial_x\psi_j &= \frac{\partial\psi_j}{\partial x} = \frac{\psi\left(x_j+h, y_j, z_j\right) - \psi\left(x_j-h, y_j, z_j\right)}{2h} \\
\partial_y\psi_j &= \frac{\partial\psi_j}{\partial y} = \frac{\psi\left(x_j, y_j+h, z_j\right) - \psi\left(x_j, y_j-h, z_j\right)}{2h}, \\
\partial_z\psi_j &= \frac{\partial\psi_j}{\partial z} = \frac{\psi\left(x_j, y_j, z_j+h\right) - \psi\left(x_j, y_j, z_j-h\right)}{2h}
\end{aligned} \tag{13}$$

where h indicates the distance between nearest neighbor model neurons, which is the size of the voxel corresponding 66μm. Plotting grey spots at positions where absolute values of orientation gradient vectors are larger than 0.01 rad/μm and those of direction gradient vectors are larger than 0.02 rad/μm, we obtain orientation-singularity lines and direction-discontinuity sheets, respectively.

The positions of orientation pinwheel centers along the model cortical surface are determined automatically as the points around which the circular integration of the orientation difference amounts to just $\pm\pi$, where the circular integration is taken in the counterclockwise direction. The counterclockwise or clockwise pinwheel centers are defined by the sign of the integral. Thus-defined pinwheel centers coincided with the position of high-gradient of preferred orientations along the cortical surface. The relative number of pinwheel centers within ocular dominance subregions is analyzed according to the previously introduced method (Hübener et al. 1997). Namely, the left- or right-eye specific subregions are defined as the domains in which model neurons are classified into the top 20% of total number of neurons. The border subregions of ocular dominance are defined as the domains in which neurons exhibit binocularity within 20%.

2.2. Simulated representation of preferred orientation and direction

We used a model visual cortex that consisted of two rectangular blocks sandwiched by two curved blocks in order to mimic the flat and curved parts of the visual cortex, respectively (Fig. 1a,b). The depth of the model cortex was 30 voxels. When we assume the depth to be 2 mm, one voxel size corresponds to 66 μm. The rectangular blocks simulate flat parts between the lateral sulcus and the crown of the lateral gyrus, whereas the curved blocks simulate the crown of the lateral gyrus. To minimize the size effect, we imposed a periodic boundary condition on the model visual cortex. In the computer simulation, we assumed the standard deviation of the dendritic arbor of cortical neurons to be 2 voxels, which corresponds to 132 μm. This implies a diameter of 264 μm, which falls in a plausible range for the tangential diameter of stellate cell dendritic arborization and pyramidal cell basal dendritic arborization in the visual cortex (290 ± 88 (SD) μm, n = 12; estimated from the data shown in Sholl, 1953).

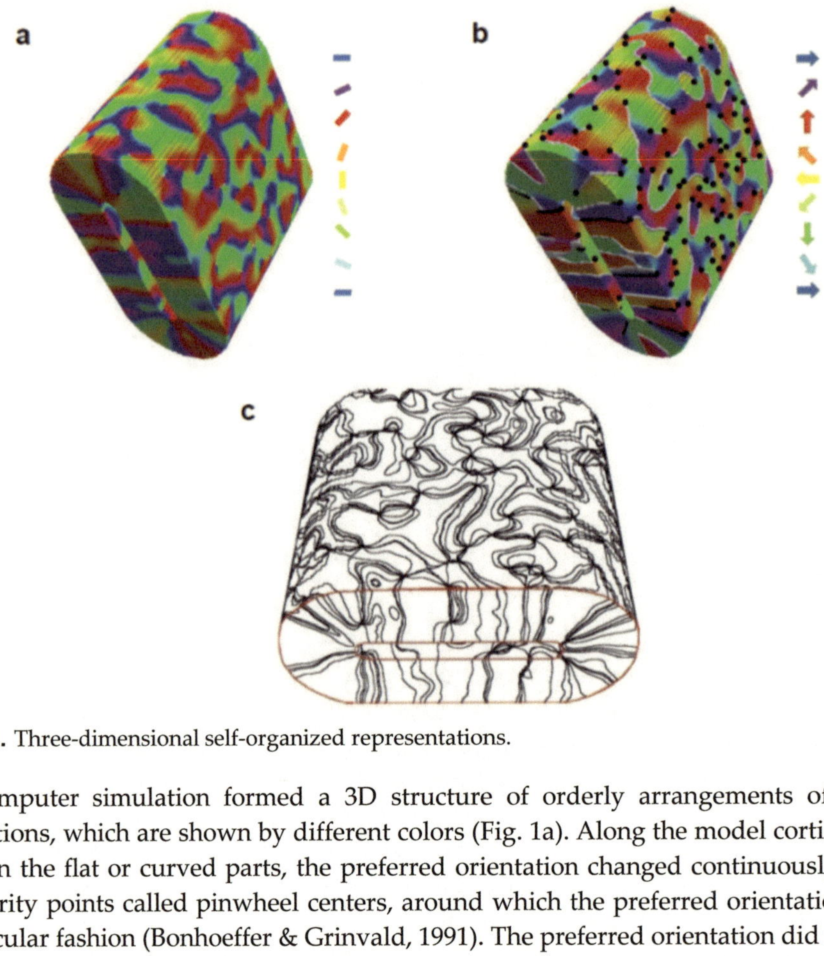

Figure 1. Three-dimensional self-organized representations.

The computer simulation formed a 3D structure of orderly arrangements of preferred orientations, which are shown by different colors (Fig. 1a). Along the model cortical surface, either in the flat or curved parts, the preferred orientation changed continuously except at singularity points called pinwheel centers, around which the preferred orientation changes in a circular fashion (Bonhoeffer & Grinvald, 1991). The preferred orientation did not change much in the depth direction of the flat parts of the model cortex, which can be seen in the sidewall of the model cortex. This indicates that preferred orientations are arranged in a columnar fashion in the flat cortical parts. On the other hand, in the curved parts of the model cortex, preferred orientations were arranged in a wedge-like structure, where the width of orientation columns became narrower from the superficial to deeper layers. It should be noted that tips of some wedge-like columns did not reach the bottom of the model visual cortex, which corresponds to the boundary between the grey and white matter.

Preferred directions were also arranged almost continuously along the cortical surface, except along discontinuity lines across which the preferred direction changed by 180° (Fig. 1b). Such direction-discontinuity lines (Kim et al., 1999) or direction fractures (Kisvarday et al., 2001; Swindale et al., 2003) are indicated by white lines. They were terminated or branched at pinwheel centers shown as black dots in Fig. 1b, which is consistent with a previous experimental finding (Kim et al., 1999; Weliky et al., 1996) and a theoretical prediction (Tanaka, 1995, 1997). Like iso-orientation domains, iso-direction domains tended to extend vertically in the flat part of the model cortex. However, there were occasions in which the preferred direction was reversed somewhere along the cortical depth.

To more clearly visualize orientation representation particularly along the cortical depth, we illustrated iso-orientation lines (Fig. 1c), where the orientation interval between adjacent lines was 15°. In the flat part of the cortex, iso-orientation lines tended to penetrate throughout the cortical depth. In contrast, in the curved part, some iso-orientation lines exhibited V-shape, although some connected the cortical surface with the bottom of the cortex, forming wedge-like orientation columns.

The present model also demonstrates the emergence of ocular dominance patches mainly in the middle layer and an orderly retinotopic arrangement of the receptive field center (for more information, see Tanaka et al., 2011).

2.3. Simulated 3D structures of orientation and direction singularities

We illustrated high-gradient regions for the preferred orientation and direction. The high-orientation-gradient regions appeared as thin rods, shown by gray rods in Figs. 2a and b. Note that these rods passed through pinwheel centers at any given layer. In the flat part of the cortex, 82 % of high-orientation-gradient rods tended to stand straight, and the other small percent (18 %) were V-shaped lines or hairpins. From visual inspection, all rods that reached the cortical surface intersected perpendicularly to the cortical surface (Fig. 2a). In contrast, in the curved part of the cortex, 34 % of high-orientation-gradient rods appeared to be hairpins whose ends were located on the cortical surface, whereas the other percent of rods (66 %) were almost straight lines connecting the cortical surface with the bottom of the cortex (Fig. 2b). The appearance of the V-shaped orientation singularity lines is due to the fact that clockwise and counterclockwise orientation pinwheel centers in a plane parallel to the cortical surface get closer and finally they are merged to vanish, as the plane moves down from the surface to deeper layers.

On the other hand, high-direction-gradient regions appeared as thin, curved and distorted sheets, shown by gray sheets in Figs. 2c and d. Figure 2c (the top view in Fig. 2a) shows the high-direction-gradient sheets in the flat part of the model visual cortex, whereas Fig. 2d illustrates the side view in Fig. 2b, showing the high-direction-gradient sheets in the curved part. From visual inspection, the high-direction-gradient sheets seemed to intersect with the cortical surface or the bottom of the cortex at right angles. The intersections formed the direction-discontinuity lines on the cortical surface, which are indicated by blue lines in Figs. 2c and d (corresponding to the white lines in Fig. 1b).

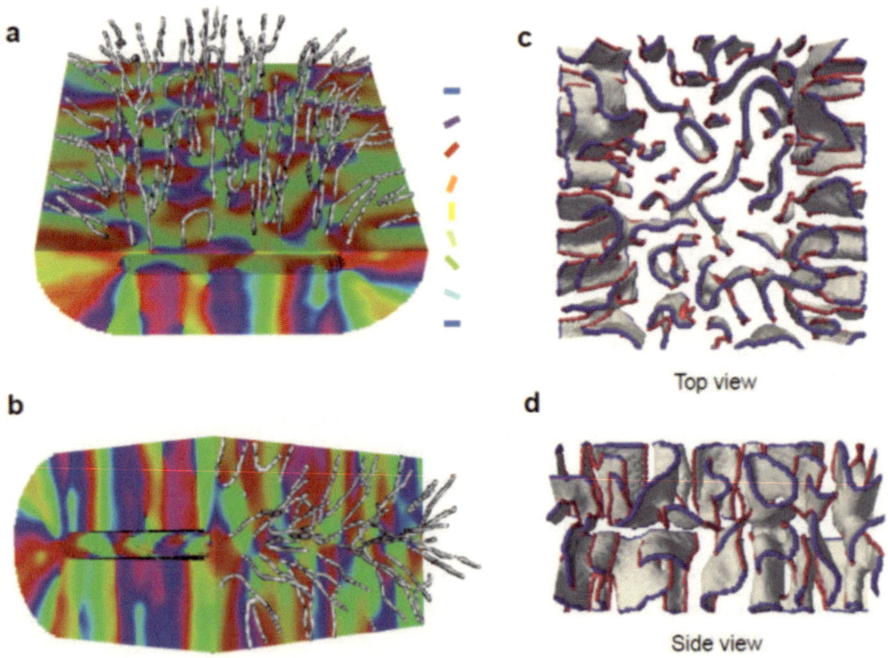

Figure 2. Orientation and direction singularities in the model cortex.

The high-direction-gradient sheets were delineated by the high-orientation-gradient rods (red rods) or the upper and lower cortical surfaces. This 3D relationship is a natural extension of the 2D relationship between pinwheel centers and direction-discontinuity lines (Figs. 1a and b). Hereafter, we refer to high-orientation-gradient rods as orientation-singularity lines and high-direction-gradient sheets as direction-discontinuity sheets. As seen in Fig. 2d, when we move radially from the cortical surface to the bottom of the cortex, the direction-discontinuity sheets became crowded. Even in the flat part (Fig. 2c), direction-discontinuity sheets covered a non-negligible area of the cortex when we see the cortex from the top. Such patterns indicate that when an electrode penetrates vertically into the visual cortex in electrophysiological recording, the preferred direction along the electrode track can reverse somewhere in the middle of the cortical depth.

To examine how the preferred orientation and direction changed in the flat and curved parts of the model cortex, we sampled 40 traces of preferred orientations and preferred directions along the cortical depth from the surface to the bottom of the cortex perpendicularly to the cortical surface. Most traces in either the curved or flat parts showed gradual changes in the preferred orientation deviating from the orientations at the cortical surface. Some traces showed large changes of preferred orientations in the middle of the cortical depth in the curved part. The mean amplitudes of changes in the preferred orientation along the depth were 35.1° and 30.5°, and the standard deviations of the amplitudes of changes in the preferred orientation were 35.0° and 16.0°, in the curved and flat parts, respectively. These values indicate that in the curved cortex, the preferred orientation changes drastically in some traces but it is rather constant in the other traces, whereas in the flat cortex, the preferred orientation changes moderately in all traces. The preferred direction in most traces showed similar changes in the preferred orientation either in the curved or flat part. Some of them, however, showed abrupt changes by 180° in the middle of the cortical depth. More reversals of preferred directions were found in the deeper layers in the curved part. We analyzed the depth-dependent probabilities to hit direction reversals in the flat and curved parts of the cortex, by sampling 14336 traces in the flat part and 14476 traces in the curved part, discarding the other traces in the transition regions between the flat and curved parts. If the direction-discontinuity sheets are flat planes, the probability to hit direction reversals is independent of the depth. However, direction reversals tended to occur more frequently midway through the cortical depth than near the cortical surface or the bottom of the cortex. This tendency reflects that direction-discontinuity sheets were wavy. The small probability to hit direction reversals near the cortical surface and the bottom of the cortex indicates that the direction-discontinuity sheets tended to intersect the cortical surface and the bottom of the cortex at right angles. In contrast, in the curved part, the preferred direction reversed more frequently in deeper layers than in superficial layers. The direction reversal in deeper layers appeared twice to three times more frequently in the curved part than in the flat part.

2.4. Multi-slice fMRI imaging of 3D orientation representation

To compare simulated results with the feature representation in the cat visual cortex, high-resolution fMRI was performed on cat visual cortex at 9.4 T (Fukuda et al., 2006; Moon et al., 2007). The cat was anesthetized with isoflurane (0.8 – 1.0%) and immobilized with pancuronium bromide (0.2 mg kg^{-1} hr^{-1}, i.v.). The imaging positions were selected in the region of dorsal surface and smaller surface veins, based on high-resolution 3D anatomical images. fMRI data were acquired using the multi-slice 2D gradient echo planner imaging sequence with the following parameters: TR = 2.0 s, TE = 10 ms, matrix = 96 × 96, and FOV = 2 × 2 cm^2, after an intravascular bolus injection of a dextran-coated monocrystalline iron oxide nanoparticles (MION) contrast agent (20 mg Fe kg^{-1} body weight). Slice thickness of 500 μm was chosen to achieve sufficient sensitivity, and an inter-slice distance of 375 μm was used to improve nominal resolution along a slice direction. Visual stimulation was given binocularly. Eight different orientations with high-contrast square-wave full-field moving gratings (0.15 cpd, 2 Hz, movement direction reversal per 0.5 s) were presented sequentially (22.5° angle increments, 10 s per angle) during the one cycle of 80 s. One stimulation cycle was repeated ten times continuously (i.e., total 800 s per run). Twenty runs were performed for signal averaging.

In the data analysis, first, we obtained single-condition maps for the 8 stimulus orientations at 8 slices according to Kalatsky & Stryker's method (Kalatsky & Stryker, 2003). We embedded each single-condition map into a rectangular solid region of 192 × 192 × 25 voxels, each of which was the size of 104 × 104 × 125 μm^3. (For more information, see Supporting Figure 1 of Tanaka et al., 2011). Then we applied the 2D Gaussian filtering with the standard deviation of 193 μm to the single-condition maps for 8 stimulus orientations at each slice. Then we applied the same filtering to these single-condition maps in the depth direction. The preferred orientation at each voxel was determined by the vector sum method

(Bonhoeffer & Grinvald, 1991), which is based on the Fourier analysis in the circular symmetric orientation dimension. Next, we calculated the orientation gradient at each voxel using Eq. (13) to show the region of orientation singularities. When we visualized high-orientation-gradient regions, we used the same threshold value as in the model.

2.5. Orientation representation reconstructed by high-resolution fMRI

Figures 3a and b, respectively, are top and coronal views reconstructed from a 3D venogram. Abbreviations of A, P, L and R for the cortical coordinate in Fig. 3a indicate anterior, posterior, left and right, respectively. Venous vessels were enhanced in the dark intensity dots and lines from tissues. The disk region of a 1.5-cm diameter with a 3.125-mm thickness surrounded by the red lines was selected for imaging. fMRI data were acquired using the multi-slice 2D gradient echo planar imaging sequence in 2 × 2 cm^2 around the lateral gyrus including areas 17 and 18 (Fig. 3a), following an intravascular bolus injection of MION. Eight 0.5-mm-thick slices were obtained from a 3.125-mm-thick slab (center-to-center distance of neighboring slices = 0.375 mm) (Fig. 3b).

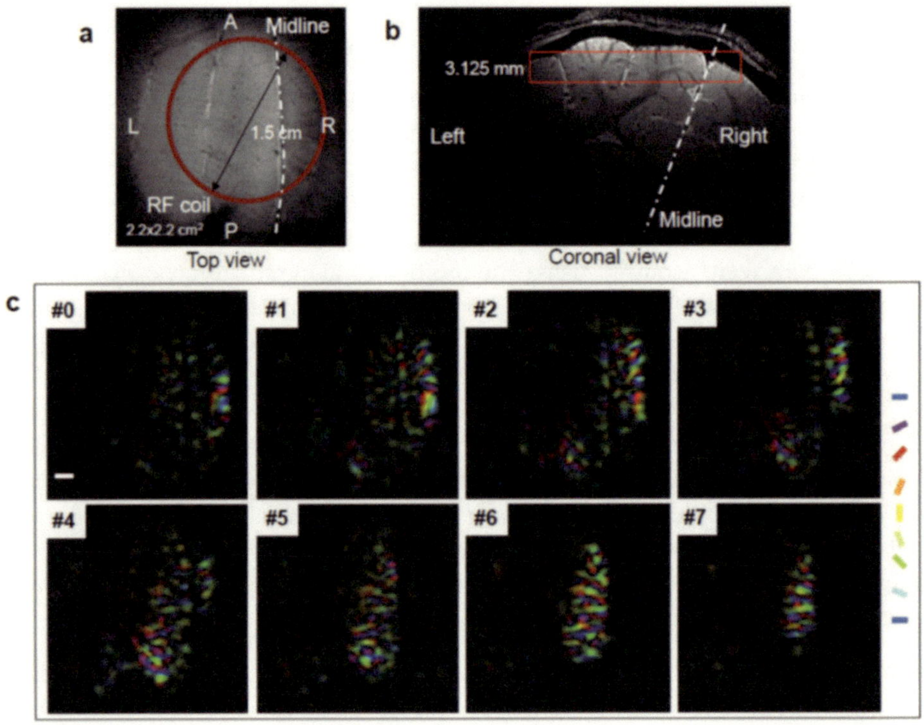

Figure 3. Multi-slice high-resolution fMRI of cat visual cortex.

Eight single-condition maps responding to binocular full-field gratings were obtained for each slice. Then, 8 orientation polar maps were calculated for different depths in the rectangular region, where color and brightness indicate the preferred orientation and orientation selectivity, respectively (Fig. 3c). The slice number is assigned from the bottom to the top in the imaging rectangular parallelepiped. The white scale bar placed at the bottom of slice #0 indicates 1 mm. Each map shows the characteristic spatial clustering of preferred orientations.

Figure 4 shows orientation representation and orientation-singularity lines in the 125-μm-thick slices, where the abbreviations for the cortical coordinates, M, L, D and V indicate, respectively, medial, lateral, dorsal and ventral, and all black scale bars indicate 1mm. In Fig. 4 in a saggital section containing the white matter, the orientation columns tended to terminate at the bottom of the grey matter at right angles with the boundary between the grey and white matter. The regions of high orientation gradient in the same section appeared as nearly straight rods, which terminated at pinwheel centers on the cortical surface (Fig. 4b). Figure 4c shows the lateral view of orientation representation in the section more medial to the section shown in Fig. 4a, which did not contain the white matter. Around the horizontal dotted line in this section, which corresponded to the bottom of the curved cortex in the medial region of recording, iso-orientation domains were not aligned vertically, different from those in Fig. 4a. Orientation-singularity lines were fractioned around there (Fig. 4d). These features imply that iso-orientation domains and singularity lines tend to run along the radial axes of the gyrus.

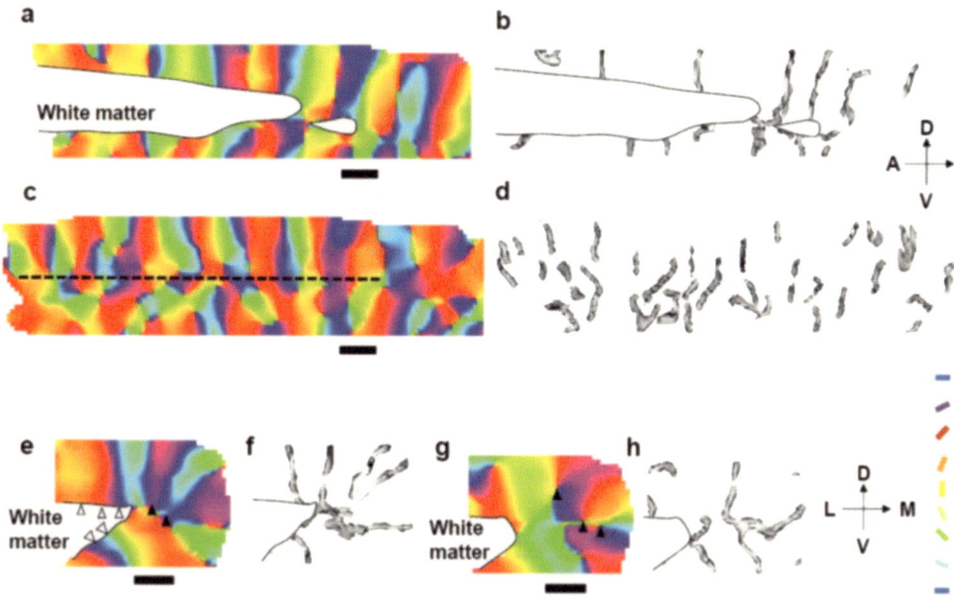

Figure 4. Orientation representations and high orientation gradients in typical sections.

In the coronal sections around the gyrus, preferred orientations were arranged in wedge-like columns rather than straight columns (Figs. 4e and g), whereas iso-orientation domains ran orthogonal to the white matter closer to the flat parts of the cortex (white arrow heads in Fig. 4e). Tips of some wedges representing single orientations (black arrow heads in Figs. 4e and g) did not reach the white matter, which indicates that orientation preferences can differ between the superficial and deep layers along the radial axes of the gyrus. Related to this feature, the orientation-singularity lines appeared as hair-pins (Figs. 4f and h).

To visualize the orientation columns around the curved and flat cortices more clearly, we illustrated iso-orientation lines in 3 slices of the coronal section and in 1 slice of the sagittal section, where the orientation interval between adjacent contour lines was set at 15° in Fig. 5. In the curved cortex, although some iso-orientation lines tended to reach the white matter, many lines were hairpins or converged to some points in the grey matter, and hence did not connect the cortical surface with the white matter (Figs. 5a-c). These characteristic features agree with the simulated results in the curved part of the model cortex (Fig. 1c). On the other hand, iso-orientation lines tended to connect the cortical surface and the white matter straightly in the flat cortex as shown in the dotted square of Fig. 5d. Interestingly, even in the flat cortex, some iso-orientation lines were hairpins or converged to points in the grey matter. This indicates that all orientation columns in the flat cortex are not necessarily straight columns.

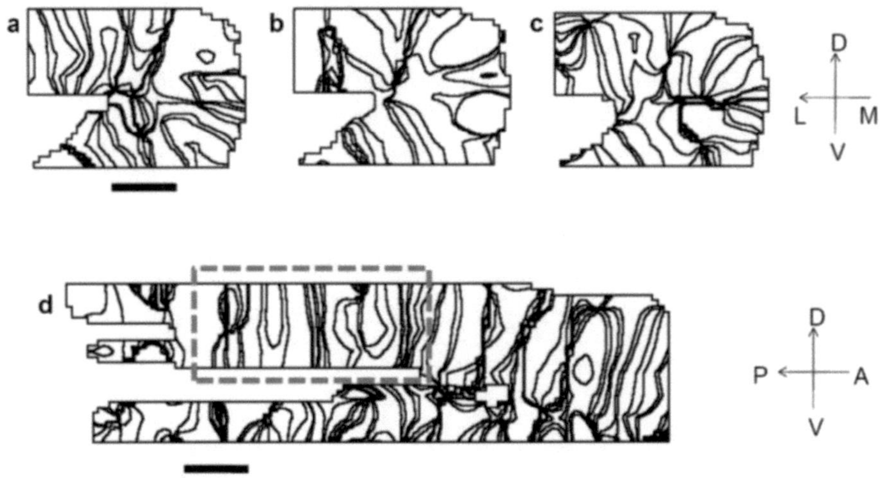

Figure 5. Iso-orientation line maps in 4 typical sections.

When the planes of the slice sections are not parallel to the straight columns that penetrate throughout the grey matter, they may appear to terminate in the middle of the cortical depth. Also, when orientation columns are wavy, even if penetrating throughout the grey matter, they may appear to terminate in the middle of the cortical depth. To examine quantitatively whether orientation columns continuously extend throughout the cortical depth at least within the imaged region, we defined the penetration index: It takes 1 when we can find a continuous path from the surface down to the white matter, keeping the same orientation within the range of 22.°, and otherwise, 0. The penetration indices were averaged in flat or curved parts both for the experimental and theoretical results. To estimate average penetration indices, we used 14336 traces (= 56 × 128 × 2 pixels) in the up- and downside of the flat parts and 14336 traces ($\cong [72 \times \pi/4] \times 128 \times 2$ pixels) in the most lateral curved parts in the simulated result, and 636 and 830 traces in the flat and curved parts, respectively, in the experimental result. The average penetration index estimated from the fMRI data was 0.87 for the flat cortex, and 0.78 for the curved cortex. These values indicate that not all orientation columns continued from the cortical surface to the white matter. However, some orientation columns reached the white matter, even if they may be wavy. The fact that the average penetration index was smaller in the curved part than in the flat part indicates that orientation columns more often terminate somewhere in the cortical depth in the curved cortex, consistent with visual inspection of Figs. 4 and 5.

On the other hand, in the simulated results, the average penetration index was 0.99 in the flat part of the cortex, and 0.89 in the curved part. It is quite likely that these values are larger than those obtained from the experiment, because detailed connectivity among different neurons and its complexity were omitted in the model. However, these two values again indicate that orientation columns in the curved cortex more frequently terminate somewhere in the cortical depth than do those in flat cortex. Taken together, the experiment and theory show that the cortical curvature partially deforms columnar organization and disrupts some columns in the middle of the cortical depth.

2.6. Effects of curvature of visual cortex

The cerebral cortex is packed into the skull and folded in a complex manner. Accordingly, most parts of the cerebral cortex are curved. It would be expected that sensory feature representation is constrained by the curvature of the cortex. Schematic pictures of columnar organization for feature representation shown in many textbooks (for example, see Kandel et al., 2000) may be too simple, particularly in the curved part of the gyrus. Hubel and Wiesel (1962) suggested that wedge-like columns appear in the apical segment of the post-lateral gyrus because the columns are parallel to the radial fiber bundles and perpendicular to cortical layers. The present simulation and fMRI data demonstrated that orientation columns are likely to appear as wedge-like columns rather than straight columns in curved parts of the cortex.

More interestingly, the columns do not necessarily extend from the cortical surface to the white matter. Related to this property, the present studies showed that orientation singularities were not necessarily straight lines penetrating from the cortical surface to the white matter. Some of them appear as hairpins, as shown in the simulation (Figs. 2a and b) and in the fMRI data from cat visual cortex (Figs. 4f and h). Since the topological constraint on the preferred orientation and direction should be valid in the bulk of the cortex either flat or curved, direction-discontinuity sheets are delimited by orientation-singularity lines. The original view of the configuration of orientation columns as the stacked-slab arrangement (Hubel et al., 1977) has been revised as a view of a pinwheel arrangement of preferred orientations (Bonhoeffer & Grinvald, 1991), retaining the concept of organization of straight columns. The present study suggests that columnar organization may be more complex than expected from the conventional hypercolumn picture: orientation columns are distorted to reconcile with the global curvature of the visual cortex. The wedge-like shape of an orientation column and the interruption of columns in the deeper layers can release the tension induced by the columnar organization in curved grey matter. Our model indicates that such a structure emerges from the competition between the tendencies of periodic arrangement and radial alignment of orientation representation in a curved cortex. Because a large part of area 17 is located near the crown of the gyrus, anatomical minicolumns arranged along the radial fiber bundle may functionally represent different orientations in superficial layers and deep layers in area 17. Moreover, the present model predicts that the preferred direction can more frequently reverse in the deeper layers around the gyrus than in the flat cortex, as reported by Berman et al. (1987). To date, it is thought that the cortical information representation obeys a columnar organization rule. The present study suggests that careful examination of functional architecture is needed, because different pieces of information can be represented in an identical anatomical minicolumn at different layers, particularly around the crowns of gyri and perhaps at fundi.

3. Orientation map plasticity in early life

To investigate the visual cortical plasticity of orientation selectivity, we need to manipulate visual experience to expose animals to restricted orientations continuously and stably. However, manipulating experienced orientations is more difficult than depriving one eye by eyelid suture for the investigation of ocular dominance plasticity (Wiesel & Hubel, 1963). For the stable orientation-restricted visual experience, we fabricated simple-structured goggles fitted with cylindrical lenses, which can be easily attached and dettached to the forhead of cats. In addition, to avoid a sampling bias problem often encountered in unit recording, we employed optical imaging of intrinsic signal to measure orientation selectivity from a wide cortical area. Some kittens were reared with head-mounted goggles to experience a single orientation in a freely moving condition inside animal cages with their mother cats and littermates for two weeks. Some other kittens were reared without goggles, while the other conditions were the same as in goggle-reared kittens. These kittens were used for a control group.

3.1. Experimental methods

The goggles were composed of planoconvex acrylic cylindrical lenses as shown in Fig. 6a (lens thickness, 10.0 mm; lens aperture diameter, 15.0 mm; lens power, +67 D). Cats on which goggles were mounted (Fig. 6b) were able to see elongated images of their environments through the goggles (Tanaka et al., 2007). For example, an image of concentric pattern is transformed to an image of vertical stripe (Figs. 6c and d). We used two types of goggles: v- and h-goggles, which elongated visual images vertically and horizontally, respectively.

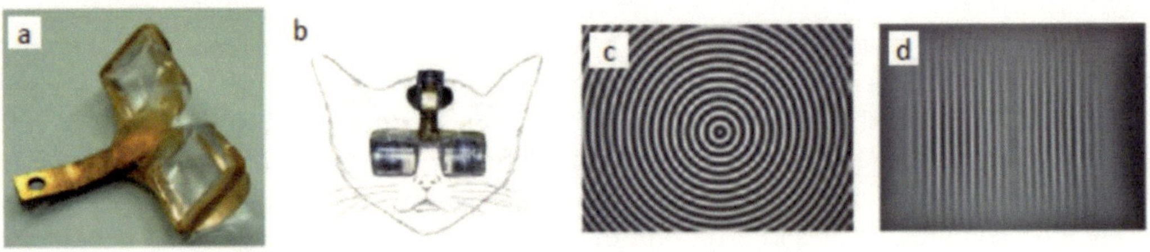

Figure 6. Cylindrical-lens-fitted goggles and visual image transformation.

Surgery was conducted according the procedure described in our previous papers (Tanaka et al., 2004, 2006). Initial anesthesia was induced using ketamine hydrochloride (5.0 mg/kg, i.m.) following sedation with medetomidine hydrochloride (0.1 mg/kg, i.m.). The animals were fixed on a stereotaxic apparatus and were artificially ventilated with a 60:40% mixture of N_2O and O_2 containing 0.5-1.0% isoflurane. Heart rate, end-tidal CO_2 concentration, and rectal temperature were continuously monitored during surgery. A metal head holder for fixing the goggles and a metal chamber for optical imaging were cemented on the animal's skull using dental resin, and the skull and dura mater covering the recording area of the lateral gyrus were removed. The cranial window (17 mm × 12 mm) was positioned approximately from P5 to A12, spanning the midline. Next, the chamber was filled with 2% agar and sealed with a polyvinylidene chloride thin film and a plastic plate. Finally, the frame of the goggles was fixed to a head holder and the position of the goggles was calibrated so that the cylindrical lenses covered the visual field as widely as possible.

Animals were anesthetized as in surgery and paralyzed with pancuronium bromide (0.1 mg/kg/h). They were artificially ventilated. Contact lenses with appropriate curvatures were used to prevent the drying of eyes. The cortex was illuminated with a 700-nm wavelength light. The focal plane was adjusted to 500 μm below the cortical surface using a tandem-lens macroscope arrangement (Ratzlaff & Grinvald, 1991). Intrinsic optical signals were measured while the animals were exposed to visual stimuli displayed on a 20-inch CRT monitor placed 30 cm in front of the animal. Images were obtained with a CCD video camera, and digitized and stored in a computer. For each stimulus presentation, the intrinsic signal was recorded for 1.0 s before and 5.0 s after the stimulus onset. A blank stimulus was presented for 15 s between successive captures of intrinsic signals. Each visual stimulus was presented once in a pseudorandom sequence in a single trial of recordings. Twenty-six to 30 trials were collected in each recording session. As visual stimuli, we used full-screen square-wave gratings, which drifted in two directions at six equally spaced orientations (interval, 30°). To functionally identify area 17, we used gratings of a spatial frequency of 0.5 c.p.d., which is optimal for area 17 neurons (Bonhoeffer et al., 1995; Movshon et al. 1978; Ohki et al., 2000). The temporal frequency of the gratings was fixed at 2.0 Hz. The optical imaging in one session was completed within 5 hours.

The analysis methods that we used were described in a previous paper (Tanaka et al., 2006). It is noteworthy to explain the methods in some detail here to show that observed map changes are attributable to biological changes rather than artificial changes originating from our analysis methods. One trial of optical imaging was composed of six frames (duration of each frame, 1 s). To extract stimulus-related intrinsic signals, we subtracted signals recorded in the first frame (without stimulus presentation) from those signals recorded in succeeding frames with stimulus presentations. Then, we averaged the subtracted signals over the 4th to 6th frames for each trial. Next, we applied the generalized indicator function method to these averaged signals (Yokoo et al., 2001), which efficiently excluded noisy signals originating from volume and oxygenation changes in thick blood vessels and spatially slowly varying fluctuations of signals inherent in the recorded intrinsic signals. It should be noted that the image data processing based on the generalized indicator function method underestimates the effects of overrepresentation of exposed orientation induced by single-orientation exposure, because the data processing method eliminates spatially slowly varying point-spread components of intrinsic signal (Gilbert et al., 1996), which may partially contain responses to the exposed orientation.

Having excluded the spatially slow noise components, we summed the stimulus-related signals over all trials for each stimulus orientation and applied Gaussian low-pass filtering with a 150-μm standard deviation to eliminate high-frequency noise. In this way, we constructed a single-condition map for each stimulus orientation. To determine the preferred orientation at each pixel inside the recorded area, we used the vector sum method (Bonhoeffer & Grinvald, 1991). Thus, at each pixel, we obtained the preferred orientation and the modulation amplitude in the second harmonic components, which is regarded as orientation selectivity. The orientation polar map was constructed with the preferred orientation and orientation selectivity as color and brightness, respectively.

For further analysis, we discarded pixels eliciting response strengths lower than a half of the response strength averaged over all pixels inside the recorded area. According to this criterion, the domains containing the remaining pixels nearly lined up with functionally defined area 17, which was exclusively activated by stimuli of a 0.5-c.p.d. spatial frequency. To construct an orientation histogram, we counted the number of pixels involved in each orientation, 30° width, and normalized them by the total number of pixels involved in all orientations.

3.2. Orientation map alteration by goggle rearing

Before examining orientation maps in goggle-reared cats, we investigated orientation maps in normally reared cats. In orientation polar maps obtained from normally reared kittens younger than P30, generally the relative size of responsive domains is largest for horizontal orientation (0° or equivalently 180°) and smallest for vertical orientation (90°). This indicates that orientation representation is biased toward the horizontal orientation for very young normal kittens. This is analogous to the innate bias toward the contralateral eye, as has been known in ocular dominance (Wiesel & Hubel, 1963). However, the sample-averaged orientation histogram across 15 normally reared kittens of P33-84 showed a weak bias toward vertical orientation.

Here, we first describe the results of goggle rearing (GR) for two weeks. Measurements in goggle-reared kittens were completed within 5 hrs after the removal of the goggles. Figure 7 shows orientation polar maps (a, c, e, g, i and k) and orientation histograms (b, d, f, h, j and l) obtained from optical imaging of functionally defined area 17 (delineated by white curves) of those kittens. In orientation polar maps, color and brightness indicate preferred orientation and orientation selectivity, respectively (scale bars: 2 mm), and in orientation histograms, the height of bins indicates the relative size of cortical domains for 6 preferred orientations, where blue horizontal lines indicate the relative size of iso-orientation domains for a uniform orientation representation. Immediately after the 2-week GR that started at P16-P17, the overrepresentation of horizontal orientation was exclusive (Figs. 7g and h), whereas that of vertical orientation was somewhat moderate (Figs. 7a and b). For GR that started at P27-P29, the overrepresentation of vertical orientation also became nearly exclusive (Figs. 7c and d). The representation of horizontal orientation was still predominant, although that of unexposed orientations appeared (Figs. 7i and j). The imbalance between vertical and horizontal orientations at P16-P17 may reflect, at least partly, the horizontal bias detected in normal kittens. When 2-week GR was started at P49-54, the induced overrepresentation of the exposed orientation, either vertical or horizontal, diminished drastically (Figs. 7e, f, k and l). A close examination of Figs. 7e and f revealed that the effect of vertical GR was reversed to a slight underrepresentation of the vertical orientation.

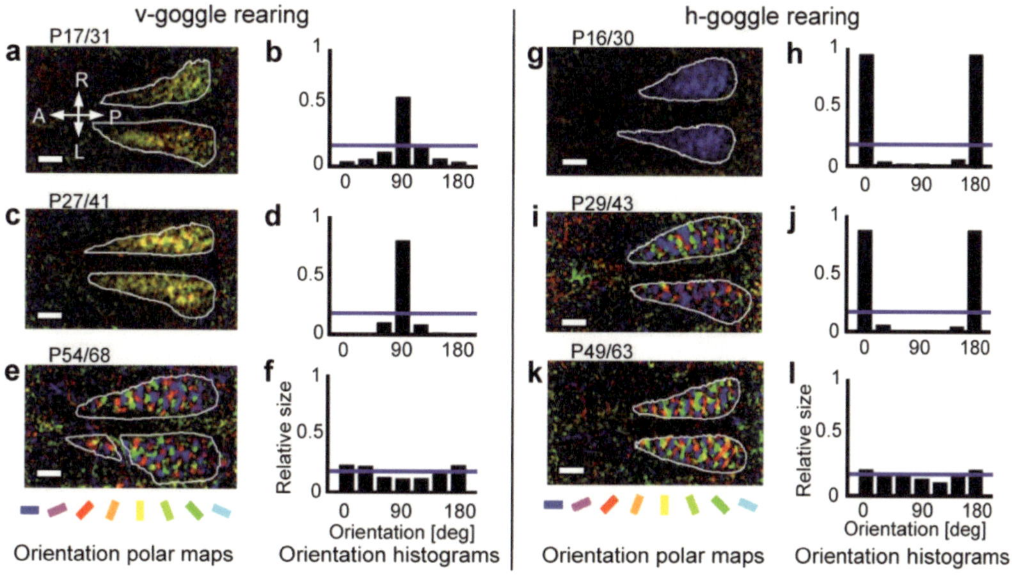

Figure 7. Orientation selectivity in kittens continuously exposed to vertical- or horizontal orientation for 2 weeks.

3.3. Critical period for orientation selectivity

Figure 8 illustrates the time profile of the sensitivity for the modification of orientation selectivity against the onset day of GR, where all data points were obtained from 18 kittens goggle-reared for 2 weeks. Here, we quantified the sensitivity as the relative size of the cortical domains for the exposed orientation, in which the average representation bias in normal kittens was subtracted at respective days of optical imaging performance (for more information, see Tanaka et al. 2007). Therefore, the positive and negative normalized relative domain size indicate the overrepresentation and underrepresentation of the exposed orientation, respectively. The sensitivity profiles for vertical- and horizontal-orientation exposures are generally consistent with each other, except for a discrepancy at 2-3 postnatal weeks. This discrepancy suggests that innate mechanisms of orientation map formation not only induce the representation bias toward horizontal orientation in normal kittens but also enhance the overrepresentation of horizontal orientation in young kittens exposed to horizontal orientation. The critical period can be defined as the postnatal period during which 2-week GR effectively causes the modification of orientation selectivity. Thus defined, the critical period starts 2 weeks after birth and lasts for 6 weeks. Note that the presently delineated critical period for orientation plasticity overlaps the most sensitive period for ocular dominance plasticity (postnatal 4-5 weeks) reported by Olson & Freeman (1980).

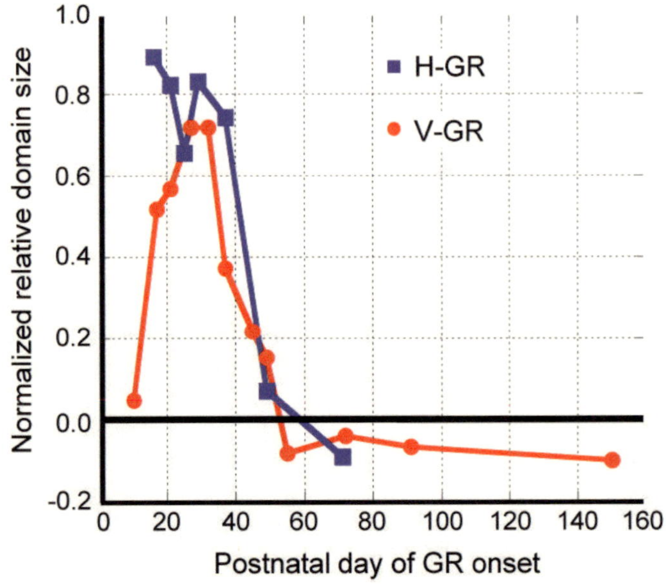

Figure 8. Sensitivity profiles for orientation plasticity.

Figure 8 also shows that the critical period is followed by a late phase of underrepresentation of the exposed orientation for GR starting between P55 and P151. We also observed the case of an adult cat reared with vertical goggles from P396 for one month; this cat showed a small relative size of cortical domains representing the exposed orientation for 90°. Therefore, continuous single-orientation exposure after the critical period, even in adulthood, leads to the underrepresentation of the exposed orientation, as consistent with previous reports on orientation plasticity in adult cats (Creutzfeldt & Heggelund, 1975; Dragoi et al., 2000).

3.4. Orientation map alteration under short- and long-term GR

Figure 9 shows how the once-induced overrepresentation of the exposed orientation changes afterwards. The normalized relative sizes of cortical domains representing exposed vertical (circles) or horizontal (squares) orientations are plotted at the end of 2-week GR (solid symbols) and also at the end of the succeeding normal viewing (hollow symbols), respectively. Plotted points for identical kittens are linked by the lines, and numerical figures indicate onset ages of GR. In 4 kittens for which 2-week GR started at P29, 32, 37 and 39, 3-day normal viewing immediately before the second optical imaging eliminated the overrepresentation: the normalized relative domain sizes returned to 0 (level of normal kittens). However, in 4 kittens in which 2-week GR started relatively earlier at P16, P21 and P25, recovery during the succeeding 3-days of normal viewing was partial.

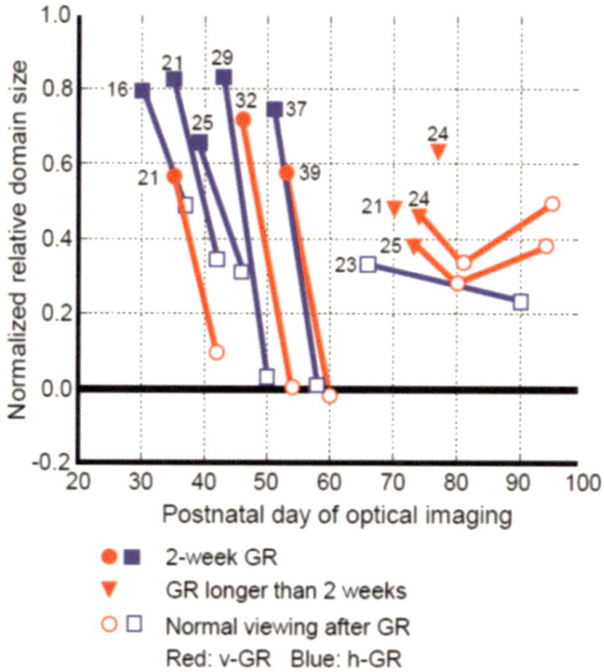

Figure 9. Effects of duration and timing of GR.

In 4 other kittens, in which long-term vertical GR for 4-6 weeks started at P21-P25 (triangles), the overrepresentation of the exposed orientation was retained at moderate levels between 0.39 and 0.64 of the normalized relative domain size in the first optical imaging. As tested in two of these kittens (P24-P73; P25-P74), the overrepresentation was preserved even after 3 weeks of normal viewing. A similar tendency was observed in another kitten in which horizontal GR started at P23 and switched to normal rearing at P51.

We can summarize normal viewing effects on GR-induced changes of orientation maps as follows:

1. When 2-week GR covers a relatively late phase of the critical period (at P29-39), normal viewing quickly eliminates the overrepresentation and restores normal orientation maps.
2. When 2-week GR covers a relatively early phase of the critical period (earlier than P29), normal viewing does not completely eliminate the overrepresentation.
3. Goggle rearing for 4 weeks or more outlasting the critical period acts to preserve the moderate overrepresentation of the exposed orientation, and reorganized orientation maps are consolidated to be robust against normal viewing thereafter.

3.5. Comparisons with previous studies

There have been two hypotheses about the effect of visual experience on orientation plasticity. One is the selection hypothesis and the other the instruction hypothesis. In the former hypothesis, after single-orientation exposure, neurons innately selective for unexposed orientations just decrease their responses to the unexposed orientations without changes of preferred orientations. In the latter hypothesis, neurons selective for unexposed orientations change their preferred orientations towards the exposed orientation. Blakemore & Cooper (1970) supported the instruction hypothesis, because they found preferred orientations of recorded units were strongly biased toward the exposed orientation in cats that had experienced striped environment. Later, Stryker et al. (1978) found that single-orientation exposure changed a large portion of units nonselective or unresponsive, although a proportion of responsive units preferring for the exposed orientation increased. Particularly, they found an orderly arrangement of selective units according to preferred orientation along the electrode tracks, as observed in normal cats, but clusters of nonselective or unresponsive units were interleaved. In our optical imaging on kittens exposed to a single orientation, stimulus-related intrinsic signals in response to unexposed orientations were reduced in cortical domains originally selective for the unexposed orientations, and a proportion of pixels without orientation selectivity tended to increase (Tanaka et al., 2006), consistently with single-unit recording by Stryker et al. (1978). However, stimulus-related intrinsic signals in response to the exposed orientation tended to increase in these domains, resulting in the changes of orientation preference.

Differences of experienced patterns during single-orientation exposure may be worth noting. Hirsch & Spinelli (1970) and Stryker et al. (1978) exposed kittens to stationary lines through their goggles. Carlson et al. (1986) also presented stationary stripe patterns with various spatial frequencies to monocularly deprived infant monkeys. To examine the effect of exposure to stationary oriented stimuli, we have reared 4 kittens with spherical-lens-fitted goggles for chronic exposure to a stationary stripe with a spatial frequency of about 0.5 and 0.15 c.p.d (Tanaka et al., 2007). Although the exposed orientation was overrepresented at the first optical imaging experiments after 2- or 3-week GR in 3 kittens, the underrepresentation of the exposed orientation occurred in the other kitten, in which the orthogonal orientation was overrepresented (data not shown). Even in the kittens showing the overrepresentation of the exposed orientation, the layouts of orientation preferences were labile during prolonged GR. In 3 of the 4 kittens, the overrepresentation disappeared or changed to the underrepresentation after long-term GR. Such labile alteration of orientation maps is characteristic of exposure to a stationary oriented pattern. This is contrasted with the finding that orientation maps altered by exposure to a dynamic single orientation through cylindrical-lens-fitted goggles are consolidated preserving the moderate overrepresentation of the exposed orientation (Fig. 9). It should be noted that the instability in orientation map alteration for stationary stripe pattern exposure was not due to the repeated optical imaging, because orientation maps altered by rearing with cylindrical-lens-fitted goggles changed gradually in successive optical imaging, and were finally stabilized at the moderate overrepresentation of the exposed orientation. The fact that Carlson et al. (1986) recorded units selective for the orthogonal orientation to the exposed orientation in the open eye may be such labile modification of orientation selectivity induced by the stationary stripe pattern exposure. The disappearance of the orientation selectivity modification for prolonged exposure to stationary oriented stimuli is suggested to have a weak impact on the structural modification of orientation maps.

The different effects of dynamic and stationary stripe exposures on orientation map alteration may be attributed to the differences in the behavioral significance of visual images through the goggles. Images transmitted through cylindrical leses contain some information on the animal's environment, in that vertically elongated stripes move associated with the movement of visual objects in the environment. It is, therefore, expected that the animal may pay attention to the images and neurons in the primary visual cortex can be sufficiently activated. Such neuronal activation consequently may have an influence on the suceptivility for orientation plasticity. In contrast, stripes exposed to by opaque lenses do not move irrespect of any dynamic changes of the environment. The animal may neglect the stripes and neurons in the primary visual cortex may not be sufficiently activated, resulting in weak or no induction of orientation plasticity. How the behavioral significance of exposed visual images affects orientation plascity is an interesting future research target.

4. Conclusion

Hubel & Wiesl's hypercolumn model successfully provides a simple view of the functional architecture of the cerebral cortex. However, our simulation of visual feature representation together with the high-resolution fMRI experiment on the cat threw a doubt about the idea of orientation columns extending from pia to white matter, especially in regions where the cortex is curved. Futhermore, the dimensionality of singularities in the orientation and direction maps was inceased by 1, when we considered the 3D visual cortex: Pinwheel centers in the orientation map appeared as point terminals of line singularities running in the 3D visual cortex at the cortical surface; direction-discontinuity lines starting or ending at pinwheel centers appeared as line crossings of direction-discontinuity sheets with the cortical surface. More extensive experiments are desired to confirm these observations.

In regrad to orientation plasticity in the developing visual cortex, it seems to be accepted that preferred orientations of neurons do not change but only responsiveness changes depending on visual experience. Our optical imaging experiments on cats, however, demonstrated that short-term single-orientation exposure dramatically altered preferred orientations until postnatal 6 weeks, which is against the current consensus. This study, on the other hand, revealed further complexity in orientation plasticity in case where animals were exposed to a single orientation for a long time or returned to a normal visual environment after single-orientation exposure. Again on this issue, further investigation is needed to obtain a better understanding of mechanisms underlying orientation plasticity in the visual cortex.

Author details

Shigeru Tanaka
The University of Electro-Communications, Japan

5. References

Albus, K., & Wolf, W. (1984). Early post-natal development of neuronal function in the kitten's visual cortex: A laminar analysis. *Journal of Physiology*, Vol. *348*, pp. 153-185

Berman, N. E., Wilkes, M. E., & Payne, B. R. (1987). Organization of orientation and direction selectivity in areas 17 and 18 of cat cerebral cortex. *Journal of Neurophysiology*, Vol. *58*, pp. 676-699

Blakemore, C., & Cooper, G. F. (1970). Development of the brain depends on visual environment. *Nature*, Vol. 228, pp. 477-478

Blakemore, C., & Van Sluyters, R. C. (1975). Innate and environmental factors in the development of the kitten's visual cortex. *Journal of Physiology*,Vol. 248, pp. 663-716

Bonhoeffer, T., & Grinvald, A. (1991). Iso-orientation domains in cat visual cortex are arranged in pinwheel-like patterns. *Nature*, Vol. 353, pp. 429-431

Bonhoeffer, T., Kim, D-S., Malonek, D., Shoham, D., & Grinvald, A. (1995). Optical imaging of the layout of functional domains in area 17 and across the area 17/18 border in cat visual cortex. *European Journal of Neuroscience*, Vol. 7, pp. 1973-1988

Carlson, M., Hubel, D. H., & Wiesel, T. N. (1986). Effects of monocular exposure oriented lines on monkey striate cortex. *Developmental Brain Research*, Vol. 25, pp. 71-81

Crair, M. C., Gillespie, D. C., & Stryker, M. P. (1998). The role of visual experience in the development of columns in cat visual cortex. *Science*, Vol. 279, pp. 566-570

Creutzfeldt, O. D., & Heggelund, P. (1975). Neural plasticity in visual cortex of adult cats after exposure to visual patterns. *Sicence*, Vol. 188, pp. 1025-127

Dragoi, V., Sharma, J., & Sur, M. (2000). Adaptation-induced plasticity of orientation tuning in adult visual cortex. *Neuron*, Vol. 28, pp. 287–298

Fukuda, M., Moon, C. H., Wang, P., & Kim, S. G. (2006). Mapping iso-orientation columns by contrast agent-enhanced functional magnetic resonance imaging: reproducibility, specificity, and evaluation by optical imaging of intrinsic signal. *Journal of Neuroscience*, Vol. 26, pp. 11821-11832

Gilbert, C. D., Das, A., Ito, M., Kapadia, M., & Westheimer, G. (1996). Spatial integration and cortical dynamics. *Proceedings of National Academy of Science USA*, Vol. 93, pp. 615-622

Hirsch, H. V., Spinelli, D. N. (1970). Visual experience modifies distribution of horizontally and vertically oriented receptive fields in cats. *Science*, Vol. 168, pp. 869-871

Hubel, D. H., & Wiesel, T. N. (1962). Receptive fields, binocular interaction and functional architecture in the cat's visual cortex. *Journal of Physiology*, Vol. 160, pp. 106-154

Hubel, D. H., & Wiesel, T. N. (1963a). Shape and arrangement of columns in cat's striate cortex. *Journal of Physiology*, Vol. 165, pp. 559-568

Hubel, D. H & Wiesel, T. N. (1963b). Receptive fields of cells in striate cortex of very young, visually inexperienced kittens. *Journal of Neurophysiology*, Vol. 26, pp. 994-1002

Hubel, D. H., Wiesel, T. N. & LeVay, S. (1977). Plasticity of ocular dominance columns in monkey striate cortex. *Philosophical Transactions of the Royal Society London B: Biological Sciences*, Vol. 278, pp. 377-409

Hübener, M., Shoham, D., Grinvald, A. & Bonhoeffer, T. (1997). Spatial relationships among three columnar systems in cat area 17. *Journal of Neuroscience*, Vol. 17, pp. 9270-9284

Kalatsky, V. A. & Stryker, M. P. (2003). New paradigm for optical imaging: temporally encoded maps of intrinsic signal. *Neuron,* Vol. 38, pp. 529-545

Kandel, E. R., Schwartz, J. H. & Jessell, T. M. (2000). *Principles of Neural Science* (4th edition), McGraw-Hill, 978-0838577011, New York

Kim, D. S., Matsuda, Y., Ohki, K., Ajima, A. & Tanaka, S. (1999). Geometrical and topological relationships between multiple functional maps in cat primary visual cortex. *Neuroreport,* Vol. 10, pp. 2515-2522

Kisvarday, Z. F., Buzas, P. & Eysel, U. T. (2001). Calculating direction maps from intrinsic signals revealed by optical imaging. *Cerebral Cortex*, Vol. 11, pp. 636-647

Moon, C. H., Fukuda, M., Park, S. H. & Kim, S. G. (2007). Neural interpretation of blood oxygenation level-dependent fMRI maps at submillimeter columnar resolution. *Journal of Neuroscience*, Vol. 27, pp. 6892-6902

Movshon, J. A., Thompson, I. D., & Tolhurst, D. J. (1978). Spatial and temporal contrast sensitivity of neurones in areas 17 and 18 of the cat's visual cortex. *Journal of Physiology,* Vol. 283, pp. 101-120

Nakagama, H. & Tanaka, S. (2004). Self-organization model of cytochrome oxidase blobs and ocular dominance columns in the primary visual cortex. *Cerebral Cortex,* Vol. 14, pp. 376–386

Ohki, K., Matsuda, Y., Ajima, A., Kim, D-S., & Tanaka, S. (2000). Arrangement of orientation pinwheel centers around area 17/18 transition zone in cat visual cortex. *Cerebral Cortex,* Vol. 10, pp. 593-601

Olson, C. R., & Freeman, R. D. (1980). Profile of the sensitive period for monocular deprivation in kittens. *Experimental Brain Research,* Vol. 39, pp. 17-21

Ratzlaff, E. H., & Grinvald, A. (1991). A tandem-lens epifluorescence macroscope: hundred-fold brightness advantage for wide-field imaging. *Journal of Neuroscience Methods,* Vol. 36, pp. 127-137

Rauschecker, J. P., & Singer, W. (1981). The effects of early visual experience on the cat's visual cortex and their possible explanation by Hebb synapses. *Journal of Physiology,* Vol. 310, pp. 215-239

Sengpiel, F., Stawinski, P., & Bonhoeffer, T. (1999). Influence of experience on orientation maps in cat visual cortex. *Nature Neuroscience,* Vol. 2, pp. 727-732

Sholl, D. A. (1953). Dendritic organization in the neurons of the visual and motor cortices of the cat. *Journal of Anatomy*, Vol. 87, pp. 387-406

Stryker, M. P., Sherk, H., Leventhal, A. G., & Hirsch, H. V. (1978). Physiological consequences for the cat's visual cortex of effectively restricting early visual experience with oriented contours. *Journal of Neurophysiology,* Vol. 1, pp. 896-909

Swindale, N. V., Grinvald, A. & Shmuel, A. (2003). The spatial pattern of response magnitude and selectivity for orientation and direction in cat visual cortex. *Cerebral Cortex,* Vol. 13, pp. 225-238

Tanaka, S. (1995). Topological analysis of point singularities in stimulus preference maps of the primary visual cortex. *The Proceedings of the Royal Society London B: Biological Science,* Vol. 261, pp. 81-88

Tanaka, S. (1997). Topology of visual cortex. *FORMA,* Vol. 12, pp. 101-106

Tanaka, S., Ribot, J., & Miyashita, M. (2004). Roles of visual experience and intrinsic mechanism in the activity-dependent self-organization of orientation maps: Theory and experiment. *Neural Networks,* Vol. 17, pp. 1363–1375

Tanaka, S., Ribot, J., Imamura, K., & Tani, T. (2006). Orientation-restricted continuous visual exposure induces marked reorganization of orientation maps in early life. *NeuroImage,* Vol. 30, pp. 462 – 477

Tanaka, S., Tani, T., Ribot, J., & Yamazaki, T. (2007). Chronically mountable goggles for persistent exposure to single orientation. *Journal of Neuroscience Methods,* Vol. 160, pp. 206-214

Tusa, R. J., Palmer, L. A., & Rosenquist, A. C. (1978). The retinotopic organization of area 17 (striate cortex) in the cat. *Journal of Comparative Neurology,* Vol. 177, pp. 213-235

Wiesel, T. N., & Hubel, D. H. (1963). Single-cell responses in striate cortex of kittens deprived of vision in one eye. *Journal of Neurophysiology,* Vol. 26, pp. 1003-1017

Yokoo, T., Knight, B. W., & Sirovich, L. (2001). An optimization approach to signal extraction from noisy multivariate data. *NeuroImage,* Vol. 14, pp. 1309-1326

Chapter 17

The Experimental Manipulation of Visual Cortex Efferents

I. Gerrikagoitia, B. Rienda and L. Martínez-Millán

Additional information is available at the end of the chapter

http://dx.doi.org/10.5772/48632

1. Introduction

The visual cortex is part of the occipital cortex that makes up the primary and secondary visual areas [1,2]. In the primary visual areas of rodents, as in other isocortical areas, two main neuronal types are present: inhibitory interneurons and projecting neurons [3,4]. The inhibitory interneurons belong to several GABAergic subpopulations, while the projection neurons are excitatory pyramidal neurons that are classically distributed in 5 layers, each of which is associated with a preferential projection area [3,4]. Accordingly, the pyramidal neurons of layers II, III and IV give rise to corticocortical connections, while those of layers V and VI project to subcortical structures. In the primary visual cortex pyramidal neurons of layer V project to superficial collicular layers and they give rise to collaterals that project to the pontine nuclei.

The aim of this review is to describe the sprouting capacities of these projecting neurons and to evaluate several strategies to enhance these capabilities in adult animals, principally considering work carried out in rodents. In the first part, we will discuss the sprouting of the corticocollicular ipsilateral connection in young animals. This connection originates in layer V pyramidal neurons and its post-lesional sprouting capacities diminish significantly after the end of the critical period (postnatal day 45). We will also discuss the use of siRNAs to knockdown the expression of molecules that inhibit post-lesional axonal sprouting in adults. Lastly, we will describe alterations in sprouting and synaptic size in the corticocortical visual connections.

2. Differential lesion responses of neonatal and adult visual cortex efferents

The visual system is widely used as a model to study plasticity, given the compartmentalized arrangement of its main stations. In rodents, most of the retinal ganglion axons cross the optic chiasm to the contralateral side [5,6]. Thus, retinal deafferentation is a convenient experimental means of investigating the plastic response mechanisms to central nervous system (CNS) lesions.

The superior colliculus (SC) is a layered mesencephalic structure that can be divided into two main compartments: the superficial strata that are mainly devoted to visual function; and the intermediate and deep strata that process multisensorial information [7-9]. The superficial layers are composed of the stratum zonale (SZ), stratum griseum superficiale (SGS), and stratum opticum (SO), and they receive their main afferent input from the retina and primary visual cortex.

In rats, virtually all retinal ganglion cells project to the contralateral SC [6,10] and the majority of optic axons reach the SC prenatally, with the remainder reaching their target in the early postnatal days [11]. Layer V pyramidal neurons of the primary visual cortex (VC1) project to the ipsilateral SC [12-14], with the first visual cortical axons that reach the SC arriving on postnatal day (P) 4/5. At this stage, the axons only appear in the SO. From P7 to P13, these projections spread out to the ventral region of the SGS and the intermediate layers, and between P13 and P19, connections are restricted to the superficial strata of the SC, ultimately forming the organizational pattern seen in adults [15]. Although both retinocollicular and corticocollicular terminals densely innervate superficial strata of the SC, the former ramify more densely in the SZ and upper SGS, while the latter project to the lower SGS and upper SO [12-14]. During development, retinal and primary visual cortex fibers undergo multiple plastic changes, which include axonal growth, target path finding, axonal pruning and projection refinement [15-17]. This results in the formation of a precisely organized topographic map that represents the visual field in the SC in a point-to-point fashion.

CNS lesions or pathologies, and the deprivation of visual stimuli, can alter the final visual corticocollicular organization, predisposing this system to phenomena of neuroplasticity [18]. The capacity to respond to CNS lesions through plastic changes varies depending on the age at which the injury takes place. Thus, during early postnatal development, while connections are being established, neuronal projections exhibit significant capacity for regeneration and reorganization in response to neuronal damage. However, this post-lesional response becomes considerably diminished in adulthood. A remarkable number of publications have described changes in the organization of neuronal connections following neonatal CNS injury. In the visual system, retinal deafferentation at birth results in severe alterations of the afferent systems that project to SC superficial layers [19]. For example, removal of SC input in neonatal rodents results in an aberrant ipsilateral retinotectal projection [20-24], whereas retinal deafferentation in adults has no such effect [25-27]. Gradual, continuous plastic changes have been described in the ipsilateral retinal axons of adult rats subjected to contralateral retinal lesions at P21, in contrast to the fast plastic response observed in neonatal rats evident within 48 hours of lesion [28].

Neonatal lesions of the visual cortex give rise to an aberrant projection to the contralateral SC [29] and expansion of the ipsilateral corticocollicular projection from the remaining unlesioned visual cortex [30]. These plastic responses during early postnatal development may occur due to axonal sprouting and/or the blockade of developmentally regulated axonal retraction. It has been suggested that axons continuously compete for postsynaptic sites in the CNS. Indeed, it is likely that during development this competition is essential for the formation and refinement of projections, although an equilibrium is reached in the mature nervous system that results in the stabilization of neuronal connections [31,32].

In previous studies, we observed an enlargement of the visual corticocollicular terminal field in rabbits after neonatal removal of contralateral retinal inputs [33], and an alteration in the plastic response to injury when the same lesion was performed in adults [34]. The anterograde axonal tracer biotin dextran amine (BDA) was used to label the corticocollicular connection emerging from layer V pyramidal neurons of the primary visual cortex in 3 different experimental groups: (i) adult rats (P60) subjected to neonatal (P1) optic nerve transection; (ii) adults rats subjected to optic nerve transection in adulthood; and (iii) control adults rats. The animals were sacrificed 10 days after BDA injection and the superior colliculi extracted for histochemical analysis. As BDA was injected into the region of the primary visual cortex that represents the lower temporal visual field [35-36], corticocollicular terminal fields were localized within the posterolateral quadrant of the SC [37] in all experimental animals. In agreement with previous studies [14,33,38], we observed a tight topographical organization of the visual corticocollicular terminal field. In control animals, the corticocollicular terminal field was column-shaped, extending from the SO up to the pial surface, and it was restricted to a small portion of the collicular surface. Fibers ascending from the SO gave rise to dense axonal networks in the lower half of SGS, and they branched to reach the upper half of this stratum and the most superficial SZ, where the fibers were oriented parallel to the collicular surface [34].

Visual deprivation in neonatal animals results in significant expansion of the corticocollicular visual terminal fields, which invaded the entire lateromedial extension of the visual collicular strata. However, the axons tended to concentrate in the posterolateral quadrant of the collicular surface, indicating that the gross topography of the connection was maintained, despite deafferentation [34]. Molecules involved in target path finding, such as ephrins and their receptors, may play a crucial role in determining retinotectal topography [39-41]. Neonatal deafferentation also significantly alters the direction of fiber projection, resulting in horizontal and oblique orientation in the majority of fibers within the SGS in deafferented animals. We previously reported a similar effect in rabbits [33]. However, the expansion of this terminal field may reflect the maintenance of collaterals during postnatal development [38,42] or active sprouting processes. Previous studies reported that in neonatal animals, corticocollicular fibers only appear in the SO [38,43]. As we observed a large density of fibers occupying almost the entire extension of the most superficial strata, SZ and SO, we can assert that an active process of axonal pruning occurred after neonatal deafferentation.

The labeled visual corticocolicular terminal fields in rats subjected to retinal deafferentation in adulthood were columnar, with no changes in extension, although staining was most intense in the upper half of the SGS and in the SZ [34]. Anterograde labeling with BDA allowed clear morphological identification of presynaptic boutons, and quantification of boutons in the terminal fields revealed a maximal density in the SGS and the SO [34]. Similar results were obtained by counting autoradiographic particles following [^{3}H]-leucine injection into the primary visual cortex [38]. Despite occurring in neonatal deafferented animals, the increase in bouton density in the absence of notable axonal arborization suggests that new synaptic terminals are formed and thus, we conclude that adult visual corticocollicular afferents maintain a certain degree of plasticity. Comparable synaptogenic responses in the adult corticorubral axons have been described following red nucleus deafferentation [44]. Cytoskeletal proteins like GAP-43 have been implicated in axonal growth [45], and GAP-43 expression in the visual cortex is abundant during postnatal development but it decreases in adulthood [46]. These observations may explain the differences in axonal branching between deafferented neonates and adults. Indeed, we also found that immature vimentin-expressing astrocytes are abundant in the neonatal SC [47], where they may induce local sprouting after retinal deafferentation.

In conclusion, our findings demonstrate that the capacity for post-lesional remodeling is partially retained by the adult central nervous system.

3. Molecular determinants involved in the dampening of the plastic response during adulthood

There is evidence accumulating that glial scar-associated molecules and myelin-derived molecules are molecular determinants that contribute to the diminished ability of adult neurons to regenerate their axons and reorganize their connections following CNS lesions. The glial scar is a meshwork composed of reactive astrocytes, oligodendrocyte precursors, meningeal fibroblasts and microglia that migrate to the lesion site to mediate tightly linked processes. Not only is it an impenetrable physical barrier to regenerating axons but it is also an important source of molecules that directly inhibit regeneration. After neuronal injury, reactive astrocytes and meningeal fibroblasts in the glial scar rapidly enhance the production and release of extracellular matrix molecules, such as the chondroitin sulfate proteoglycans (CSPGs), which are important inhibitors of axonal growth [48-49]. In addition, molecules involved in axonal path finding, such as ephrins and ephrin A4 receptor [50,51], semaphorin 3A [52-54] and Slit proteins [55], have been implicated in the mechanisms by which the gliar scar prevents axonal growth [56].

Myelin also mediates the inhibition of axonal growth in the CNS and for 30 years, post-lesional products of CNS myelin have been known to specifically inhibit axonal extension [57]. Subsequent studies confirmed that CNS myelin and mature oligodendrocytes contain molecular components that restrict axonal regeneration [58-61]. Several proteins expressed by oligodendrocytes have been identified as myelin-associated inhibitors on the basis of their ability to inhibit neurite outgrowth and induce growth cone collapse. Of these, Nogo [62-64], myelin associated glycoprotein (MAG) [65,66], and oligodendrocyte myelin glycoprotein (OMgp) [67] are considered the main contributors to the inhibitory effects of CNS myelin.

NgR, a GPI-linked protein with multiple leucine-rich repeats, is the receptor for Nogo-66, and it mediates the signaling cascade that inhibits axonal growth [68]. More recent studies have shown that MAG and OMgp can also bind to NgR to exert their inhibitory actions [69-71]. The neurotrophin receptor p75 ($p75^{NTR}$) forms a complex with NgR that mediates axonal growth inhibition and that initiates the signaling cascade triggered by myelin derived inhibitors [67,71,72]. $p75^{NTR}$ is not ubiquitously expressed in the adult brain, whereas almost all mature CNS neurons respond to inhibition by myelin. Thus, it is likely that other proteins assume the function of $p75^{NTR}$. TROY is an orphan member of the tumor necrosis factor receptor (TNFR) superfamily that is widely expressed by both embryonic and adult neurons [73,74], and it has been identified as a functional homolog of $p75^{NTR}$ that may contribute to the inhibitory effects of myelin [75,76]. Nonetheless, the role of TROY as a signal transducing receptor in the inhibition of axonal growth remains unclear, as its expression has not been consistently demonstrated in the adult CNS [77]. Lingo-1, the third component of this receptor complex [78], belongs to a large family of proteins that contain leucine-rich repeats and immunoglobulins [79]. Physical association of Lingo-1, NgR and $p75^{NTR}$ results in the formation of a tripartite receptor complex that mediates the inhibitory signaling triggered by myelin inhibitors [78], and the intracellular signaling cascade this complex activates alters the Rac1/RhoA balance in growth cones. RhoA, Rac1 and Cdc42 are widely expressed members of the small GTPase family that regulate actin dynamics and microtubule assembly. Rac1 and RhoA exert antagonistic effects on growth cone dynamics via their effector-kinases, PAK1 and ROCK, stimulating growth cone motility and inducing collapse, respectively. In the damaged nervous system, myelin-derived inhibitors alter the Rac1 and RhoA signaling equilibrium, augmenting RhoA activity at the expense of Rac1 activity [80, 81]. RhoA activation activates the sequential ROCK/LIM kinase/cofilin signaling cascade, resulting in the depolymerization of actin filaments and subsequent growth cone collapse [82]. This intracellular mechanism can be influenced by several molecules, including MAG, Nogo, OMgp, Netrin-1, ephrins and CSPGs, and it has been proposed as the convergence point of several inhibitors of axonal growth that exert similar functions [78,80,83-85].

4. Strategies to promote corticocollicular sprouting after visual deafferentation in adulthood

Several strategies have been described to promote the regeneration and reorganization of neuronal connections following CNS injury. Regeneration of mature damaged axons has been demonstrated using antibodies against myelin-derived inhibitors. For example, treatment of adult rats with anti-Nogo-A IN-1 after spinal cord lesions promotes significant axonal sprouting and regeneration over long distances caudal to the lesion site, accompanied by motor improvements and restoration of sensorial function [86-88]. Similarly, in animal models of spinal cord injury and stroke, the intrathecal administration of antibodies that effectively neutralize Nogo-A activity enhances regeneration of the corticospinal tract fibers, restoring damaged neuronal circuits and promoting functional recovery [89,90]. In support of these findings, the intrathecal administration of anti-Nogo-A antibodies in monkeys subjected to cervical spinal cord hemisection promotes extensive functional recovery, increased sprouting and regenerative axonal elongation [91].

Other strategies to promote axonal regeneration and reorganization following adult CNS lesions have been described in transgenic animal models. Nogo-A single knockout and Nogo-A/B double knockout mice exhibit dramatic increases in axonal sprouting and extension after spinal cord injury, accompanied by substantial locomotor recovery [92,93]. While no increase in axon regeneration was observed in another study in either Nogo-A/B double knockout or Nogo-A/B/C triple knockout mice [94], a more recent study using the optic nerve crush model in Nogo-A/B/C triple knockout mice reported significant axon regeneration [95], suggesting Nogo influences in axon regeneration *in vivo*.

Blockade of RhoA and ROCK activation with C3 transferase and Y-27632 antagonists, respectively, enhances axonal growth in myelin substrates *in vitro* [83,84,96] and *in vivo* [83,84]. However, the effectiveness of these antagonists appears to depend on their mode of administration, as C3 transferase was not effective in all *in vivo* studies [96]. Since the discovery of RNA interference [97], numerous studies have focused on inhibiting target molecules using siRNAs that specifically silence the expression of target mRNAs [98]. Several studies have reported the promotion of neurite outgrowth *in vitro* following siRNA administration. For example, siRNAs against $p75^{NTR}$ disinhibit dorsal root ganglia neurite outgrowth in the presence of MAG [99]. Likewise, siRNA-mediated silencing of components of the inhibitory signaling cascade, including $p75^{NTR}$, NgR and RhoA mRNA, enhances dorsal root ganglia neurite outgrowth in the presence of CNS myelin, with RhoA knockdown exerting the strongest effect [100]. A recent study using a murine model of multiple sclerosis demonstrated that systematic administration of siRNAs against Nogo-A promotes functional recovery accompanied by a significant increase of GAP43 expression, a protein expressed in growing axons. Based on these findings, the authors suggested that axonal repair may underlie the improved clinical outcome in mice treated with siRNAs against Nogo-A [101].

5. Disinhibition of axonal growth by small interfering RNAs against the Nogo Receptor and RhoA

Given the essential role of myelin-derived molecules in the inhibition of neurite outgrowth, we studied the effect of NgR and RhoA knockdown, key mediators of the signaling cascade that promotes actin depolymerization and subsequent growth cone collapse, and that triggers inhibition of axon growth [82]. We investigated whether these interventions result in the expansion of the corticocollicular connection in rats subjected to unilateral retinal deafferentation in adulthood, a response that normally only occurs when this lesion is induced neonatally. To this end, we administered a single injection of siRNAs against NgR or RhoA into the left primary visual cortex immediately after the enucleation of the right eye in two-month-old Sprague Dawley rats. After four days, the animals received a microinjection of the anterograde tracer BDA 10,000 at the site of siRNA administration. Seven days later the animals were perfused and the nervous tissue processed for histochemical analysis. Control rats received the same siRNA injections into the primary visual cortex. The effect of the siRNAs on NgR and RhoA mRNA levels were measured by qRT-PCR in the cortex beneath the injection site.

Microinjection of siRNAs against NgR and RhoA into the primary visual cortex of adult enucleated rats promoted a mild expansion of the ipsilateral visual corticocollicular terminal field, although in both cases the centre of the field presented a characteristic column-like shape extending from the SO up to the pial surface, a similar pattern to that seen in non-siRNA treated animals. Likewise, following siRNA injection, many fibers were observed running parallel to the pial surface, mainly located within the ventral half of the SGS and running away from the terminal field center towards the middle line. Moreover, several growth cone-bearing axons were observed in these cases, suggesting active axonal growth (Fig. 1, 2).

To confirm the inhibitory effect of siRNAs on NgR and RhoA mRNA expression in the primary visual cortex, and hence the involvement of these molecules in the reorganization of the visual corticocollicular field in adult rats subjected to retinal deafferentation, relative mRNA levels were quantified by qRT-PCR 24 hours after siRNA injection. This revealed significant decreases in NgR and RhoA mRNA levels (44.8 ± 7.3% and 21.67 ± 10.53%, respectively, relative to controls: Fig. 3).

These results demonstrate that siRNA-mediated abolition of the expression of key mediators of axonal growth inhibition, such as NgR and more notably RhoA, promotes axonal outgrowth after adult CNS injury. Indeed, recent studies using different approaches to reduce the expression of molecules involved in axonal growth inhibition have reported similar beneficial effects on axonal growth. For example, the administration of monoclonal antibodies or peptide antagonists improves axonal and functional regeneration in rats subjected to spinal cord lesions [102-104]. An increase in the number of regenerated retinal ganglion cells axons passing through and growing beyond the injured optic nerve has also been described in an NgR double negative mutant model [105]. Recent studies also demonstrated that siRNA knockdown of $p75^{NTR}$ increases dorsal root ganglia neurite outgrowth in the presence of MAG [99], while the reduction of NgR expression levels using small hairpin RNAs augments axonal growth in neuronal cultures [106].

Several authors have reported increased neurite outgrowth following RhoA inactivation, both *in vitro* [80,83,84,96,100,107] and *in vivo* [83,84]. In our study RhoA knockdown resulted in a greater expansion of the visual corticocollicular terminal field. Similarly, siRNA knockdown of $p75^{NTR}$, NgR and most significantly, RhoA, was shown to disinhibit dorsal root ganglia neurite outgrowth in the presence of myelin [100]. It was suggested that in addition to myelin-derived inhibitory ligands, which act by binding to NgR, other neurite growth inhibitors including ephrins, semaphorins and CSPGs, may converge on the RhoA signaling pathway leading to growth cone collapse [108,109]. Thus, NgR knockdown may block the inhibitory action of myelin derived ligands alone, with no influence on other inhibitory ligands. Nonetheless, RhoA knockdown could block the convergent signaling from all inhibitory ligands.

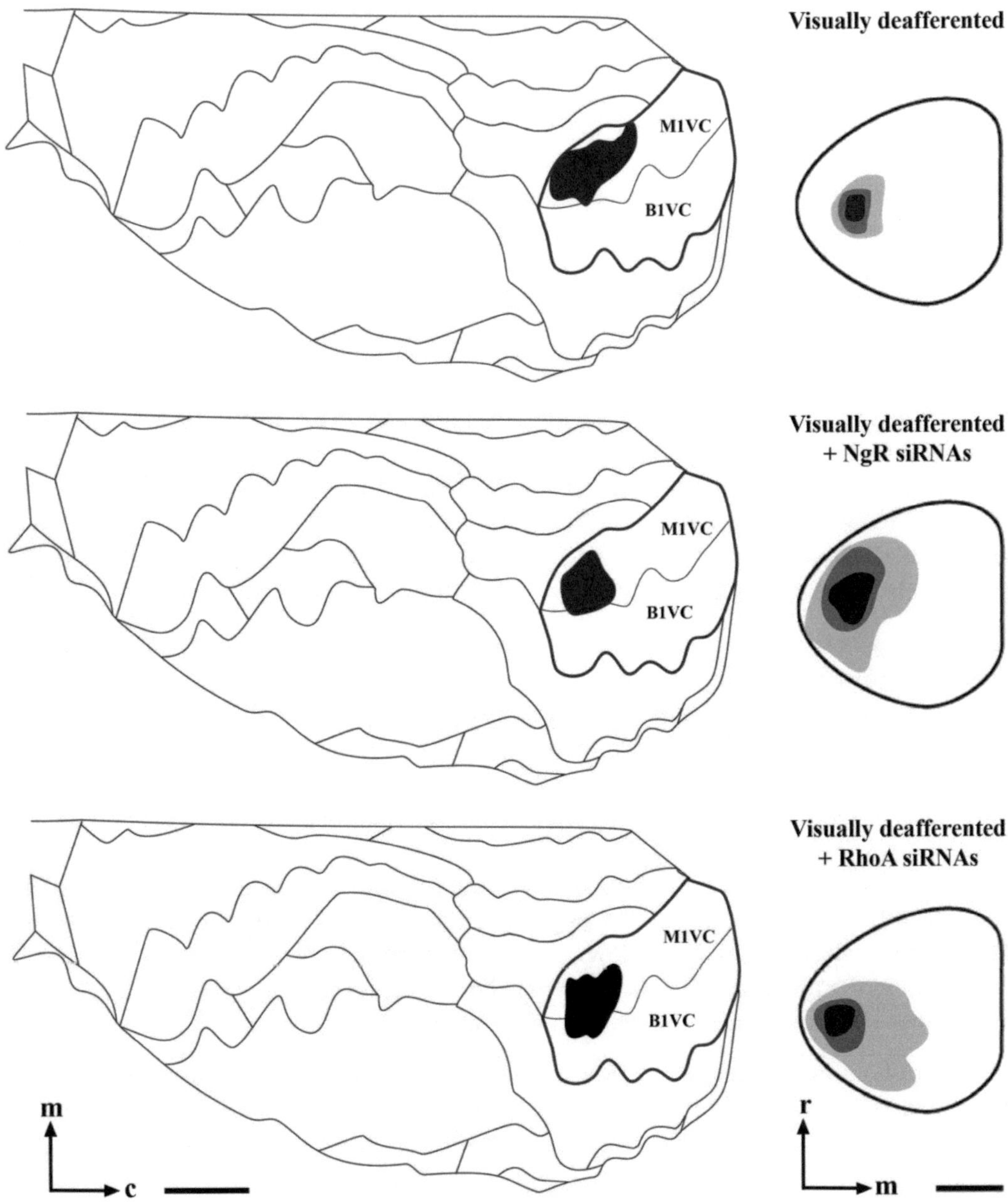

Figure 1. Scheme showing a dorsal view of the site of BDA injection into the primary visual cortex (left) and the projection site in the superior colliculus (right) in different experimental conditions. The administration of siRNAs against NgR and RhoA led to the expansion of the visual corticocollicular terminal field in animals subjected to retinal deafferentation in adulthood. The black areas in the SC denote regions with the greatest density of fibers, while the grey shaded areas denote regions of decreasing axonal density. M1VC, monocular primary visual cortex; B1VC, binocular primary visual cortex; c, caudal; m, medial; r, rostral. Scale bars = 2 mm (left) and 1 mm (right).

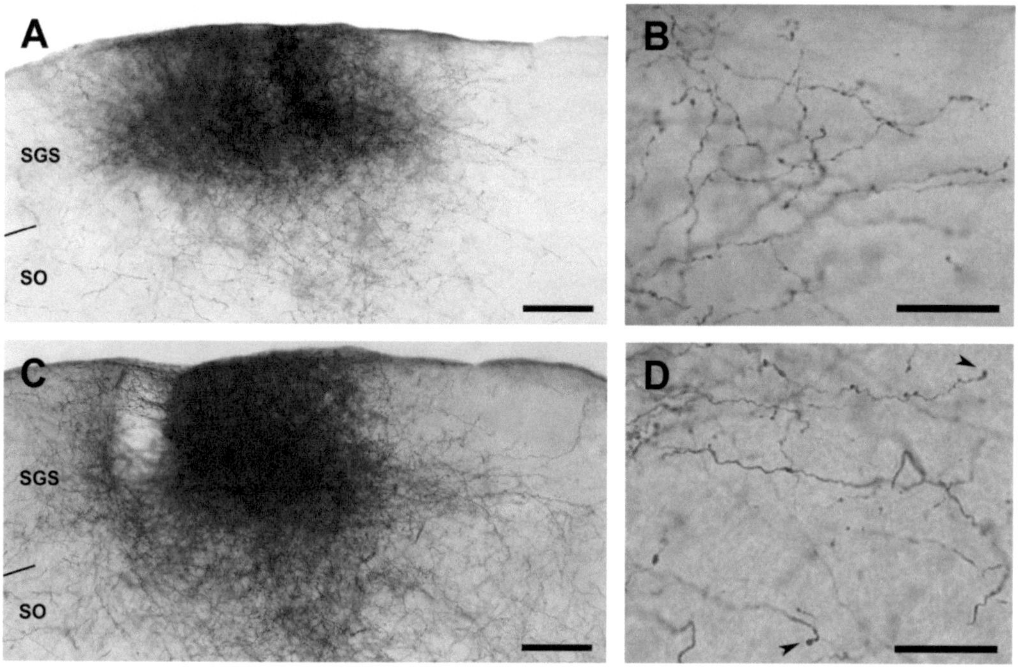

Figure 2. Photomicrographs of BDA-labeled visual corticocollicular terminal fields following administration of siRNAs against NgR (A,B) and RhoA (C,D) in rats visually deafferented in adulthood. (A,C) The microinjection of siRNAs in the primary visual cortex, the projection origin, evoked an increase in terminal field extension, with fibers running towards the lateral SC and the medial edge. (B,D) Detail of axons in the SGS running away from the terminal field, some exhibiting terminal thickening (arrowheads), which may indicate the presence of vestigial growth cone. SGS, stratum griseum superficiale; SO, stratum opticum. Scale bars = 100 μm (A,C) and 30 μm (B,D).

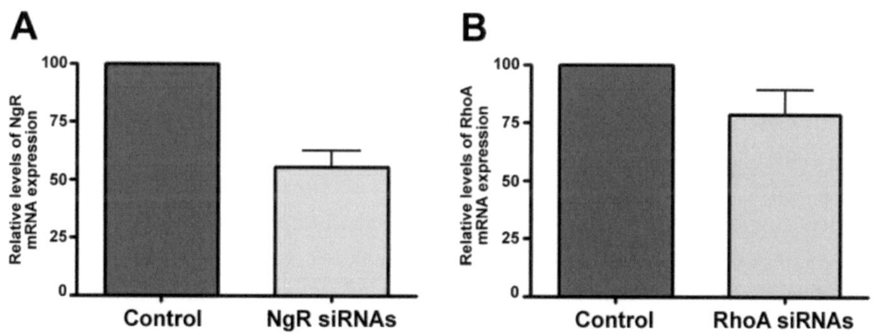

Figure 3. Relative expression of Nogo Receptor (A) and RhoA (B) mRNA in the primary visual cortex following administration of their corresponding siRNAs. Weaker NgR and RhoA mRNA expression in the siRNA-treated groups than in the untreated controls was detected. The relative mRNA levels are normalized to YWHAZ and TATA box binding protein reference genes.

In summary, our *in vivo* results strongly support the use of siRNAs to silence inhibitors of axonal growth, promoting reorganization and axonal outgrowth of the visual corticocollicular connection in adult enucleated rats following a single siRNA injection.

6. Does guanosine enhance corticocortical synaptogenesis?

Considerable effort has been directed towards identifying the specific molecules that guide axonal growth and subsequent synaptogenesis during development, some of which are inductive glial factors [110,111]. Evidence gathered over the last decade has attributed a fundamental role to astrocytes in regulating synaptogenesis and modulating synaptic plasticity during critical periods in different sensory and motor systems [112]. During postnatal development, astrocytes are strongly involved in the formation of synaptic contacts in the CNS, participating in each of the 3 stages of synaptogenesis: (i) the establishment of contacts between neurons; (ii) the formation of the synapse; and (iii) synaptic stabilization or elimination [113]. The role of astrocytes in regulating the synaptic stability of retinal ganglion cells (RGCs) has been studied in detail by culturing purified RGCs in the presence or absence of astrocytes [114]. Astrocytes promote an increase in the number of RGC synapses, although this effect is reversible since when cultured for one week after removing the glia there is a significant reduction in the number of synaptic puncta. The regulatory role of astrocytes in synaptogenesis has also been demonstrated through ultrastructural and physiological studies *in vivo*. Once retinocollicular afferents reach the collicular superficial strata, the synaptic arrangement is closely correlated with the growth and differentiation of astrocytes at the end of the first postnatal week in rats [114], or from P30-P40 in opposums [115].

Matricellular proteins are extracellular regulatory factors secreted by astrocytes that mediate cell-matrix interactions. This is heterogeneous group of proteins includes thrombospondins [116,117], HEVIN [118] and cholesterol [119], which are strongly expressed during development and in response to injury [120,121]. In addition, these matricellular proteins interact with different matrix constituents, growth factors, integrins and other cell surface receptors [122]. Co-culture of purified glutamatergic RGCs with astrocytes results in the secretion of cholesterol by glia, which promotes synaptogenesis [122]. The absence of glial cells from these cultures, or a reduction in the cholesterol content of glia-conditioned medium, diminishes both the number of synapses and GluR2/3 expression by RGCs [123]. While cholesterol production within the CNS is necessary for growth and survival, lipid raft signaling, synaptic vesicle formation and synaptic function [124], increased synaptogenesis and axon pruning requires additional cholesterol production [122]. Recent *in vitro* studies indicate that guanosine increases the efflux of cholesterol from astrocytes [125], the primary source of cholesterol in the nervous system. Moreover, binding of cholesterol to apolipoprotein E (ApoE) promotes synapse formation in RGC cultures [122]. We assessed the synaptogenic effect of guanosine administration *in vivo*, having anterogradely labeled the visual corticocortical connection in young adult male Sprague-Dawley rats by injecting BDA into the primary visual cortex. After BDA administration (24 hr), an osmotic pump was implanted at the site of BDA injection to administer guanosine (300 μM) and 2 weeks after tracer injection, the animals were sacrificed and the nervous tissue analyzed histochemically. While a clear corticocortical projection from primary to secondary visual areas was observed in all cases, guanosine administration significantly increases the number and size of the presynaptic boutons along the axonal branches that reach the secondary visual areas, while the pattern of visual corticocortical projections was preserved. Laterally running fibers emerged at several different levels, white matter fibers ran close to layer VI, while at the level of layers VI and V, afferent fibers gave off divergent branches to form a dense plexus. A smaller contingent of corticocortical fibers ran horizontally along layers IV and V, and a very superficial group of fibers ran laterally at the level of layer I [126].

We observed 2 plexuses in this efferent connection, a deep plexus in layer IV-VI and another in the superficial layer I, both of which were connected by ascending fibers that gave off scarce divergent branches containing irregularly distributed presynaptic boutons. Treatment with guanosine either increased the number or altered the orientation of the axonal branches of the visual corticocortical connection. Moreover, the number and size of synaptic boutons was significantly higher in these animals, and most were more rounded/oval than those in control animals. Guanosine administration significantly increased bouton density (number/200 μm^2), which was 1.3-fold higher in treated versus control rats ($p<0.02$). Moreover, while the average size of small synaptic boutons did not appear to be affected by guanosine (0.57 ± 0.07 μm^2 vs. 0.47 ± 0.05 μm^2 in control animals; $p<0.002$), the larger boutons were significantly larger on average in guanosine-treated rats (3.76 ± 0.06 μm^2 vs. 2.26 ± 0.1 μm^2 in control rats; $p<0.002$). These data highlight the synaptogenic specificity of the astrocytic factors elicited by guanosine (Fig. 4) [126].

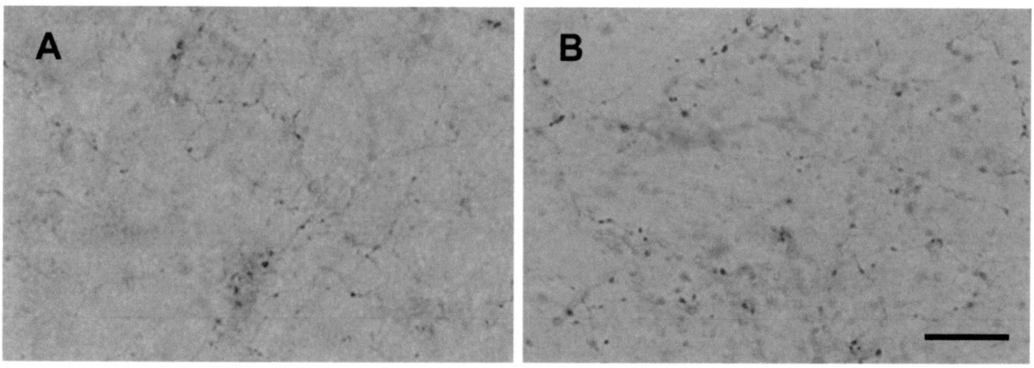

Figure 4. Representative photomicrographs of BDA-labeled visual corticocolicular terminal fields in control (A) and guanosine-treated rats (B). Note the markedly higher density of labeled presynaptic boutons in the guanosine-treated rat than in the control animals. Scale bar = 20 μm.

We propose that synaptogenesis induced by the local application of guanosine *in vivo* may be mediated by factors such as cholesterol, ApoE and pleiotropic factors secreted by astrocytes. Guanosine administration increases both cholesterol and ApoE efflux from astrocytes *in vitro,* supporting a pharmacological role of guanosine in the modulation of cholesterol homeostasis in the brain [125]. Moreover, astrocytes that release guanosine can exert neurotrophic effects and promote neuritogenesis, possibly via MAP-kinase and PI3-

kinase signaling pathways [127]. Previous studies failed to report an increase in synapse number in response to cholesterol administration *in vitro* [116], despite a strong enhancement in synaptic efficacy [119]. However, guanosine increased both the number or size of synaptic boutons in our *in vivo* model. These morphological changes were observed at least one week after 7 days of local guanosine administration and it is likely that this effect progressively diminishes over subsequent days, as is usually observed in nervous structures following lesion. Nonetheless, the synaptogenic effects promoted by reactive astrocytes in denervated terminal fields can last for months [34]. The larger synaptic boutons generated following guanosine administration may reflect the accumulation of presynaptic components such as mitochondria, synaptic vesicles and presynaptic receptors, elements that could eventually exert a modulatory effect upon functional aspects of neurotransmission, such as transmitter release or presynaptic potentiation. It remains unclear whether the proportion of synapses that contact neurons varies after guanosine administration, as astrocytes promote cholesterol-mediated glutamatergic synaptogenesis but they induce GABAergic synaptogenesis via a different mechanism [128], raising the possibility that the majority of new synapses are glutamatergic. Changes in the proportion of inhibitory and excitatory synapses may trigger homeostatic mechanisms [129] that maintain the synaptic activity of the connection within certain functional limits.

Synaptogenesis occurs both during development and adult life. In addition to the aforementioned factors, several other factors promote synaptogenesis in mature nervous systems, including GDNF (glial derived neurotrophic factor) and sex hormones, particularly in areas that display strong synaptic plasticity [130,131]. *In vivo* studies of the neocortex [132,133] revealed the ongoing growth and retraction of dendritic spines, accompanied by the elimination and formation of synapses. While we have only examined labeled projecting axons, synaptogenic effects may also extend to axons emerging from interneurons. Therefore, it may be of interest to analyze GABAergic synaptogenesis in the area surrounding the site of implantation of the osmotic pump that supplies guanosine in this experimental paradigm.

The increase in the number and size of a significant proportion of synapses after guanosine administration indicates a potentiation of axon growth that may promote reinnervation after partial experimental lesion of a neural pathway, or after elimination of a specific afferent connection projecting to a given brain region. We are currently investigating other strategies to inhibit molecules that restrict axonal sprouting and regeneration, including the injection of siRNAs against the p75 receptor and LINGO-1 into the contralateral visual cortex following monocular retinal deafferentation, with encouraging preliminary results.

7. Conclusion

In contrast to the classical dogma of neuronal regeneration, the results presented here indicate that both corticocortical and corticosubcortical connections can be manipulated in adult animals. We focused specifically on two connections, namely corticocollicular and corticocortical projections emerging from the primary visual cortex, and we demonstrate significant post-lesional sprouting of these neurons following specific siRNA knockdown of molecules that inhibit axon regeneration. This strategy is particularly efficacious on a broad range of potential targets. The combination of this knockdown approach with strategies to promote axonal growth by trophic stimuli may be particularly promising for the therapeutic modulation of specific neuronal connections in the future.

Author details

I. Gerrikagoitia, B. Rienda and L. Martínez-Millán*
Dept. of Neurosciences, Faculty of Medicine, University of the Basque Country, Leioa, Bizkaia, Spain

Acknowledgement

Grant sponsors: Fondo de Investigaciones Sanitarias (Ministerio de Sanidad y Consumo) PI05/2046 and PS09/00476; Universidad del País Vasco/Euskal Herriko Unibertsitatea GIU06/15; Gobierno Vasco SA-2010/00095 and GIC10/113; UPV/EHU Predoctoral Fellowship PIFA/01/2006/042.

Technical and human support from SGIker is gratefully acknowledged.

8. References

[1] Zilles K, Zilles B, Schleicher A (1980) A Quantitative Approach to Cytoarchitectonics. VI. The Areal Pattern of the Cortex of Albino Rat. Anat. embryol. 159: 335-360.
[2] Zilles K, Wree A (1995) Cortex: Areal and Laminar Structure. In: Paxinos G, editors. The Rat Nervous System. San Diego: Academic press. pp. 649-685.
[3] Dreher B, Thong IG, Shameem N, McCall MJ (1985) Development of Cortical Afferents and Cortico-tectal Efferents of the Mammalian (Rat) Primary Visual Cortex. Aust. n. z. j. ophthalmol. 13: 251-261.
[4] Martínez-García F, González-Henández T, Martínez-Millán L (1994) Pyramidal and Non Pyramidal Callosal Cells in the Striate Cortex of the Adult Rat. J. comp. neurol. 350: 439-451.
[5] Dräger UC, Olsen JF (1980) Origins of Crossed and Uncrossed Retinal Projections in Pigmented and Albino Mice. J. comp. neurol. 191: 383-412.
[6] Dreher B, Sefton AJ, Ni SYK, Nisbett G (1985) The Morphology, Number, Distribution and Central Projections of Class I Retinal Ganglion Cells in Albino and Hooded Rats. Brain behave. evol. 26: 10-48.
[7] Huerta MF, Harting JK (1984) Connectional Organization of the Superior Colliculus. Trends Neurosci. 7: 286-289.

* Corresponding Author

[8] Huerta MF, Harting JK (1984) The Mammalian Superior Colliculus: Studies of its Morphology and Connections. In: Vanegas H, editors. Comparative Neurology Of The Optic Tectum. New York: Plenum Press. pp. 687-773.

[9] Stein BE, Meredith MA (1993) Multisensory Convergence Patterns. The Merging of the Senses. Cambridge: The MIT Press. pp. 117-122

[10] Linden R, Perry VH (1983) Massive Retinotectal Projection in Rats. Brain res. 272: 145-149.

[11] Dallimore EJ, Cui Q, Beazley LD, Harvey AR (2002) Postnatal Innervation of the Rat Superior Colliculus by Axons of Late-Born Retinal Ganglion Cells. Eur. j. neurosci. 16: 1295-1304.

[12] Lund RD (1966) The Occipitotectal Pathway of the Rat. J. anat. 100: 51-62.

[13] Lund RD (1969) Synaptcis Patterns of the Superficial Layers of the Superior Colliculus of the Rat. J. comp. neurol. 135: 179-208.

[14] Harvey AR, Worthington DR (1990) The Projection from Different Visual Cortical Areas to the Rat Superior Colliculus. J. comp. neurol. 298: 281-292.

[15] Thong IG, Dreher B (1987) The Development of the Corticotectal Pathway in the Albino Rat: Transient Projections from the Visual and Motor Cortices. Neurosci. lett. 80: 275-282.

[16] Land PW, Lund RD (1979) Development of the Rat Uncrossed Retinotectal Pathway and its Relation to Plasticity Studies. Science. 205: 698-700.

[17] Simon DK, O'Leary DDM (1992) Development of Topographic Order in the Mammalian Retinocollicular Projection. J. neurosci. 12: 1212-1232.

[18] Navarro X, Vivó M, Valero-Cabré A (2007) Neural Plasticity after Peripheral Nerve Injury and Regeneration. Prog. neurobiol. 82: 163-201.

[19] Toldi J, Fehér O, Wolff JR (1996) Neuronal Plasticity Induced by Neonatal Monocular (and Binocular) Enucleation. Prog. neurobiol. 48: 191-218.

[20] Chow KL, Mathers LH, Spear PD. (1973) Spreading of Uncrossed Retinal Projection in Superior Colliculus of Neonatally Enucleated Rabbits. J. comp. neurol. 151: 307-322.

[21] Lund RD, Land PW, Boles J (1980) Normal and Abnormal Uncrossed Retinotectal Pathways in Rats: An HRP Study in Adults. J. comp. neurol. 189: 711-720.

[22] Insausti R, Blakemore C, Cowan WM (1985) Postnatal Development of the Ipsilateral Retinocollicular Projection and the Effects of Unilateral Enucleation in the Golden Hamster. J. comp. neurol. 23: 393-409.

[23] Ostrach LH, Crabtree JW, Chow KL (1986) The Ipsilateral Retinocollicular Projection in the Rabbit: An Autoradiographic Study of Neonatal Development and Effects of Unilateral Enucleation. J. comp. neurol. 254: 369-381.

[24] Chan SO, Jen LS (1988) Enlargement of Uncrossed Retinal Projections in the Albino Rat: Additive Effects of Neonatal Eye Removal and Thalamectomy. Brain res. 461: 163-168.

[25] Lund RD, Cunningham TJ, Lund JS (1973) Modified Optic Projections after Unilateral Eye Removal in Young Rats. Brain behav. evol. 8: 51-72.

[26] Lund RD, Lund JS (1976) Plasticity in the Developing Visual System: The Effects of Retinal Lesions Made in Young Rats. J. comp. neur. 169: 133-154.

[27] Shen CL (1987) Retinofugal Sprouting of Ipsilateral Projections in Rat. Proc. natl. sci. counc. Repub. China B. 11: 282-288.

[28] Serfaty CA, Campello-Costa P, Linden R (2005) Rapid and Long-Term Plasticity in the neonatal and Adult Retinotectal Pathways Following a Retinal Lesion. Brain res. bull. 66: 128-134.

[29] Rhoades RW, Chalupa LM (1978) Functional and Anatomical Consequences of Neonatal Visual Cortical Damage in the Superior Colliculus of the Golden Hamster. J. neurophysiol. 41: 1466-1494.

[30] Rhoades RW (1981) Expansion of the Ipsilateral Visual Corticotectal Projection in Hamsters Subjected to Partial Lesions of the Visual Cortex During Infancy: Anatomical Experiments. J. comp. neurol. 197: 425-445.

[31] Purves D, Licthman JW (1983) Specific Connections between Nerve Cells. Annu. rev. physiol. 45: 553-565.

[32] Chiaia NL, Zhang S, King TD, Rhoades RW (1994) Evidence for Prenatal Competition Among the Central Arbors of Trigeminal Primary Afferent Neurons: Single Axon Analysis. J. comp. neurol. 345: 303-313.

[33] García del Caño G, Gerrikagoitia I, Goñi O, Martínez-Millán L (1997) Sprouting of the Visual Corticocollicular Terminal Field after Removal of Contralateral Retinal Inputs in Neonatal Rabbits. Exp. brain res. 117: 399-410.

[34] García del Caño G, Gerrikagoitia I, Martínez-Millán (2002) Plastic Reaction of the Rat Visual Corticocollicular Connection after Contralateral Retinal Deafferentation at the Neonatal or Adult Stage: Axonal Growth Versus Reactive Synaptogenesis. J comp. neurol. 446: 166-178.

[35] Thomas HC, Espinoza SG (1987) Relationships between Interhemispheric Cortical Connections and Visual Areas in Hooded Rats. Brain res. 417: 214-224.

[36] Dreher B, Dehay C, Bullier J (1990) Bihemispheric Collateralization of Cortical Afferents and Subcortical Efferents to the Rat Visual Cortex. Eur. j. neurosci. 2: 317-331.

[37] Siminoff R, Schwassmann Ho, Kruger L (1996) An Electrophysiological Study of the Visual Projection to the Superior Colliculus of the Rat. J. comp. neurol. 127: 435-444.

[38] López-Medina A, Bueno-López Jl, Reblet C (1989) Postnatal Development of the Occipitotectal Pathway in the Rat. Int. j. dev. biol. 33: 277-286.

[39] Marcus RC, Gale NW, Morrison ME, Mason CA, Yancopoulos GD (1996) Eph Family Receptors and their Ligands Distribute in Opposing Gradients in the Developing Mouse Retina. Dev. biol. 180: 786-789.

[40] Zhang JH, Cerretti DP, Yu T, Flanagan JG, Zhou R (1996) Detection of Ligands in Regions Anatomically Connected to Neurons Expressing The Eph Receptor Bsk: Potential Roles in Neuron-Target Interactions. J. neurosci. 16: 7182-7192.

[41] Frisén J, Yates PA, Mclaughlin T, Friedman GC, O'leary DDM, Barbacid M (1998) Ephrin-A5 (Al-1/Rags) Is Essential for Proper Retinal Axon Guidance and Topographic Mapping in the Mammalian Visual System. Neuron. 20: 235-243.

[42] Plummer Kl, Behan M (1992) Postnatal Development of the Corticotectal Projection in Cats. J. comp. neurol. 315: 178-199.

[43] Thong IG, Dreher B (1986) The Development of the Corticotectal Pathway in the Albino Rat. Brain res. 390: 227-238.

[44] Tsukahara N, Hultborn N, Murakami F, Fujito Y (1975) Electrophysiological Study of Formation of New Synapses and Collateral Sprouting in Red Nucleus Neurons after Partial Denervation. J. neurophysiol. 38: 1359-1372.

[45] Tetzlaff W, Alexander SW, Miller FD, Bisby MA (1991) Response of Facial and Rubrospinal Neurons to Axotomy: Changes in mRNA Expression for Cytoskeletal Proteins and Gap-43. J. neurosci. 11: 2528-2544.

[46] Mower Gd, Rosen Km (1993) Developmental and Environmental Changes in Gap-43 Gene Expression in Cat Visual Cortex. Brain res. mol. brain res. 20: 254-258.

[47] Pulido-Caballero J, Jiménez Sampedro F, Echevarria-Aza D, Martínez-Millán L (1994) Postnatal Development of Vimentin-Positive Cells in the Rabbit Superior Colliculus. J. comp. neural. 343: 102-112.

[48] Fawcett JW, Asher RA (1999) The Glial Scar and Central Nervous System Repair. Brain res. bull. 49: 377-391.

[49] Morgenstern DA, Asher RA, Fawcett JW (2002) Chondroitin Sulphate Proteoglycans in the CNS Injury Response. Prog. brain res. 137: 313-332.

[50] Willson CA, Irizarry-Ramírez M, Gaskins HE, Cruz-Orengo L, Figueroa JD, Whittemore SR, Miranda JD (2002) Upregulation of Epha Receptor Expression in the Injured Adult Rat Spinal Cord. Cell transplant. 11: 229-239.

[51] Bundesen LQ, Scheel TA, Bregman BS, Kromer LF (2003) Ephrin-B2 and EphB2 Regulation of Astrocyte-Meningeal Fibroblast Interactions in Response to Spinal Cord Lesions in Adult Rats. J. neurosci. 23: 7789-7800.

[52] Pasterkamp RJ, Anderson PN, Verhaagen J (2001) Peripheral Nerve Injury Fails to Induce Growth of Lesioned Ascending Dorsal Column Axons into Spinal Cord Scar Tissue Expressing the Axon Repellent Semaphorin3A. Eur. j. neurosci. 13: 457-471.

[53] De Winter F, Oudega M, Lankhorst AJ, Hamers FP, Blits B, Ruitenberg MJ, Pasterkamp RJ, Gispen WH, Verhaagen J (2002) Injury-Induced Class 3 Semaphorin Expression in the Rat Spinal Cord. Exp. neurol. 175: 61-75.

[54] Kaneko S, Iwanami A, Nakamura M, Kishino A, Kikuchi K, Shibata S, Okano HJ, Ikegami T, Moriya A, Konishi O, Nakayama C, Kumagai K, Kimura T, Sato Y, Goshima Y, Taniguchi M, Ito M, He Z, Toyama Y, Okano H (2006) A Selective Sema3A Inhibitor Enhances Regenerative Responses and Functional Recovery of the Injured Spinal Cord. Nat. med. 12: 1380-1389.

[55] Hagino S, Iseki K, Mori T, Zhang Y, Hikake T, Yokoya S, Takeuchi M, Hasimoto H, Kikuchi S, Wanaka A (2003) Slit and Glypican-1 mRNAs are Coexpressed in the Reactive Astrocytes of the Injured Adult Brain. Glia. 42: 130-138.
[56] Silver J, Miller JH (2004) Regeneration Beyond the Glial Scar. Nat. rev. neurosci. 5: 146-156.
[57] Berry M (1982) Post-Injury Myelin-Breakdown Products Inhibit Axonal Growth: An Hypothesis to Explain the Failure of Axonal Regeneration in the Mammalian Central Nervous System. Bibl. anat. 1-11.
[58] Caroni P, Schwab ME (1988) Antibody Against Myelin-Associated Inhibitor of Neurite Growth Neutralizes Nonpermissive Substrate Properties of CNS White Matter. Neuron. 1: 85-96.
[59] Savio T, Schwab ME (1989) Rat CNS White Matter, but not Gray Matter, is Nonpermissive for Neuronal Cell Adhesion and Fibre Outgrowth. J. neurosci. 9: 1126-1133.
[60] Bandtlow C, Zachleder T, Schawb ME (1990) Oligodendrocytes Arrest Neurite Growth by Contact Inhibition. J. neurosci. 10: 3837-3848.
[61] Moorman SJ (1996) The Inhibition of Motility that Results from Contact between Two Oligodendrocytes in vitro can be Blocked by Pertussis Toxin. Glia. 16: 257-265.
[62] Chen MS, Huber AB, Van Der Haar ME, Frank M, Schnell L, Spillmann AA, Christ F, Schwab ME (2000) Nogo-A is a Myelin-Associated Neurite Outgrowth Inhibitor and an Antigen for Monoclonal Antibody IN-1. Nature. 403: 434-439.
[63] Grandpré T, Nakamura F, Vartanian T, Strittmatter SM (2000) Identification of the Nogo Inhibitor of Axon Regeneration as a Reticulon Protein. Nature. 403: 439-444.
[64] Prinjha R, Moore SE, Christie G, Michalovich D, Simmons DL, Walsh FS (2000) Inhibitor of Neurite Outgrowth in Humans. Nature. 403: 383-384.
[65] Mckerracher L, David S, Jackson DL, Kottis V, Dunn RJ, Braun PE (1994) Identification of Myelin-Associated Glycoprotein as a Major Myelin Derived Inhibitor of Neurite Growth. Neuron. 13: 805-811.
[66] Mukhopadhyay G, Doherty P, Walsh FS, Crocker PR, Filbin MT (1994) A Novel Role for Myelin-Associated Glycoprotein as an Inhibitor of Axonal Regeneration. Neuron. 13: 757-767.
[67] Wang KC, Koprivica V, Kim JA, Sivasankaran R, Guo Y, Neve RL, He Z (2002) Oligodendrocyte-Myelin Glycoprotein is a Nogo Receptor Ligand that Inhibits Neurite Outgrowth. Nature. 417: 941-944.
[68] Fournier AE, Grandpré T, Strittmatter SM (2001) Identification of a Receptor Mediating Nogo-66 Inhibition of Axonal Regeneration. Nature. 409: 341-346.
[69] Domeniconi M, Cao Z, Spencer T, Sivasankaran R, Wang KC, Nikulina E, Kimura N, Cai H, Deng K, Gao Y, He Z, Filbin MT (2002) Myelin-Associated Glycoprotein Interacts with the Nogo-66 Receptor to Inhibit Neurite Outgrowth. Neuron. 35: 283-290.
[70] Liu PB, Fournier A, Grandpré T, Strittmatter SM (2002) Myelin-Associated Glycoprotein as a Functional Ligand for the Nogo-66 Receptor. Science. 297: 1190-1193.

[71] Wong ST, Henley JR, Kanning KC, Huang KH, Bothwell M, Poo MM (2002) A p75 (NTR) and Nogo Receptor Complex Mediates Repulsive Signaling by Myelin Associated Glycoprotein. Nat. neurosci. 5: 1302-1308.

[72] Yamashita T, Higuchi H, Tohyama M (2002) The P75 Receptor Transduces the Signal from Myelin-Associated Glycoprotein to Rho. J. cell biol. 157: 565-570.

[73] Kojima T, Morikawa Y, Copeland NG, Gilbert DJ, Jenkins NA, Senba E, Kitamura T (2000) TROY, a Newly Identified Member of the Tumor Necrosis Factor Receptor Superfamily, Exhibits a Homology with Edar and is Expressed in Embryonic Skin and Hair Follicles. J. biol. chem. 275: 20742-20747.

[74] Hisaoka T, Morikawa Y, Kitamura T, Senba E (2003) Expression of a Member of Tumor Necrosis Factor Receptor Superfamily, TROY, in the Developing Mouse Brain. Brain res. dev. brain res. 143: 105-109.

[75] Park JB, Yiu G, Kaneko S, Wang J, Chang J, He XL, García KC, He Z (2005) A TNF Receptor Family Member, TROY, is a Coreceptor with Nogo Receptor in Mediating the Inhibitory Activity of Myelin Inhibitors. Neuron. 45: 345-351.

[76] Shao Z, Browning JL, Lee X, Scott ML, Shulga-Morskaya S, Allaire N, Thill G, Levesque M, Sah D, Mccoy JM, Murray B, Jung V, Pepinsky RB, Mi S (2005) TAJ/TROY, an Orphan TNF Receptor Family Member, Binds Nogo-66 Receptor 1 and Regulates Axonal Regeneration. Neuron. 45: 353-359.

[77] Barrette B, Vallieres N, Dube M, Lacroix S (2007) Expression Profile of Receptors for Myelin-Associated Inhibitors of Axonal Regeneration in the Intact and Injured Mouse Central Nervous System. Mol. cell. neurosci. 34: 519-538.

[78] Mi S, Lee X, Shao Z, Thill G, Ji B, Relton J, Levesque M, Allaire N, Perrin S, Sands B, Crowell T, Cate RL, McCoy JM, Pepinsky RB (2004) LINGO-1 is a Component of the Nogo-66 Receptor/P75 Signaling Complex. Nat. neurosci. 7: 221-228.

[79] Carim-Todd L, Escarceller M, Estivill X, Sumoy L (2003) LRRN6A/LERN1 (Leucine-Rich Repeat Neuronal Protein 1), a Novel Gene with Enriched Expression in Limbic System and Neocortex. Eur. j. neurosci. 18: 3167-3182.

[80] Niederöst B, Oertle T, Fritsche J, Mckinney RA, Bandtlow CE (2002) Nogo-A and Myelin-Associated Glycoprotein Mediate Neurite Growth Inhibition by Antagonistic Regulation of RhoA and D Rac1. J. neurosci. 22: 10368-10376.

[81] Chaudhry N, Filbin MT (2006) Myelin-Associated Inhibitory Signaling and Strategies to Overcome Inhibition. J. cereb. blood flow metab. 27: 1096-1107.

[82] Maekawa M, Ishizaki T, Boku S, Watanabe N, Fujita A, Iwamatsu A, Obinata T, Ohashi K, Mizuno K, Narumiya S (1999) Signaling from Rho to the Actin Cytoskeleton Through Protein Kinases ROCK and LIM-Kinase. Science. 285: 895-898.

[83] Lehmann M, Fournier A, Selles-Navarro I, Dergham P, Sebok A, Leclerc N, Tigyi G, Mckerracher L (1999) Inactivation of Rho Signalling Pathway Promotes CNS Axon Regeneration. J. neurosci. 19: 7537-7547.

[84] Dergham P, Ellezam B, Essagian C, Avedissian H, Lubell WD, Mckerracher L (2002) Rho Signaling Pathway Targeted to Promote Spinal Cord Repair. J. neurosci. 22: 6570-6577.

[85] Monnier PP, Sierra A, Schwab JM, Henke-Fahle S, Mueller BK (2003) The Rho/ ROCK Pathway Mediates Neurite Growth-Inhibitory Activity Associated with the Chondroitin Sulfate Proteoglycans of the CNS Glial Scar. Mol. cell neurosci. 22: 319-330.

[86] Schnell L, Schwab ME (1990) Axonal Regeneration in the Rat Spinal Cord Produces by an Antibody Against Myelin-Associated Neurite Growth Inhibitors. Nature. 343: 269-272.

[87] Bregman BS, Kunkel-Bagden E, Schnell L, Dai HN, Gao D, Schwab ME (1995) Recovery from Spinal Cord Injury Mediated by Antibodies to Neurite Growth Inhibitors. Nature. 378: 498-501.

[88] Thallmair M, Metz GAS, Z'Graggen WJ, Raineteau O, Kartje GL, Schwab ME (1998) Neurite Growth Inhibitors Restrict Structural Plasticity and Functional Recovery Following Corticospinal Tract Lesions. Nat. neurosci. 1: 124-131.

[89] Liebscher T, Schnell L, Schnell D, Scholl J, Schneider R, Gullo M, Fouad K, Mir A, Rausch M, Kindler D, Hamers FP, Schwab ME (2005) Nogo-A Antibody Improves Regeneration and Locomotion of Spinal Cord-Injured Rats. Ann. neurol. 58: 706-719.

[90] Mullner A, Gonzenbach RR, Weinmann O, Schnell L, Liebscher T, Schwab ME (2008) Lamina-Specific Restoration of Serotonergic Projections after Nogo-A Antibody Treatment of Spinal Cord Injury in Rats. Eur. neurosci. 27: 326-333.

[91] Freund P, Schmidlin E, Wannier T, Bloch J, Mir A, Schwab ME, Rouiller EM (2006) Nogo-A-Specific Antibody Treatment Enhances Sprouting and Functional Recovery after Cervical Lesion in Adult Primates. Nat. med. 12: 790-792.

[92] Kim JE, Li S, Grandpré T, Qiu D, Strittmatter SM (2003) Axon Regeneration in Young Adult Mice Lacking Nogo-A/B. Neuron. 38: 187-199.

[93] Simonen M, Pedersen V, Weinmann O, Schnell L, Buss A, Ledermann B, Christ F, Sansig G, Van Der PH, Schwab ME (2003) Systemic Deletion of the Myelin-Associated Outgrowth Inhibitor Nogo-A Improves Regenerative and Plastic Responses after Spinal Cord Injury. Neuron. 38: 201-211.

[94] Zheng B, Ho C, Li S, Keirstead H, Steward O, Tessier-Lavigne M (2003) Lack of Enhanced Spinal Regeneration in Nogo-Deficient Mice. Neuron. 38: 213-224.

[95] Su Y, Wang F, Zhao SG, Pan SH, Liu P, Teng Y, Cui H (2008) Axonal Regeneration after Optic Nerve Crush in Nogo-A/B/C Knockout Mice. Mol. vis. 14: 268-273.

[96] Fournier AE, Takizawa BT, Strittmatter SM (2003) Rho Kinase Inhibition Enhances Axonal Regeneration in the Injured CNS. J. neurosci. 23: 1416-1423.

[97] Fire A, Xu S, Montgomery MK, Kostas SA, Driver SE, Mello CC (1998) Potent and Specific Genetic Interference by Double-Stranded RNA in Caenorhabditis Elegans. Nature. 391: 806-811.

[98] Elbashir SM, Lendeckel W, Tuschl T (2001) RNA Interference is Mediated by 21- And 22-Nucleotide RNAs. Genes. dev. 15: 188-200.

[99] Higuchi H, Yamashita T, Yoshikawa H, Tohyama M (2003) Functional Inhibition of the P75 Receptor Using a Small Interfering RNA. Biochem. biophys. res. commun. 301: 804-809.

[100] Ahmed Z, Dent RG, Suggate EL, Barrett LB, Seabright RJ, Berry M, Logan A (2005) Disinhibition of Neurotrophin-Induced Dorsal Root Ganglion Cell Neurite Outgrowth on CNS Myelin by siRNA-Mediated Knockdown of NgR, p75^{NTR} and Rho-A. Mol. cell neurosci. 28: 509-523.

[101] Yang Y, Liu Y, Wei P, Peng H, Winger R, Hussain RZ, Ben LH, Cravens PD, Gocke AR, Puttaparthi K, Racke MK, Mctigue DM, Lovett-Racke AE (2010) Silencing Nogo-A Promotes Functional Recovery in Demyelinating Disease. Ann. neurol. 67: 498-507.

[102] Grandpré T, Li S, Strittmatter SM (2002) Nogo-66 Receptor Antagonist Peptide Promotes Axonal Regeneration. Nature. 417: 547-551.

[103] Li S, Strittmatter SM (2003) Delayed Systemic Nogo-66 Receptor Antagonist Promotes Recovery from Spinal Cord Injury. J. neurosci. 23: 4219-4227.

[104] Lee JK, Kim JE, Sivula M, Strittmatter SM (2004) Nogo Receptor Antagonism Promotes Stroke Recovery by Enhancing Axonal Plasticity. J. neurosci. 24: 6209-6217.

[105] Fischer D, He Z, Benowitz LI (2004) Counteracting the Nogo Receptor Enhances Optic Nerve Regeneration if Retinal Ganglion Cells are in an Active Growth State. J. neurosci. 24: 1646-1651.

[106] Xu S, Liu M, Zhang T, Lv B, Liu B, Yuan W (2011) Effect of Lentiviral shRNA of Nogo Receptor on Rat Cortex Neuron Axon Outgrowth. Can. j. neurol. sci. 38: 133-138.

[107] Bryan B, Cai Y, Wrighton K, Wu G, Feng XH, Liu M (2005) Ubiquitination of RhoA by Smurf1 Promotes Neurite Outgrowth. Febs. lett. 579: 1015-1019.

[108] Hunt D, Coffin RS, Anderson PN (2002) The Nogo Receptor, its Ligands and Axonal Regeneration in the Spinal Cord; A Review. J. neurocytol. 31: 93-120.

[109] Sandvig A, Berry M, Barrett LB, Butt A, Logan, A (2004) Myelin-, Reactive Glia-, and Scar-Derived CNS Axon Growth Inhibitors: Expression, Receptor Signaling, and Correlation with Axon Regeneration. Glia. 46: 25-251.

[110] Bork T, Schabtach E, Grant P (1987) Factors Guiding Optic Fibres in Developing Xenopus Retina. J. comp. neurol. 264: 147-158.

[111] Rangarajan R, Gong Q, Gaul U (1999) Migration and Function of Glia in the Developing Drosophila Eye. Development. 126: 3285-3292.

[112] Ullian EM, Christopherson KS, Barres BA (2004) Role for Glia in Synaptogenesis. Glia. 47: 209-216.

[113] Slezak M, Pfrieger FW (2003) New Roles for Astrocytes: Regulation of CNS Synaptogenesis. Trends Neurosci. 26: 531-535.

[114] Ullian EM, Sapperstein SK, Christopherson KS, Barres BA (2001) Control of Synapse Number by Glia. Science. 291: 657-61.

[115] Correa-Gillieron EM, Cavalcante LA (1999) Synaptogenesis in Retino-Receptive Layers of the Superior Colliculus of the Opossum Didelphis Marsupialis. Brain behav. evol. 54: 71-84.

[116] Christopherson KS, Ullian EM, Stokes CC, Mullowney CE, Hell JW, Agah A, Lawler J, Mosher DF, Bornstein P, Barres BA (2005) Thrombospondins are Astrocyte-Secreted Proteins that Promote CNS Synaptogenesis. Cell. 120: 421-433.

[117] Faissner A, Pyka M, Geissler M, Sobik T, Frischknecht R, Gundelfinger ED, Seidenbecher C (2010) Contributions of Astrocytes to Synapse Formation and Maturation-Potential Functions of the Perisynaptic Extracellular Matrix. Brain res. rev. 63: 26-38.

[118] Kucukderelia H, Allenb NJ, Leea AT, Fenga A, Ozlua MI, Conatsera LM, Chakrabortyb C, Workmanc G, Weaverc M, Sagec EH, Barresb BE, Eroglua C (2011) Control of Excitatory CNS Synaptogenesis by Astrocyte-Secreted Proteins Hevin and SPARC. Proc. natl. acad. Sci. 108: E440-E449.

[119] Bornstein P (2001) Thrombospondins as Matricellular Modulators of Cell Function. J. clin. invest. 107: 929-934.

[120] Bornstein P, Sage EH (2002) Matricellular Proteins: Extracellular Modulators of Cell Function. Curr. opin. cell biol. 14: 608-616.

[121] Mauch DH, NäGler K, Schumacher S, Göritz C, Müller EC, Otto A, Pfrieger FW (2001) CNS Synaptogenesis Promoted by Glia-Derived Cholesterol. Science 294: 1354-1357.

[122] Cáceres M, Suwyn C, Maddox M, Thomas JW, Preuss TM (2007) Increased Cortical Expression of Two Synaptogenic Thrombospondins in Human Brain Evolution. Cereb. cortex. 17: 2312-2321.

[123] Göritz C, Mauch DH, Pfrieger FW (2005) Multiple Mechanisms Mediate Cholesterol-Induced Synaptogenesis in a CNS Neuron. Mol. cell. neurosci. 29: 190-201.

[124] Thiele C, Hannah MJ, Fahrenholz F, Huttner WB (2000) Cholesterol Binds to Synaptophysin and is Required for Biogenesis of Synaptic Vesicles. Nat. cell biol. 2: 42-49.

[125] Ballerini P, Ciccarelli R, Di Iorio P, Buccella S, D'Alimonte I, Giuliani P, Masciulli A, Nargi E, Beraudi A, Rathbone MP, Caciagli F. 2006. Guanosine Effect on Cholesterol Efflux and Apolipoprotein E Expression in Astrocytes. Purinergic Signal. 2: 637-649.

[126] Gerrikagoitia I, Martínez-Millán L (2009) Guanosine-induced Synaptogenesis in the Adult Brain in vivo. Anat. rec. (Hoboken). 292: 1968-1975.

[127] Rathbone M, Pilutti L, Caciagli F, Jiang S (2008) Neurotrophic Effects of Extracellular Guanosine. Nucleosides nucleotides nucleic acids. 27: 666-672.

[128] Hughes EG, Elmariah SB, Balice-Gordon RJ (2010) Astrocyte Secreted Proteins Selectively Increase Hippocampal Gabaergic Axon Length, Branching, and Synaptogenesis. Mol. cell. neurosci. 43: 136.

[129] Turrigiano GG. 1999. Homeostatic Plasticity in Neuronal Networks: The More Things Change, the More They Stay the Same. Trends neurosci. 22: 221-227.

[130] Ledda F, Paratcha G, Sandoval-Guzmán T, Ibáñez CF (2007). GDNF and Gfralpha1 Promote Formation of Neuronal Synapses by Ligand-Induced Cell Adhesion. Nat. neurosci. 10: 293-300.

[131] Leranth C, Hajszan T, Szigeti-Buck K, Bober J, Maclusky NJ (2008) Bisphenol A Prevents the Synaptogenic Response to Estradiol in Hippocampus and Prefrontal Cortex of Ovariectomized Nonhuman Primates. Proc. natl. acad. sci. USA. 105: 14187-14191.

[132] Holtmaat A, De Paola V, Wilbrecht L, Knott GW (2008) Imaging of Experience-Dependent Structural Plasticity in the Mouse Neocortex in vivo. Behav. brain res. 192: 20-25.

[133] Knott G, Holtmaat A (2008) Dendritic Spine Plasticity-Current Understanding from in vivo Studies. Brain res. rev. 58: 282-289.

Chapter 18

Role of Feedforward and Feedback Projections in Figure-Ground Responses

Marina Arall, August Romeo and Hans Supèr

Additional information is available at the end of the chapter

http://dx.doi.org/10.5772/47753

1. Introduction

In the visual brain incoming sensory information is first decomposed into elementary features in low-level areas and then transferred to high-level areas. There the features are grouped into coherent perceptual representations. Recent findings, however, have established that stimulus evoked responses in the primary visual cortex are modulated by surrounding stimuli. The modulated responses depend on proper recurrent interactions between different, separate visual regions. These extra-classical receptive field responses combine local visual signals with more global information from the visual scene and often reflect relatively high-level perceptual attributes of the stimuli. One of the fundamental problems to be solved by the visual system is the segregation of figure from ground (see Figure 1). A key factor in the figure-ground process is the combination of local with global information. Therefore, contextual influences on neuronal activity have been interpreted as the neural substrate of figure-ground perception.

2. Feedforward projections in the visual system

The visual brain is considered to be hierarchically structured. From the retina most information flows to the primary visual cortex (also referred to as striate cortex, V1, or E17) through the thalamic lateral geniculate nucleus (LGN). In V1 neurons extract simple, rather abstract features (e.g. orientation) within a small part of the visual scene. The feature information is further conveyed to surrounding extra-striate areas and from there to the higher level visual areas. In fact, the feedforward projection is dichotomized into two streams. Axons projecting towards areas in the temporal lobe define the ventral pathway (also called as the "what" or "perception" stream) and projections to the parietal areas form the dorsal pathway (also called the "where" or "action" stream). Information flowing to the ventral pathway relates to objects and shapes whereas information conveyed to the dorsal pathway relates to attention and space (see Figure 2).

Figure 1. Figure-Ground: Classical psychophysical experiments highlighted that figures emerge from its parts, being perceived as single shapes. Many very well known cases of ambiguity (such as the Rubin vase) exemplify this fact. In these images at any given moment we can perceive as the figure only one of the alternative interpretations, the other becoming the background. The neurophysiological correlates of this phenomenon are discussed here.

The neurons in these latter areas have large receptive fields in order to integrate the elementary visual features. A classical receptive field is defined as the region of the visual scene from which a neuronal cell receives direct information by way of feedforward connections. Then, these cells responses to feedforward inputs are more closely related to our daily experience of the external visual world than are the responses in lower order areas since their selectivity is to more elaborated shapes of an object such as a face. That is, what Hubel and Wiesel advanced in 1968 is essentially true: receptive fields of cells at one level of the visual system are formed from inputs by cells at a lower level. In this way, small, simple receptive fields combine to form large, complex receptive fields.

Feedforward projections are therefore the anatomical substrate for the initial transient response of a neuron to a stimulus, and determine the size and tuning properties of the stimulus evoked response. For instance, the orientation tuning of V1 neurons is predominantly determined by feedforward inputs (Miller, 2003) and by the biophysical membrane properties of the cells (Cardin et al., 2007). The spatial arrangement of the receptive fields of cells in the primary visual cortex follows a retino-topical organization and provides a topographic map of the visual world. Simple cells have an elongated receptive field structure, with an excitatory central oval and an inhibitory surrounding region (Hubel & Wiesel, 1968). In order to excite these cells stimuli need to have a particular orientation or direction. In the case of V1 complex cells, the receptive fields have no clear separation of excitatory and inhibitory regions. To excite these cells an oriented stimulus may need to move in a particular direction and might also need to be of a particular length. Beside excitatory neurons, inhibitory cells are also tuned to orientation and spatial frequency (Cardin et al., 2007). Thus, V1 cells respond selectively to simple, rather abstract features that make up an object within a small part of the visual scene mainly by reason of their connections with striate projecting neurons.

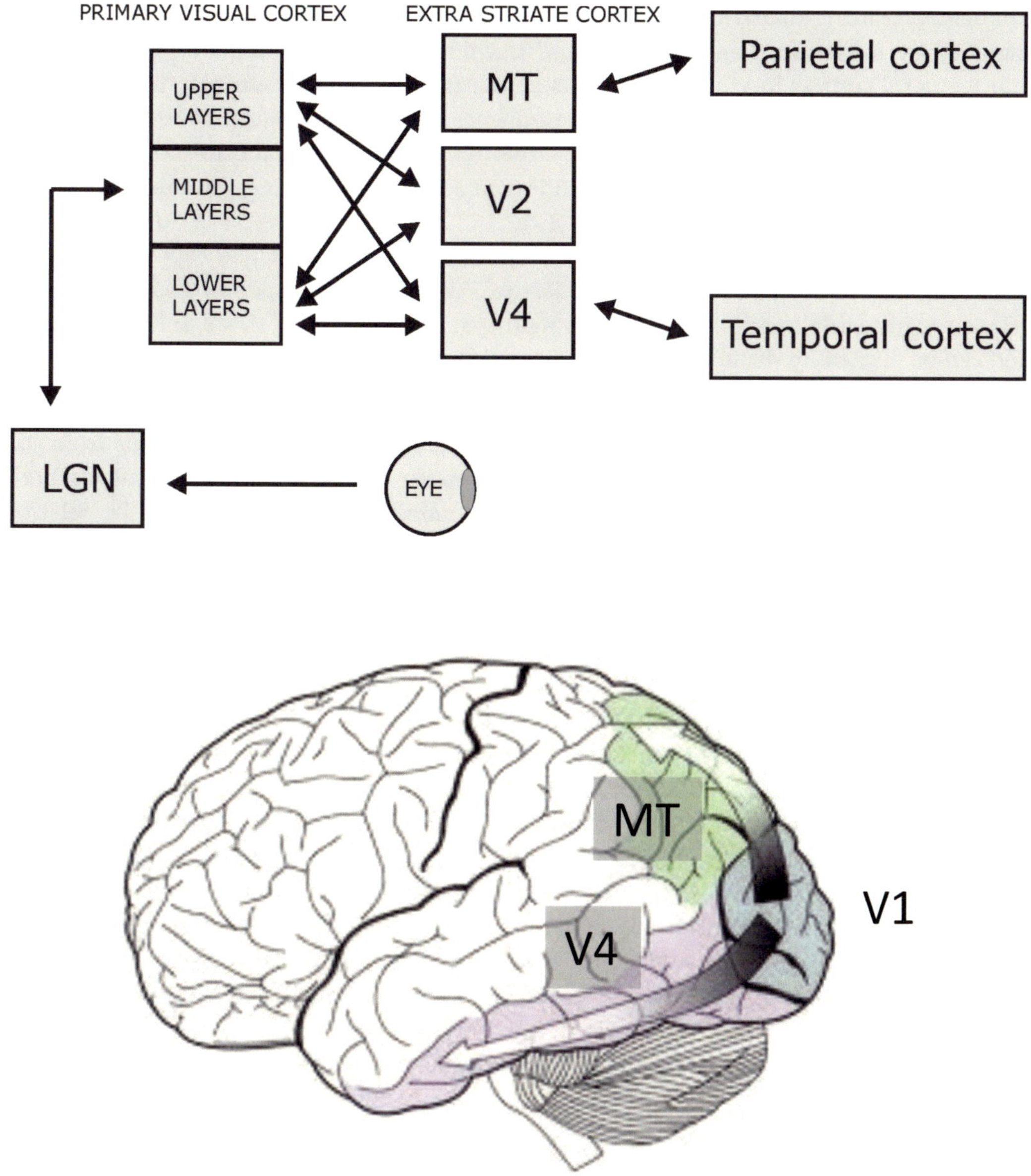

Figure 2. Schematic representation of the main information pathways of the visual system and its anatomical location. Sensory information is conveyed from the retina to the primary visual cortex (V1) from where it is distributed across the higher visual areas via the extra-striate areas. The dorsal stream begins with V1, goes through visual area V2, then to the dorsomedial area and visual area MT (also known as V5) and to the posterior parietal cortex. The ventral stream begins with V1, goes through visual area V2, then through visual area V4, and to the inferior temporal cortex. Top-down information from high-level visual areas towards low-level areas is mediated by feedback connections.

3. Contextual modulation of classical receptive field responses

The feedforward established response property of visual neurons is not fixed. It can be modified by factors such as experience and learning, or, more importantly, by the spatial and temporal context in which a stimulus is presented. The latter strongly influences the stimulus evoked response of a cell. The prominence of contextual information processing is reflected by the fact that the majority of neurons in the primary visual cortex are sensitive to such contextual influences from surrounding regions. Surrounding stimuli outside the classical receptive field do not activate the cell but modulate the response to the stimulus that falls within it. This modulation by the extra classical receptive field signals contextual information to the cell which adds to the classical receptive field response. Such modulation effects are primarily seen for stimuli with high spatial frequencies (Meese & Holmes, 2007) and can be elicited by distal stimulus configurations at distances of up to 30mm within the primary visual cortex (Alexander & Wright, 2006).

The effects of surrounding stimuli on a centre stimulus are complex and signals from the surround have been reported both to be suppressive and facilitatory, as well as both selective and unselective. The way modulation interacts in V1 depends on the relative position and orientation of the centre and surrounding stimuli. For example, for static lines neuronal facilitation is observed when a near threshold stimulus inside the classical receptive field is flanked by high contrast collinear elements located in the surrounding regions of visual space when compared to a single presentation of the low threshold line (Polat et al., 1998). In contrast, when the flanked lines differ in their orientation or are not collinearly aligned suppression of neural activity to the target line is observed (Kapadia et al., 2000). For drifting gratings, surround influence is mainly suppressive and suppression tends to be stronger when the surround grating also moves in the neurons preferred direction. When the surround is 90 degrees from the preferred orientation (orthogonal), suppression becomes weaker and sometimes results in response facilitation (Jones et al., 2001). For an orthogonal surround grating suppression is strongest on the flanks (Cavanaugh et al., 2002). Similar accounts for surround suppression have been reported in optical imaging studies (Grinvald et al., 1994) and in the cat visual cortex (Walker et al., 1999). Context modulation is not only a robust feature of neurons in the primary visual cortex, it is also observed in high visual areas of the monkey, for instance for MT (middle temporal) neurons in the motion domain and for V4 neurons in the color domain (Allman et al., 1985).

Surround stimuli not only have an effect on cortical neurons but also on thalamic relay cells. For example, surround stimuli used for neurons in the primary visual cortex suppress the classical receptive field response of neurons in the lateral geniculate nucleus (LGN) suggesting that contextual interactions alter the transfer of thalamocortical information. Similar effects are also observed in the cat where surround suppression is not primarily attributable to intra-cortical inhibition but to a reduction of thalamocortical inputs (Ozeki et al., 2004). A modification in the feedforward signal by non-classical receptive field stimulation in the cat visual cortex is also seen to enhance orientation tuning selectivity (Chen et al., 2005). Context modulation seems thus to be a very general phenomenon throughout the visual brain allowing the comparison of the sensory patterns inside and outside the receptive field.

4. Contextual modulation in figure-ground segmentation

Most of these contextual modulations are described for stimulations by a single bar with surrounding bars. Visual perception, however, requires the grouping of such individual features into coherent and meaningful objects. For example, for a figure-ground texture the orientated line segments are grouped in such a way that they generate the percept of a textured figure overlying a homogeneous background (see Figure 3). Thus, to form a neural representation of the figure the individual encoded line segments of the figure need to be grouped and to be segregated from line segments from the background. In the primary visual cortex, this grouping operation is likely implemented by the same mechanisms as for contextual modulation (Kapadia et al., 2000).

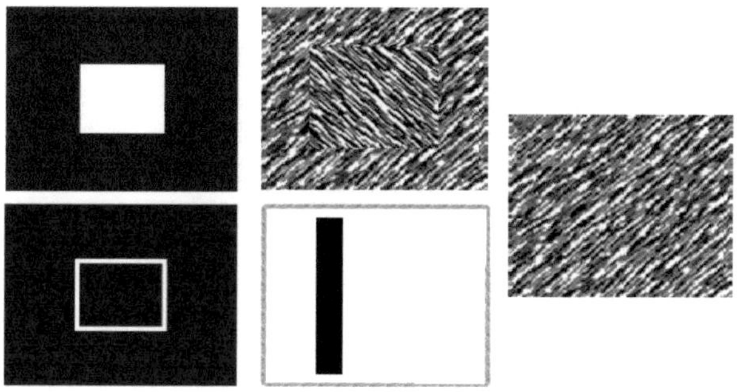

Figure 3. Four different types of figure-ground stimuli and a background in isolation. The figure is defined either by a difference in contrast, in the orientation of its texture lines or in the color of its borders.

While stimulating with such a figure-ground texture and recording neural spike activity in the primary visual cortex, two stages of neural processing after stimulus onset can be discerned. One dominated by the early (<100 msec) response transient, another occurring at relatively longer latencies (> 100 msec). The early stage is associated with feedforward processing and early feature extraction (e.g. stimulus orientation), the later stage has been related to recurrent processing and high level visual processes such as perceptual grouping and segmentation (Lamme & Roelfsema, 2000)(see Figure 4).

For example, at a latency of about 100 msec, (Lamme, 1995; Zipser et al., 1996), when a neuron has its receptive field on the figure location, the cell's activity is enhanced compared to the activity when its receptive field is located on the background. The neural segmentation signals the figure as a whole. Indeed, it is found to be present at the borders as well as at the centre of a textured defined figure (Lamme et al., 1999). This type of contextual modulation is referred to as figure-ground modulation. A study (Rossi et al., 2001) implied the absence of figure-ground based contextual modulation in macaque visual cortex, but it is possible that the authors underestimated the extent of modulation (Corthout & Supèr, 2004).

The delay in the onset of extra-classical receptive field modulation is independent of the time at which the receptive field itself was first stimulated and is not a side effect of the recent history of receptive field stimulation. Zisper et al. (Zipser et al., 1996) showed this by using a two-step procedure in which they first present a homogeneous texture display (thereby generating the initial burst of neural activity) and then subsequently modifying only the extra receptive field stimulus so that a textured-defined figure appeared. After the initial burst, the response strength settled into a steady state of activity. However, between 80 and 100 msec after the display changed to the figure configuration, the response rate rebounded to a more elevated level of activity.

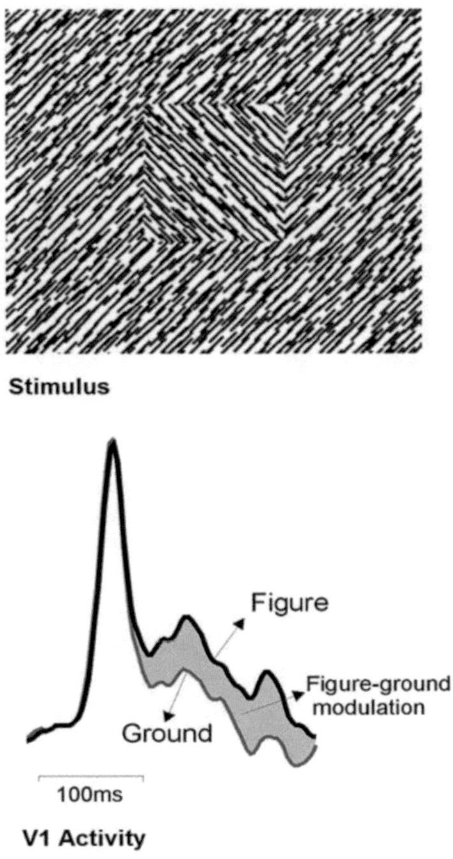

Figure 4. Late V1 responses signal figure-ground context (shaded area). Traces represent the strength of spiking activity over time. When a texture is presented to the eye neurons in the visual cortex respond robustly (= first peak of activity). After approximately 100 ms. responses differ according to the context of the classical receptive field stimulus. In the figure case responses are enhanced (black trace) compared to the homogeneous or ground condition (grey trace). This enhanced neural activity is referred to figure-ground modulation.

Neurophysiological observations show that figure-ground modulation occurs first at the border of the figure followed by modulation for the center region of the textured figure (Lamme et al., 1999; Marcus & Van Essen, 2002; Huang & Paradiso, 2008). These findings can be interpreted as a filling-in process or, alternatively, as two independent processes of border detection and a grouping operation where surface responses simply lag behind the responses to the border.

The finding that surface signals and not boundary signals are reduced by extra-striate lesions (Lamme et al., 1999) argues for two distinct mechanisms. Also, the finding that the onset of the modulated responses across the whole surface is the same (Lamme et al, 1999) argues against a gradual filling-in process of textured stimuli over time and favors independent mechanisms for boundary and surface detection. In Supèr et al. 2010, by means of computational modeling it was shown that the whole figure pops-out instantaneously and no filling-in process of the figural region takes place. Therefore, the model data also fit the idea of two independent mechanisms for local border and surface detection.

Lamme showed onset latencies for figure-ground modulation of 60-120 ms after stimulus onset, or 30-60 ms after response onset (Lamme et al., 1999). General, non-specific surround suppression, in contrast, is an earlier contextual effect which takes about 7 ms to develop after response onset (Knierim & Van Essen, 1992). This authors also found that the orientation specific modulation of responses to centre-surround stimuli occurs a bit later, around 15-20ms after the response onset (Knierim & Van Essen, 1992). In another study, early textured figure–ground segregation was seen to occur at 40-80 ms after stimulus onset (Marcus & Van Essen, 2002) and was not different between V1 and V2 neurons.

5. Figure-ground activity as a neural correlate of visual perception

So far we have described how by modulating the classical receptive field activity extra-classical receptive field effects combine local signals with more global information from the visual scene. Such extra classical respective field responses, therefore, will reflect in our brain relatively high-level perceptual attributes of the stimuli that fall within the neuron's small receptive field.

Several studies show that the influences of various contextual patterns on neuronal activity in the primary visual cortex of awake, behaving monkeys resemble in many respects with the influences of the same contextual stimuli on human perception (Li et al., 2000; Kapadia et al., 2000). For example, when an oriented line is embedded in similar lines within similar orientation, it will be less salient than when the surrounding lines have an orthogonal orientation. Correspondingly, contextual modulation is stronger in the latter case than in the first case. Furthermore, presence of surround features result in neuronal response suppression and also in perceptual masking (Li et al., 2000). This masking can be relieved by a difference in orientation between the target and surrounding features (Van der Smagt et al., 2005). Similarly, contextual modulation has been interpreted as the neural substrate of many perceptual phenomena, like pop-out (Knierim & Van Essen 1992), perceived brightness (Rossi et al., 1996), figure-ground segmentation (Lamme, 1995; Zisper et al., 1996), detection of focal orientation discontinuity (Sillito et al., 1995), tilt illusion (Gilbert & Wiesel, 1990), and perceptual grouping (Kapadia et al., 2000).

In figure-ground perception, neurons in the primary visual cortex not only provide border information from illusory contours (Von der Heydt et al., 1984; Grosof et al., 1993; Lee & Nguyen, 2001), they also carry information about surface perception. As we stated before the figure seems to pop-out: when, for example, a surface area is perceived neurons in the primary visual cortex are activated throughout the region topographically corresponding to the perceived surface and not restricted to the region representing the border of the surface (Komatsu, 2007). Similarly, they correlate with perceived surface lightness (MacEvoy & Paradiso, 2001).

But a direct link between the figure-ground modulation and the animal's percept of the figure was not found before a study by Supèr et al. (Supèr et al., 2001a) showing that figure-ground responses are present when the animal perceives the figure and absent when the animal does not perceive the figure. It also proves that the early stimulus driven activity (0-100 ms) does not relate to whether the figure is seen or not seen but exclusively the late figure-ground modulation (see Figure 5).

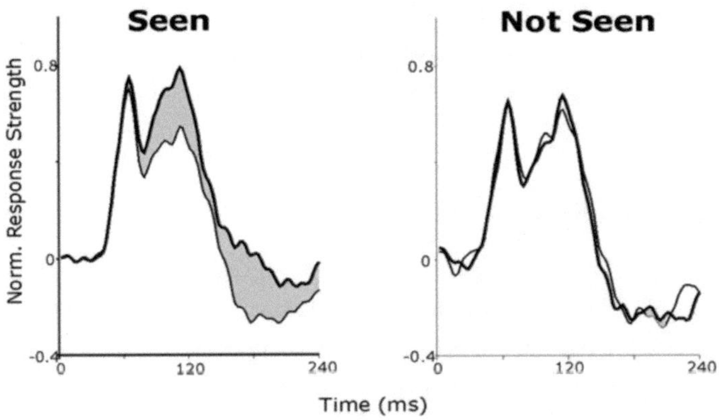

Figure 5. Figure-ground modulation (shaded areas) is present for perceived stimuli (left panel) and absent for not perceived (right panel) figures. Note that in both condition neurons are equally well activated by the feedforward projections, i.e. the first peak responses (adapted from Supèr et al 2001a).

Similarly, figure-ground modulation is selectively suppressed in anesthetized animals, while responses remain selective for low-level features such as orientation of texture bars (Lamme et al., 1998). Also backward masking of figure-ground textures rendering the figure invisible abolishes figure-ground modulation (Lamme et al., 2002), and figure-ground perception is severely impaired when feedback information from extra-striate areas is removed (Supèr & Lamme, 2007a). Finally, figure-ground modulation represents a neural correlate of working memory (Supèr et al., 2001b) and becomes part of the motor preparation (Supèr et al., 2003b, 2004; Supèr & Lamme, 2007b).

6. Feedback connections to primary visual cortex

Most, perhaps all, feedforward connections from V1 to higher visual areas are reciprocated by strong feedback projections. V1 connects with at least 12 subdivisions of the visual cortex. It receives projections from the following extra-striate visual areas: V2, V3, V3A, V4, V4t, MT (V5), parieto-occipital sulcus (PO) and posterior intraparietal area (PIP) (Felleman & Van Essen, 1991). Feedback pathways to V1 carry mainly excitatory input and project preferentially to pyramidal cells (see Figure 6).

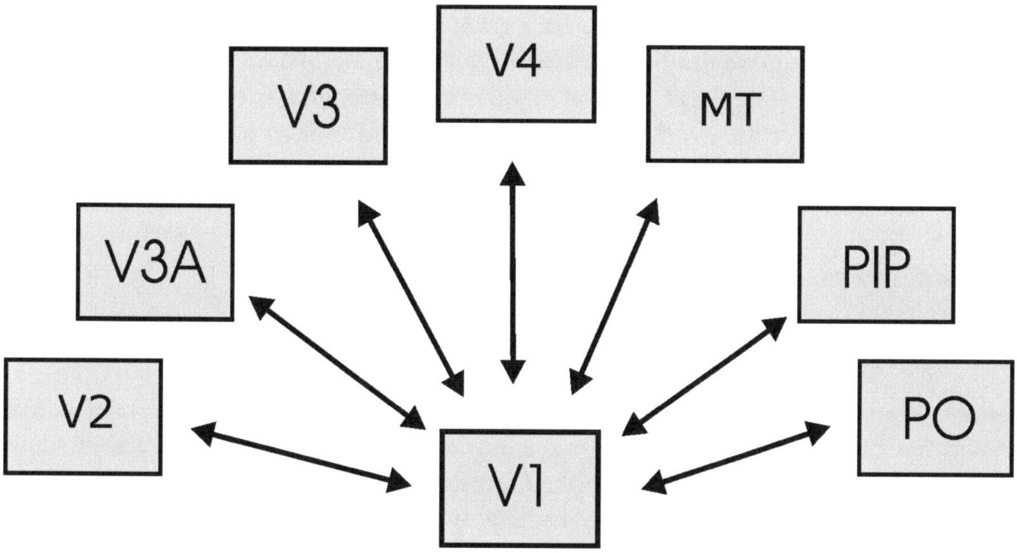

Figure 6. Main feedforward and feedback projections between V1 and extra-striate areas.

Being the number of feedback axons significant, the cortico-cortical connections generate a lower mean-amplitude excitatory post-synaptic potential (PSP) than either thalamo-cortical or feedforward cortico-cortical connections (Shao & Burkhalter, 1996). Conceivably these weak synaptic connections indicate a modulatory role for feedback to V1 neurons since it does not suffice to activate its otherwise silent cells.

In fact, feedback connections show an orderly topographic organization and terminate in discrete patches within V1. The patchy feedback terminations overlap with patches of V1 feedforward projecting neurons (Angelucci et al., 2002), tend to target alike tuned cells (Budd, 1998), and correlate with ocular dominance, iso-orientation columns, and the so called Cytochrome Oxidase-rich blobs (neurons assembled in cylindrical shapes) (Sincich & Horton, 2005).

What's more, the distribution patterns of feedback axons follow a laminar segregation (Felleman & Van Essen, 1991). Feedback axons terminate in upper layers 1, 2/3, 4B and lower layers 5/6, whereas the granular layer is excluded from feedback projections. Some layers appear to have reciprocal connections: projections from primary visual cortex to MT originate from layers 4B and 6. Feedback from MT is predominantly to layers 4B and 6.

Similarly, feedforward projection to V2 and V3 comes mainly from layers 2/3, which also receive most feedback from V2 and V3. Besides feedback to V1, the striate cortex also feeds back to the LGN. Feedback to the LGN is retinotopically organized, and the cells in layer 6 of the visual cortex that provide the feedback arise from differently distributed cell groups, which have functionally selective visual-response properties.

On the other hand, conduction velocities of feedback connections are just as fast as those of feedforward connections (~3-10 m/sec). Apparently, feedback acts on the early part of the stimulus evoked response (Hupé et al., 2001) which suggests that feedback signals are present in V1 all together with feedforward signals from the thalamus. The role of feedback in the early stage response can be seen specifically in the fact that inactivation of areas V2 and MT reduces the response of neurons in V1 to visual stimulation of their receptive field center. It also reduces the suppressive effect of surround motion stimulation. Moreover, feedback-enhanced centre-surround antagonism influences the stimulus driven synchronization. For instance, orientation tuning curves are much broader in the absence of feedback. Thus, retinal stimulation not solely determines the responses of V1 neurons but they are deeply influenced by extensive top-down information.

7. Horizontal connections

Intrinsic horizontal connections that link surrounding neurons convey information from beyond the classical receptive field representing an alternative to feedback for providing contextual information of the target stimulus (Angelucci et al., 2002; Cudeiro and Sillito, 2006). In V1 they are intra-laminar projections made by excitatory neurons in layers 1, 2/3, 4B, and 5/6. Horizontal connections are frequently reciprocal and project locally (short; limited to a few hundreds of microns) up to several millimeters (long) within the primary visual cortex. The distribution of horizontal axonal projections is not globular but tends to be co-aligned with the shape of the receptive fields where axons project collinearly (Angelucci et al., 2002). Moreover, the termination of horizontal axons appears to be patchy indicating that these axons specifically select neighboring cells to contact. For instance, horizontal connections preferentially interconnect columns of similar ocular dominance and cells with similar orientation preference. Interestingly, the excitatory inputs from lateral connections and also from feedback pathways can suppress activity of neurons in the column.

It has been proposed that short horizontal connections shape the spatial summation properties of V1 neurons at low contrast. One example of such "short-range" surround modulation is the enhancement of the receptive field center response to an optimally oriented low-contrast stimulus by flanking co-oriented and co-axial high-contrast stimuli; a phenomenon thought to underlie perceptual grouping of contour elements named co-linear facilitation. A further reason why short horizontal connections may be the underlying anatomical substrate of this phenomenon is that GABA inactivation of laterally displaced V1 sites reduces co-linear facilitation. Horizontal axons have slow velocity conductance (typically 0.1-0.2 m/sec), i.e. about 30-50 times slower than feedforward and feedback connections (Girard et al., 2001). Since it has been shown that contextual suppressive effects come from large regions (4-7mm), the limited horizontal spread of axons (up to 3.5-4.5 mm radius in V1 monkey) together with the already mentioned slow conductance velocities of these fibers cast doubt on a role for horizontal connections in perceptual integration (See Supèr et al., 2010).

8. Role of feedback in figure-ground

Feedback projections from higher visual areas to lower areas are more suitable to provide the contextual information necessary for figure-ground segmentation since they have high conductance velocity (~3-10 m/sec), have large spread in V1 and influence surround mediated responses in it.

Figure-ground segregation may start with a boundary detection process followed by filling-in the surface between these boundaries. Psychophysical studies where detection is initiated at the boundaries between surfaces (Motoyoshi, 1999) lead to such an interpretation. Discriminating local discontinuities in texture elements suffices for border detection, which in principle can be accomplished by horizontal projections. Surface detection, however, is likely an expression of more global influences. Neurophysiological data show that surface signals, and not boundary signals, are abolished by extra-striate lesions (see Lamme et al., 1999) and support such as role for feedback.

Not all feedback may contribute to figure-ground segmentation; although inactivation of V2 does decrease the neuronal response to the single bar, it has no effect on centre-surround interactions of neurons in the primary visual cortex (Hupé et al., 2001). This may mean that figure-ground segmentation occurs in parts of the cortex that do not receive feedback, at least from V2. Indeed, the exact role of feedback in figure-ground segregation is not clear. For instance, has feedback a decisive role in the occurrence of figure-ground activity or a more modulatory role in controlling the strength of the figure-ground signal? Many arguments are inconsistent with a leading role of feedback projections in producing either contextual effects or directly figure-ground segmentation. A lesion study provides further evidence showing that after removing most of the feedback (including V3, V4, MT, MST, but not V2) to V1 detection of textured figure-ground stimuli presented in the lesioned field was not affected (Supèr & Lamme, 2007a).

However, consistent with the modulatory role, visual context presumably transmitted by feedback may activate non-stimulated regions of V1 (Smith & Muckli, 2010), and in agreement with TMS experiments (Pascual-Leone & Walsh, 2001; Silvanto et al., 2005; Corthout, 1999), patient studies demonstrate that V1 alone is not sufficient for simple figure-ground segregation (Allen et al., 2009) suggesting that feedback is required. Yet, as stated before, inactivation of V2, which is the main contributor of feedback to the primary visual cortex, has no effect on centre-surround interactions of V1 neurons (Hupé et al., 2001).

Alternatively, feedback may enhance the response modulation of the figure as a whole. Feedback has been shown to have a push-pull effect where the responses to centre stimulus are enhanced and the responses to surrounding stimuli suppressed (Cudeiro & Sillito, 2006).

A sort of push-pull operation also takes place during figure-ground segregation. Compared to responses to homogeneous textures, responses to figure elements are enhanced and responses to ground elements, where a figure is presented outside the receptive field, are weakened. In this case, feedback acts as a kind of attention mechanism by pulling the figure signal and pushing the ground responses and so enhancing stimulus contrast (De Weerd et al., 1999; Hayes & Merigan 2007). Note that this does not mean that figure-ground activity represents a neural correlate of attention. Figure enhancement is observed when attention is divided or directed away from the figure (Landman et al., 2003b). Shifting attention away from the figure location by presenting a pop-out stimulus outside the receptive field produces a suppressive effect for both 'figure' and 'ground' responses, but not necessarily abolish the figure-ground signal (Supèr et al., 2001b).

9. Arguments against a prominent role of feedback in figure-ground

Several more arguments are inconsistent with a leading role of feedback projections in producing contextual effects and figure-ground segmentation. Surround effects are primarily suppressive but blockade of intra-cortical inhibition does not reduce significantly surround suppression (Ozeki et al., 2004). Surround suppression is fast and may arrive even earlier than the feedforward triggered excitatory classical receptive fields response (Bair et al., 2003; Webb et al. 2005). This timing is inconsistent with contextual modulation by late feedback. Also surround suppression in the monkey LGN emerges too fast for an involvement from cortical feedback (Alitto & Usrey, 2008).

Moreover, Supèr and Lamme results in 2007(a), where by removing feedback (but not V2) to V1 figure-ground perception was impaired though visual detection of textured figure-ground stimuli was not affected, imply that figure-ground segmentation occurs without feedback from these extra-striate areas and without producing visual awareness. This agrees with the belief that figure-ground organization is an automatic process (Qiu et al., 2007). For example, preserved figure-ground segregation is observed in neglect patients (Driver et al., 1992) and surface segregation signals evolve independent of attention (Landman et al., 2003b). Similarly, the assignment of border-ownership precedes object recognition and the deployment of attention (Qiu et al., 2007; Von der Heydt et al., 2004). Furthermore, the short onset latencies and sometimes incomplete cue invariance suggest that border-ownership assignment is not generated in higher level visual areas but within the lower visual areas (Zhou et al., 2000).

In addition, figure-ground segmentation depends on the size of the figure region and drops with increasing figure sizes (>8^0-12^0). This size dependency argues against segregation by feedback since termination fields of feedback projections cover large regions of visual space in V1. Finally, an intriguing finding is that contextual neural interactions corresponding to perception are observed at sub-cortical levels in the LGN and even in the retina (Rossi & Paradiso, 1999) and that competition for object awareness is fully resolved in monocular visual cortex (Tong & Engel, 2001). So, there is considerable evidence against a major role of feedback in figure-ground segregation.

10. Feedforward segregation of figure-ground

Recently it has been demonstrated that figure-ground segregation can be achieved in a purely feedforward manner (Supèr et al., 2010). By means of a computational model (see Figure 7) and using biological plausible spiking neurons surround inhibition was the key factor. The feedforward segregation of figure from ground was robust. A decrease of the input contrast by 80% still yielded figure-ground segregation. Figure-ground segregation occurred for very small figures (even for the size of 1x1 pixel) and for large figures. Since the surround inhibition depended on stimulus size, figure-ground segregation failed when the figure size approximated the background size. This agrees with human figure-ground perception, where small stimuli are interpreted as figures and larger ones as background. When figure and background have the same size the assignment of figure and ground became ambiguous (Barenholtz & Feldman, 2006).

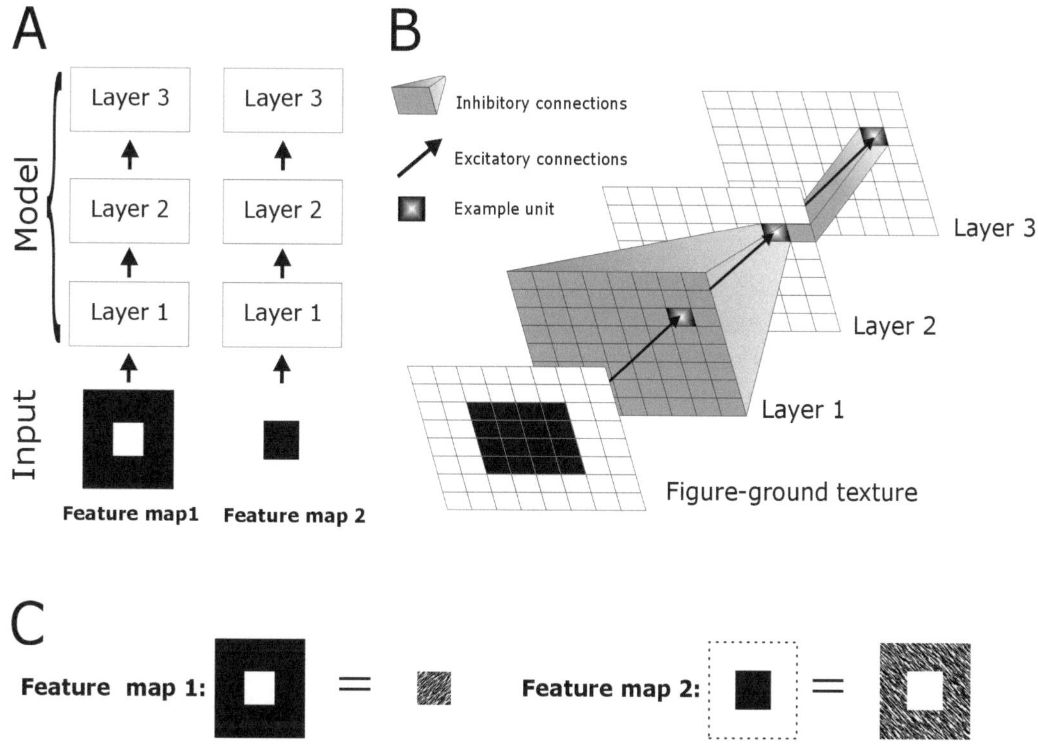

Figure 7. A) Model architecture. It was a three layered model of spiking neurons. B) Connectivity. Local excitation was combined with global inhibition. C) Equivalence between the used feature maps and the original figure-ground textured stimuli.

Feedback has a direct consequence on the activity of the ascending neurons where it lowers the responses to figure elements in layer 1. Despite the inhibitory nature, feedback enhances the figure-ground signal in layer 2. Feedback accomplishes this by a differential effect on neural activity; it enhances figure responses and lowers background responses (Supèr & Romeo, 2011). Such push-pull effect is also observed in neurons of the visual cortex responding to figure-ground textures (Supèr et al., 2001a; Landman et al., 2003a; Scholte et al., 2008). Moreover, the model shows that feedback especially enhances figure-ground signal when the feedforward input is relatively weak. So feedback acts as a kind of attention mechanism enhancing stimulus contrast (De Weerd et al., 1999; Hayes & Merigan, 2007). In accordance, feedback improves stimulus response precision (Andolina et al., 2007) and feature contrast (Huang et al., 2007), and enhances figure-ground discrimination (Hupé et al., 1998) and top-down attention may enhance both feedforward responses in the LGN (McAlonan et al., 2008) and figure-ground modulatory responses in early cortex (Scholte et al., 2006; Roelfsema et al., 2007; Qiu et al., 2007). Therefore, instead of generating the contextual effects needed for figure-ground segmentation, it is speculated that inhibitory feedback boosts the feedforward generated figure-ground activity. Markedly, feedforward inhibition decreases the figure-ground signal (Supèr et al., 2010) whereas inhibition through feedback increases the figure-ground signal (Supèr & Romeo, 2011). Further studies are needed to understand the dynamics that lead to such a difference.

11. Cortical state, attention, and figure-ground segmentation

The strength of figure-ground modulation depends on the momentary state of the visual cortex (Supèr et al., 2003a, 2003b; Van der Togt et al., 2006. See Figure 8). A proper state is characterized by low-frequency correlated neural firing. Absence or deficiency in such synchronous firing prohibits figure-ground segregation resulting in the occasionally failure to detect a stimulus (Supèr et al., 2003a). Supèr & Romeo (2011) showed that feedback affects the strength of figure-ground activity by changing the cortical state, i.e. changing the firing from low-frequency bursting mode (9Hz) to a tonic firing pattern, which is consistent with the observations that feedback shifts neural responses in the thalamus from a bursting mode into a tonic mode (Sherman, 2001).

Low frequency or busting activity is generally associated with less attentive states. For example, in the thalamic LGN of the awake animal, bursting is more common during periods of drowsiness and is largely restricted to episodes lasting a few seconds with most of the episodes showing rhythmic bursting activity in the delta (0.5-4Hz) frequency (Weyland et al., 2001). In accordance, other studies report that the state of vigilance is associated with single or tonic firing patterns whereas rhythmic bursting at alpha frequencies (8-12Hz) relates to periods of low vigilance (Steriade et al., 1999; Llinás & Steriade, 2006). Furthermore, tonic firing increases the signal-to-noise ratio (Sherman, 2001). Similarly to the dynamical changes in cortical state, fast temporal changes in EEG activity have also been associated with changes in attention and discrimination (Vogel & Luck, 2000; Arnott et al., 2001; Bastiaansen & Brunia, 2001). Putting these findings together it is reasonable to assume that moments of high vs. low vigilance, so to say, have different strength of figure-ground modulation because of the different firing pattern of the ascending neurons (see also Supèr et al., 2003a).

Such an explanation may also be relevant for the observed discrepancy on attentional effects in V1. Whereas single-unit studies of attention in monkeys have repeatedly revealed relatively modest attentional modulations in V1, human functional magnetic resonance imaging studies demonstrate a large attentional enhancement of the blood oxygen level-dependent (BOLD) signal in V1. A recent report shows that the neuronal metabolic rate differs between low frequency oscillatory bursting and more random or aperiodic (tonic) neural firing where the former gives smaller BOLD responses (Parkes et al., 2004). If one considers that attention, carried by top-down feedback, affects besides spike rate also the firing pattern (bursting versus tonic) fMRI recordings will measure a stronger attentional signals than single cell recordings. Finally, it has been shown that cognitive processing of sensory stimuli, like attention is represented by spike rate as well as by spike timing (synchrony). The finding that feedback changes spike rate by changing spike timing may shed some new light on the debate about the neural correlates of cognitive processing.

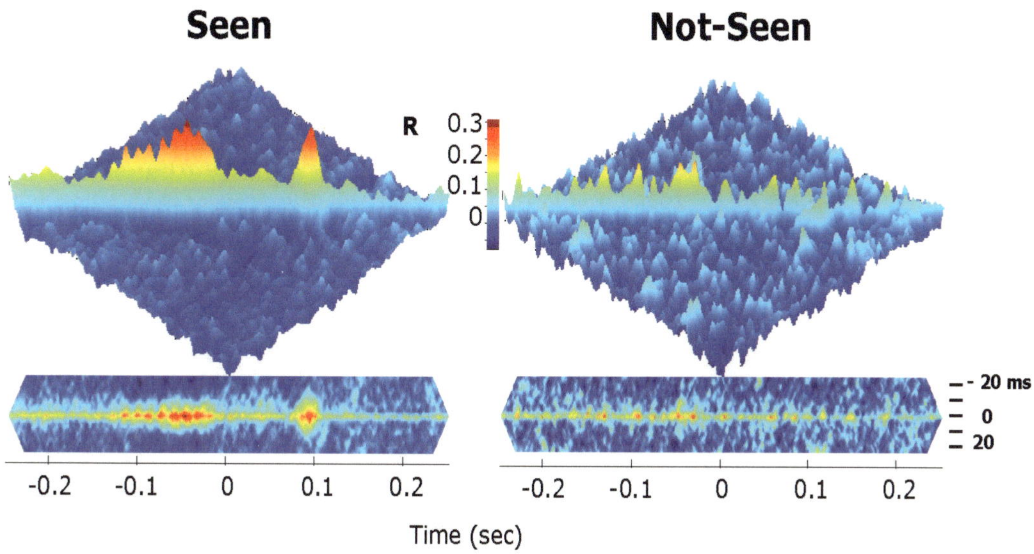

Figure 8. Synchronized V1 activity over time during a figure-ground perception task. Seen condition corresponds to those trials where the animal correctly detected the stimulus and Not-Seen condition corresponds to the trials where the animal failed to perceive the stimulus. A side and a top view are shown of these correlations. Color indicate correlation strength. Time is from onset of figure-ground texture (adapted from Van der Togt et al., 2006).

The states of arousal and attention are strongly linked with the natural release of neuromodulators, in particular acetylcholine, which influence recurrent processing. The neuromodulator acetylcholine reduces the efficacy of feedback and intra-cortical connections via the activation of muscarinic receptors (Kimura & Baughman, 1997). It also increases the efficacy of feedforward connections via the activation of nicotinic receptors (Disney et al., 2007). Application of acetylcholine in the primary visual cortex reduces the extent of spatial integration and enhances the neuronal responses especially in the later (sustained) part of the response (Roberts et al., 2005). Neuromodulators may also modify orientation tuning and improve signal-to-noise ratio of neural responses in the primary visual cortex (Zinke et al., 2006).

The finding that for a perceived figure the strength of neural activity and the functional connectivity (synchrony) between neurons in the primary visual cortex *prior* the textured figure-ground presentation is stronger than for a not perceived figure (Supèr at el., 2003a), exemplifies a role of cortical state in stimulus perception. In other words, activity immediately (~100 msec and not earlier) preceding the onset of the figure-ground stimulus relates to the animal's perception of the figure. Apparently, the visual cortex has to quickly attain an appropriate state before the sensory information enters the cortex. It appears that the different states of the brain preceding stimulus onset (receptive vs. unreceptive, so to say) have little or no effect on the early activity that is evoked by the stimulus, but are specifically associated with the occurrence of later recurrent interactions between areas (Supèr et al., 2003a).

During the later stages when figure-ground modulation develops the characteristics of synchronous activity changes. Still, it does not show an increase or a difference in high frequency components for figure and ground responses. This means that synchrony does not represent a neural correlate of figure-ground segregation, which is consistent with psychophysical (Kiper et al., 1996; Farid & Adelson, 2001), and other neurophysiological studies (Lamme & Spekreijse, 1998; Shadlen & Movshon, 1999; Bair et al, 2001; Thiele & Stoner, 2003). It is inconsistent, however, with a substantial amount of literature suggesting that synchronous activity has a role in high level processes such as perceptual organization, attention, sensory-motor binding, and consciousness (see Engel & Singer, 2001). The modulations in high frequency synchrony relate to perceptual grouping of local feature combinations, which in a figure-ground stimulus are similar for figure and ground textures. In other words the receptive fields of the recorded cells that are located in the centre of the figure are covered on average by identical local features as when they are located on the background. Thus no differences are expected in high frequency synchrony which may provide a plausible explanation for the absence of synchrony modulation in figure-ground task.

12. Conclusion

To sum up, the visual system uses feedforward suppression for figure-ground segmentation. It turns out that global inhibition is an important ingredient for figure-ground organization although it includes also a feedback component. The latter controls figure-ground segregation by influencing the neural firing patterns of feedforward projecting neurons, enhancing figure responses and further suppressing background responses which results in a stronger figure-ground signal.

Author details

Marina Arall, August Romeo and Hans Supèr
Faculty of Psychology, University of Barcelona (UB), Institute for Brain, Cognition and Behavior (IR3C), Catalan Institution for Research and Advanced Studies (ICREA), Spain

Acknowledgement

This work was supported by grants to HS (SEJ2006-15095, PSI2010-18139 & SAF2009-10367) from the Spanish Ministry of Education and Science (MICINN) and (2009-SGR-308) from Catalan government (AGAUR).

13. References

Alexander DM, & Wright JJ (2006) The maximum range and timing of excitatory contextual modulation in monkey primary visual cortex. *Vis. Neurosci.* 23: 721-728.

Alitto HJ, & Usrey, WM (2008) Origin and dynamics of extraclassical suppression in the lateral geniculate nucleus of the macaque monkey. *Neuron* 57: 135-146.

Allman JM, Mienzin F, & McGuiness E (1985) Stimulus specific responses from beyond the classical receptive field: neurophysiological mechanisms for localglobal comparisons in visual neurons. *Ann. Rev. Neurosci.* 8: 407-430.

Allen HA, Humphreys GW, Colin J, & Neumann H (2009) Ventral extra-straiate cortical areas are required for human visual texture segmentation. *J. Vision* 9: 1-14

Andolina IM, Jones HE, Wang W, & Sillito AM (2007) Corticothalamic feedback enhances stimulusresponse precision in the visual system. *Proc. Natl. Acad. Sci. U A* 104: 1685-1690.

Angelucci A, Levitt JB, Waltan EJS, Hupé J-M, Bullier J, & Lund JS (2002) Circuits for local and global signal integration in primary visual cortex. *J. Neurosci.* 22: 8633-8646.

Arnott SR, Pratt J, Shore DI, & Alain C (2001) Attentional set modulates visual areas: an event-related potential study of attentional capture. *Cogn. Brain Res.* 12: 383-395.

Bair W, Zohary E, & Newsome WT (2001) Correlated firing in macaque visual area MT: Time scales and relationship to behavior. *J. Neurosci.* 21: 1676-1697.

Bair W, Cavanaugh JR, & Movshon, JA (2003) Time course and time-distance relationships for surround suppression in macaque V1 neurons. *J. Neurosci.* 23: 7690-7701.

Barenholtz E, & Feldman, J (2006) Determination of visual figure and ground in dynamically deforming shapes. *Cognition* 101: 530-544.

Bastiaansen MC, & Brunia CH. (2001) Anticipatory attention: an event-related desynchronization approach. *Int. J. Psychophysiol.* 43: 91-107.

Budd, JML (1998) Extrastriate feedback to primary visual cortex in primates: a quantitative analysis of connectivity. *Proc. R. Soc. Lond. B.* 265: 1037-1044.

Cardin JA, Palmer LA, & Contreras D (2007) Stimulus feature selectivity in excitatory and inhibitory neurons in primary visual cortex. *J. Neurosci.* 27: 10333-10344.

Cavanaugh JR, Bair W, & Movshon JA (2002). Selectivity and spatial distribution of signals from the receptive field surround in macaque V1 neurons. *J. Neurophysiol.* 88: 2547–2556.

Chen G, Dan Y, & Li C-Y (2005) Stimulation of non-classical receptive field enhances orientation selectivity in the cat. *J. Physiol.* 564: 233-243.

Corthout E, Uttl B, Ziemann U, Cowey A, & Hallett M (1999) Two periods of processing in the (circum)striate visual cortex as revealed by transcranial magnetic stimulation. *Neuropsychologia* 37: 137-145.

Corthout E, & Supèr H (2004) Contextual modulation in V1: the Rossi-Zipser controversy. *Exp. Brain Res.* 156: 118–123.

Cudeiro J, and Sillito AM, (2006) Looking back: corticothalamic feedback and early visual processing. *Trends Neurosci.* 29: 298-306.

De Weerd P, Peralta III MR, Desimone R, & Ungerleider LG (1999) Loss of attentional stimulus selection after extrastraite cortical lesions in macaques. *Nature Neurosci.* 2: 753-758.

Disney AA, Aoki C, & Howken MJ (2007) Gain modulation by nicotine in macaque V1. *Neuron* 56: 701- 713.

Driver J, Baylis GC, & Rafal RD (1992) Preserved figure-ground segregation and symmetry perception in visual neglect. *Nature* 360: 73-75

Engel AK, & Singer W (2001) Temporal binding and the neural correlates of sensory awareness. *Trends Cogn. Sci.* 5: 16-25.

Farid H, & Adelson EH (2001) Synchrony Does Not Promote Grouping in Temporally Structured Displays. *Nat. Neurosci.* 4: 875-876.

Felleman DJ, & Van Essen DC (1991) Distributed hierarchical processing in the primate cerebral cortex. *Cerebral Cortex* 1: 1-47.

Gilbert CD, & Wiesel TN (1990) The influence of contextual stimuli on the orientation selectivity of cells in primary visual cortex of the cat. *Vision Res.* 30: 1689–1701.

Girard P, Hupe, JM, & Bullier J (2001) Feedforward and feedback connections between areas V1 and V2 of the monkey have similar rapid conduction velocities. *J. Neurophysiol.* 85: 1328-1331.

Grinvald A, Lieke EE, Frostig RD, & Hildesheim R (1994) Cortical point-spread function and long-range lateral interactions revealed by real-time optical imaging of macaque monkey primary visual cortex. *J. Neurosci.* 14: 2545–2568.

Grosof DH, Shapely RM, & Hawken MJ (1993) Macaque V1 neurons can signal 'illusory' contours. *Nature* 365: 550-552.

Hayes RD, & Merigan WH (2007) Mechanisms of sensitivity loss due to visual cortex lesions in humans and macaques. *Cerebral Cortex* 17: 1117-1128.

Huang JY, Wang C, & Dreher B (2007) The effects of reversible inactivation of postero-temporal visual cortex on neuronal activities in cat's area 17. *Brain Res.* 1138: 111-1128.

Huang X, & Paradiso MA (2008) V1 response timing and surface filling-in. *J. Neurophysiol.* 100: 539-47.

Hubel DH, & Wiesel TN (1968) Receptive fields and functional architecture of monkey striate cortex. *J. Physiol. (Lond.)* 195: 215-243.

Hupé JM, James AC, Payne BR, Lomber SG, & Girard P, et al. (1998) Cortical feedback improves discrimination between figure and background by V1, V2 and V3 neurons. *Nature* 394: 784-787.

Hupé JM, James AC, Girard P, & Bullier J (2001) Response modulations by static texture surround in area V1 of the macaque monkey do not depend on feedback connections from V2. *J. Neurophysiol.* 85: 146-163.

Jones HE, Grieve KL, Wang W, & Sillito AM (2001) Surround suppression in primate V1. *J. Neurophysiol.* 86: 2011-2028.

Kapadia MK, Westheimer G, & Gilbert, CD (2000) Spatial distribution of contextual interactions in primary visual cortex and in visual perception. *J. Neurophysiol.* 84: 2048-2062.

Kimura F, & Baughman RW (1997) GABAergic Transcallosal Neurons in Developing Rat Neocortex. *Europ. J. Neurosci.* 11: 3597-3609.

Kiper DC, Gegenfurtner KR, & Movshon A (1996) Cortical oscillations do not affect visual segmentation. *Vision Res.* 36: 539-544.

Knierim JJ, & Van Essen DC (1992) Visual cortex: cartography, connectivity, and concurrent processing. *Curr. Opin. Neurobiol.* 2: 150-155.

Komatsu H (2007) The neural mechanisms of perceptual filling-in. *Nat. Neurosci. Rev.* 7: 220-231.

Lamme VAF (1995) The neurophysiology of figure-ground segregation in primary visual cortex. *J. Neurosci.* 15: 1605-1615.

Lamme VAF, & Spekreijse H (1998) Neuronal synchrony does not represent texture segregation. *Nature* 396: 362-366.

Lamme VAF, Zipser K, & Spekreijse H (1998) Figure-ground activity in primary visual cortex is suppressed by anesthesia. *Proc. Natl. Acad. Sci. USA.* 95: 3263-8.

Lamme VAF, Rodriguez-Rodriguez V, & Spekreijse H (1999) Separate processing dynamics for texture elements, boundaries and surfaces in primary visual cortex of the macaque monkey. *Cerebral Cortex* 9: 406-13.

Lamme VAF, & Roelfsema, PR (2000) The distinct modes of vision offered by feedforward and recurrent processing. *Trends Neurosci.* 23: 571-9.

Lamme VAF, Zipser K, & Spekreijse H (2002) Masking interrupts figure–ground signals in V1. *J. Cogn. ÇNeurosci.* 14: 1044–1053.

Landman R, Spekreijse H, & Lamme VAF (2003a) Set size effects in the macaque striate cortex. *J. Cogn. Neurosci.* 15: 873-882.

Landman R, Spekreijse H, Lamme, VAF (2003b) Relationship between change detection and post- change activity in visual area V1. *Neuroreport* 15: 2211-2214.

Lee TS, & Nguyen M (2001) Dynamics of subjective contour formation in the early visual cortex. *Proc. Natl. Acad. Sci. USA.* 98: 1907–1911.

Li W, Thier P, & Wehrhahn C (2000) Contextual influence on orientation discrimination of humans and responses of neurons in V1 of alert monkeys. *J. Neurophysiol.* 83: 941-54.

Llinás RR, & Steriade M (2006) Bursting of thalamic neurons and states of vigilance. *J. Neurophysiol.* 95: ç 3297-308.

MacEvoy SP, & Paradiso MA (2001) Lightness constancy in primary visual cortex. *Proc. Natl. Acad. Sci. ç USA.* 98: 8827-8831.

Marcus DS, & Van Essen DC (2002) Scene segmentation and attention in primate cortical areas V1 and V2. *J. Neurophysiol.* 88: 2648-58.

McAlonan K, Cavanaugh J, & Wurtz RH (2008) Guarding the gateway to cortex with attention in visual thalamus. *Nature* 456: 391-394.

Meese TS, & Holmes D, (2007) Spatial and temporal dependencies of cross-orientation suppression in human vision. *Proc. Biol. Sci.* 274: 127-136.

Miller KD (2003) Understanding layer 4 of the cortical circuit: A model based on cat V1. *Cerebral Cortex* 13: 73-82.

Motoyoshi I (1999) Texture filling-in and texture segregation revealed by transient masking. *Vision Res.* 39: 1285-1291.

Ozeki H, Sadakane O, Akasaki T, Naito T, & Shimegi S, et al. (2004) Relationship between excitation and inhibition underlying size tuning and contextual response modulation in the cat primary visual cortex. *J. Neurosci.* 24: 1428-1438.

Parkes LM, Fries P, Kerskens cm, & Norris DG (2004) Reduced BOLD response to periodic visual stimulation. *NeuroImage* 21: 236-243.

Pascual-Leone A, & Walsh V (2001) Fast back projections from the motion to the primary visual area necessary for visual awareness. *Science* 292: 510-512.

Polat U, Mizobe K, Pettet MW, Kasamatsu T, & Norcia AM (1998) Collinear stimuli regulate visual responses depending on Cell's contrast threshold. *Nature* 391: 580-584.

Qiu FT, Sugihara T, & von der Heydt R (2007) Figure-ground mechanisms provide structure for selective attention. *Nat. Neurosci.* 10: 1492-1499.

Roberts MJ, Zinke W, Guo K, Robertson R, McDonald JS, & Thiele A (2005) Acetylcholine Dynamically Controls Spatial Integration in Marmoset Primary Visual Cortex. *J. Neurophysiol.* 93: 2062-2072.

Roelfsema PR, Tolboom M, & Khayat, PS (2007) Different processing phases for features, figures, and selective attention in the primary visual cortex. *Neuron* 56: 785-792.

Rossi AF, Rittenhouse CD, & Paradiso M (1996) The representation of brightness in primary visual cortex. *Science* 273: 1104-1107.

Rossi AF, & Paradiso, MA (1999) Neural correlates of perceived brightness in the retina, lateral geniculate nucleus, and striate cortex. *J. Neurosci.* 19: 6145-56.

Rossi AF, Desimone R, & Ungerleider LG (2001) Contextual modulation in primary visual cortex of macaques. *J. Neurosci.* 21: 1698-709.

Scholte HS, Witteveen SC, Spekreijse H, & Lamme VA (2006) The influence of inattention on the neural correlates of scene segmentation. *Brain Res.* 1076: 106-115.

Scholte HS, Jolij J, Fahrenfort JJ,& Lamme VA (2008) Feedforward and recurrent processing in scene segmentation: electroencephalography and functional magnetic resonance imaging. *J. Cogn. Neurosci.* 20: 2097-109.

Shadlen MN, & Movshon, JA (1999) Synchrony unbound: a critical evaluation of the temporal binding hypothesis. *Neuron* 24: 67-77.

Shao Z, & Burkhalter A (1996) Different balance of excitation and inhibition in forward and feedback circuits of rat visual cortex. *J. Neurosci.* 16: 7353-65.

Sherman M (2001) Tonic and burst firing: dual modes of thalamocortical relay. *Trends Neurosci.* 24: 122- 126.

Sillito AM, Grieve KL, Jones HE, Cudeiro J, & Davis J (1995) Visual cortical mechanisms detecting focal orientation discontinuities. *Nature* 378: 492-496.

Silvanto J, Cowey A, Lavie N, & Walsh V (2005) Striate cortex (V1) activity gates awareness of motion. *Nat. Neurosci.* 8: 143-154.

Sincich LC, & Horton JC (2005) The circuitry of V1 and V2: integration of color, form, and motion. *Annu. Rev. Neurosci.* 28: 303-326.

Smith FW, & Muckli L (2010) Nonstimulated early visual areas carry information about surrounding context. *Proc. Natl. Acad. Sci. USA.* 107: 20099-20103.

Steriade M, McCormick DA, & Sejnowski TJ (1999) Thalamocortical oscillations in the sleeping and aroused brain. *Science* 262: 679-685.

Supèr H, Spekreijse H,& Lamme VAF (2001a) Two distinct modes of sensory processing observed in the monkey primary visual cortex (V1). *Nat. Neurosci.* 4: 304-310.

Supèr H, Spekreijse H, & Lamme VAF (2001b) A neural correlate of working memory in the monkey primary visual cortex. *Science* 293: 120-124.

Supèr H, Van der Togt C, Spekreijse H, & Lamme VAF (2003a) Internal state of the monkey primary visual cortex predicts figure-ground perception. *J. Neurosci.* 23: 3407-3414.

Supèr H, Spekreijse H, & Lamme VAF (2003b) Figure-ground activity in primary visual cortex (V1) of the monkey matches the speed of behavioral response. *Neurosci. Lett.* 344: 75-78.

Supèr H, van der Togt C, Spekreijse H, & Lamme VAF (2004) Correspondence of presaccadic activity in the monkey primary visual cortex with saccadic eye movements. *Proc. Natl. Acad. Sci. USA* 101: 3230-3235.

Supèr H,& Lamme VAF (2007a) Altered figure-ground perception in monkeys with an extra-striate lesion. *Neuropsychologia* 45: 3329-3334.

Supèr H, & Lamme VAF (2007b) Strength of Figure-Ground Activity in Monkey Primary Visual Cortex Predicts Saccadic Reaction Time in a Delayed Detection Task. *Cerebral Cortex* 17: 1468-1475.

Supèr H, Romeo A, & Keil M (2010) Feed-Forward Segmentation of Figure-Ground and Assignment of Border-Ownership. *PLoS ONE* 5(5): e10705.

Supèr H, & Romeo A (2011) Feedback Enhances Feedforward Figure-Ground Segmentation by Changing Firing Mode. *PLoS ONE* 6(6): e21641.

Thiele A, & Stoner G (2003) Neural synchrony does not correlate with motion coherence in cortical area MT. *Nature* 421: 366-370.

Tong F, & Engel SA (2001) Interocular rivalry revealed in the human cortical blind-spot representation. *Nature,* 411: 195-199.

Van der Smagt MJ, WehrHahn C, & Albright TD (2005) Contextual Masking of Oriented Lines: Interaction Between Surface Segmentation Cues. *J. Neurophysiol.* 94: 576-589.

Van der Togt C, Kalitzin S, Spekreijse H, Lamme VAF, & Supèr H (2006) Synchrony dynamics in monkey V1 predicts success in visual detection. *Cerebral Cortex* 16: 136-148.

Vogel EK, & Luck SJ (2000) The visual N1 component as an index of a discrimination process. *Psychophysiology* 37: 190-203.

Von der Heydt R, Peterhans E, & Baumgartner G (1984) Illusory contours and cortical neuron responses. *Science* 224: 1260-1262.

Von der Heydt R, Sugihara T, & Qiu, FT (2004) Border ownership and attentional modulation in neurons of the visual cortex. *Perception* 33:46.

Walker GA, Ohzawa I, & Freeman RD (1999) Asymmetric suppression outside the classical receptive field of the visual cortex. *J. Neurosci.* 19: 10536-10553.

Webb BS, Tinsley CJ, Vincent CJ, & Derrington AM (2005) Spatial distribution of suppressive signals outside the classical receptive field in lateral geniculate nucleus. *J. Neurophysiol.* 94: 1789-1797.

Weyland TG, Boudreaux M, & Guido W (2001) Burst and tonic response modes in thalamic neurons during sleep and wakefulness. *J. Neurophysiol.* 85: 1107-1118.

Zinke W, Roberts MJ, Guo K, McDonald JC, Robertson R, & Thiele A (2006) Cholinergic modulation of response properties and orientation tuning of neurons in primary visual cortex of anesthetized marmoset monkeys. *Europ. J. Neurosci.* 24: 314-328.

Zipser K, Lamme VAF, Schiller PH (1996) Contextual modulation in primary visual cortex. *J. Neurosci.* 16: 7376–7389.

Zhou H, Friedman HS, Von der Heydt R (2000) Coding of border ownership in monkey visual cortex. *J. Neurosci.* 20: 6594-6611.